Cellular and Molecular Mechanisms Underlying the Pathogenesis of Hepatic Fibrosis

Cellular and Molecular Mechanisms Underlying the Pathogenesis of Hepatic Fibrosis

Special Issue Editor

Ralf Weiskirchen

MDPI • Basel • Beijing • Wuhan • Barcelona • Belgrade • Manchester • Tokyo • Cluj • Tianjin

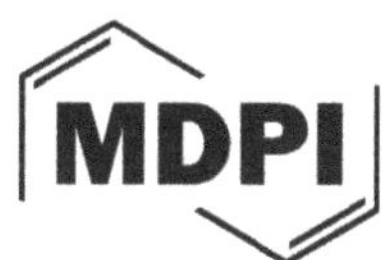

Special Issue Editor
Ralf Weiskirchen
University Hospital RWTH Aachen
Germany

Editorial Office
MDPI
St. Alban-Anlage 66
4052 Basel, Switzerland

This is a reprint of articles from the Special Issue published online in the open access journal *Cells* (ISSN 2073-4409) (available at: https://www.mdpi.com/journal/cells/special_issues/hepatic_fibrosis).

For citation purposes, cite each article independently as indicated on the article page online and as indicated below:

LastName, A.A.; LastName, B.B.; LastName, C.C. Article Title. *Journal Name* **Year**, *Article Number*, Page Range.

ISBN 978-3-03936-188-5 (Hbk)
ISBN 978-3-03936-189-2 (PDF)

Cover image courtesy of Ralf Weiskirchen.

Contents

About the Special Issue Editor

Ralf Weiskirchen, Professor, Ph.D. was born in 1964 Bergisch Gladbach, North Rhine-Westphalia (Germany). After his school education, he studied Biology and completed his Ph.D. at the University of Cologne (Germany). Thereafter, he worked as Research Associate at the Institute of Biochemistry at the University of Innsbruck (Austria). Back in Germany, he habilitated at the RWTH University Hospital Aachen and became a Professor in 2007. Presently, he is head of the Institute of Molecular Pathobiochemistry, Experimental Gene Therapy and Clinical Chemistry (IFMPEGKC) in Aachen. His major research focus is the analysis of the molecular mechanisms underlying the pathogenesis of hepatic fibrosis. In the past, he has intensively studied general aspects of cytokine and chemokine activities and their signaling pathways in models of hepatic inflammation, fibrosis/cirrhosis and hepatocellular carcinoma. In addition, he has isolated and established novel biomarkers or predisposition traits (SNPs, haplotypes) that allow determining the outcome of liver disease. The long-term objective of Professor Weiskirchen's studies is to translate experimental findings into novel diagnostic or therapeutic strategies. Ralf Weiskirchen has authored over 400 articles in peer-reviewed journals and has given a large number of presentations and lectures at medical and scientific conferences. He is editorial board member of a wealth of journals, and an active member of the German Association for the Study of the Liver (GASL) and the European Association for the Study of the Liver (EASL).

Preface to "Cellular and Molecular Mechanisms Underlying the Pathogenesis of Hepatic Fibrosis"

Liver fibrosis is an important chronic disease considered one of the leading causes of death worldwide. It is characterized by progressive accumulation of extracellular matrix in the liver which destroys the physiological architecture and results in functional impairments. Based on the high medical and economic burden associated with hepatic fibrosis and associated complications, there is an urgent need to understand the pathogenetic mechanisms of this disease and to improve present diagnostic and therapeutic options. Undoubtedly, the evolution of understanding the functional role of cells and mediators contributing to the progression and outcome of liver fibrogenesis has been remarkable during the last years. Nevertheless, well-accepted anti-fibrotic therapies are still missing.

Key issues, current perspectives, and novel experimental findings in liver fibrosis research were recently summarized by over 300 leading experts from 25 countries in a Special Issue of Cells entitled "Cellular and Molecular Mechanisms Underlying the Pathogenesis of Hepatic Fibrosis". The respective collection of articles covers general mechanistic concepts of liver fibrosis, provide information about disease mediators, highlight important aspects relevant in disease progression and discuss therapeutic and diagnostic consequences resulting thereof.

The present book contains a small selection of 12 articles of the mentioned Special Issue. These reports highlight different aspects of liver fibrosis research and exemplarily show how this fascinating discipline has made conceptual advances during the last years. They further document how basic researchers and clinicians work together in understanding the pathogenesis of hepatic fibrosis and how this knowledge can be used to establish novel therapeutic or diagnostic options.

I would like to thank all authors again for providing excellent and stimulating contributions to the mentioned Special Issue and this book project. Moreover, I would like to acknowledge the excellent and efficient work of the expert reviewers that helped in realizing this project by reviewing submissions in a timely, fair, and constructive manner.

I am grateful to the Multidisciplinary Digital Publishing Institute (MDPI), which enabled the Special issue and the production of this book.

At the end, I wish the reader of this book pleasant reading and hope that she/he will be inspired to download additional articles of the Special Issue that are freely available at: https://www.mdpi.com/journal/cells/special_issues/hepatic_fibrosis.

Ralf Weiskirchen
Special Issue Editor

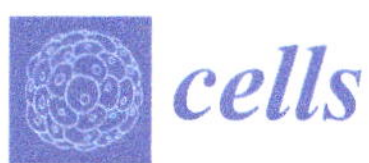

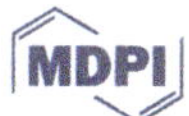

Review

Current Status in Testing for Nonalcoholic Fatty Liver Disease (NAFLD) and Nonalcoholic Steatohepatitis (NASH)

Hannah K. Drescher [1,*], Sabine Weiskirchen [2] and Ralf Weiskirchen [2,*]

1 Gastrointestinal Unit and Liver Center, Massachusetts General Hospital, Harvard Medical School, Boston, MA 02114, USA

2 Institute of Molecular Pathobiochemistry, Experimental Gene Therapy and Clinical Chemistry (IFMPEGKC), RWTH University Hospital, 52074 Aachen, Germany

* Correspondence: hdrescher@mgh.harvard.edu (H.K.D.); rweiskirchen@ukaachen.de (R.W.)

Received: 23 July 2019; Accepted: 6 August 2019; Published: 7 August 2019

Abstract: Nonalcoholic fatty liver disease (NAFLD) is the most common chronic liver disease in Western countries with almost 25% affected adults worldwide. The growing public health burden is getting evident when considering that NAFLD-related liver transplantations are predicted to almost double within the next 20 years. Typically, hepatic alterations start with simple steatosis, which easily progresses to more advanced stages such as nonalcoholic steatohepatitis (NASH), fibrosis and cirrhosis. This course of disease finally leads to end-stage liver disease such as hepatocellular carcinoma, which is associated with increased morbidity and mortality. Although clinical trials show promising results, there is actually no pharmacological agent approved to treat NASH. Another important problem associated with NASH is that presently the liver biopsy is still the gold standard in diagnosis and for disease staging and grading. Because of its invasiveness, this technique is not well accepted by patients and the method is prone to sampling error. Therefore, an urgent need exists to find reliable, accurate and noninvasive biomarkers discriminating between different disease stages or to develop innovative imaging techniques to quantify steatosis.

Keywords: nonalcoholic steatohepatitis; fibrosis; grading; staging; imaging; algorithms; scores; biomarkers

---

1. Introduction

In the 1990s, nonalcoholic steatohepatitis (NASH) was considered to be a relatively uncommon disease, only occurring in obese women with type 2 diabetes. Things changed quickly after a study came up in 1996 describing NASH the second most commonly occurring liver disease in patients after acute and chronic viral hepatitis infection [1]. Even more important for the field of NASH was a review in 1998 highlighting that fibrosis and cirrhosis are complications associated with NASH in more than 15–50% of all cases [2]. In the same article, Day and James postulated the two-hit hypothesis according to which the pathogenesis of NASH is initiated by a first hit predominantly caused by accumulating lipids in hepatocytes leading to apoptosis of these cells and excessive oxidative stress. Steatosis then sensitizes the liver to develop advanced NASH by a potential second hit driven by infiltrating immune cells, which release inflammatory mediators such as cytokines. This shift to an inflammatory milieu can finally lead to fibrotic tissue remodeling which can easily progress to end stage liver disease such as cirrhosis and the development of hepatocellular carcinoma (HCC). Today, this hypothesis is considered to be inadequate to explain the multiple and complex disease drivers to nonalcoholic fatty liver disease (NAFLD). Lately the multiple-hit hypothesis is better framing the variable circumstances implicating disease development and progression [3]. However, studies show that disease progression is not always linear and it is not fully clear who is more likely to progress to more advanced stages [4]. Considered as the hepatic manifestation of metabolic syndrome, NAFLD is in most cases associated with type 2 diabetes and dyslipidemia (Figure 1) [5].

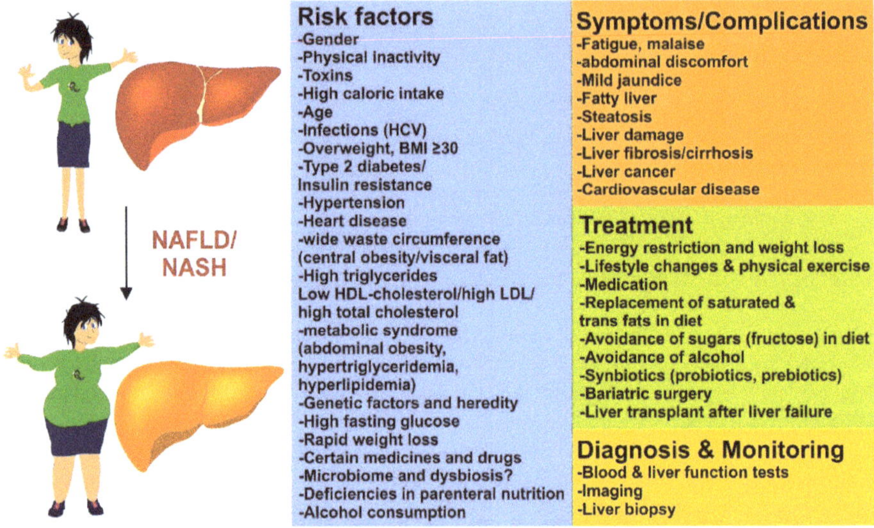

Figure 1. Risk factors, symptoms, diagnosis, and treatment of nonalcoholic liver disease. Predisposition and disease progression in NAFLD/NASH is influenced by comorbidities [6], genetic determinants [7], and environmental factors including drugs and toxins [8]. The range of resulting symptoms and complication of NAFLD/NASH can vary from very mild to life-threating. Diagnosis and monitoring of disease can be done by blood tests [9], liver function tests [10] and imaging [11]. However, a liver biopsy should be performed based on an individualized decision and is still the gold standard in scoring and grading of steatosis, inflammation, and fibrosis [12]. Although an ultimate therapy is still missing, beneficial effects on NAFLD/NASH progression are energy restriction, lifestyle changes, improved diets, and elevated physical activity [13]. In addition, in biopsy-proven NASH and fibrosis, medication with antiglycemic drugs, insulin sensitizers, synbiotics, or compounds interfering with fat metabolism or preventing oxidative stress have favorable effects on disease outcome [13,14]. Surgical procedures, including bariatric surgery, to treat obesity and liver transplant after liver failure are extreme forms in NAFLD/NASH treatment [15].

Taking the direct association with insulin resistance and obesity into account, NAFLD is a global health burden with rising impact [16,17]. It is known that almost 25% of the global population is affected by NAFLD and/or its complications, making it the most common chronic and progressive liver disease especially in industrialized countries [18]. Models even predict a prevalence of NAFLD in adults of more than 30% of the total population with around 20% being diagnosed as NASH. Looking at these developments, calculations show that the incidence of HCC and NASH-related liver transplantation will be doubled until 2030 [19–21].

Up-to-date weight loss and lifestyle changes are still the only possible ways to overcome NAFLD. Regrettably, very few patients successfully achieve long term weight reduction. Therefore, there is an urgent need for the development of a pharmacological treatment for patients with NASH and fibrosis. NASH and fibrosis typically develop asymptomatic till they progress to end-stage liver disease at which liver transplantation is the only cure available. At present, first guidelines consent to the use of pioglitazone, vitamin E and pentoxifylline in patients with NASH to reduce steatosis, but they still have many potential side-effects or have low efficiency [22–25]. Other agents such as obeticholic acid, cenicriviroc, elafibranor and selonsertib are actually in clinical trial phase III (Figure 2) [26]. Although these various clinical trials show promising results to target NAFLD and NASH therapeutically, there is no approved pharmacological treatment available yet [27–31].

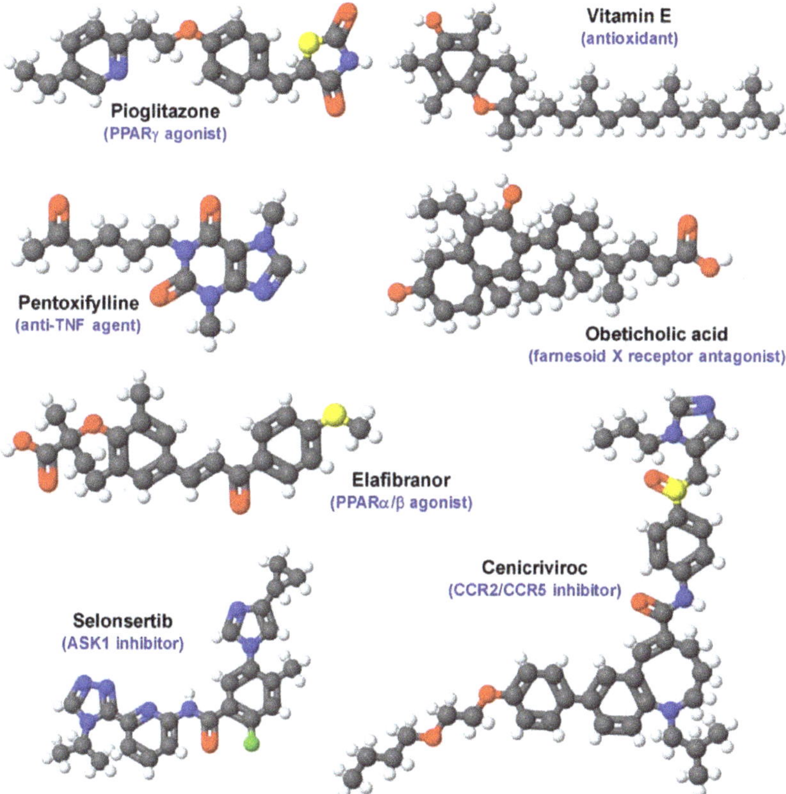

Figure 2. Established compounds and drug candidates evaluated for the treatment of NAFLD/NASH in clinical trial phase III. Pioglitazone (PPARγ agonist), vitamin E (antioxidant), pentoxifylline (anti tumor necrosis factor-α (TNF-α) agent). Obeticholic acid (farnesoid X receptor antagonist), cenicriviroc (CCR2/CCR5 inhibitor), elafibranor (PPARα/δ agonist), and selonsertib (ASK1 inhibitor) have different molecular targets. The different biological activities of the drugs point to the complexity of NAFLD/NASH, having a large variety of potential therapeutic drug targets. The depicted structures were generated with the open source molecule viewer Jmol using data deposited in the PubChem compound database with CIDs: 4829, 14985, 4740, 447715, 11285792, 9864881, and 71245288). For more details about the biological activity of each drug refer to [32].

On the basis of different imaging techniques and the combination of clinical factors the presence of NASH in an individual can be strongly suspected. However, the gold standard to diagnose NASH is still an invasive liver biopsy [4]. This is not only less accepted and harmful to the patient, but also often leading to late diagnoses at the point of end-stage liver disease due to the fact that NAFLD is in most cases asymptomatic prior to the transition to NASH. In addition, not all researchers agree with the view that there exists a necessity of differentiating by histology the so-called simply or benign fatty liver from NASH. This is due to the fact that NAFLD may be less benign than it is currently thought to be and that there exists a high degree of heterogeneity of NAFLD [33].

Twenty to thirty percent of all NAFLD patients progress to NASH-fibrosis. Therefore, there is an urgent need to find reliable noninvasive biomarkers and screening techniques to diagnose NAFLD and NASH and monitor patients at an earlier time point at which lifestyle changes and potential newly developed drugs can be used purposefully.

In addition, other less common conditions can cause similar clinical and histological phenotypes like NAFLD and NASH [34]. There is common sense that the primary causes for the development of NAFLD are obesity, type II diabetes, dyslipidemia, insulin resistance and some genetic disorders [34]. However, there are other less common conditions in which NAFLD is the consequence of secondary causes, including specific disorders of lipid metabolism (abetalipoproteinemia, hypobetalipoproteinemia, familial combined hyperlipidemia, glycogen storage disease, Weber–Christian syndrome, lipodystrophy), total parenteral nutrition, hepatitis C infection, severe surgical weight loss, medications (amiodarone, tamoxifen, methotrexate, corticosteroids, highly active antiretroviral therapy), starvation, Wilson's disease, environmental toxicity, and celiac disease [34].

Some other conditions associated with metabolic syndrome that can lead to NAFLD are the obstructive sleep apnea syndrome (OSAS), polycystic ovary syndrome (PCOS), and non-obese NAFLD. OSAS is a common sleep disorder, which is associated with chronic intermittent hypoxia and increased proinflammatory cytokine production [35]. OSAS and obesity often coexist and the chronic hypoxia induces hyperglycemia, insulin resistance, and hepatic lipid peroxidation, which are hallmarks of the metabolic syndrome [35]. Similarly, PCOS is a frequent endocrine disease in women associated with a number of metabolic consequences, including obesity, dyslipidemia, insulin resistance, type 2 diabetes, and low-grade inflammation [36]. Therefore, it is not surprising that PCOS patients are prone to develop NAFLD. Interestingly, NAFLD can also occur in non-obese individuals. Although these patients have a normal body mass index (BMI), they have metabolic abnormalities similar to those characteristically associated with obesity [37]. Consequently, these normal weight or lean individuals displaying obesity-related features are called metabolically obese but normal weight (MONW) patients [37]. Although the pathways and pathophysiological mechanisms driving NAFLD and NASH in non-obese persons are not completely understood, it is speculated that major risk factors are dysfunctional fat, decreased muscle mass, genetic factors, different patterns of the gut microbiota, and epigenetic changes occurring early in life [38].

To avoid diagnostic pitfalls in the distinction of NAFLD provoked by traditional risk factors of metabolic disease and secondary causes of NAFLD, it is essential that clinicians comprehensively evaluate the patient, because both conditions vary considerably and will require different therapeutic regimens [34,39].

This review summarizes the current screening methods used to complement the overall appearance of NAFLD/NASH and provides an outlook on potential upcoming candidates to replace the need of taking liver biopsies.

2. Blood and Serum Tests

Liver biopsy is still the standard procedure to diagnose NASH. Besides the risk of complications during surgery, it involves a lot of bias because only a little specimen of the liver is taken, which not always represent the actual status of the entire liver [40]. This runs the risk to underestimate disease severity in many cases [41]. Finding reliable biomarkers which can be measured with less or even noninvasive techniques is therefore of urgent need.

However, NAFLD and NASH are complex multi factorial diseases and therefore no single surrogate marker is likely to be omniscient to predict clinical outcome or benefits of a therapy. Despite the fact that all biomarkers and scores have their limitations, interest is increasing rapidly in the use of these markers to predict information about progression and outcome of the disease. Therefore, respective surrogate biomarker and scores offered by the market should be used with much care and limited to situations where it has been demonstrated robust ability in disease management.

In addition, there is an urgent need to improve standardization in the usage of these operations. On the other site, it is obvious that the surrogate markers can be extremely helpful when handled correctly. This was very recently demonstrated in a study using telemedicine-based comprehensive, continuous care intervention (CCl) together with carbohydrate restriction-induced ketosis and behavior changes. The respective study showed that a NAFLD liver fat score (i.e., N-LFS) was reduced in the CCl group, whereas it was not changed in a group of patients receiving usual care [42]. This exemplarily demonstrates that surrogate markers can provide good measurement for the efficacy of a specific therapy.

Here we will summarize blood and serum biomarkers, which are already available and discuss their benefits and shortcomings in the diagnosis and management of NASH and NAFLD.

2.1. Steatosis

Hepatic steatosis is the key feature of NAFLD. Steatosis is diagnosed when more than 5% of hepatocytes contain fat or when the total amount of intrahepatic triglycerides is bigger than 5.5% without having any other liver disease in the patient's history [23,24]. Today there is no specific serum marker to assess hepatic steatosis available. However, several reproducible blood biomarker panels and scores were developed to help diagnose NAFLD (Table 1).

Table 1. Blood biomarker panels to identify inflammatory liver disease.

Panel	Parameters Included	Reference
NAFLD ridge score	ALT, HDL, cholesterol, triglycerides, HbA1c, leukocyte count, hypertension	[43,44]
NAFLD Liver Fat Score (NLFS)	Liver fat content, metabolic syndrome, type 2 diabetes, AST, AST:ALT, fasting insulin level	[45]
Hepatic Steatosis Index (HIS)	AST:ALT, BMI, diabetes, sex	[46]
Fatty liver index (FLI)	BMI, waist circumference, triglycerides, γ-GT	[47,48]
Lipid accumulation product (LAP) index	sex, triglycerides, weight circumference	[49]
Fatty Liver Inhibition of Progression (FLIP) algorithm	histological steatosis, disease activity, fibrosis score	[50]
CHeK score	age, HbA1c, γ-GT, adiponectin, M30	[51]
NAFLD Fibrosis Score (NFS)	AST:ALT, albumin, platelet count, age, BMI, hyperglycemia (impaired fasting glucose)	[52]
Fibrosis-4 Score (FIB-4)	AST, ALT, platelet count, age	[53]
AST to Platelet Ratio Index (APRI)	AST:platelet count	[54]
BARD Score	BMI, AST:ALT, diabetes	[55]
Enhanced Liver Fibrosis panel (ELF)	Age, TIMP-1, PIIINP, HA	[56]
Hepascore	bilirubin, γ-GT, HA, α_2M, age, gender	[57]
FibroTest-FibroSURE/ActiTest	α_2M, haptoglobin, γ-GT, total bilirubin, apolipoprotein A1, ALT, age, gender	[58]
FibroMeter NAFLD index (FibroMeter^{VCTE})	platelet count, prothrombin index, ferritin, AST, ALT, body weight, age, liver stiffness determined by vibration controlled transient elastography (VCTE)	[59,60]

Abbreviations used are: α_2M, α_2-macroglobulin; γ-GT, γ-glutamyltransferase; ALT, alanine aminotransferase; AST, aspartate aminotransferase; BMI, body mass index; HA, hyaluronic acid; HbA1c, glycated hemoglobin; HDL, high-density lipoprotein; M30, antigen of the serum cytokeratin 18; PIIINP, amino-terminal propeptide of type III procollagen; TIMP-1, tissue inhibitor of metalloproteinases 1.

Most of these multiparametric panels include biochemical markers indicating liver damage or dysfunction (AST, ALT, bilirubin, γ-GT, platelet count, haptoglobin), lipid metabolism disorders (cholesterol, triglycerides), diabetes (HbA1c, fasting insulin level), inflammation (α_2M, ferritin), or provide information about matrix expression and turnover (TIMP-1, PIIINP, HA) (Figure 3).

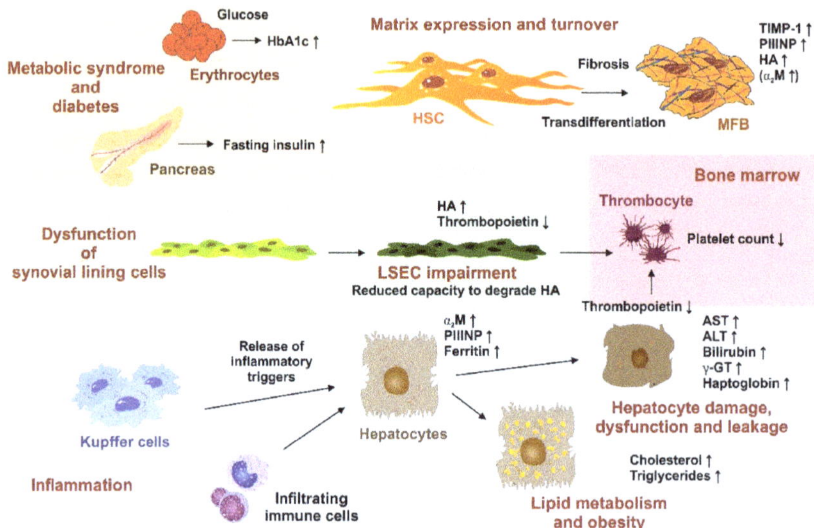

Figure 3. Significance of laboratory parameters in the diagnosis NAFLD and NASH. In the scheme, the biological source and alteration of individual biochemical markers during progression of NAFLD/NASH are indicated. High caloric intake and elevated quantities of fat result in hepatic steatosis, triggering steatohepatitis. The inflammatory response is triggered by infiltrating immune cells and liver-resident Kupffer cells releasing a plenitude of inflammatory triggers. As a consequence, the expression of acute phase response proteins (α_2 macroglobulin (α_2M) and ferritin) is increased in hepatocytes. In addition, the increase of cholesterol and triglycerides provokes cellular fat accumulation, damage, and cellular leakage of hepatocytes. This is indicated by elevated quantities of aspartate aminotransferase (AST), alanine aminotransferase (ALT), bilirubin, and γ-glutamyltransferase (γ-GT). Subsequently, the overall capacity of these cells to synthesize typical liver proteins (haptoglobuin, thrombopoietin) decreases. Lower quantities of thrombopoietin results in reduced formation of platelets within the bones. Dysfunction of synovial lining cells (reduced capacity to degrade hyaluronic acid (HA)) and ongoing fibrogenesis lead to elevated levels of HA. In addition, the transdifferentiation of hepatic stellate cells (HSC) to myofibroblast (MFB) is associated with the occurrence of typical biomarkers (tissue inhibitor of matrix metalloproteinase-1 (TIMP-1), amino-terminal propeptide of type III procollagen (PIIINP)), which correlate to extracellular matrix formation and/or turnover. The metabolic syndrome associated with NAFLD/NASH results in higher quantities of fasting insulin and basal glucose triggering the non-enzymatic formation of glycated hemoglobin (HbA1c). All these parameters are diagnostically relevant in the diagnosis or scoring of NAFLD/NASH and are the basis of various blood biomarker panels to identify inflammatory liver disease.

With an AUROC (area under the receiver-operating characteristic curve) accuracy value of 0.87, the NAFLD ridge score is currently one of the most efficient panel based on laboratory parameters. The NAFLD ridge score was developed as a machine learning algorithm facilitating registry research. It includes serum levels of alanine aminotransferase (ALT), high-density lipoprotein (HDL) cholesterol, triglycerides, hemoglobin A1c (HbA1c), leukocyte count, and the presence of hypertension [43,44]. With proton magnetic resonance spectroscopy (H-MRS) as reference, the NAFLD ridge score has a negative predictive value of 96%. However, this score is good to detect NAFLD but yet limited to the research setting and does not give the opportunity to distinguish between different steatosis grades or to assess changes during the development of steatosis over time.

A quantitative and by this more sensitive score to be calculated is the NAFLD Liver Fat Score (NLFS). This score includes the measurement of the liver fat content as determined by H-MRS, the presence or absence of the metabolic syndrome together with type 2 diabetes mellitus, aspartate aminotransferase (AST) levels, the AST:ALT ratio, and the fasting insulin serum level. With a sensitivity of 86% and a specificity of 71% the NLFS defines a liver fat content of more than 5.56% [45]. A recent study from Ruiz-Tovar and colleagues tested the accuracy of the NLFS in patients one year after bariatric surgery and considered it to be the most accurate biochemical score to assess liver steatosis at the moment [61]. The Hepatic Steatosis Index (HIS) also considers the AST/ALT ratio, BMI, diabetes and sex and has a sensitivity of 66% and a specificity of 69% [46].

The fatty liver index (FLI) includes BMI, waist circumference and serum levels of triglycerides and the γ-glutamyltransferase (γ-GT). It could be shown that the FLI significantly correlates with insulin resistance [47,48]. The major drawback when rating HIS and FLI is that ultrasonography is used as the reference standard to diagnose fatty liver. This technique is in general dependent on the operator and thereby to some extent biased and insensitive if only mild steatosis is present. The lipid accumulation product index (LAP) first established by Bedogni et al. takes into account sex, serum triglyceride levels and weight circumference to evaluate lipid overaccumulation [49].

A comparison of the accuracy in predicting NAFLD in a cross-sectional NAFLD cohort showed that NLFS is the best score to reliably predict NAFLD with an AUC of 0.771 [62]. Although the presented scores are capable to indicate the presence of hepatic steatosis, there are several limitations given. To be critically considered are the facts that using these indices it is not possible to distinguish between different steatosis grades and detect and trace changes over time is not possible.

2.2. Steatohepatitis

The transition from simple hepatic steatosis to NASH is the most crucial step during the development of severe liver disease with poor prognosis and the higher risk to get fibrosis and progress to end-stage liver disease. Thus, the assessment of NASH and the possibility to distinguish between the dynamic changes from NAFLD to NASH are ongoing challenges. Precise diagnosis still depends on liver biopsy with huge variability between pathologists. For that reason, Bedossa et al. developed the Fatty Liver Inhibition of Progression (FLIP) algorithm, which requires pathologists to follow generalized criteria for scoring. The FLIP algorithm considers histologically steatosis, disease activity and fibrosis scores [50]. Very recently, Canbay and colleagues established a novel machine learning approach to assess the severity of NAFLD and distinguish between NAFLD and NASH. In this study NAFLD was defined as the NAFLD activity score (NAS) ≤ 4 and NASH as NAS ≥ 4. With the help of an ensemble feature selection approach (EFS) they identified age, HbA1c, γ-GT, adiponectin and the apoptosis marker M30 to be the biomarkers highly associated with the prediction of NAFLD. The developed CHeK score, which is available at http://CHek.heiderlab.de is not only able to detect NASH, but also to monitor the development from NAFLD to NASH and can be used to screen patients in a long-term follow up during disease progression or therapy [51].

Besides histological scoring, the development from NAFLD to NASH involves a variety of different molecular, cellular and hormonal changes. Numerous blood biomarker and panels were investigated and developed trying to detect and reflect disease severity and underlying pathways. The apoptosis marker cytokeratin 18 (CK18) is a very well-studied individual blood biomarker so far. NASH patients show a significant increase of plasma CK18 indicating hepatocyte death through apoptosis and necroptosis compared to NAFLD patients [63]. CK18 is the main intermediate filament protein in hepatocytes and is released upon the initiation of cell death [64]. While the whole length CK18 is predominantly released upon hepatic necrosis, caspase cleaved CK18 (M30) is mainly produced by apoptotic cells [65]. Although CK18 is considered to be one of the most promising biomarkers, several studies showed that the sensitivity to predict NASH is 66%, while the specificity is 82% [66,67]. In addition, the ability of M30 to predict NASH and distinguish between NAFLD and NASH was calculated as 0.82 [68]. To increase the reliability of CK18 as a noninvasive biomarker for NASH a study shows that the combination with serum levels of the apoptosis-mediating surface antigen FAS (sFAS) further increases the accuracy [69]. However, the optimal cut-off serum concentrations still vary between different studies and require further investigation.

NASH is predominantly characterized by pathological alterations in glucose and lipid metabolism. These alterations include modifications in adipokines (such as leptin, adiponectin and resistin) and liver-derived lipid hormones like the fibroblast growth factor 21 (FGF21), which is secreted upon peroxisome proliferator-activated receptor-α (PPARα) activation [70,71]. FGF21 was found to be significantly elevated in patients with mild to moderate hepatic steatosis. Serum levels were directly linked to increased intrahepatic triglyceride accumulation and liver damage [72,73]. However, FGF21 is known to also increase in sepsis and systemic inflammation [74]. Further, adipokines were shown also to reflect visceral adiposity leading to a moderate specificity value of 62% with a specificity of 78% [68]. Further studies even show a drop of FGF21 levels with increasing liver inflammation [75].

The most evident difference between simple steatosis and advanced steatohepatitis is the absence of an inflammatory infiltrate. As a hallmark of NASH, a variety of inflammatory markers are elevated in patients with NASH, while disease is progressing. Increasing serum levels of C-reactive protein (CRP), tumor necrosis factor-α (TNF-α) and several interleukins such as, IL-6 and IL-8 were proposed as clinical markers. Although, they all correlate with the observed inflammatory status in NASH, none of them reached statistically significant values adjusted by the FDR on univariable analysis to be approved as a diagnostic marker yet because of their insensitivity to NASH specific inflammatory changes.

Recently, the transcription factor forkhead box protein A (FOXA1), also known as hepatocyte nuclear factor 3-α, was described as a potential new biomarker as it is involved in mediating homeostasis and metabolism by targeting genes in liver, adipose tissue and pancreas [76]. Moya et al. could show that FOXA1 acts anti-steatotic by lowering fatty acid uptake and is suppressed in patients with NAFLD and insulin resistance [77]. Therefore, the authors proposed this protein as sensitive noninvasive biomarker of liver fat accumulation, mitochondrial membrane potential and the production of reactive oxygen species (ROS). The limitation coming along with using a transcription factor as biomarker is, that FOXA1 is not secreted into the serum.

Oxidative stress, which is indicated by excessive ROS production, is one of the most important mechanisms underlying the disease pathogenesis of NASH finally leading to lipid oxidation and inflammation [78]. Based on changes in lipid catabolism and de novo lipogenesis the oxNASH score was calculated including the linoleic acid:13-hydroxyoctadecadienoic acid (13-HODA) ratio together with the patient characteristics age, BMI and AST level. This score reached diagnostic accuracy with an AUROC 0.74–0.83 [79]. Because mass spectroscopy is needed for the measurement of the described parameters, the oxNASH score is not commonly used today. In line with biomarkers targeting products, which are secreted due to an altered lipid metabolism, insulin-like growth factor binding protein 1 (IGFBP-1) was recently suggested as a potential serum marker for NAFLD and NAFLD-related fibrosis. It is exclusively upregulated in the liver in response to hepatic inflammation and oxidative stress and regulated by insulin [80]. On this basis, Regué et al. could show that the global deletion of the insulin-like growth factor 2 mRNA-binding protein 2 (IGF2BP2 or IGF2 mRNA-binding protein 2, IMP-2) lead to a resistance to obesity and fatty liver in mice treated with a high fat diet (HFD) due to reduced adiposity [81]. A limitation of those markers is that elevations might be not exclusively related to NAFLD-induced conditions, but also the metabolic syndrome and insulin resistance in general. Anyhow this is an interesting starting point for future investigations also in regard to therapeutic interventions and the understanding of the mechanisms that lead to steatosis.

The expression of ferritin is generally known to be increased in patients with NAFLD and metabolic syndrome. It was further shown to be independently associated with increased steatosis grades, NASH and NASH fibrosis with an AUROC of 0.62 [82,83]. This accuracy can be increased to an AUROC of 0.81 when including AST, BMI, type 2 diabetes, presence or absence of hypertension and platelet count to ferritin levels [84]. The broad and long-lasting search for novel biomarkers to diagnose NASH, which are modestly accurate, show the multiple factors involved in NAFLD and the complexity of disease mechanisms. To date the combination of several biomarkers drastically increases diagnostic preciseness. Especially for NASH, panels like the Nash Test (NT) include baseline patient characteristics such as age, gender, height, weight and serum levels of triglycerides, cholesterol, transaminases, total bilirubin, α_2-macroglobulin, haptoglobin, apolipoprotein A1, γ-GT [85].

Overall, most of the actual biomarkers and panels need further validation on cohorts with patients, including several different ethnicities and various starting points and outcomes. Up to now most validation studies work with patients undergoing bariatric surgery. Also choosing the best cut-off value for the specific serum markers is still not optimal. This points to the urgent need of basic research studies to help better understanding the underlying mechanisms and key molecules involved in the development of NAFLD and progression to NASH and end-stage liver disease.

2.3. Fibrosis

Studies show that the F2 stage of fibrosis is one of the most critical points in the progression from NASH and NASH fibrosis to end-stage liver disease, making it a crucial step for therapeutic intervention [86,87]. The risk of liver-specific mortality at stages F3 and F4 fibrosis is shown to increase by 50–80%. Thus, diagnosis and monitoring patients with noninvasive strategies is a major focus of actual research. Effective clinical NASH treatment is achieved when fibrosis progression is prevented and/or fibrosis is improved.

Most biomarkers do not measure fibrogenesis or fibrinolysis directly. Thus, those indirect surrogate markers show a low accuracy leading to the necessity of biomarker panels to improve their reliability on the discrimination between different fibrosis stages. The most common scores that combine several clinical parameters are the NAFLD Fibrosis Score (NFS), the Fibrosis-4 Score (FIB-4), the AST to Platelet Ratio Index (APRI) and the BARD Score, which includes BMI, AST:ALT ratio and diabetes.

The NFS includes several generally measured parameters and is well-studied in regards to its accuracy [45]. Simple online calculation of the respective score can be done free of charge at http://www.nafldscore.com/. Taking into account the AST:ALT ratio, albumin, platelet count, age, BMI and hyperglycemia, the NFS has a high predictive value, thereby avoiding the need of liver biopsy in many patients [45]. Nevertheless, there are two different cutoff level described to either exclude or diagnose advanced fibrosis. This is leading to the problem that patients who end up with scores in between the two cutoff levels are not classified properly.

The FIB-4 index described in 2010 by McPherson et al. has an accuracy of AUROC 0.86 for advanced fibrosis and relies on the AST, ALT, platelet count and age [53]. With a high negative predictive value of more than 90% and a positive predictive value of 82% the FIB-4 index is one of the reliable fibrosis scores to avoid liver fibrosis for diagnosis. Also, for the FIB-4 index there are two different cutoff level, i.e., a score <1.45 for moderate and >3.25 for advanced fibrosis [88]. Both, the NFS and FIB-4 scores have been shown to be capable to predict decompensation in patients with NAFLD and NASH [89,90].

Modified by the diagnosis of chronic hepatitis C is the APRI index calculating the AST/platelet ratio. Based on its simplicity to be calculated the APRI index has a comparably low accuracy with AUROC 0.788 to predict advanced fibrosis but is highly feasible as few and very common markers are used [54]. An online tool for calculating and interpretation of APRI index results can be found at: https://www.hepatitisc.uw.edu/go/evaluation-staging-monitoring/evaluation-staging/calculating-apri.

The BARD score, including the presence of type II diabetes, BMI and the AST:ALT ratio, comes with an AUROC of 0.81 to detect F3 fibrosis. Developed by Harrison et al. in 2008, this score has a high negative predictive value of 96% whereas the positive predictive value is modest [55].

Very recently the MACK-3 was proposed as a marker for fibrotic NASH. MACK-3 includes the HOMA insulin resistance, AST and CK18 serum level. With an AUROC of 0.80 and a negative predictive value of 100% for fibrotic NASH and 74% for active NASH MACK-3 seems to be a promising score for future investigation and validation [91].

Taken together, the scores that are actually available still have only moderate sensitivity and further investigation on noninvasive markers is urgently needed. Although all scores have comparable high negative predictive values and use common parameters measured during the general blood work so that they are easy to calculate and are definitely useful to screen patients, which are at risk to develop NAFLD related fibrosis and end-stage liver disease.

The measurement of specific fibrosis biomarkers in serum such as hyaluronic acid [92], procollagen III amino-terminal peptide (PIIINP) type IV collagen [93], TIMP-1 (tissue inhibitor of metalloproteinase 1) [94] or laminin [95] did not reach clinical routine, although they correlate with NASH and fibrosis with AUROC ranging from 0.87 (for hyaluronic acid) to 0.97 (for TIMP-1) [96]. The reason for that is most likely that measurement is cost-intensive and technically complex.

Further developments in the field combine different serum parameters in complex algorithms such as the Enhanced Liver Fibrosis panel (ELF) [56], FibroTest/FibroSURE/ActiTest [58], FibroMeter NAFLD index [59,60], Hepascore [57], and many others show very promising results to diagnose and distinguish patients with F0-F2 fibrosis from those with F3-F4 fibrosis. Those algorithms have to be validated in the clinics and have to be further developed and simplified to be able to make them widely applicable.

For the validation of a new diagnostic test method, the STARD checklist (Standards of Reporting of Diagnostic Accuracy Studies) was established and published by 13 journals in 2003 and modified to also meet the criteria needed for the evaluation of liver fibrosis in 2015. This Liver-FibroSTARD checklist should help to reach consent on the requirements for new noninvasive fibrosis markers [97,98].

However, it is obvious that the prediction of NASH severity by a noninvasive fibrosis marker, score, a diagnostic test, or an algorithm incorporating a panel of biomarkers is not necessarily capable of making a comprehensive statement of the disease outcome. Confounding factors, comorbidities, or simple blood parameters can significantly impact the progression or overall outcome of NASH. This was recently documented in a cross-sectional study in which 100 obese patients suffering from hepatic steatosis were analyzed for the occurrence of atherosclerosis [99]. Interestingly, the authors found that a lowered copper bioavailability is linked to atherosclerosis, which is the main complication of NAFLD. In line, reduced hepatic copper concentrations were found in human NAFLD patients and associated with higher degrees of hepatic steatosis in rats fed with low dietary copper [100].

3. Imaging

Although histological evaluation of liver biopsies and calculation of values that are based on the determination of serum markers and measurement of body features are extremely helpful to get information on inflammation and fibrosis, these methods have also some limitation. In particular, liver biopsy is invasive, relative costly and associated with relevant biopsy-related complications including bleeding, pain and infections. Moreover, it has been known for decades that the procedure has a high inter-observer variability and may not be representative for the whole organ [101]. In addition, it is impossible to apply liver biopsy to monitor changes in fibrosis stages because this would require multiple repetition of the procedure. Similarly, single or combination of biomarker measurements, which meet all the diagnostic criteria required for widespread, cost-effective, and reliable use are not available. A major pitfall in all these measurements is that the evaluation of any new biomarker is hindered by the lack of reference tests and the inter-technique analytical variability and performance of individual parameters. Therefore, individual biomarkers or multiparametic panels of biomarkers have reached only limited clinical application. Imaging techniques, providing direct information about the health status of the liver, have therefore emerged as attractive alternatives to assess steatosis, steatohepatitis, fibrosis, cirrhosis or hepatic cancer. In the following we will briefly summarize of imaging-based methods for diagnosing NASH and NAFLD.

3.1. *Ultrasound*

Historically, the first report on using ultrasonography as a diagnostic tool in hepatic steatosis and steatohepatitis was published in 1981, in which patients suffering from alcohol-related disease were analyzed for parenchymal alterations, fatty infiltration, dilatation of hepatic veins and ascites [102].

Later studies have shown that the sensitivity of this radiologic modality is somewhat limited when the content of hepatic steatosis is below a certain threshold [103]. However, by use of this imaging technique, it was demonstrated in a prospective study investigating a cohort of 400 patients that the overall prevalence of NAFLD and NASH is significantly higher than originally estimated [104]. Based on these findings, the method is a significant diagnostic add-on for screening of patients at risk for NAFLD and NASH, in particular when liver enzymes are elevated. In line with this assumption, a very recent descriptive, cross-sectional study categorizing 109 patients into different grades of NAFLD by ultrasonography showed that ultrasound is still an important, cheap, and easy-to-use imaging tool for the diagnosis and grading of fatty liver diseases [105]. In addition, the authors could demonstrate that ultrasound is ideally suited to manage patients with fatty liver in follow-ups, because of its significant association with deranged lipid profiles and the lack of any side effects.

Contrast-enhanced ultrasound (CEUS) allowing to monitor not only qualitatively, but also quantitative analysis of lesion microcirculation has helped to establish diagnostic procedures for detection of focal and diffuse liver pathologies and to assess a differential diagnosis between benign and malignant liver lesions [106].

3.2. Ultrasound-Based Elastography Techniques

In 2005, it was demonstrated that the propagation and velocity of low-frequency pulsed shear waves in real time in biological tissue is directly correlated to the amount of extracellular matrix [107]. Respective methods relying on the velocity of shear waves, introduced as "transient elastography", "vibration-controlled transient elastography (VCTE)" or "real-time shear wave elastography (SWE)" are particularly suited to detect liver cirrhosis by high stiffness in which it has a diagnostic specificity of 99% [108]. It is noteworthy, that a VCTE device such as the FibroScan introduced by Echosens SA can be performed as a point-of-care (POCT) test at the place of patient care enabling test results to be immediately shared instantly with care providers or patients. Unfortunately, the device has potential technical limitations in patients suffering from ascites, high quantities of chest wall fat, and in individuals who are morbidly obese [109].

In acoustic radiation force impulse elastography (ARFI) measuring beam passes over a standardized region of interest of the liver, obesity as defined by a BMI of larger 30 kg/m^2 or ascites are not considered obstacles [110]. However, ARFI imaging was found to have a poor diagnostic performance in patients with BMI larger than 35 kg/m^2 [111]. Other ultrasound real-time imaging modalities for soft tissue elasticity mapping are SWE or supersonic shear imaging (SSI) [104]. In these measurements, the propagation of the waves is stored in small video clips from which the elasticity of the analyzed tissue can be mapped quantitatively [112]. Although, these methods have good to excellent performance for the noninvasive staging of fibrosis in hepatitis B infected patients, data on other liver disease cohorts are still needs to be established [113].

However, in some disease conditions, the combination of elastography techniques with special NAFLD scores composed of simple measures of patient characteristics and clinical chemistry parameters increase the overall accuracy in assessment of clinically significant liver fibrosis in NAFLD [114]. The combination of various methods is therefore potentially relevant to better identify patients in which a liver biopsy is appropriately indicated.

3.3. Controlled Attenuation Parameter

The controlled attenuation parameter (CAP) was developed specifically for the FibroScan device to allow detection of hepatic steatosis in patients with about 10% of fatty hepatocyte degeneration without being influenced by liver fibrosis or cirrhosis. This threshold is clinically highly relevant because the diagnosis of steatosis is generally made when hepatic lipid content exceeds 5–10% by weight [115]. A significant correlation of the CAP signal and steatosis was first demonstrated in 2010 [116]. This study showed that CAP can efficiently separate grades of steatosis with AUROC values of 0.91 and 0.95 for the detection of more than 10% and 33% of steatosis. However, although these characteristics are diagnostically promising, it should be critically mentioned that CAP increases after a meal across all stages of fibrosis, potentially leading to misclassification of patients when the operator does not adhere to preanalytical necessities [117].

3.4. Magnetic Resonance Imaging in NASH and NAFLD

Magnetic resonance imaging (MRI) provides another possibility to quantify hepatic fat content with high spatial resolution. Like the other imaging techniques mentioned before, MRI scans do not require or emit ionizing radiation. However, the generation of meaningful MRI images in high resolution requires long imaging times that can be shortened by intravenous administration of gadolinium(III)-based contrast agents [11]. Advanced MRI techniques such as MRI proton density fat fraction (MRI-PDFF) were developed to specifically detect the presence of hepatic steatosis and to assess liver fat over the entire liver [118]. In this analysis, the PDFF is given as an absolute percentage ranging from 0% to 100% and defined as the ratio of density of mobile protons from fat (i.e., triglycerides) and the total density of protons from mobile triglycerides and mobile water [119]. Based on its robustness, practicability, reproducibility PDFF was proposed as the best-suited quantitative MR-based quantitative MR-based biomarker of tissue fat concentration for large-scale research endeavors and widespread clinical implementation [120]. Several independent studies analyzing NAFLD patients showed that MRP-PDFF performed better than CAP for diagnosing all stages of steatosis and had an overall better diagnostic accuracy [121–123].

3.5. Magnetic Resonance Elastography

A meta-analysis including retrospective studies showed that magnetic resonance elastography (MRE) is particularly useful to determine liver stiffness and has high accuracy for the diagnosis of significant or advanced fibrosis and cirrhosis [124]. Therefore, this imaging modality may be highly suitable to detect progression and treatment response in patients with chronic liver disease. This imaging technique is complementary to ultrasound-based elastography techniques and is highly accurate in diagnosing advances fibrosis in patients suffering from NAFLD [125]. This was documented in a prospective study in which the accuracy of 3D-MRE and 2D-MRE was compared in a cohort of 100 consecutive patients with biopsy-proven NAFLD [126]. This study further revealed that 3D-MRE is significantly more accurate than 2D-MRE for diagnosis of advanced fibrosis in NAFLD patients.

MRE was also found to be more accurate than ultrasound-based transient elastography in a cross-sectional study of more than 100 NAFLD patients in which fibrosis were detected with an AUROC of 0.82 (95% confidence interval, 0.74–0.91) [122]. Also, for classification of steatosis and necroinflammtory activity, MRE showed higher diagnostic performance than transient elastography in patients with NAFLD [121,127].

4. Genetic Tests

Genome wide association studies increased our knowledge and understanding of genetic and genomic alterations and components during NASH development and progression leading to the identification of several potential target genes, not only for therapeutic intervention, but also for the prediction of risk patients. The most abundant alterations are genetic variations in form of single nucleotide polymorphisms (SNPs). As very common alterations in NASH variants of the genes encoding patatin-like phospholipase domain-containing protein 2 (*PNPLA3*), transmembrane 6 superfamily member 2 (*TM6SF2*), membrane-bound O-acetyltransferase domain-containing protein 7 (*MBOAT7*) and glucokinase regulatory protein (*GCKR*) were identified. These genes are spread across the human genome (Figure 4).

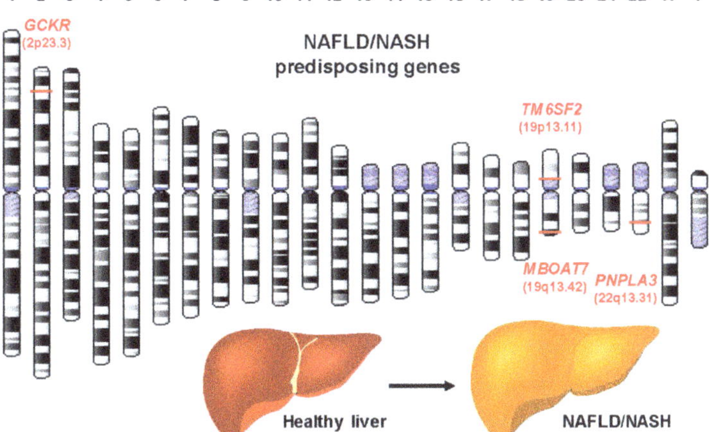

Figure 4. Gene alterations in NASH. Gene alterations/modifications associated with the pathogenesis of NASH affect the *GCKR*, *TM6SF2*, *PNPLA3*, and *MBOAT7* genes. The chromosomal location of respective genes is depicted in the ideogram. Gene annotations were done with the Genome Decoration Page (https://www.ncbi.nlm.nih.gov/genome/tools/gdp) and genomic coordinates deposited in the Online Mendelian Inheritance in Man (OMIM) database under accession no. 609567 (*PNPLA3*, 22q13.31), 606563 (*TM6SF2*, 19p13.11), 606048 (*MBOAT7*, 19q13.42), and 600842 (*GCKR*, 2p23.3).

The patatine-like phospholipase domain-containing protein 3 gene (*PNPLA3*) encodes for the triacylglycerol lipase adiponutrin that mediates the hydrolysis of triacylglycerol in adipocytes and hepatocytes. One of the most abundant DNA sequence variations associated with NAFLD and NASH is the isoleucine to methionine substitution in the *PNPLA3* gene at position 148 (PNPLA3-148M variant) [128,129]. This leads to a loss-of-function ending up in the accumulation of mutated 148M in hepatocytes and hepatic stellate cells where it further leads to the malignant storage of triglycerides [130]. Respective patients that are homozygous and carrying this variant have a tenfold increased risk to develop NAFLD-related HCC.

Transmembrane 6 superfamily member 2 (*TM6SF2*) is generally expressed in the liver and in the small intestine. It regulates the secretion of triglycerides and the content of lipid droplets as it is involved in VLDL (very low-density lipoprotein) secretion. The most frequent SNP is known in the *TM6SF2* gene is the E167K variant. This polymorphism is a loss-of-function mutation triggered by the replacement of glutamic acid by lysine at position 167. This mutation leads to the accumulation of triglycerides in hepatocytes and at the same time lowers the systemic lipoprotein levels [131].

A mutation leading to the replacement of cysteine by threonine is a common variant within the membrane bound O-acyltransferase domain-containing 7 (*MBOAT7*) gene. Recent investigations link this variant with a decrease in systemic and intrahepatic phosphatidyl-inositol containing arachidonic acid, thereby leading to an increased risk of getting NAFLD, NASH, and related end-stage liver diseases [132]. Another genetic variant, which was shown to be directly associated with the development of NAFLD by influencing the regulation of *de novo* lipogenesis and hepatic glucose uptake is the P446L mutation in the *GCKR* gene encoding for the glucokinase regulatory protein [133].

Besides those mentioned above, further genome-wide analysis show other gene variants associated with a higher risk of developing NAFLD and progress to related end-stage diseases. In this context, genetic polymorphisms of ethanol metabolizing enzymes (e.g., alcohol dehydrogenase) and cytochrome p450 2E1 (*CYP2E1*) activation triggering oxidative biotransformation and ROS formation, which is relevant in generating lipid peroxides, and their interference with the outcome of alcohol-induced liver disease and NASH has been discussed [134]. In particular, there are several clinical studies showing that alterations in *CYP2E1* activity are observed under various conditions, including obesity rendering respective persons more susceptible to liver injury [134,135]. Getting more knowledge about the exact effects influenced by those gene variations can be beneficial in the development of new therapeutic options and drug targets to treat NASH in the future.

More recently, several exploratory studies conducted in preclinical models identified circulating levels of non-coding RNA (ncRNA) such as microRNA and long ncRNA (lncRNA) to be associated with the pathogenesis and progression of various liver diseases [136]. In particular, several microRNAs representing a new class of highly conserved small non-coding RNA were shown to be critically involved in the regulation of complex gene networks in almost all acute and chronic liver disease [137]. As an example, profiling in diet-induced NASH progression and regression models identified the upregulation of a signature composed of six defined microRNA in NASH mice that allowed accurate distinguishing of NASH from lean mice [138]. However, in view of the large number of reported preclinical studies on miRNA, only a few have entered clinical trials and precise information about their diagnostic and prognostic value for human liver disease is still missing.

5. Screening for NAFLD and NASH

Identification of pre-symptomatic individuals or patients at risk would be the best to enable earlier disease intervention and management. There is a large number of early signs or symptoms indicating the onset of NAFLD, including central obesity, elevated serum triglyceride, and impaired fasting glucose. In addition, anorexia, nausea, vomiting, malaise, headache, or even epigastric and right upper quadrant abdominal pain, mild jaundice, and thrombocytopenia can already hint to initiation of NAFLD. Therefore, it was proposed that the potential of simple steatosis to progress into severe NAFLD necessitates timely detection of risk stratification in community-based healthcare settings [139]. However, despite multiple research reports demonstrating amazing promises, most of the proposed early protein or nucleic acid biomarkers are presently characterized by low sensitivity, low stability, and limited specificity [139]. In addition, screening programs, analyzing diagnostic panels are costly. Last but not least, NAFLD may be less benign than currently thought [33]. Therefore, there are limitations in defining diagnostic starting points for the management of prodomic phases of NAFLD. This is potentially the reason, why Scientific Societies such as the American Association for the Study of Liver Diseases (AASLD), the European Association for the Study of Liver Diseases (EASL), the National Institute for Health and Care Excellence (NICE), and the Asia-Pacific Working Party do not support a NAFLD screening program or only recommend screening programs in high-risk groups [140].

6. Other Factors in NAFLD and NASH

Most recently, first reports described that exosomes carrying a variety of cargoes, including proteins, fats, and various kinds of nucleic acids (mRNAs, microRNAs, other noncoding RNAs) have fundamental implications in liver pathobiology [141–144]. Although the precise mechanisms by which they contribute to NAFLD and NASH are still somewhat enigmatic, there are first reports proposing defined exosomal microRNAs such as miR-192 released from injured hepatocytes as potential new biomarkers to evaluate the progression from simple steatosis to NASH [145]. First encouraging studies have generated significant interest in exosomes as targets for biomarkers development [144].

Other researchers focus on potential roles of the adipose tissue in NAFLD. In particular, adipose tissue macrophages were proposed as key players in NAFLD [146]. There is a general consensus that a large set of signaling molecules such as lipids, microRNAs, adipokines and immune-related compounds are released from adipose tissue into the portal vein triggering hepatic inflammation [146]. In particular, the release of fatty acids from dysfunctional adipocytes results in liver parenchymal cell toxicity, which causes the ectopic accumulation of triglyceride-derived toxic metabolites increasing the activity of inflammatory pathways [147]. However, all these mechanisms are presently only partially understood and the impact of different macrophage phenotypes on the formation of NAFLD and NASH needs additional studies.

Another recent focus discussed in NAFLD and NASH research is the occurrence of quantitative and qualitative changes of the intestinal flora. Such a dysbiosis can result from altered food metabolism, intoxication, or increased permeability of the intestinal barrier. There is nowadays increasing evidence suggesting a critical role for the gut microbiome in the pathogenesis of obesity and metabolic syndrome [148]. The gut microbiota contributes to liver steatosis by modulating the uptake, bio-processing, fermentation, and synthesis of several effector molecules such as short-chain fatty acids, bile acids, cholines, and many other substances [149]. Moreover, it is intensively discussed at present if the microbiome composition can be used as a biomarker to differentiate between NAFLD and NASH [148]. However, standardized test systems or microbiota-targeted personalized treatment approaches for NAFLD and NASH are still not available.

7. Conclusions

Worldwide, NAFLD and NASH as well as NAFLD-related diseases (OSAS, PCOS, non-obese NAFLD), have emerged as leading causes of chronic liver disease in the last decades. The pathogenesis of respective diseases is complex and influenced by genetic factors, patients' characteristics, and a variety of risk factors. Although the factors and involved pathways triggering initiating and progression of NAFLD and NASH are reasonably well known, there is an urgent clinical need to establish reliable, noninvasive biomarkers, tests or algorithms that avoid the need of liver biopsy and allow to differentiate between disease stages. During the last decades, a great variety of multiparametric panels and parameter combinations (NFLS, HIS, FLI, LAP index, FLIP, CHeK, NFS, APRI, BARD, ELF, Hepascore) taking into account serum markers (e.g., ALT, AST, bilirubin, Hb1Ac, HDL, α_2M, platelet counts), patient characteristics (sex, gender, BMI), or comorbidities (diabetes) were established. However, all these diagnostic panels have limitations and alone are not suitable to replace liver biopsy. Nowadays, high-resolution imaging modalities such as ultrasound, MRI, elastography, and CAP have been established. Several of these techniques, such as MRI-PDFF, which can specifically detect the presence of hepatic steatosis and assess liver fat over the entire liver, might be useful to substitute biopsies and greatly assist the objective follow-up of therapeutic trials. Finally, liver-derived exosomes released into the systemic circulation and toxic lipids are in focus as targets for biomarkers development in liquid liver biopsies.

Author Contributions: Conceptualization, H.K.D. and R.W.; writing—original draft preparation, H.K.D. and R.W.; writing—review and editing, H.K.D., R.W. and S.W.; visualization, S.W.; funding acquisition, R.W.

Funding: This research was funded by the German Research Foundation (SFB/TRR57).

Conflicts of Interest: The authors declare no conflicts of interest.

References

1. Byron, D.; Minuk, G.Y. Clinical hepatology: Profile of an urban, hospital-based practic. *Hepatology* **1996**, *24*, 813–815. [CrossRef] [PubMed]
2. James, O.F.; Day, C.P. Non-alcoholic steatohepatitis (NASH): A disease of emerging identity and importance. *J. Hepatol.* **1998**, *29*, 495–501. [CrossRef]
3. Buzzetti, E.; Pinzani, M.; Tsochatzis, E.A. The multiple-hit pathogenesis of non-alcoholic fatty liver disease (NAFLD). *Metabolism* **2016**, *65*, 1038–1048. [CrossRef] [PubMed]
4. Wong, T.; Wong, R.J.; Gish, R.G. Diagnostic and treatment implications of nonalcoholic fatty liver disease and nonalcoholic steatohepatitis. *Gastroenterol. Hepatol.* **2019**, *15*, 83–89.
5. Angulo, P. Obesity and nonalcoholic fatty liver disease. *Nutr. Rev.* **2007**, *65*, 57–63. [CrossRef]
6. Younossi, Z.M.; Marchesini, G.; Pinto-Cortez, H.; Petta, S. Epidemiology of nonalcoholic fatty liver disease and nonalcoholic steatohepatitis: Implications for liver transplantation. *Transplantation* **2019**, *103*, 22–27. [CrossRef] [PubMed]
7. Sookoian, S.; Pirola, C.J. Genetics of nonalcoholic fatty liver disease: From pathogenesis to therapeutics. *Semin. Liver Dis.* **2019**, *39*, 124–140. [CrossRef] [PubMed]

8. Allard, J.; Le Guillou, D.; Begriche, K.; Fromenty, B. Drug-induced liver injury in obesity and nonalcoholic fatty liver disease. *Adv. Pharmacol.* **2019**. [CrossRef]
9. Poynard, T.; Munteanu, M.; Charlotte, F.; Perazzo, H.; Ngo, Y.; Deckmyn, O.; Pais, R.; Mathurin, P.; Ratziu, V. FLIP consortium, the FibroFrance-CPAM group; FibroFrance-Obese group. Impact of steatosis and inflammation definitions on the performance of NASH tests. *Eur. J. Gastroenterol. Hepatol.* **2018**, *30*, 384–391. [CrossRef]
10. Lykke Eriksen, P.; Sørensen, M.; Grønbæk, H.; Hamilton-Dutoit, S.; Vilstrup, H.; Thomsen, K.L. Non-alcoholic fatty liver disease causes dissociated changes in metabolic liver functions. *Clin. Res. Hepatol Gastroenterol.* **2019**, 13. [CrossRef]
11. Weiskirchen, R.; Tacke, F. The role of radiologic modalities in diagnosing nonalcoholic steatohepatitis (NASH) and fibrosis. *Curr. Hepatol. Rep.* **2018**, *17*, 324–335. [CrossRef]
12. Ratziu, V.; Bellentani, S.; Cortez-Pinto, H.; Day, C.; Marchesini, G. A position statement on NAFLD/NASH based on the EASL 2009 special conference. *J. Hepatol.* **2010**, *53*, 372–384. [CrossRef]
13. Schon, H.-T.; Weiskirchen, R. Exercise-induced release of pharmacologically active substances and their relevance for therapy of hepatic injury. *Front. Pharmacol.* **2016**, *7*, 1101. [CrossRef]
14. Jeznach-Steinhagen, A.; Ostrowska, J.; Czerwonogrodzka-Senczyna, A.; Boniecka, I.; Shahnazaryan, U.; Kuryłowicz, A. Dietary and pharmacological treatment of nonalcoholic fatty liver disease. *Medicina* **2019**, *55*, 166. [CrossRef]
15. Diwan, T.S.; Rice, T.C.; Heimbach, J.K.; Schauer, D.P. Liver transplantation and bariatric surgery: Timing and outcomes. *Liver Transplant.* **2018**, *24*, 1280–1287. [CrossRef]
16. Conway, B.N.; Han, X.; Munro, H.M.; Gross, A.L.; Shu, X.-O.; Hargreaves, M.K.; Zheng, W.; Powers, A.C.; Blot, W.J. The obesity epidemic and rising diabetes incidence in a low-income racially diverse southern US cohort. *PLoS ONE* **2018**, *13*, e0190993. [CrossRef]
17. Hirode, G.; Vittinghoff, E.; Wong, R.J. Increasing clinical and economic burden of nonalcoholic fatty liver disease among hospitalized adults in the United States. *J. Clin. Gastroenterol.* **2019**, *10*, 1097. [CrossRef]
18. Younossi, Z.M.; Koenig, A.B.; Abdelatif, D.; Fazel, Y.; Henry, L.; Wymer, M. Global epidemiology of nonalcoholic fatty liver disease-meta-analytic assessment of prevalence, incidence, and outcomes. *Hepatology* **2016**, *64*, 73–84. [CrossRef]
19. Estes, C.; Razavi, H.; Loomba, R.; Younossi, Z.; Sanyal, A.J. Modeling the epidemic of nonalcoholic fatty liver disease demonstrates an exponential increase in burden of disease. *Hepatology* **2018**, *67*, 123–133. [CrossRef]
20. Estes, C.; Anstee, Q.M.; Arias-Loste, M.T.; Bantel, H.; Bellentani, S.; Caballeria, J.; Colombo, M.; Craxi, A.; Crespo, J.; Day, C.P.; et al. Modeling NAFLD disease burden in China, France, Germany, Italy, Japan, Spain, United Kingdom, and United States for the period 2016-2030. *J. Hepatol* **2018**, *69*, 896–904. [CrossRef]
21. Cholankeril, G.; Wong, R.J.; Hu, M.; Perumpail, R.B.; Yoo, E.R.; Puri, P.; Younossi, Z.M.; Harrison, S.A.; Ahmed, A. Liver transplantation for nonalcoholic steatohepatitis in the US: Temporal trends and outcomes. *Dig. Dis. Sci.* **2017**, *62*, 2915–2922. [CrossRef]
22. Bril, F.; Kalavalapalli, S.; Clark, V.C.; Lomonaco, R.; Soldevila-Pico, C.; Liu, I.C.; Orsak, B.; Tio, F.; Cusi, K. Response to pioglitazone in patients with nonalcoholic steatohepatitis with vs. without type 2 diabetes. *Clin. Gastroenterol. Hepatol.* **2018**, *16*, 558–560. [CrossRef]
23. Chalasani, N.; Younossi, Z.; Lavine, J.E.; Charlton, M.; Cusi, K.; Rinella, M.; Harrison, S.A.; Brunt, E.M.; Sanyal, A.J. The diagnosis and management of nonalcoholic fatty liver disease: Practice guidance from the American Association for the Study of Liver Diseases. *Hepatology* **2018**, *67*, 328–357. [CrossRef]
24. EASL–EASD–EASO Clinical Practice Guidelines for the management of non-alcoholic fatty liver disease. *J. Hepatol.* **2016**, *64*, 1388–1402. [CrossRef]
25. Sharma, B.C.; Kumar, A.; Garg, V.; Reddy, R.S.; Sakhuja, P.; Sarin, S.K. A Randomized controlled trial comparing efficacy of pentoxifylline and pioglitazone on metabolic factors and liver histology in patients with non-alcoholic steatohepatitis. *J. Clin. Exp. Hepatol.* **2012**, *2*, 333–337. [CrossRef]
26. Wong, V.W.-S.; Chitturi, S.; Wong, G.L.-H.; Yu, J.; Chan, H.L.-Y.; Farrell, G.C.; Chitturi, S. Pathogenesis and novel treatment options for non-alcoholic steatohepatitis. *Lancet Gastroenterol. Hepatol.* **2016**, *1*, 56–67. [CrossRef]
27. Friedman, S.L.; Neuschwander-Tetri, B.A.; Rinella, M.; Sanyal, A.J. Mechanisms of NAFLD development and therapeutic strategies. *Nat. Med.* **2018**, *24*, 908–922. [CrossRef]

28. Townsend, S.; Newsome, P.N. Non-alcoholic fatty liver disease in 2016. *Br. Med Bull.* **2016**, *119*, 143–156. [CrossRef]
29. Neuschwander-Tetri, B.A.; Loomba, R.; Sanyal, A.J.; Lavine, J.E.; Van Natta, M.L.; Abdelmalek, M.F.; Chalasani, N.; Dasarathy, S.; Diehl, A.M.; Hameed, B.; et al. Farnesoid X nuclear receptor ligand obeticholic acid for non-cirrhotic, non-alcoholic steatohepatitis (FLINT): A multicentre, randomised, placebo-controlled trial. *Lancet* **2015**, *385*, 956–965. [CrossRef]
30. Brunt, E.M.; Wong, V.W.-S.; Nobili, V.; Day, C.P.; Sookoian, S.; Maher, J.J.; Bugianesi, E.; Sirlin, C.B.; Neuschwander-Tetri, B.A.; Rinella, M.E. Nonalcoholic fatty liver disease. *Nat. Rev. Dis. Prim.* **2015**, *1*, 15080. [CrossRef]
31. Neuschwander-Tetri, B.A. Lifestyle modification as the primary treatment of NASH. *Clin. Liver Dis.* **2009**, *13*, 649–665. [CrossRef]
32. Tacke, F.; Weiskirchen, R. An update on the recent advances in antifibrotic therapy. *Expert Rev. Gastroenterol. Hepatol.* **2018**, *12*, 1–10. [CrossRef]
33. Haas, J.T.; Francque, S.; Staels, B. Pathophysiology and mechanisms of nonalcoholic fatty liver disease. *Annu. Rev. Physiol.* **2016**, *78*, 181–205. [CrossRef]
34. Kneeman, J.M.; Misdraji, J.; Corey, K.E. Secondary causes of nonalcoholic fatty liver disease. *Therap. Adv. Gastroenterol.* **2012**, *5*, 199–207. [CrossRef]
35. Paschetta, E.; Belci, P.; Alisi, A.; Liccardo, D.; Cutrera, R.; Musso, G.; Nobili, V. OSAS-related inflammatory mechanisms of liver injury in nonalcoholic fatty liver disease. *Mediat. Inflamm.* **2015**, *2015*, 815721. [CrossRef]
36. Macut, D.; Božić-Antić, I.; Bjekić-Macut, J.; Tziomalos, K. Management of endocrine disease: Polycystic ovary syndrome and nonalcoholic fatty liver disease. *Eur. J. Endocrinol.* **2017**, *177*, R145–R158. [CrossRef]
37. Kim, D.; Kim, W.R. Nonobese fatty liver disease. *Clin. Gastroenterol. Hepatol.* **2017**, *15*, 474–485. [CrossRef]
38. Younes, R.; Bugianesi, E. NASH in lean individuals. *Semin. Liver Dis.* **2019**, *39*, 86–95. [CrossRef]
39. Koch, L.K.; Yeh, M.M. Nonalcoholic fatty liver disease (NAFLD): Diagnosis, pitfalls, and staging. *Ann. Diagn. Pathol.* **2018**, *37*, 83–90. [CrossRef]
40. Ratziu, V.; Charlotte, F.; Heurtier, A.; Gombert, S.; Giral, P.; Bruckert, E.; Grimaldi, A.; Capron, F.; Poynard, T. Sampling variability of liver biopsy in nonalcoholic fatty liver disease. *Gastroenterology* **2005**, *128*, 1898–1906. [CrossRef]
41. McGill, D.B.; Rakela, J.; Zinsmeister, A.R.; Ott, B.J. A 21-year experience with major hemorrhage after percutaneous liver biopsy. *Gastroenterology* **1990**, *99*, 1396–1400. [CrossRef]
42. Vilar-Gomez, E.; Athinarayanan, S.J.; Adams, R.N.; Hallberg, S.J.; Bhanpuri, N.H.; McKenzie, A.L.; Campbell, W.W.; McCarter, J.P.; Phinney, S.D.; Volek, J.S.; et al. Post hoc analyses of surrogate markers of non-alcoholic fatty liver disease (NAFLD) and liver fibrosis in patients with type 2 diabetes in a digitally supported continuous care intervention: An open-label, non-randomised controlled study. *BMJ Open* **2019**, *9*, e023597. [CrossRef]
43. Yip, T.C.-F.; Ma, A.J.; Wong, V.W.-S.; Tse, Y.-K.; Chan, H.L.-Y.; Yuen, P.-C.; Wong, G.L.-H.; Yip, T.C.; Wong, V.W.; Tse, Y.; et al. Laboratory parameter-based machine learning model for excluding non-alcoholic fatty liver disease (NAFLD) in the general population. *Aliment. Pharmacol. Ther.* **2017**, *46*, 447–456. [CrossRef]
44. Yip, T.C.-F.; Wong, V.W.-S.; Yip, T.C.; Wong, V.W. How to identify patients with advanced liver disease in the community? *Hepatology* **2017**, *66*, 7–9. [CrossRef]
45. Kotronen, A.; Peltonen, M.; Hakkarainen, A.; Sevastianova, K.; Bergholm, R.; Johansson, L.M.; Lundbom, N.; Rissanen, A.; Ridderstråle, M.; Groop, L.; et al. Prediction of non-alcoholic fatty liver disease and liver fat using metabolic and genetic factors. *Gastroenterology* **2009**, *137*, 865–872. [CrossRef]
46. Lee, J.-H.; Kim, D.; Kim, H.J.; Lee, C.-H.; Yang, J.I.; Kim, W.; Kim, Y.J.; Yoon, J.-H.; Cho, S.-H.; Sung, M.-W.; et al. Hepatic steatosis index: A simple screening tool reflecting nonalcoholic fatty liver disease. *Dig. Liver Dis.* **2010**, *42*, 503–508. [CrossRef]
47. Bedogni, G.; Bellentani, S.; Miglioli, L.; Masutti, F.; Passalacqua, M.; Castiglione, A.; Tiribelli, C. The fatty liver index: A simple and accurate predictor of hepatic steatosis in the general population. *BMC Gastroenterol.* **2006**, *6*, 33. [CrossRef]
48. Calori, G.; Lattuada, G.; Ragogna, F.; Garancini, M.P.; Crosignani, P.; Villa, M.; Bosi, E.; Ruotolo, G.; Piemonti, L.; Perseghin, G. Fatty liver index and mortality: The cremona study in the 15th year of follow-up. *Hepatology* **2011**, *54*, 145–152. [CrossRef]

49. Bedogni, G.; Kahn, H.S.; Bellentani, S.; Tiribelli, C. A simple index of lipid overaccumulation is a good marker of liver steatosis. *BMC Gastroenterol.* **2010**, *10*, 98. [CrossRef]
50. Bedossa, P. Utility and appropriateness of the fatty liver inhibition of progression (FLIP) algorithm and steatosis, activity, and fibrosis (SAF) score in the evaluation of biopsies of nonalcoholic fatty liver disease. *Hepatology* **2014**, *60*, 565–575. [CrossRef]
51. Canbay, A.; Kälsch, J.; Neumann, U.; Rau, M.; Hohenester, S.; Baba, H.A.; Rust, C.; Geier, A.; Heider, D.; Sowa, J.-P. Non-invasive assessment of NAFLD as systemic disease—A machine learning perspective. *PLoS ONE* **2019**, *14*, e0214436. [CrossRef]
52. Angulo, P.; Hui, J.M.; Marchesini, G.; Bugianesi, E.; George, J.; Farrell, G.C.; Enders, F.; Saksena, S.; Burt, A.D.; Bida, J.P.; et al. The NAFLD fibrosis score: A noninvasive system that identifies liver fibrosis in patients with NAFLD. *Hepatology* **2007**, *45*, 846–854. [CrossRef]
53. McPherson, S.; Henderson, E.; Stewart, S.F.; Burt, A.D.; Day, C.P. Simple non-invasive fibrosis scoring systems can reliably exclude advanced fibrosis in patients with non-alcoholic fatty liver disease. *Gut* **2010**, *59*, 1265–1269. [CrossRef]
54. Kruger, F.C.; Daniels, C.R.; Kidd, M.; Swart, G.; Brundyn, K.; Van Rensburg, C.; Kotze, M. APRI: A simple bedside marker for advanced fibrosis that can avoid liver biopsy in patients with NAFLD/NASH. *S. Afr. Med. J.* **2011**, *101*, 477–480.
55. Harrison, S.A.; Oliver, D.; Arnold, H.L.; Gogia, S.; A Neuschwander-Tetri, B. Development and validation of a simple NAFLD clinical scoring system for identifying patients without advanced disease. *Gut* **2008**, *57*, 1441–1447. [CrossRef]
56. Rosenberg, W.M.; Voelker, M.; Thiel, R.; Becka, M.; Burt, A.; Schuppan, D.; Hubscher, S.; Roskams, T.; Pinzani, M.; Arthur, M.J. Serum markers detect the presence of liver fibrosis: A cohort study. *Gastroenterology* **2004**, *127*, 1704–1713. [CrossRef]
57. Adams, L.A.; Bulsara, M.; Rossi, E.; DeBoer, B.; Speers, D.; George, J.; Kench, J.; Farrell, G.; McCaughan, G.W.; Jeffrey, G.P. Hepascore: An accurate validated predictor of liver fibrosis in chronic hepatitis C Infection. *Clin. Chem.* **2005**, *51*, 1867–1873. [CrossRef]
58. Poynard, T.; Imbert-Bismut, F.; Munteanu, M.; Ratziu, V. FibroTest-FibroSURE™: Towards a universal biomarker of liver fibrosis? *Expert Rev. Mol. Diagn.* **2005**, *5*, 15–21. [CrossRef]
59. Cales, P.; Oberti, F.; Michalak, S.; Rousselet, M.-C.; Konaté, A.; Gallois, Y.; Ternisien, C.; Chevailler, A.; Lunel, F.; Hubert-Fouchard, I.; et al. A novel panel of blood markers to assess the degree of liver fibrosis. *Hepatology* **2005**, *42*, 1373–1381. [CrossRef]
60. Boursier, J.; Guillaume, M.; Leroy, V.; Irlès, M.; Roux, M.; Lannes, A.; Foucher, J.; Zuberbuhler, F.; Delabaudière, C.; Barthelon, J.; et al. New sequential combinations of non-invasive fibrosis tests provide an accurate diagnosis of advanced fibrosis in NAFLD. *J. Hepatol.* **2019**, *71*, 389–396. [CrossRef]
61. Ruiz-Tovar, J.; Zubiaga, L. Validation of biochemical scores for liver steatosis before and 1 year after sleeve gastrectomy. *Surg. Obes. Relat. Dis.* **2019**. [CrossRef]
62. Cheung, C.-L.; Lam, K.S.; Wong, I.C.; Cheung, B.M. Non-invasive score identifies ultrasonography-diagnosed non-alcoholic fatty liver disease and predicts mortality in the USA. *BMC Med.* **2014**, *12*, 154. [CrossRef]
63. Feldstein, A.E.; Wieckowska, A.; Lopez, A.R.; Liu, Y.-C.; Zein, N.N.; McCullough, A.J. Cytokeratin-18 fragment levels as noninvasive biomarker for nonalcoholic steatohepatitis: A multicenter validation study. *Hepatology* **2009**, *50*, 1072–1078. [CrossRef]
64. Eguchi, A.; Wree, A.; Feldstein, A.E. Biomarkers of liver cell death. *J. Hepatol.* **2014**, *60*, 1063–1074. [CrossRef]
65. Church, R.J.; Watkins, P.B. The transformation in biomarker detection and management of drug-induced liver injury. *Liver Int.* **2017**, *37*, 1582–1590. [CrossRef]
66. Malik, R.; Chang, M.; Bhaskar, K.; Nasser, I.; Curry, M.; Schuppan, D.; Byrnes, V.; Afdhal, N. The clinical utility of biomarkers and the nonalcoholic steatohepatitis CRN liver biopsy scoring system in patients with nonalcoholic fatty liver disease. *J. Gastroenterol. Hepatol.* **2009**, *24*, 564–568. [CrossRef]
67. Kwok, R.; Tse, Y.K.; Wong, G.L.; Ha, Y.; Lee, A.U.; Ngu, M.C.; Chan, H.L.; Wong, V.W. Systematic review with meta-analysis: Non-invasive assessment of non-alcoholic fatty liver disease–the role of transient elastography and plasma cytokeratin-18 fragments. *Aliment. Pharmacol. Ther.* **2014**, *39*, 254–269. [CrossRef]
68. He, L.; Deng, L.; Zhang, Q.; Guo, J.; Zhou, J.; Song, W.; Yuan, F. Diagnostic value of CK-18, FGF-21, and related biomarker panel in nonalcoholic fatty liver disease: A systematic review and meta-analysis. *BioMed Res. Int.* **2017**, *2017*, 9729107. [CrossRef]

69. Tamimi, T.I.A.-R.; Elgouhari, H.M.; Alkhouri, N.; Yerian, L.M.; Berk, M.P.; Lopez, R.; Schauer, P.R.; Zein, N.N.; Feldstein, A.E. An apoptosis panel for nonalcoholic steatohepatitis diagnosis. *J. Hepatol.* **2011**, *54*, 1224–1229. [CrossRef]
70. Jarrar, M.H.; Baranova, A.; Collantes, R.; Ranard, B.; Stepanova, M.; Bennett, C.; Fang, Y.; Elariny, H.; Goodman, Z.; Chandhoke, V.; et al. Adipokines and cytokines in non-alcoholic fatty liver disease. *Aliment. Pharmacol. Ther.* **2008**, *27*, 412–421. [CrossRef]
71. Wu, G.; Li, H.; Fang, Q.; Zhang, J.; Zhang, M.; Zhang, L.; Wu, L.; Hou, X.; Lu, J.; Bao, Y.; et al. Complementary Role of fibroblast growth factor 21 and cytokeratin 18 in monitoring the different stages of nonalcoholic fatty liver disease. *Sci. Rep.* **2017**, *7*, 5095. [CrossRef]
72. Li, H.; Fang, Q.; Gao, F.; Fan, J.; Zhou, J.; Wang, X.; Zhang, H.; Pan, X.; Bao, Y.; Xiang, K.; et al. Fibroblast growth factor 21 levels are increased in nonalcoholic fatty liver disease patients and are correlated with hepatic triglyceride. *J. Hepatol.* **2010**, *53*, 934–940. [CrossRef]
73. Yilmaz, Y.; Eren, F.; Yonal, O.; Kurt, R.; Aktas, B.; Celikel, C.A.; Özdoğan, O.; Imeryuz, N.; Kalayci, C.; Avsar, E.; et al. Increased serum FGF21 levels in patients with nonalcoholic fatty liver disease. *Eur. J. Clin. Investig.* **2010**, *40*, 887–892. [CrossRef]
74. Gariani, K.; Drifte, G.; Dunn-Siegrist, I.; Pugin, J.; Jornayvaz, F.R. Increased FGF21 plasma levels in humans with sepsis and SIRS. *Endocr. Connect.* **2013**, *2*, 146–153. [CrossRef]
75. Yan, H.; Xia, M.; Chang, X.; Xu, Q.; Bian, H.; Zeng, M.; Rao, S.-X.; Yao, X.; Tu, Y.; Jia, W.; et al. Circulating fibroblast growth factor 21 levels are closely associated with hepatic fat content: A cross-sectional study. *PLoS ONE* **2011**, *6*, e24895. [CrossRef]
76. Lau, H.H.; Ng, N.H.J.; Loo, L.S.W.; Jasmen, J.B.; Teo, A.K.K. The molecular functions of hepatocyte nuclear factors – In and beyond the liver. *J. Hepatol.* **2018**, *68*, 1033–1048. [CrossRef]
77. Moya, M.; Benet, M.; Guzmán, C.; Tolosa, L.; García-Monzón, C.; Pareja, E.; Castell, J.V.; Jover, R. Foxa1 reduces lipid accumulation in human hepatocytes and is down-regulated in nonalcoholic fatty liver. *PLoS ONE* **2012**, *7*, e30014. [CrossRef]
78. Ramadori, P.; Drescher, H.; Erschfeld, S.; Schumacher, F.; Berger, C.; Fragoulis, A.; Schenkel, J.; Kensler, T.W.; Wruck, C.J.; Trautwein, C.; et al. Hepatocyte-specific Keap1 deletion reduces liver steatosis but not inflammation during non-alcoholic steatohepatitis development. *Free. Radic. Boil. Med.* **2016**, *91*, 114–126. [CrossRef]
79. Feldstein, A.E.; Lopez, R.; Tamimi, T.A.-R.; Yerian, L.; Chung, Y.-M.; Berk, M.; Zhang, R.; McIntyre, T.M.; Hazen, S.L. Mass spectrometric profiling of oxidized lipid products in human nonalcoholic fatty liver disease and nonalcoholic steatohepatitis. *J. Lipid Res.* **2010**, *51*, 3046–3054. [CrossRef]
80. Hagström, H.; Stål, P.; Hultcrantz, R.; Brismar, K.; Ansurudeen, I. IGFBP-1 and IGF-I as markers for advanced fibrosis in NAFLD – a pilot study. *Scand. J. Gastroenterol.* **2017**, *52*, 1427–1434. [CrossRef]
81. Regué, L.; Minichiello, L.; Avruch, J.; Dai, N. Liver-specific deletion of IGF2 mRNA binding protein-2/IMP2 reduces hepatic fatty acid oxidation and increases hepatic triglyceride accumulation. *J. Boil. Chem.* **2019**, *294*, 11944–11951. [CrossRef]
82. Kowdley, K.V.; Belt, P.; Wilson, L.A.; Yeh, M.M.; Neuschwander-Tetri, B.A.; Chalasani, N.; Sanyal, A.J.; Nelson, J.E.; Network, N.C.R. Serum ferritin is an independent predictor of histologic severity and advanced fibrosis in patients with nonalcoholic fatty liver disease. *Hepatology* **2012**, *55*, 77–85. [CrossRef]
83. Maliken, B.D.; Nelson, J.E.; Klintworth, H.M.; Beauchamp, M.; Yeh, M.M.; Kowdley, K.V. Hepatic reticuloendothelial system cell iron deposition is associated with increased apoptosis in nonalcoholic fatty liver disease. *Hepatology* **2013**, *57*, 1806–1813. [CrossRef]
84. Ajmera, V.; Perito, E.R.; Bass, N.M.; Terrault, N.A.; Yates, K.P.; Gill, R.; Loomba, R.; Diehl, A.M.; Aouizerat, B.E.; Network, N.C.R. Novel plasma biomarkers associated with liver disease severity in adults with nonalcoholic fatty liver disease. *Hepatology* **2017**, *65*, 65–77. [CrossRef]
85. Poynard, T.; Ratziu, V.; Charlotte, F.; Messous, D.; Munteanu, M.; Imbert-Bismut, F.; Massard, J.; Bonyhay, L.; Tahiri, M.; Thabut, D.; et al. Diagnostic value of biochemical markers (NashTest) for the prediction of non alcoholo steato hepatitis in patients with non-alcoholic fatty liver disease. *BMC Gastroenterol.* **2006**, *6*, 34. [CrossRef]

86. Angulo, P.; Kleiner, D.E.; Dam-Larsen, S.; Adams, L.A.; Bjornsson, E.S.; Charatcharoenwitthaya, P.; Mills, P.R.; Keach, J.C.; Lafferty, H.D.; Stahler, A.; et al. Liver fibrosis, but no other histologic features, is associated with long-term outcomes of patients with nonalcoholic fatty liver disease. *Gastroenterology* **2015**, *149*, 389–397. [CrossRef]
87. Ekstedt, M.; Hagström, H.; Nasr, P.; Fredrikson, M.; Stål, P.; Kechagias, S.; Hultcrantz, R. Fibrosis stage is the strongest predictor for disease-specific mortality in NAFLD after up to 33 years of follow-up. *Hepatology* **2015**, *61*, 1547–1554. [CrossRef]
88. Sterling, R.K.; Lissen, E.; Clumeck, N.; Sola, R.; Correa, M.C.; Montaner, J.; Sulkowski, M.S.; Torriani, F.J.; Dieterich, D.T.; Thomas, D.L.; et al. Development of a simple noninvasive index to predict significant fibrosis in patients with HIV/HCV coinfection. *Hepatology* **2006**, *43*, 1317–1325. [CrossRef]
89. Kim, D.; Kim, W.R.; Kim, H.J.; Therneau, T.M. Association between non-invasive fibrosis markers and mortality among adults with non-alcoholic fatty liver disease in the United States. *Hepatology* **2013**, *57*, 1357–1365. [CrossRef]
90. Cheah, M.C.; McCullough, A.J.; Goh, G.B.-B. Current modalities of fibrosis assessment in non-alcoholic fatty liver disease. *J. Clin. Transl. Hepatol.* **2017**, *5*, 261–271. [CrossRef]
91. Chuah, K.-H.; Yusoff, W.N.I.W.; Sthaneshwar, P.; Mustapha, N.R.N.; Mahadeva, S.; Chan, W.-K. MACK-3 (combination of hoMa, Ast and CK18): A promising novel biomarker for fibrotic non-alcoholic steatohepatitis. *Liver Int.* **2019**, *39*, 1315–1324. [CrossRef]
92. Lydatakis, H.; Hager, I.P.; Kostadelou, E.; Mpousmpoulas, S.; Pappas, S.; Diamantis, I. Non-invasive markers to predict the liver fibrosis in non-alcoholic fatty liver disease. *Liver Int.* **2006**, *26*, 864–871. [CrossRef]
93. Tanwar, S.; Trembling, P.M.; Guha, I.N.; Parkes, J.; Kaye, P.; Burt, A.D.; Ryder, S.D.; Aithal, G.P.; Day, C.P.; Rosenberg, W.M. Validation of terminal peptide of procollagen III for the detection and assessment of nonalcoholic steatohepatitis in patients with nonalcoholic fatty liver disease. *Hepatology* **2013**, *57*, 103–111. [CrossRef]
94. Abdelaziz, R.; Elbasel, M.; Esmat, S.; Essam, K.; Abdelaaty, S. Tissue inhibitors of metalloproteinase-1 and 2 and obesity related non-alcoholic fatty liver disease: Is there a relationship? *Digestion* **2015**, *92*, 130–137. [CrossRef]
95. Santos, V.N.; Leite-Mór, M.M.; Kondo, M.; Martins, J.R.; Nader, H.; Lanzoni, V.P.; Parise, E.R. Serum laminin, type IV collagen and hyaluronan as fibrosis markers in non-alcoholic fatty liver disease. *Braz. J. Med. Biol. Res.* **2005**, *38*, 747–753. [CrossRef]
96. Wong, V.W.-S.; Adams, L.A.; De Lédinghen, V.; Wong, G.L.-H.; Sookoian, S. Noninvasive biomarkers in NAFLD and NASH—Current progress and future promise. *Nat. Rev. Gastroenterol. Hepatol.* **2018**, *15*, 461–478. [CrossRef]
97. Boursier, J.; De Lédinghen, V.; Poynard, T.; Guechot, J.; Carrat, F.; Leroy, V.; Wong, G.L.-H.; Friedrich-Rust, M.; Fraquelli, M.; Plebani, M.; et al. An extension of STARD statements for reporting diagnostic accuracy studies on liver fibrosis tests: The Liver-FibroSTARD standards. *J. Hepatol.* **2015**, *62*, 807–815. [CrossRef]
98. Guechot, J.; Boursier, J.; De Lédinghen, V.; Poynard, T.; Carrat, F.; Leroy, V.; Wong, G.L.-H.; Friedrich-Rust, M.; Fraquelli, M.; Plebani, M.; et al. Liver-FibroSTARD checklist and glossary: Tools for standardized design and reporting of diagnostic accuracy studies of liver fibrosis tests. *Clin. Chem. Lab. Med.* **2015**, *53*, 1135–1137. [CrossRef]
99. Tarantino, G.; Porcu, C.; Arciello, M.; Andreozzi, P.; Balsano, C. Prediction of carotid intima-media thickness in obese patients with low prevalence of comorbidities by serum copper bioavailability. *J. Gastroenterol. Hepatol.* **2018**, *33*, 1511–1517. [CrossRef]
100. Aigner, E.; Strasser, M.; Haufe, H.; Sonnweber, T.; Hohla, F.; Stadlmayr, A.; Solioz, M.; Tilg, H.; Patsch, W.; Weiss, G.; et al. A role for low hepatic copper concentrations in nonalcoholic fatty liver disease. *Am. J. Gastroenterol.* **2010**, *105*, 1978–1985. [CrossRef]
101. Myers, R.P.; Fong, A.; Shaheen, A.A.M. Utilization rates, complications and costs of percutaneous liver biopsy: A population-based study including 4275 biopsies. *Liver Int.* **2008**, *28*, 705–712. [CrossRef]
102. Taylor, K.J.; Gorelick, F.S.; Rosenfield, A.T.; A Riely, C. Ultrasonography of alcoholic liver disease with histological correlation. *Radiology* **1981**, *141*, 157–161. [CrossRef]
103. Mishra, P.; Younossi, Z.M. Abdominal ultrasound for diagnosis of nonalcoholic fatty liver disease (NAFLD). *Am. J. Gastroenterol.* **2007**, *102*, 2716–2717. [CrossRef]

104. Williams, C.D.; Stengel, J.; Asike, M.I.; Torres, D.M.; Shaw, J.; Contreras, M.; Landt, C.L.; Harrison, S.A. Prevalence of nonalcoholic fatty liver disease and nonalcoholic steatohepatitis among a largely middle-aged population utilizing ultrasound and liver biopsy: A prospective study. *Gastroenterology* **2011**, *140*, 124–131. [CrossRef]
105. Khanal, U.P.; Paudel, B.; Gurung, G.; Hu, Y.S.; Kuo, C.W. Correlational study of nonalcoholic fatty liver disease diagnosed by ultrasonography with lipid profile and body mass index in adult Nepalese population. *J. Med. Ultrasound* **2019**, *27*, 19–25. [CrossRef]
106. Battaglia, V.; Cervelli, R. Liver investigations: Updating on US technique and contrast-enhanced ultrasound (CEUS). *Eur. J. Radiol.* **2017**, *96*, 65–73. [CrossRef]
107. Sandrin, L.; Tanter, M.; Catheline, S.; Fink, M. Shear modulus imaging with 2-D transient elastography. *IEEE Trans. Ultrason. Ferroelectr. Freq. Control.* **2002**, *49*, 426–435. [CrossRef]
108. Poynard, T.; Munteanu, M.; Luckina, E.; Perazzo, H.; Ngo, Y.; Royer, L.; Fedchuk, L.; Sattonnet, F.; Pais, R.; Lebray, P.; et al. Liver fibrosis evaluation using real-time shear wave elastography: Applicability and diagnostic performance using methods without a gold standard. *J. Hepatol.* **2013**, *58*, 928–935. [CrossRef]
109. Afdhal, N.H. Fibroscan (Transient Elastography) for the measurement of liver fibrosis. *Gastroenterol. Hepatol.* **2012**, *8*, 605–607.
110. Palmeri, M.L.; Wang, M.H.; Rouze, N.C.; Abdelmalek, M.F.; Guy, C.D.; Moser, B.; Diehl, A.M.; Nightingale, K.R. Noninvasive evaluation of hepatic fibrosis using acoustic radiation force-based shear stiffness in patients with nonalcoholic fatty liver disease. *J. Hepatol.* **2011**, *55*, 666–672. [CrossRef]
111. Karlas, T.; Dietrich, A.; Peter, V.; Wittekind, C.; Lichtinghagen, R.; Garnov, N.; Linder, N.; Schaudinn, A.; Busse, H.; Prettin, C.; et al. Evaluation of transient elastography, acoustic radiation force impulse imaging (ARFI), and enhanced liver function (ELF) score for detection of fibrosis in morbidly obese patients. *PLoS ONE* **2015**, *10*, e0141649. [CrossRef]
112. Bercoff, J.; Tanter, M.; Fink, M. Supersonic shear imaging: A new technique for soft tissue elasticity mapping. *IEEE Trans. Ultrason. Ferroelectr. Freq. Control.* **2004**, *51*, 396–409. [CrossRef]
113. Herrmann, E.; de Ledinghen, V.; Cassinotto, C.; Chu, W.C.; Leung, V.Y.; Ferraioli, G.; Filice, C.; Castera, L.; Vilgrain, V.; Ronot, M.; et al. Assessment of biopsy-proven liver fibrosis by two-dimensional shear wave elastography: An individual patient data-based meta-analysis. *Hepatology* **2018**, *67*, 260–272. [CrossRef]
114. Alkhouri, N.; Sedki, E.; Alisi, A.; Lopez, R.; Pinzani, M.; Feldstein, A.E.; Nobili, V. Combined paediatric NAFLD fibrosis index and transient elastography to predict clinically significant fibrosis in children with fatty liver disease. *Liver Int.* **2013**, *33*, 79–85. [CrossRef]
115. Reddy, J.K.; Rao, M.S. Lipid metabolism and liver inflammation. II. Fatty liver disease and fatty acid oxidation. *Am. J. Physiol. Liver Physiol.* **2006**, *290*, G852–G858. [CrossRef]
116. Sasso, M.; Beaugrand, M.; De Lédinghen, V.; Douvin, C.; Marcellin, P.; Poupon, R.; Sandrin, L.; Miette, V. Controlled Attenuation Parameter (CAP): A novel VCTE™ guided ultrasonic attenuation measurement for the evaluation of hepatic steatosis: Preliminary study and validation in a cohort of patients with chronic liver disease from various causes. *Ultrasound Med. Biol.* **2010**, *36*, 1825–1835. [CrossRef]
117. Kjærgaard, M.; Thiele, M.; Jansen, C.; Madsen, B.S.; Görtzen, J.; Strassburg, C.; Trebicka, J.; Krag, A. High risk of misinterpreting liver and spleen stiffness using 2D shear-wave and transient elastography after a moderate or high calorie meal. *PLoS ONE* **2017**, *12*, e0173992. [CrossRef]
118. Caussy, C.; Reeder, S.B.; Sirlin, C.B.; Loomba, R. Non-invasive, quantitative assessment of liver fat by MRI-PDFF as an endpoint in NASH trials. *Hepatology* **2018**, *68*, 763–772. [CrossRef]
119. Reeder, S.B.; Hu, H.H.; Sirlin, C.B. Proton Density Fat-Fraction: A Standardized MR-Based Biomarker of Tissue Fat Concentration. *J. Magn. Reson. Imaging* **2012**, *36*, 1011–1014. [CrossRef]
120. Wang, X.; Hernando, D.; Reeder, S.B. Sensitivity of chemical shift-encoded fat quantification to calibration of fat MR spectrum. *Magn. Reson. Med.* **2016**, *75*, 845–851. [CrossRef]
121. Imajo, K.; Kessoku, T.; Honda, Y.; Tomeno, W.; Ogawa, Y.; Mawatari, H.; Fujita, K.; Yoneda, M.; Taguri, M.; Hyogo, H.; et al. Magnetic resonance imaging more accurately classifies steatosis and fibrosis in patients with nonalcoholic fatty liver disease than transient elastography. *Gastroenterology* **2016**, *150*, 626–637. [CrossRef]
122. Park, C.C.; Nguyen, P.; Hernandez, C.; Bettencourt, R.; Ramirez, K.; Fortney, L.; Hooker, J.; Sy, E.; Alquiraish, M.; Valasek, M.A.; et al. Magnetic resonance elastography vs transient elastography in detection of fibrosis and noninvasive measurement of steatosis in patients with biopsy-proven nonalcoholic fatty liver disease. *Gastroenterology* **2017**, *152*, S70. [CrossRef]

123. Runge, J.H.; Smits, L.P.; Verheij, J.; Depla, A.; Kuiken, S.D.; Baak, B.C.; Nederveen, A.J.; Beuers, U.; Stoker, J. MR spectroscopy-derived proton density fat fraction is superior to controlled attenuation parameter for detecting and grading hepatic steatosis. *Radiology* **2018**, *286*, 547–556. [CrossRef]
124. Singh, S.; Venkatesh, S.K.; Wang, Z.; Miller, F.H.; Motosugi, U.; Low, R.N.; Hassanein, T.; Asbach, P.; Godfrey, E.M.; Yin, M.; et al. Diagnostic performance of magnetic resonance elastography in staging liver fibrosis: A systematic review and meta-analysis of individual participant data. *Clin. Gastroenterol. Hepatol.* **2015**, *13*, 440–451. [CrossRef]
125. Castera, L.; Friedrich-Rust, M.; Loomba, R. Noninvasive assessment of liver disease in patients with nonalcoholic fatty liver disease. *Gastroenterology* **2019**, *156*, 1264–1281. [CrossRef]
126. Loomba, R.; Cui, J.; Wolfson, T.; Haufe, W.; Hooker, J.; Szeverenyi, N.; Ang, B.; Bhatt, A.; Wang, K.; Aryafar, H.; et al. Novel 3D magnetic resonance elastography for the noninvasive diagnosis of advanced fibrosis in NAFLD: A prospective study. *Am. J. Gastroenterol.* **2016**, *111*, 986–994. [CrossRef]
127. Costa-Silva, L.; Ferolla, S.M.; Lima, A.S.; Vidigal, P.V.T.; Ferrari, T.C.D.A. MR elastography is effective for the non-invasive evaluation of fibrosis and necroinflammatory activity in patients with nonalcoholic fatty liver disease. *Eur. J. Radiol.* **2018**, *98*, 82–89. [CrossRef]
128. Eslam, M.; Valenti, L.; Romeo, S. Genetics and epigenetics of NAFLD and NASH: Clinical impact. *J. Hepatol.* **2018**, *68*, 268–279. [CrossRef]
129. Romeo, S.; Kozlitina, J.; Xing, C.; Pertsemlidis, A.; Cox, D.; Pennacchio, L.A.; Boerwinkle, E.; Cohen, J.C.; Hobbs, H.H. Genetic variation in PNPLA3 confers susceptibility to nonalcoholic fatty liver disease. *Nat. Genet.* **2008**, *40*, 1461–1465. [CrossRef]
130. Pingitore, P.; Pirazzi, C.; Mancina, R.M.; Motta, B.M.; Indiveri, C.; Pujia, A.; Montalcini, T.; Hedfalk, K.; Romeo, S. Recombinant PNPLA3 protein shows triglyceride hydrolase activity and its I148M mutation results in loss of function. *Biochim. Biophys. Acta (BBA) Mol. Cell Biol. Lipids* **2014**, *1841*, 574–580. [CrossRef]
131. Luukkonen, P.K.; Zhou, Y.; Haridas, P.N.; Dwivedi, O.P.; Hyötyläinen, T.; Ali, A.; Juuti, A.; Leivonen, M.; Tukiainen, T.; Ahonen, L.; et al. Impaired hepatic lipid synthesis from polyunsaturated fatty acids in TM6SF2 E167K variant carriers with NAFLD. *J. Hepatol.* **2017**, *67*, 128–136. [CrossRef]
132. Donati, B.; Dongiovanni, P.; Romeo, S.; Meroni, M.; McCain, M.; Miele, L.; Petta, S.; Maier, S.; Rosso, C.; De Luca, L.; et al. MBOAT7 rs641738 variant and hepatocellular carcinoma in non-cirrhotic individuals. *Sci. Rep.* **2017**, *7*, 4492. [CrossRef]
133. Beer, N.L.; Tribble, N.D.; McCulloch, L.J.; Roos, C.; Johnson, P.R.; Orho-Melander, M.; Gloyn, A.L. The P446L variant in GCKR associated with fasting plasma glucose and triglyceride levels exerts its effect through increased glucokinase activity in liver. *Hum. Mol. Genet.* **2009**, *18*, 4081–4088. [CrossRef]
134. Teschke, R. Alcoholic liver disease: Alcohol metabolism, cascade of molecular mechanisms, cellular targets, and clinical aspects. *Biomedicines* **2018**, *6*, 106. [CrossRef]
135. Joshi-Barve, S.; Kirpich, I.; Cave, M.C.; Marsano, L.S.; McClain, C.J. Alcoholic, nonalcoholic, and toxicant-associated steatohepatitis: Mechanistic similarities and differences. *Cell. Mol. Gastroenterol. Hepatol.* **2015**, *1*, 356–367. [CrossRef]
136. Roy, S.; Trautwein, C.; Luedde, T.; Roderburg, C. A General Overview on non-coding RNA-based diagnostic and therapeutic approaches for liver diseases. *Front. Pharmacol.* **2018**, *9*, 805. [CrossRef]
137. Schueller, F.; Roy, S.; Vucur, M.; Trautwein, C.; Luedde, T.; Roderburg, C. The role of miRNAs in the pathophysiology of liver diseases and toxicity. *Int. J. Mol. Sci.* **2018**, *19*, 261. [CrossRef]
138. Liu, J.; Xiao, Y.; Wu, X.; Jiang, L.; Yang, S.; Ding, Z.; Fang, Z.; Hua, H.; Kirby, M.S.; Shou, J. A circulating microRNA signature as noninvasive diagnostic and prognostic biomarkers for nonalcoholic steatohepatitis. *BMC Genom.* **2018**, *19*, 188. [CrossRef]
139. Turchinovich, A.; Baranova, A.; Drapkina, O.; Tonevitsky, A. Cell-free circulating nucleic acids as early biomarkers for NAFLD and NAFLD-associated disorders. *Front. Physiol.* **2018**, *9*, 9. [CrossRef]
140. Leoni, S.; Tovoli, F.; Napoli, L.; Serio, I.; Ferri, S.; Bolondi, L. Current guidelines for the management of non-alcoholic fatty liver disease: A systematic review with comparative analysis. *World J. Gastroenterol.* **2018**, *24*, 3361–3373. [CrossRef]
141. Masyuk, A.I.; Masyuk, T.V.; LaRusso, N.F. Exosomes in the pathogenesis, diagnostics and therapeutics of liver diseases. *J. Hepatol.* **2013**, *59*, 621–625. [CrossRef]
142. Sato, K.; Meng, F.; Glaser, S.; Alpini, G. Exosomes in liver pathology. *J. Hepatol.* **2016**, *65*, 213–221. [CrossRef]

143. Sung, S.; Kim, J.; Jung, Y. Liver-derived exosomes and their implications in liver pathobiology. *Int. J. Mol. Sci.* **2018**, *19*, 3715. [CrossRef]
144. Eguchi, A.; Feldstein, A.E. Extracellular vesicles in non-alcoholic and alcoholic fatty liver diseases. *Liver Res.* **2018**, *2*, 30–34. [CrossRef]
145. Lee, Y.-S.; Kim, S.Y.; Ko, E.; Lee, J.-H.; Yi, H.-S.; Yoo, Y.J.; Je, J.; Suh, S.J.; Jung, Y.K.; Kim, J.H.; et al. Exosomes derived from palmitic acid-treated hepatocytes induce fibrotic activation of hepatic stellate cells. *Sci. Rep.* **2017**, *7*, 3710. [CrossRef]
146. Korf, H.; Boesch, M.; Meelberghs, L.; Van Der Merwe, S. Macrophages as key players during adipose tissue–liver crosstalk in nonalcoholic fatty liver disease. *Semin. Liver Dis.* **2019**, *39*, 291–300. [CrossRef]
147. Mendez-Sanchez, N.; Cruz-Ramon, V.C.; Ramirez-Perez, O.L.; Hwang, J.P.; Barranco-Fragoso, B.; Cordova-Gallardo, J. New aspects of lipotoxicity in nonalcoholic steatohepatitis. *Int. J. Mol. Sci.* **2018**, *19*, 2034. [CrossRef]
148. Jayakumar, S.; Loomba, R. Review article: Emerging role of the gut microbiome in the progression of nonalcoholic fatty liver disease and potential therapeutic implications. *Aliment. Pharmacol. Ther.* **2019**, *50*, 144–158. [CrossRef]
149. Kolodziejczyk, A.A.; Zheng, D.; Shibolet, O.; Elinav, E. The role of the microbiome in NAFLD and NASH. *EMBO Mol. Med.* **2019**, *11*, e9302. [CrossRef]

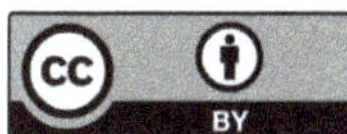

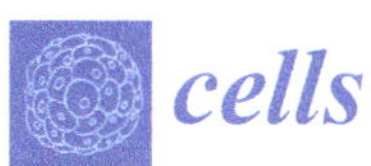
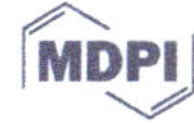
Article

Dynamic Changes in Function and Proteomic Composition of Extracellular Vesicles from Hepatic Stellate Cells during Cellular Activation

Xinlei Li [1], Ruju Chen [1], Sherri Kemper [1] and David R Brigstock [1,2,*]

[1] Center for Clinical and Translational Research, The Abigail Wexner Research Institute, Nationwide Children's Hospital, Columbus, OH 43205, USA; Xinlei.Li@NationwideChildrens.org (X.L.); Ruju.Chen@NationwideChildrens.org (R.C.); Sherri.Kemper@Nationwidechildrens.org (S.K.)

[2] Department of Surgery, Wexner Medical Center, The Ohio State University, Columbus, OH 43210, USA

* Correspondence: David.Brigstock@NationwideChildrens.Org; Tel.: +1-614-355-2824; Fax: +1-614-722-5892

Received: 8 January 2020; Accepted: 23 January 2020; Published: 25 January 2020

Abstract: During chronic liver injury, hepatic stellate cells (HSC) undergo activation and are the principal cellular source of collagenous scar. In this study, we found that activation of mouse HSC (mHSC) was associated with a 4.5-fold increase in extracellular vesicle (EV) production and that fibrogenic gene expression (CCN2, Col1a1) was suppressed in Passage 1 (P1; activated) mHSC exposed to EVs from Day 4 (D4; relatively quiescent) mHSC but not to EVs from P1 mHSC. Conversely, gene expression (CCN2, Col1a1, αSMA) in D4 mHSC was stimulated by EVs from P1 mHSC but not by EVs from D4 mHSC. EVs from Day 4 mHSC contained only 46 proteins in which histones and keratins predominated, while EVs from P1 mHSC contained 337 proteins and these were principally associated with extracellular spaces or matrix, proteasome, collagens, vesicular transport, metabolic enzymes, ribosomes and chaperones. EVs from the activated LX-2 human HSC (hHSC) line also promoted fibrogenic gene expression in D4 mHSC in vitro and contained 524 proteins, many of which shared identity or had functional overlap with those in P1 mHSC EVs. The activation-associated changes in production, function and protein content of EVs from HSC likely contribute to the regulation of HSC function in vivo and to the fine-tuning of fibrogenic pathways in the liver.

Keywords: extracellular vesicle; hepatic stellate cell; hepatic fibrosis; exosome; microvesicle; liver

1. Introduction

Hepatic fibrosis is the result of chronic liver injury and is characterized by the deposition of collagen and other insoluble extracellular matrix components [1]. The major fibrosis-causing cells in the liver are hepatic stellate cells (HSC) that reside in the Space of Disse [1–3]. Under normal conditions, HSC are quiescent pericyte-like cells that store large amounts of vitamin A in cytoplasmic lipid droplets. However, in response to liver injury. HSC undergo a phenotypic activation whereby they become contractile collagen-producing myofibroblasts that function either transiently in acute injury to produce a provisional matrix that supports hepatocyte repopulation or persistently in chronic injury to unrelentingly produce fibrotic material that causes scarring and exacerbates impaired liver function. These properties arise due to increased production and/or response by HSC of molecules involved in fibrogenesis, survival and inflammation [4]. The central role of HSC in fibrosis has spawned intense effort to target either key molecular mediators of fibrosis or the activated cells themselves (e.g., using cytotoxic agents) in a quest to develop new therapies for liver fibrosis [5,6]. While hepatic fibrosis is a major cause of morbidity and mortality and is a significant contributing factor to cirrhosis, which accounts for 32,000 deaths in the US and more than 1 million deaths globally each year [7], there is a severe lack of approved anti-fibrotics for improving patient outcomes [8,9]. Rational therapeutic strategies are being developed by leveraging our knowledge of the molecular mechanisms that regulate fibrosis and this has already led to the identification of a considerable number and variety of targets that are at various stages of pre-clinical or clinical testing [10,11]. Success in this area may most likely be achieved by combining anti-fibrotic strategies with other modalities that target hepatocyte injury or inflammation [10,12], but even so will require diligent design of clinical trials that have historically been vexed with difficulties and setbacks for reasons that include differences in fibrosis reversibility between humans and animal models, role of genetic background on fibrosis penetrance, protracted time-course of fibrosis development and influence of disease etiology on drug effectiveness [10,13,14]. Continued research of HSC biology is necessary to improve our understanding of the cellular and molecular aspects of fibrosis and to optimize development of new therapeutic options.

The biological activities of HSC occur as a result of their orchestrated interactions with other cells in the liver [12,15]. Recently, a new hepatic signaling network has been identified that involves the shuttling of molecular information between different liver cells by extracellular vesicles (EVs) [16–20]. EVs are membranous nanovesicles (50–500 nm) that comprise principally exosomes and microvesicles which are liberated from cells by, respectively, fusion of multivesicular bodies with the plasma membrane or budding off from the plasma membrane [21,22]. Despite many early reports that exosomes and microvesicles can be distinguished by size and/or the presence of marker proteins, it has recently been emphasized [23] that these features do not allow such discrimination. Thus, the use of the terms "exosome" or "microvesicle" firstly infers knowledge of specific EV biogenetic pathways that are extremely difficult to ascertain given current tools and technical limitations and, secondly, fails to take into account the innate heterogeneity of EVs in biological samples. Accordingly, since current recommendations for operationally defining EVs include reference to the cell of origin [23], in this report we have used "EVs from HSC" or 'HSC EVs" to describe the population of EVs that we recovered from HSC-conditioned culture medium using the stated enrichment methods. Irrespective of the precise EV subtypes involved, accumulating data suggest that a complex EV network exists in the liver whereby quiescent or activated HSC exchange EV cargo molecules (proteins, mRNAs, microRNAs) with one another or with cells such as hepatocytes or liver sinusoidal endothelial cells [24–32]. This bi-directional molecular transfer ensures that normal homeostatic functions or injury-associated responses in the liver are fine-tuned and synchronized at the cellular level.

An area of growing interest is the manner in which the EV cargo content varies according to the phenotypic status of their cells of origin. In view of the highly distinct functions of quiescent versus activated HSC, we hypothesized that the EVs from these cells exhibit fundamental differences in their biological properties and/or molecular payload. In this report we provide evidence for such differences in terms of their respective actions on cultured HSC and their protein cargo as assessed by mass spectrometry and proteomic analysis. We also provide a comparative proteomic analysis of EVs from activated mouse and human HSC and show substantial overlap in their constituent protein content and their predicted functional roles.

2. Material and Methods

2.1. Animals and Primary Mouse HSC (mHSC) Culture

Animal procedures were conducted using protocol 04504AR approved by the Institutional Animal Care and use Committee of the Research Institute at Nationwide Children's Hospital (Columbus, OH, USA). Mouse HSC (mHSC) isolation was accomplished using standard procedures. Briefly, wild-type male Swiss Webster mice (4–5 wks old; $n = 5$) underwent systemic perfusion with 20–30 mL HBSS under deep anesthesia followed by two steps of perfusion with 15 mL Dulbecco's Modified Eagle's Medium (DMEM) containing 2 mg/mL pronase or 0.5 mg/mL collagenase I, respectively. After this 40 min perfusion technique, livers were removed, diced with scissors and digested in 0.33 mg/mL pronase and 166 U/mL DNase I in DMEM at 37 °C for 10 min. mHSC were collected by Optiprep density centrifugation, counted using a hemocytometer, and plated at 10^6 cells/mL in DMEM/F12 medium containing 20% fetal bovine serum for 1 h. For short-term culture, primary mHSC were switched to serum-free Hyclone™ SFM4MegaVir medium (Thermo Fisher Scientific, Waltham, MA, USA) one day after initial seeding and the medium was collected 3 days later (i.e., on Day 4) for EV isolation. For long-term culture, the medium on Day 1 primary mHSC was replaced with fresh DMEM/F12/fetal bovine serum (FBS) and the cells were cultured until Day 10 whereupon they were split 1:5 and the resulting passage 1 (P1) cells were grown in DMEM/F12/FBS cells for 5 days. On Day 15, the medium was removed and replaced with SFM4MegaVir medium which was then collected 2 days later (i.e., on Day 17) for EV isolation.

2.2. Mouse HSC Characterization

D4 or P1 mHSC cultures were analyzed for auto-fluorescence upon excitation at 405 nm and emission at 450 nm to detect vitamin A-positive oil droplets using a LSM 510 confocal microscope (Carl Zeiss Microscopy Inc., Thornwood, NY, USA) and the incidence of positive cells was established by comparison to the number of cells observed with the same instrument by bright field microscopy. mHSC were fixed with 4% paraformaldehyde for 15 min at room temperature and incubated with anti-αSMA (1:500; Invitrogen, Waltham MA) or anti-reelin (1:200; R&D Systems, Minneapolis, MN, USA) for 1 h and developed with, respectively, Alexa Fluor 488 goat anti-mouse IgG (Invitrogen) or Alexa Fluor 568 donkey anti-goat IgG (Invitrogen). The frequency of αSMA- or reelin positive cells was determined by comparison to the number of cells that were positive for DAPI nuclear staining Quantitative real time polymerase chain reaction (qRT-PCR) was used to evaluate gene expression in primary mHSC within 4 days of plating or after passage to P1 as described below.

2.3. Human LX-2 CELLS

The human HSC (hHSC) line, LX-2, (a kind gift from Dr Scott Friedman, Icahn School of Medicine at Mount Sinai, New York, NY, USA) was cultured in DMEM/10% FBS. Cells were seeded at 10^7 cells/mL and allowed to grow to 90% confluency. For harvesting of EVs, spent medium was removed and replaced with serum-free DMEM which was then collected 2 days later.

2.4. EV Isolation

EVs from primary mHSC or human LX-2 hHSC were enriched from their respective serum-free conditioned media by sequential centrifugation of the supernatant obtained after 300× g for 15 min, 2000× g for 20 min, 10,000× g for 30 min and ultracentrifugation at 100,000× g for 70 min at 4 °C (T-70 i fixed-angle rotor; Beckman Coulter, Brea, CA, US, USA). The pellet from the latter step was dispersed in phosphate-buffered saline (PBS) and underwent a repeat round of ultracentrifugation. The use of differential ultracentrifugation is consistent with current recommendations for EV enrichment and is the technique most commonly used by researchers for primary EV separation and concentration [23]. The resulting pellet was dispersed in PBS and the constituent EVs were characterized as described below.

2.5. Nanoparticle Tracking Analysis (NTA)

A Nanosight 300 instrument (Malvern Instruments, Westborough, MA) was calibrated with 100 nm polystyrene latex microspheres (Magsphere Inc., Pasadena, CA, USA) and used to analyze HSC EVs that were diluted to 10^7–10^8 particles/mL in PBS. Each EV sample was analyzed in duplicate and mean particle concentration and size were estimated with v3.2 analytical software (Malvern Instruments). Recordings were performed at room temperature with a camera gain of 15 and a shutter speed of 4.13 ms. The detection threshold was set to 6.

2.6. Western Blotting

Proteins were detergent-extracted from EVs and subjected to sodium dodecyl polyacrylamide gel electrophoresis (SDS-PAGE; 10 μg/lane) and transferred to nitrocellulose membrane for Western blot detection using antibodies to CD9 (1:500; Abcam, Cambridge, MA, USA), flotillin-1 (1:200; BD Biosciences, San Jose, CA, USA), Tsg101 (1:500; Thermo Fisher Scientific), fibronectin (FN1) (1:1000; Abcam), FN1 EDA domain (1:250; Sirius Biotech, Genoa, Italy), FN1 EDB domain (1:100; Sirius Biotech), pan-keratin (1:500; Cell Signaling Technology, Danvers, MA, USA), proteasome subunit alpha type-6 (PSMA6, 1:500; ABclonal Inc, Woburn, MA, USA) or ribosomal protein S27a (RPS27A, 1:500; ABclonal). Blots were developed using IRDye 800 CW secondary antibodies (LI-COR Biosciences, Lincoln, NE, USA) in conjunction with Odyssey CLx Imaging (LI-COR Biosciences).

2.7. Gene Expression in HSC

Gene expression was evaluated in primary mHSC on Day 4 or after passage to P1. To assess EV bioactivity, D4 or P1 mHSC were switched overnight to medium containing 2% exosome-depleted serum and then treated for 48 h with 8 μg/mL EV from D4 mHSC, P4 mHSC, or LX-2 hHSC. Total RNA was extracted from the cells using a miRNeasy mini kit (Qiagen) and reverse transcribed using a miScript II RT kit (Qiagen) according to the manufacturer's protocols. Transcripts for common fibrosis-related molecules (e.g., collagen 1a1, cellular communication network factor 2 (CCN2), αSMA) or that corresponded to proteins which were determined by MS to be differentially expressed in EVs from D4 versus P1 mHSC (see below) were evaluated by qRT-PCR using an Eppendorf Mastercycler System and SYBR Green Master Mix (Eppendorf, Hauppauge, NY). Each reaction was run in duplicate, and samples were normalized to 18S ribosomal RNA. Negative controls were a non-reverse transcriptase reaction and a non-sample reaction. Primers are shown in Supplemental Table S1.

2.8. EV Protein Extraction and Digestion

EV pellets were resuspended in 100 μL 50 mM ammonium bicarbonate containing 0.1% Rapigest (Waters Corp., Milford, MA, USA), sonicated twice for 10 s and incubated with shaking for 1 h at room temperature. Extracts were clarified at 13,000 rpm in a microcentrifuge and protein concentration was determined using a Qubit assay kit (Thermo Fisher Scientific). Dithiothreitol was added to a final concentration of 5 mM and the sample was incubated at 65 °C for 30 min. Iodoacetamide was then added to a final concentration of 15 mM and the sample was incubated in the dark, at room temperature for 30 min. Sequencing grade trypsin (Promega Corp, Madison, WI, USA) was added at a 1:30 ratio and the sample was digested overnight at 37 °C. Trifluoroacetic acid was then added to a final concentration of 0.5% and sample was incubated at 37 °C for 30 min to precipitate the Rapigest. The sample was clarified at 13,000 rpm for 5 min in a microcentrifuge, dried in a vacufuge and resuspended in 20 μL 50 mM acetic acid. Peptide concentration was determined at 280 nm using a nanodrop spectrophotometer (Thermo Fisher). Five separate D4 EV preparations and three separate P1 EV preparations, all from different mHSC isolations, were individually prepared in this manner for mass spectrometry.

2.9. Mass Spectrometry (MS)

EV protein identification was performed using nano-liquid chromatography-nanospray tandem mass spectrometry (LC/MS/MS) on a Thermo Scientific Q Exactive mass spectrometer equipped with an EASY-Spray™ Sources operated in positive ion mode. Each sample was injected into a μ-Precolumn Cartridge (Thermo Scientific) and desalted with 0.1% formic acid in water for 5 min. Samples were then separated on an easy spray nano column (Pepmap™ RSLC, C18 3μ 100 A, 75 μm × 150 mm, Thermo Scientific) using a two-dimensional (2D) RSLC high-performance liquid chromatography system (Thermo Scientific). Mobile phase A was 0.1% formic acid in water and mobile phase B was acetonitrile/0.1% formic acid. Peptide elution was achieved with a multi-linear gradient comprising 2–35% B over 225 min, 35–55% B over 35 min, 55–90% B over 10 min and then 90% B isocratic for 5 min. After each run, the column was equilibrated in 2% B for 20 min before the next sample injection.

The MS/MS method was a Top10 method: the analysis was programmed for a full scan recorded between *m/z* 400–1600 and an MS/MS scan to generate product ion spectra to determine amino acid sequence in consecutive scans starting from the most abundant peaks in the spectrum, and then selecting the next nine most abundant peaks. To achieve high mass accuracy MS determination, the full scan was performed at a resolution setting of 70,000. The AGC target ion number for full scan was set at 3×10^6 ions, maximum ion injection time was set at 100 ms. MS/MS was performed using a stepped normalized CE of 25, 30, and 35, acquired at a resolution of 17,500 with an AGC target of 1×10^5 ions and a maximum injection time of 50 ms. Dynamic exclusion was enabled with a repeat count of 1 within 30 s.

Sequence information from the MS/MS data was processed by converting the raw files into a merged file (.mgf) using MS convert (ProteoWizard). The resulting mgf files were searched using Mascot Daemon by Matrix Science version 2.6.0 (Boston, MA, USA) and the database searched against Uniprot Mouse database. The mass accuracy of the precursor ions was set to 10 ppm, and accidental inclusion of 1 13C peaks was also included into the search. The fragment mass tolerance was set to 0.05 Da. Four missed cleavages for the enzyme were permitted. A decoy database was also searched to determine the false discovery rate (FDR) and peptides were filtered according to the FDR. Proteins with less than 1% FDR as well as a minimal of two significant peptides detected were considered as valid proteins. Proteomics data was summarized in scaffold to allow for spectral counting analysis. Complete MS datasets are available in the Supplemental Data section as Tables S2–S4.

2.10. Gene Ontology, Pathway Enrichment, and Protein-Protein Interaction Networks

Grouping of EV proteins into cellular components was accomplished using Gene Ontology (GO) analysis (http://geneontology.org/) and the Funrich database (https://FunRich.org). EV protein functions and utilities were determined using DAVID ((https://david.ncifcrf.gov/) analysis of The Kyoto Encyclopedia of Genes and Genomes (KEGG; https://www.genome.jp/kegg/). Search Tool for the Retrieval of Interacting Genes (STRING, https://string-db.org/) was employed to determine interactions among EV proteins using a minimum interaction score of 0.4 for the D4 mHSC EV dataset, and 0.9 for the P1 mHSC or LX-2 EV datasets. The Markov Cluster Algorithm method with an inflation parameter of 2 was applied for clustering. These analyses were each performed with a criterion FDR < 0.05.

2.11. Statistical Analysis

Experiments were performed at least twice in duplicate, with data expressed as mean ± S.E.M. qRT-PCR data were analyzed by student's *t*-test using Sigma plot 11.0 software (SPSS Inc., Chicago, IL, USA). A p value < 0.05 was considered statistically significant.

3. Results

3.1. Characterization of Primary mHSC

Autofluorescence for vitamin A, which is stored in cytoplasmic oil droplets in HSC and is useful for identifying or characterizing HSC, was detected in 91.3 ± 3.4% of D4 mouse cells and 85.4 ± 8.0% of P1 mouse cells (Figure 1A). Staining for αSMA, a marker of HSC activation, was detectable in only 3.3 ± 0.7% of D4 cells but in 93.3 ± 5.0% of P1 cells demonstrating the high degree of activation of P1 cells as compared to D4 cells (Figure 1B). Staining for reelin, which is preferentially expressed in quiescent HSC but not in other hepatic cell types [33], was detected in 98.4 ± 1.6% of D4 mHSC and 13.1 ± 1.2% of P1 mHSC (Figure 1C). This is consistent with previous findings showing that reelin expression declines during HSC activation [33] and also argues that our early (and hence later) primary HSC cultures were essentially devoid of contaminating cells that might otherwise confound analysis. Since absolute quiescence is not feasible because HSC start to autonomously activate after isolation, the above staining data nonetheless led us to conclude that D4 (the earliest time point at which we could reproducibly harvest sufficient numbers of EVs for detailed analysis) represented a relatively quiescent state as compared to P1 cells which were highly activated, thus validating our subsequent comparative EV analysis.

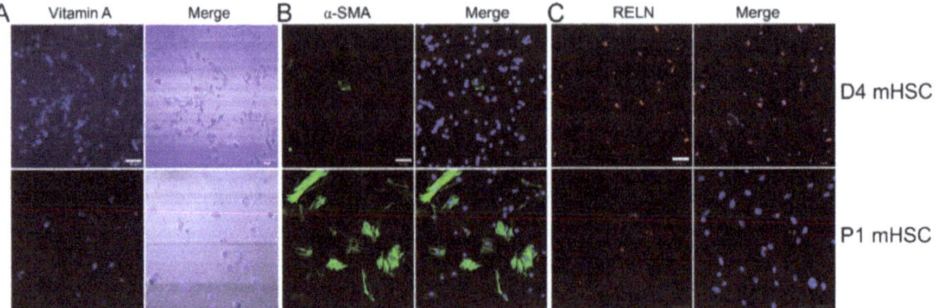

Figure 1. Characterization of primary mouse HSC. (**A**) Primary D4 or P1 mHSC were evaluated for vitamin A autofluorescence (left) or examined by phase contrast (right), and imaged by confocal microscopy. Based on six fields, Vitamin A was positive in 91.3 ± 3.4% of D4 mHSC and 85.4 ± 8.0% of P1 mHSC. (**B**) D4 or P1 mHSC were stained with anti-αSMA (left) which was then merged with DAPI (right). Based on three fields, α SMA was positive in 3.3 ± 0.7% of D4 mHSC and 93.3 ± 5.0% of P1 mHSC. (**C**) D4 or P1 mHSC were stained with anti-reelin (left) which was then merged with DAP1 (right). Based on two fields, the frequency of reelin-positive cells was 98.4 ± 1.6% for D4 mHSC and 13.1 ± 1.2% for P1 mHSC. Bars: 50 μm for A and C; 100 μm for B.

3.2. Physico-Chemical and Biological Properties of EVs from mHSC or hHSC

Serial low speed centrifugation and ultracentrifugation of serum-free medium from each cell type resulted in a significantly greater yield (4.5-fold) of EVs from P1-P2 mHSC than D4 mHSC showing that EV production was positively correlated with mHSC activation (Figure 2A). EVs from D4 mHSC or P1 mHSC were very similar in terms of mean size (144.3 ± 3.2 nm and 133.5 ± 20.61 nm, respectively) and size range (approx. 50–500 nm) (Figure 2B). Western blot revealed that EVs from either D4 or P1 mHSC were positive for proteins such as CD9, Tsg101 and flotillin-1 that are commonly associated with or enriched in EVs from other systems (Figure 2C). Thus, EVs from D4 or P1 mHSC exhibited shared physical properties and expression of key EV proteins. Additional characterization of mHSC EVs including conventional or cryogenic transmission electron microscopy and dynamic light scattering have been reported by us previously [25].

We have previously demonstrated and characterized the binding interactions between target HSC and EVs from mHSC or hHSC, including functional delivery of specific EV payload components [24,25,27,28,34]. When added to P1 mHSC, EVs from D4 mHSC caused expression of CCN2 or Col1a1 to be suppressed in the cells (Figure 2D), an observation that is consistent with our earlier reports that EVs from quiescent mHSC suppress fibrogenic gene expression as well as levels of proteins such as αSMA [25,27,28]. We extended these findings by showing that EVs from P1 mHSC did not alter expression of these genes in P1 mHSC (Figure 2D), yet they stimulated expression of CCN2, Col1a1 or αSMA in D4 mHSC (Figure 2E), the latter of which is consistent with our prior demonstration that αSMA mRNA or protein in HSC is stimulated by EVs from activated HSC or by EVs carrying an enriched CCN2 payload [24]. By contrast, EVs from D4 mHSC had no significant effect on gene expression in D4 mHSC (Figure 2E). We previously conducted transmission electron microscopy and cell binding assays of EVs purified from LX-2 hHSC [24,25] and expanded those data in this study by using NTA to show that they were of similar size as those from mHSC (151.9 ± 5.8 nm; size range 50–500 nm), contained EV-associated proteins such as flotillin-1 and CD63 (Figure 2F), and, like EVs from P1 mHSC, were able to stimulate gene expression in D4 mHSC (Figure 2E).

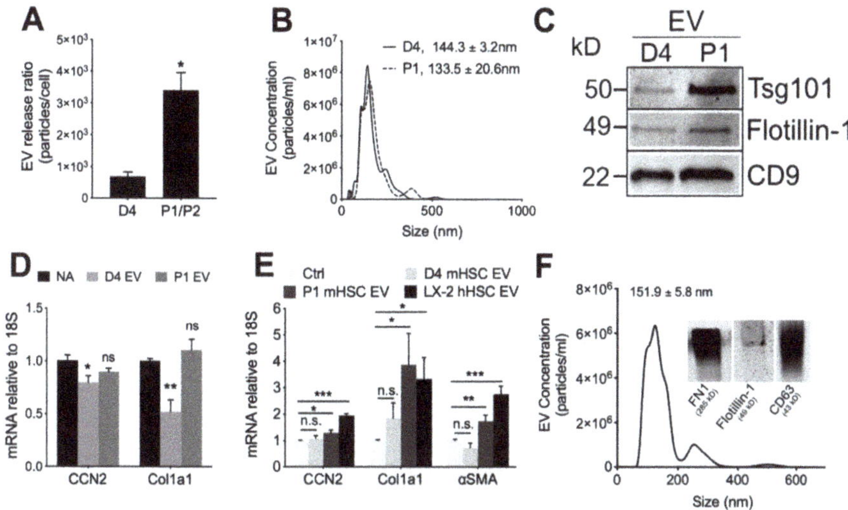

Figure 2. Characterization of EVs from mouse HSC. NTA was performed on EVs that had been purified by differential centrifugation of 2-day serum-free conditioned medium from D4 HSC or P1-P2 HSC, with particle number expressed as a function of (**A**) cell number or (**B**) particle size (mean ± S.E.M. for particle diameter (nm) is indicated). (**C**) Western blot analysis of D4 or P1 EVs (25 µg EV protein per lane) showing the presence of common EV proteins. (**D**) P1 HSC or (**E**) D4 HSC were treated for 48 h with 8 µg/mL EVs from D4 mHSC, P1 mHSC or LX-2 hHSC after which expression for the indicated transcripts was determined by qRT-PCR. (**F**) EVs purified from LX-2 hHSC under serum-free conditions were analyzed by NTA or Western blot (inset). *, $p < 0.05$; **, $p < 0.01$; ***, $p < 0.005$; n.s., not significant.

3.3. Proteomic Analysis of EVs from mHSC

Mass spectrometry for mHSC EVs revealed striking qualitative and quantitative differences of proteins in EVs from D4 mHSC versus EVs from P1 mHSC (Supplemental Tables S2 and S3). Analysis of five separate EV samples from D4 mHSC or three separate EV samples from P1 mHSC resulted in the identification of between, respectively, 31 and 58 proteins or 426 and 504 proteins (Figure 3A). Subsequent analysis of these data was focused on 46 proteins that were present in at least three EV samples from D4 mHSC and on 337 proteins that were common to all 3 EV samples from P1 mHSC. Of these, 19 proteins were unique to D4 mHSC EVs, 310 proteins were unique to P1 mHSC EVs and 27 proteins were shared between D4 and P1 mHSC EVs (Figure 3B). With respect to the 19 D4-specific proteins, the most abundant (quantitative value ~100) included three histones (H15, H10, H11) and ezrin (EZR1), a membrane-bound cytoskeleton linker protein (Figure 3C). Of the shared proteins, 11 proteins were present at significantly higher levels in EVs from D4 mHSC compared to EVs from P1 mHSC and six of these (H4, H13, H2B1F, H14, K2C1, H2A1B) were the most abundant proteins (quantitative value ~100–1000) in EVs from D4 mHSC (Figure 3D). No D4 mHSC-specific EV protein had this level of abundance (Figure 3C) but three proteins (FN1 (also termed FINC), FBLN2, PGBM) reached a comparable abundance level among the proteins specific to P1 mHSC EVs (Figure 3E). Western blot analysis was used to confirm the high abundance of keratin in EVs from D4 mHSC and of FN1 in EVs from P1 mHSC (Figure 4A). Western blot and MS analysis demonstrated the presence of EDA and EDB sequences in the FN1 protein showing that it was the cell-associated form as opposed to the plasma form which lacks these domains (Supplemental Figure S1). For the 21 proteins that were differentially expressed in EVs from D4 versus P1 cells, analysis of the producer cells by RT-PCR showed that their corresponding cellular transcripts were comparably differentially expressed for only eight candidates (H10, K2C8, K2C1, ACTG, EZR1, TSPAN8, RAI3, AQP1) with the rest showing no significant difference in expression except H2B1F which showed inverse cellular mRNA expression (P1 > D4) as compared to EV protein level (D4 > P1) (Figure 4B).

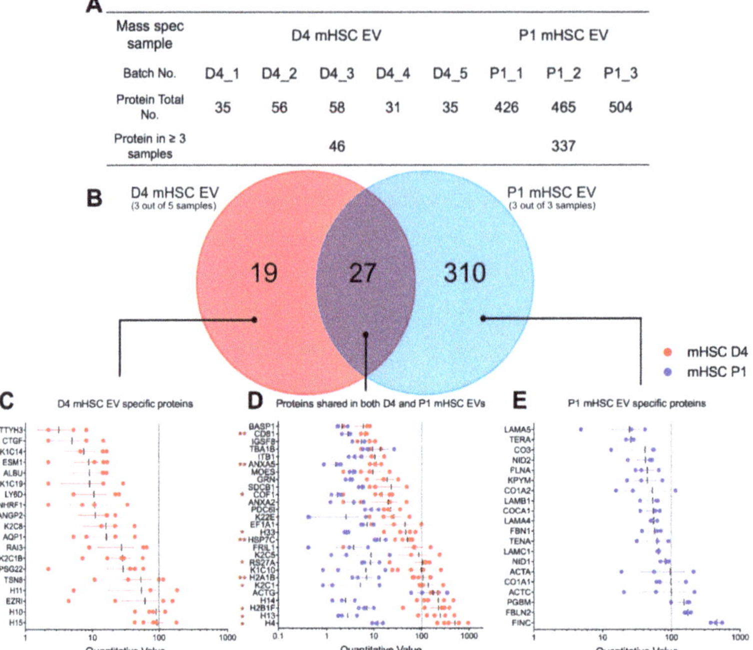

Figure 3. Proteomic composition of mHSC EVs. (**A**) Summary of quantitative features of EV proteins analyzed from five D4 mHSC EV samples or three P1 mHSC EV samples. (**B**) Venn diagram showing distribution of proteins between EVs from D4 versus P1 mHSC. The figure also shows the identities and quantifications of (**C**) the 19 proteins specific for D4 mHSC EVs; (**D**) the 27 proteins shared by both groups for which 11 proteins were significantly enriched in EVs from D4 mHSC (*, $p < 0.05$, **, $p < 0.01$) and (**E**) the 20 most abundant proteins specific for EVs from P1 mHSC.

When all D4 mHSC EV proteins or all P1 mHSC EV proteins were analyzed using GO/Funrich, the 20 most highly represented components were generally differentially expressed, with proteasome complex and collagen trimer being unique to P1 mHSC EVs (Figure 5A). The 27 proteins common to EVs from both D4 and P1 mHSC shared enrichment for components that included exosomes, membranes, cytoplasm, extracellular space, focal adhesion, ECM, microparticles, vesicles, cytoskeleton and cell-cell adherins (Figure 5B), many of which were shared with proteins that were P1-specific (Figure 5C). Proteins in D4-specific EVs included some of the same components (exosomes, vesicles) but in there was an absence of extracellular or adhesion components and instead a concentration of membraneous (apical, aipicolateral or microvillus membrane, sarcolemma), nuclear (chromosome, euchromatin) and structural-functional (dystrophin glycoprotein complex, costamere) components (Figure 5D).

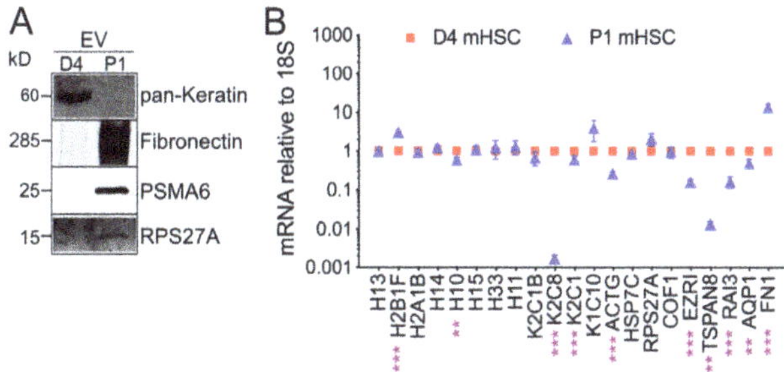

Figure 4. EV Western blot and cellular transcript levels for differentially expressed EV proteins. (**A**) Western blots of EVs from D4 mHSC or P1 mHSC to verify differential levels of representative proteins identified by MS. (**B**) qRT-PCR was performed on RNA from D4 or P1 mHSC using primers designed to amplify mRNA corresponding to proteins that were more highly expressed in EVs from D4 mHSC than in EVs from P1 mHSC (see Figure 3C,D). Data are mean ± S.E.M. for duplicate determinations performed twice individually. **, $p < 0.01$, ***, $p < 0.005$.

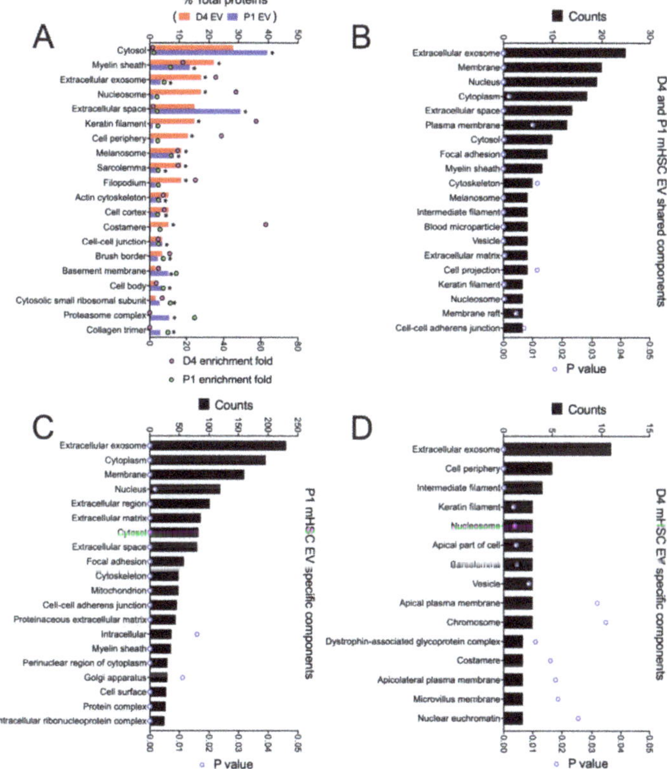

Figure 5. Cellular component analysis of proteins in EVs from D4 and/or P1 mHSC. GO analysis was performed using the Funrich database to identify EV proteins with significant enrichment versus the Uniprot database. The figure shows the 20 most highly ranked cellular components for proteins that were (**A**) in the entire mHSC EV proteome from D4 cells compared to those from P1 cells; (**B**) shared between EVs from D4 and P1 mHSC; (**C**) specific to P1 mHSC EVs. (**D**) Components specific to D4 mHSC EVs. Only cellular components with significant enrichment (* $p < 0.05$) are shown.

KEGG pathway analysis of all 46 proteins in D4 mHSC EVs and all 337 proteins in P1 mHSC EVs revealed one unique pathway for D4 mHSC EVs (alcoholism, involving 8% of the proteins), four shared pathways for D4 and P1 mHSC EVs (regulation of actin cytoskeleton, leucocyte transendothelial migration, systemic lupus erythematosus, and proteoglycans in cancer, each involving 3–11% of the proteins) and 33 unique pathways for P1 mHSC EVs (for which focal adhesion, PI3K-Akt signaling, proteasome, ECM-receptor interaction and pathways in cancer each involved the highest proportion (8–10%) of the proteins) (Figure 6A). While no KEGG pathway was identified for the 19 D4 mHSC-specific EV proteins, most of the these pathways were, respectively, prominent for either the 27 proteins that were shared between D4 and P1 mHSC EVs (regulation of actin cytoskeleton, leucocyte transendothelial migration, systemic lupus erythematosus, alcoholism) (Figure 6B) or the P1 mHSC EV-specific proteins (focal adhesion, PI3K-Akt signaling, proteasome, ECM-interactions, pathways in cancer) (Figure 6C).

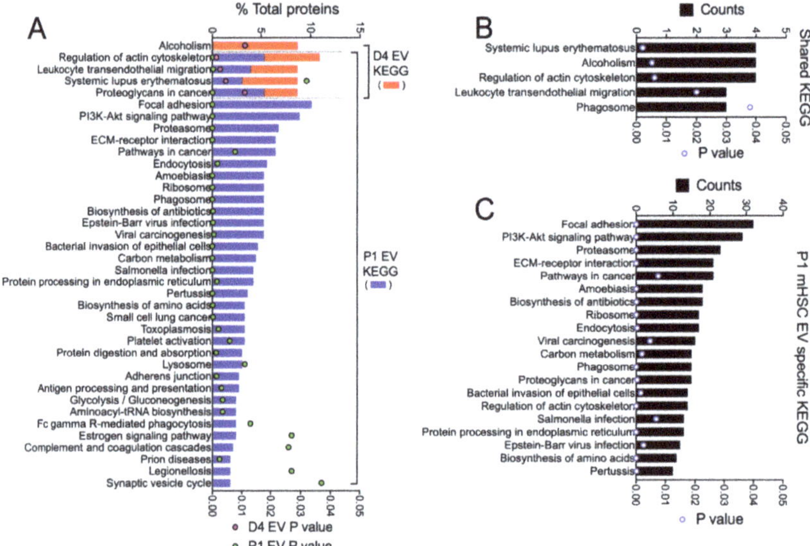

Figure 6. KEGG pathway analysis of proteins in EVs from D4 and/or P1 mHSC. EV proteins were analyzed online using DAVID v6.8 software for KEGG pathway analysis. The figure shows pathways that were (**A**) in the entire mHSC EV proteome from D4 mHSC versus P1 mHSC; (**B**) shared between EVs from D4 and P1 mHSC; or (**C**) specific to P1 mHSC EVs (top 20 pathways shown). Only pathways with significant enrichment ($p < 0.05$) are shown.

STRING analysis of the proteomic data to identify principal protein interactions and functions revealed striking differences between each type of EV. Whereas the proteins in D4 mHSC EVs were organized into a simple network comprising nodes that included keratins and histones (Supplemental Figure S2), those in P1 mHSC EVs demonstrated much more complex interactions with principal nodes containing proteins associated with collagens, ECM, vesicular transport, metabolic enzymes, proteasomes, ribosomes, chaperones and tRNA ligase (Supplemental Figure S3). Representative proteins from key nodes in each network were verified by Western blot as being specific for D4 mHSC EVs (keratin) or P1 mHSC EVs (PSMA6, RPS27A) (Figure 4A).

3.4. *Proteomic Analysis of EVs from hHSC*

We next used MS to investigate the protein components in EVs from LX-2 hHSC (Supplemental Table S4). Analysis of three separate LX-2 hHSC EV samples resulted in the identification of between

567 and 762 proteins, 524 of which were common to all three samples (Figure 7A). In light of the profibrogenic actions of EVs from activated mHSC or hHSC (Figure 2E), it was interesting that of the 524 LX-2 hHSC EV proteins, 206 were shared with the 337 proteins in EVs from P1 mHSC (Figure 7B). Only 26 LX-2 hHSC proteins were shared with EVs from D4 mHSC, (Figure 7B). All three types of EVs had 21 proteins in common with one another (Figure 7B). Quantitative analysis (Figure 7C–F) showed that when proteins in each group were ranked based on expression levels in LX-2 EVs, those shared with EVs from D4 mHSC but not P1 mHSC had the lowest expression (five proteins; quantitative value range = 8–80), while those shared with EVs from P1 mHSC but not with EVs from D4 mHSC had the highest expression (185 proteins; quantitative range = 100–1000 for the top 20) (Figure 7C,F). The most abundant protein was FN1 (Figure 7F), the presence of which was confirmed in LX-2 hHSC EVs by Western blot analysis (Figure 2F). Top-ranked proteins specific to LX-2 hHSC EVs had an intermediate level of expression (313 proteins; quantitative value 50–200 for the top 20) while the proteins in LX-2 hHSC EVs that were shared with EVs from both D4 and P1 mHSC were very variably expressed (21 proteins; quantitative range 5–500) (Figure 7D,E).

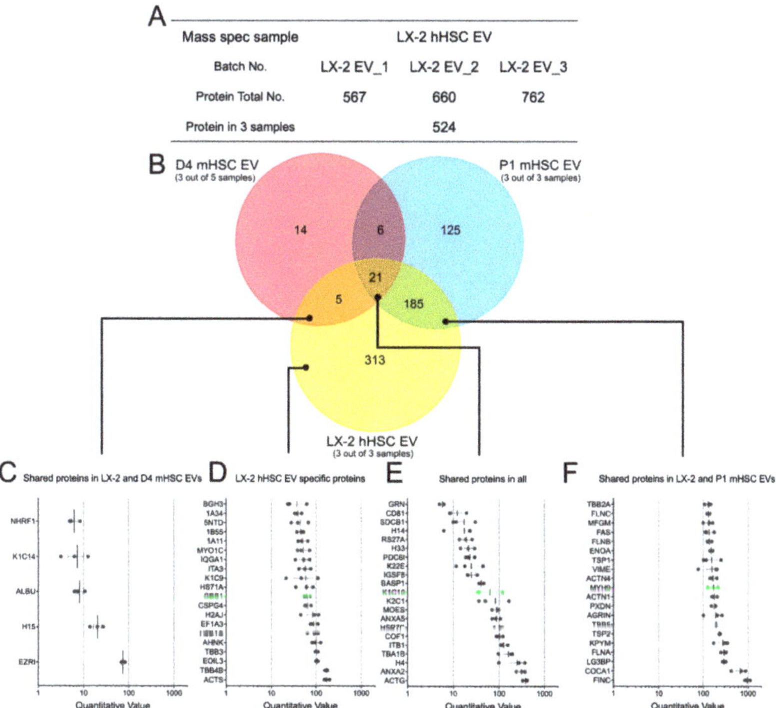

Figure 7. Proteomic composition of EVs from LX-2 hHSC and/or D4 or P1 mHSC. (**A**) Summary of quantitative features of EV proteins analyzed from LX-2 hHSC EV samples. (**B**) Venn diagram showing distribution of proteins between EVs from LX-2 hHSC, D4 mHSC and P1 mHSC. Also shown are the identities and quantifications of (**C**) the five proteins shared between LX-2 hHSC EVs and D4 mHSC EVs; (**D**) the 20 most abundant proteins specific to EVs from LX-2 hHSC; (**E**) the 21 proteins shared by EVs from all three cell types; and (**F**) the 20 most abundant proteins shared by EVs from LX-2 hHSC and P1 mHSC.

GO analysis was performed on the total proteins identified in EVs from activated human or mouse HSC, as well as those that were shared or not shared between them (Figure 8). For the entire EV proteome from LX-2 cells, the principal components were related to exosome, cytoplasm, cytosol, membrane, nucleus, ECM, focal adhesion, extracellular space, cell surface, cell-cell adherins, perinuclear region of cytoplasm, mitochondrion, nucleoplasm and myelin sheath (Figure 8A). Many of these components were shared with P1 mHSC EVs but additional components in this shared group included melansome, actin cytoskeleton and proteosome complex (Figure 8B). The same or highly similar components were represented by the proteins that were unique to EVs from either LX-2 cells (Figure 8C) or P1 mHSC (Figure 8D). The outcome of this component analysis was largely reflected in the KEGG analysis of the respective EV protein groups (Figure 9). For example, the top 20 KEGG pathways for the complete LX-2 hHSC EV proteome (Figure 9A) showed substantial overlap with the pathways for the P1 mHSC EV proteome (Figure 6A) and included focal adhesion, PI3K-Akt signaling, regulation of actin cytoskeleton, pathways in cancer, proteoglycans in cancer, ribosome, phagosome, leukocyte transendothelial migration, protein processing in the ER and carbon metabolism. These pathways were also predominant for the 206 proteins shared between LX-2 hHSC EVs and P1 mHSC EVs (Figure 9B). Some of the same or related components were evident for LX-2 hHSC EV-specific proteins (regulation of cytoskeleton, pathways in cancer, ribosome, PI3k-AKT signaling, proteoglycans in cancer, phagosome, focal adhesion, cell adhesion molecules, alcoholism) (Figure 9C) or for P1 mHSC EV-specific proteins (proteasome, ECM-receptor interactions) (Figure 9D) but the remaining components in these groups were quite dissimilar and diverged from those typically noted above. Finally, STRING analysis of the entire LX-2 hHSC EV proteome (Supplemental Figure S4) or of the EV proteins shared between LX-2 cells and P1 mHSC (Supplemental Figure S5) revealed major interactions between nodes associated with collagens, ECM, metabolic enzymes, vesicular transport, chaperones or ribosomes and these were very similar to those for the entire P1 mHSC EV proteome (Supplemental Figure S3).

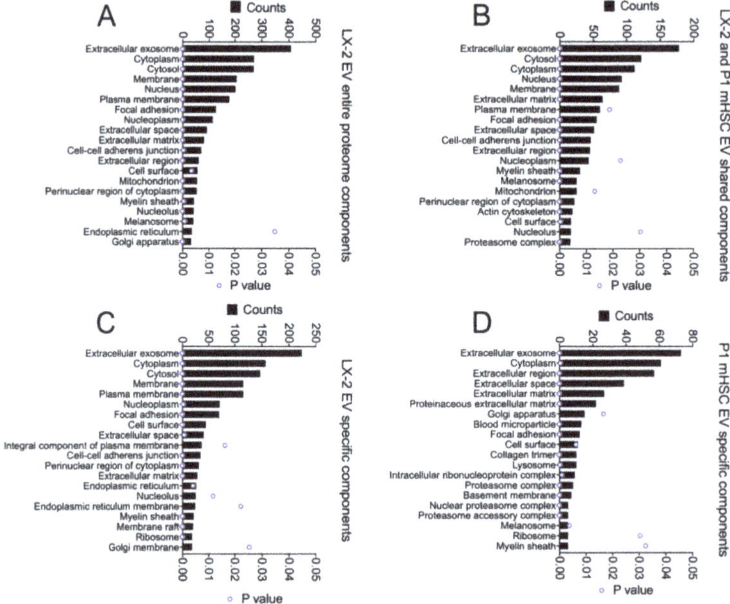

Figure 8. Cellular component analysis of proteins in EVs from LX-2 hHSC and/or P1 mHSC. GO analysis was performed on proteins in EVs from LX-2 hHSC as in Figure 5. The figure shows the 20 most highly ranked cellular components for proteins that were (**A**) in the entire LX-2 HSC EV proteome; (**B**) shared between EVs from LX-2 hHSC and P1 mHSC; (**C**) specific to LX-2 hHSC EVs; or (**D**) specific to P1 mHSC EVs. Only cellular components with significant enrichment ($p < 0.05$) are shown.

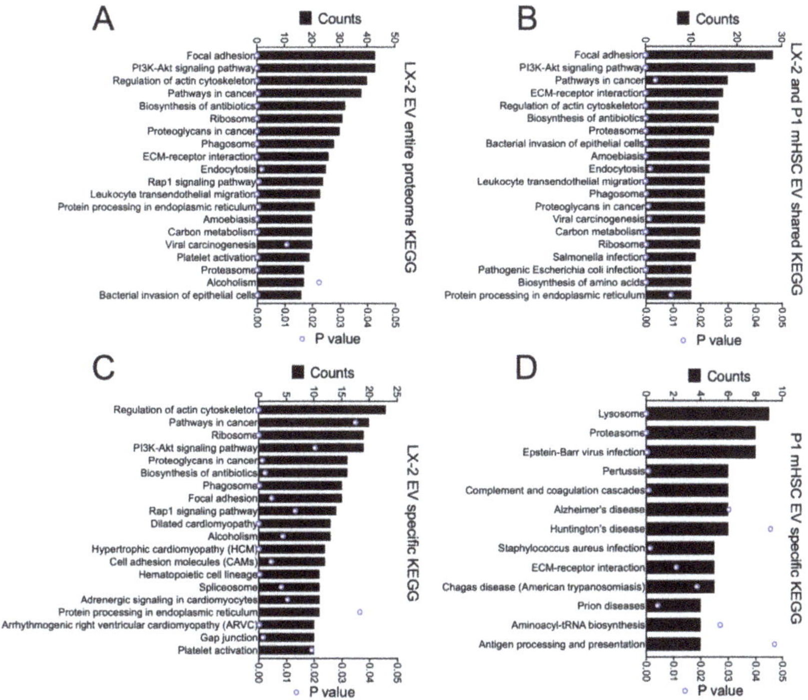

Figure 9. KEGG pathway analysis of proteins in EVs from LX-2 hHSC and/or P1 mHSC. EV proteins were analyzed as in Figure 6. The figure shows the top 20 pathways identified for (**A**) the entire LX-2 hHSC EV proteome; (**B**) proteins shared between LX-2 hHSC EVs and P1 mHSC EVs; or (**C**) proteins unique to LX-2 hHSC EVs. (**D**) Pathways identified for EV proteins that were specific to P1 mHSC. Only pathways with significant enrichment ($p < 0.05$) are shown.

4. Discussion

EVs have attracted considerable attention for the role they likely play in mediating cell-cell communication throughout the body. In the liver, EVs are proposed to regulate hepatic homeostasis or to contribute to pathophysiogical processes such as viral spread, non-alcoholic steatohepatitis, alcoholic liver disease, and cancer [16,17]. A large body of research has shown that hepatocytes infected with hepatitis B or C viruses or that have been exposed to agents such as alcohol, carbon tetrachloride or palmitate produce EVs that stimulate macrophage activation and immune function which are common features of numerous liver diseases and often associated with fibrotic pathology [30,35–40]. HSC fibrogenesis is stimulated by these types of hepatocyte-derived EVs [29,32,41], while other phenotypic features of activated HSC such as migration and AKT phosphorylation have been shown to be enhanced by EVs from liver sinusoidal endothelial cells [42]. On the other hand, EVs from healthy hepatocytes [43], various stem cells [44–51] or the serum of healthy mice [52] have the ability to inhibit experimental liver fibrosis, largely by suppressing inflammatory responses and/or pathways of activation or fibrogenesis in HSC. The recognition that HSC are EV targets has highlighted an important new mechanism by which fibrogenic pathways in the liver are modulated and has given a new lead for novel anti-fibrotic therapies based on suppressing the action of pro-fibrotic EVs or harnessing the actions of EVs that are intrinsically anti-fibrotic.

As shown in this report, HSC themselves are also EV producers but relatively little is known about this phenomenon. Whereas the physico-chemical properties of HSC EVs were quite consistent whether their producer cells were activated or not, we found that the HSC EV production rate, biological properties and protein composition were highly dependent on HSC activation status. Specifically, our results showed, firstly, that fibrogenic gene expression was suppressed upon exposure of activated HSC to EVs from relatively quiescent HSC but not to EVs from activated HSC and, secondly, that gene expression in relatively quiescent HSC was stimulated upon exposure of the cells to EVs from activated HSC but not to EVs from relatively quiescent cells. Thus, pathways of EV communication between HSC may be either stimulatory or inhibitory and are manifest principally when the activation status of the EV producer HSC is different to that of the EV recipient HSC. We also showed that HSC activation is associated with a 4.5-fold increase in EV release and that EVs from activated HSC contained considerably more proteomic information than their quiescent counterparts: there were 337 proteins in EVs from P1 mHSC but only 46 proteins in EVs from D4 mHSC. Generally, EVs from D4 mHSC exhibited a high abundance and high proportion of histones and keratins, while EVs from P1 mHSC contained proteins principally associated with extracellular spaces, ECM, proteasome complexes, collagens, ECM, vesicular transport, metabolic enzymes, ribosomes and chaperones. These differences reflected the distinct phenotypes and functions of their respective EV producer cells: quiescent HSC are resting vitamin-A storing cells whereas activated HSC are contractile myofibroblasts that interact with various immune cells, are highly proliferative and migratory, are metabolically very active, have high energy requirements and produce numerous cytokines, chemokines and extracellular matrix components. Even so, it will be important in future studies to evaluate the molecular payload of EVs from HSC that have been activated in vitro by cytokines (e.g., TGF-β) or in vivo due to liver injury as there may be qualitative or quantitative differences that have functional impact as compared to the EVs in this study that were from HSC that had autonomously activated in culture.

It is interesting that FN1 was expressed exclusively in EVs from P1 HSC and was the most abundant protein overall in EVs from activated or quiescent HSC. FN1 exists either as a soluble plasma form that lacks EDA and EDB domains and is produced principally by hepatocytes or as a cell-associated form which contains the EDA and EDB domains and is produced by numerous cell types. Analysis of the FN1 protein in P1 mHSC EVs showed it to be the cell-associated form because sequencing identified a near-complete EDA domain as well as a partial N-terminal EDB domain, consistent with its detection using FN1 antibodies directed to the EDA or EDB regions. We have previously reported that HSC EVs use cell surface integrins as receptors, including integrin $\alpha5\beta1$, which is a receptor for FN1 [34]. In activated HSC, FN1-integrin $\alpha5\beta1$ interactions are important for the regulation of cell adhesion, survival, cytoskeletal rearrangements or expression of matrix metalloproteases or collagen I [53–57], but this interaction may also underlie the binding of EVs to target HSC, the extent of which will be dependent on activation-associated changes in cellular integrin expression and EV FN1 levels. Importantly, EV FN1 may also directly participate in downstream pro-fibrogenic actions of HSC EVs in light of recent studies showing, firstly, that FN1 in cancer cell microvesicles mediates their ability to confer transformation characteristics on fibroblasts and epithelial cells [58] and, secondly, that exosomal FN1 mediates the mitogenic activity of exosomes from mesenchymal stem cells [59]. Such functions may also be conserved in EVs from hHSC, since we showed FN1 to be the most abundant component of EVs from LX-2 cells in these studies. Indeed, an important feature that emerged from the current investigation was the recognition that EVs from activated hHSC have the same pro-fibrogenic properties and share many of the same proteins as their mouse counterparts resulting in considerable overlap in the components and pathways in which they are involved. The 206 proteins that were common to both species represented approximately 40% of all 524 proteins in EVs from activated hHSC and 61% of all 337 proteins in EVs from activated mHSC. The incorporation of these shared proteins into EVs from activated HSC of mice and humans suggests that their functional roles were under strong selective pressure during evolution.

It remains to be determined what other constituents (protein, RNA or miRNA or combinations thereof) in the EV molecular payload might be relevant to the relative suppressive or stimulatory actions of EVs from, respectively, quiescent or activated HSC. Even so, it is striking that the proteomic payloads of EVs from activated human or mouse HSC correspond to cellular components that are well characterized for their involvement in HSC activation and/or fibrogenesis (i.e., ECM, proteasome complexes, collagens, metabolic enzymes, ribosomes, chaperones) and it is tempting to speculate that the EV counterparts have similar functions. Although we have previously used a transfection approach to show that HSC-derived EVs can shuttle GFP-CCN2 intercellularly [24], this overexpression system may not have faithfully mimicked native mechanisms because CCN2 was not detected in EVs from P1 mHSC in this study. With respect to the anti-fibrogenic actions of EVs from D4 mHSC, the high prevalence of keratins or histones in the relatively small proteome suggests that structural elements or nucleosomal regulation may underlie the suppressive activities. However, preliminary transfection studies in which activated HSC were transfected with cDNAs encoding single D4 mHSC-specific or -enriched EV histones (H4, H10, H11, H13, H14, H15, H2B1F) did not result in an attenuation of fibrogenic markers even though each over-expressed protein was detected by Western blot (X.L. and D.R.B., unpublished data), suggesting that these proteins are not anti-fibrogenic at least when tested individually, but additional combinatorial testing of these and other candidates (e.g., keratins) must be undertaken in the future. For a variety of differentially expressed mHSC EV proteins, we found that the levels of their corresponding cellular transcripts were quite variable, ranging from concordant to discordant with their respective EV protein levels, suggesting that there is selectivity in the post-transcriptional or post-translational mechanisms by which a given protein is incorporated into the EVs.

Apart from proteins, the EV molecular payload contains miRs and mRNAs that may also contribute to EV-mediated regulation of fibrogenesis. For example, we previously showed that inhibition of pro-fibrogenic CCN2 in quiescent HSC is achieved by targeting of the CCN2 3′ untranslated region by Twist-1-miR-199a-miR-214 and that all three components of this axis can be delivered in EVs to activated HSC in which CCN2 expression is then suppressed [25,27,28]. Even so, one must recognize that while these types of reductionist strategies to understand EV bioactivity have been widely pursued in the EV research field in general, they do not take account of EV heterogeneity at the single vesicle and systems level and the importance of adopting a more global view of EV cargo as it relates to functional aspects of EV biology has recently been emphasized [60]. Thus, a holistic approach may be preferable for understanding the combinatorial actions of EV cargo constituents in mediating EV biological actions [60]. We expect that detailed comparative studies between EVs from quiescent versus activated HSC of their respective miRnomes and RNAnomes, together with their proteomes as accomplished in this study, will provide a foundation for the identification of EV components and their corresponding cellular targets that accounts for their distinct biological actions. Whatever the factors involved, it is interesting to speculate that the suppressive actions of EVs from quiescent HSC may help to protect the liver from overt HSC activation, especially in cases of mild or acute injury.

In conclusion, mHSC activation is associated with an increase in EV production, a switch in EV bioactivity whereby EV-mediated suppression of mHSC fibrogenic gene expression gives way to EV-mediated stimulation of the same, and a dramatic increase in the complexity of the EV proteome. Activated hHSC produce EVs that exhibit profibrogenic activities and have similar protein components and functions as EVs from activated mHSC. We thus propose that activation-associated changes in production, function and protein content of EVs from HSC may contribute to the regulation of HSC function in vivo and to the fine-tuning of fibrogenic pathways in the liver.

Supplementary Materials: The following are available online at http://www.mdpi.com/2073-4409/9/2/290/s1: Figure S1. Fibronectin in EVs from P1 mHSC; Figure S2. String analysis for entire proteome in EVs from D4 mHSC; Figure S3. String analysis for entire proteome in EVs from P1 mHSC; Figure S4. String analysis for entire proteome in EVs from LX-2 hHSC; Figure S5. String analysis for proteins shared in EVs from P1 mHSC and LX-2 hHSC; Table S1. qRT-PCR primers used for mouse gene detection; Table S2. MS datasets for D4 mHSC proteome; Table S3. MS datasets for P1 mHSC proteome; Table S4. MS datasets for LX-2 hHSC proteome.

Author Contributions: Conceptualization, X.L. and D.R.B.; Data curation, X.L., R.C. and S.K.; Formal analysis, X.L., R.C. and D.R.B.; Funding acquisition, D.R.B.; Investigation, X.L., R.C. and S.K.; Methodology, X.L., R.C. and S.K.; Project administration, D.R.B.; Writing – original draft, X.L. and D.R.B.; Writing – review and editing, X.L., R.C., S.K. and D.R.B. All authors have read and agreed to the published version of the manuscript.

Funding: This research was funded by NIH grants R21 AA025974 and R21 AA023626.

Acknowledgments: We thank the staff of the Proteomics Shared Resource of the OSU Campus Chemical Instrument Center for help with Mass Spectrometry which was supported by NIH grant P30 CA016058.

Conflicts of Interest: The authors declare no conflict of interest.

References

1. Hernandez-Gea, V.; Friedman, S.L. Pathogenesis of liver fibrosis. *Annu. Rev. Pathol.* **2011**, *6*, 425–456. [CrossRef]
2. Lee, U.E.; Friedman, S.L. Mechanisms of hepatic fibrogenesis. *Best Pr. Res. Clin. Gastroenterol.* **2011**, *25*, 195–206. [CrossRef]
3. Puche, J.E.; Saiman, Y.; Friedman, S.L. Hepatic stellate cells and liver fibrosis. *Compr. Physiol.* **2013**, *3*, 1473–1492. [CrossRef] [PubMed]
4. De Oliveira da Silva, B.; Ramos, L.F.; Moraes, K.C.M. Molecular interplays in hepatic stellate cells: Apoptosis, senescence, and phenotype reversion as cellular connections that modulate liver fibrosis. *Cell Biol. Int.* **2017**, *41*, 946–959. [CrossRef] [PubMed]
5. Higashi, T.; Friedman, S.L.; Hoshida, Y. Hepatic stellate cells as key target in liver fibrosis. *Adv. Drug Deliv. Rev.* **2017**, *121*, 27–42. [CrossRef] [PubMed]
6. Ezhilarasan, D.; Sokal, E.; Najimi, M. Hepatic fibrosis: It is time to go with hepatic stellate cell-specific therapeutic targets. *Hepatobiliary Pancreat Dis. Int.* **2018**, *17*, 192–197. [CrossRef]
7. Mokdad, A.A.; Lopez, A.D.; Shahraz, S.; Lozano, R.; Mokdad, A.H.; Stanaway, J.; Murray, C.J.; Naghavi, M. Liver cirrhosis mortality in 187 countries between 1980 and 2010: A systematic analysis. *BMC Med.* **2014**, *12*, 145. [CrossRef]
8. Cohen-Naftaly, M.; Friedman, S.L. Current status of novel antifibrotic therapies in patients with chronic liver disease. *Ther. Adv. Gastroenterol.* **2011**, *4*, 391–417. [CrossRef]
9. Ghiassi-Nejad, Z.; Friedman, S.L. Advances in antifibrotic therapy. *Expert Rev. Gastroenterol. Hepatol.* **2008**, *2*, 803–816. [CrossRef]
10. Lemoinne, S.; Friedman, S.L. New and emerging anti-fibrotic therapeutics entering or already in clinical trials in chronic liver diseases. *Curr. Opin. Pharm.* **2019**, *49*, 60–70. [CrossRef]
11. Bansal, R.; Nagorniewicz, B.; Prakash, J. Clinical Advancements in the Targeted Therapies against Liver Fibrosis. *Mediat. Inflamm.* **2016**, *2016*, 7629724. [CrossRef] [PubMed]
12. Rockey, D.C. Translating an understanding of the pathogenesis of hepatic fibrosis to novel therapies. *Clin. Gastroenterol. Hepatol.* **2013**, *11*, 224–231. [CrossRef] [PubMed]
13. Schuppan, D.; Pinzani, M. Anti-fibrotic therapy: Lost in translation? *J. Hepatol.* **2012**, *56* (Suppl. 1), S66–S74. [CrossRef]
14. Trautwein, C.; Friedman, S.L.; Schuppan, D.; Pinzani, M. Hepatic fibrosis: Concept to treatment. *J. Hepatol.* **2015**, *62*, S15–S24. [CrossRef] [PubMed]
15. Friedman, S.L. Molecular regulation of hepatic fibrosis, an integrated cellular response to tissue injury. *J. Biol. Chem.* **2000**, *275*, 2247–2250. [CrossRef] [PubMed]
16. Szabo, G.; Momen-Heravi, F. Extracellular vesicles in liver disease and potential as biomarkers and therapeutic targets. *Nat. Rev. Gastroenterol. Hepatol.* **2017**, *14*, 455–466. [CrossRef]
17. Maji, S.; Matsuda, A.; Yan, I.K.; Parasramka, M.; Patel, T. Extracellular vesicles in liver diseases. *Am. J. Physiol. Gastrointest Liver Physiol.* **2017**, *312*, G194–G200. [CrossRef]
18. Lemoinne, S.; Thabut, D.; Housset, C.; Moreau, R.; Valla, D.; Boulanger, C.M.; Rautou, P.E. The emerging roles of microvesicles in liver diseases. *Nat. Rev. Gastroenterol. Hepatol.* **2014**, *11*, 350–361. [CrossRef]
19. Hirsova, P.; Ibrahim, S.H.; Verma, V.K.; Morton, L.A.; Shah, V.H.; LaRusso, N.F.; Gores, G.J.; Malhi, H. Extracellular vesicles in liver pathobiology: Small particles with big impact. *Hepatology* **2016**, *64*, 2219–2233. [CrossRef]
20. Cai, S.; Cheng, X.; Pan, X.; Li, J. Emerging role of exosomes in liver physiology and pathology. *Hepatol. Res.* **2017**, *47*, 194–203. [CrossRef]
21. Kowal, J.; Arras, G.; Colombo, M.; Jouve, M.; Morath, J.P.; Primdal-Bengtson, B.; Dingli, F.; Loew, D.; Tkach, M.; Thery, C. Proteomic comparison defines novel markers to characterize heterogeneous populations of extracellular vesicle subtypes. *Proc. Natl. Acad. Sci. USA* **2016**, *113*, E968–E977. [CrossRef] [PubMed]

22. Thery, C. Exosomes: Secreted vesicles and intercellular communications. *F1000 Biol. Rep.* **2011**, *3*, 15. [CrossRef] [PubMed]
23. Thery, C.; Witwer, K.W.; Aikawa, E.; Alcaraz, M.J.; Anderson, J.D.; Andriantsitohaina, R.; Antoniou, A.; Arab, T.; Archer, F.; Atkin-Smith, G.K.; et al. Minimal information for studies of extracellular vesicles 2018 (MISEV2018): A position statement of the International Society for Extracellular Vesicles and update of the MISEV2014 guidelines. *J. Extracell. Vesicles* **2018**, *7*, 1535750. [CrossRef] [PubMed]
24. Charrier, A.; Chen, R.; Chen, L.; Kemper, S.; Hattori, T.; Takigawa, M.; Brigstock, D.R. Exosomes mediate intercellular transfer of pro-fibrogenic connective tissue growth factor (CCN2) between hepatic stellate cells, the principal fibrotic cells in the liver. *Surgery* **2014**, *156*, 548–555. [CrossRef]
25. Chen, L.; Charrier, A.; Zhou, Y.; Chen, R.; Yu, B.; Agarwal, K.; Tsukamoto, H.; Lee, L.J.; Paulaitis, M.E.; Brigstock, D.R. Epigenetic regulation of connective tissue growth factor by MicroRNA-214 delivery in exosomes from mouse or human hepatic stellate cells. *Hepatology* **2014**, *59*, 1118–1129. [CrossRef]
26. Chen, L.; Chen, R.; Kemper, S.; Brigstock, D.R. Pathways of production and delivery of hepatocyte exosomes. *J. Cell Commun. Signal.* **2018**, *12*, 343–357. [CrossRef]
27. Chen, L.; Chen, R.; Kemper, S.; Charrier, A.; Brigstock, D.R. Suppression of fibrogenic signaling in hepatic stellate cells by Twist1-dependent microRNA-214 expression: Role of exosomes in horizontal transfer of Twist1. *Am. J. Physiol. Gastrointest Liver Physiol.* **2015**, *309*, G491–G499. [CrossRef]
28. Chen, L.; Chen, R.; Velazquez, V.M.; Brigstock, D.R. Fibrogenic Signaling Is Suppressed in Hepatic Stellate Cells through Targeting of Connective Tissue Growth Factor (CCN2) by Cellular or Exosomal MicroRNA-199a-5p. *Am. J. Pathol.* **2016**, *186*, 2921–2933. [CrossRef]
29. Devhare, P.B.; Sasaki, R.; Shrivastava, S.; Di Bisceglie, A.M.; Ray, R.; Ray, R.B. Exosome-Mediated Intercellular Communication between Hepatitis C Virus-Infected Hepatocytes and Hepatic Stellate Cells. *J. Virol.* **2017**, *91*. [CrossRef]
30. Seo, W.; Eun, H.S.; Kim, S.Y.; Yi, H.S.; Lee, Y.S.; Park, S.H.; Jang, M.J.; Jo, E.; Kim, S.C.; Han, Y.M.; et al. Exosome-mediated activation of toll-like receptor 3 in stellate cells stimulates interleukin-17 production by gammadelta T cells in liver fibrosis. *Hepatology* **2016**, *64*, 616–631. [CrossRef]
31. Povero, D.; Panera, N.; Eguchi, A.; Johnson, C.D.; Papouchado, B.G.; de Araujo Horcel, L.; Pinatel, E.M.; Alisi, A.; Nobili, V.; Feldstein, A.E. Lipid-induced hepatocyte-derived extracellular vesicles regulate hepatic stellate cell via microRNAs targeting PPAR-gamma. *Cell. Mol. Gastroenterol. Hepatol.* **2015**, *1*, 646–663. [CrossRef] [PubMed]
32. Lee, Y.S.; Kim, S.Y.; Ko, E.; Lee, J.H.; Yi, H.S.; Yoo, Y.J.; Je, J.; Suh, S.J.; Jung, Y.K.; Kim, J.H.; et al. Exosomes derived from palmitic acid-treated hepatocytes induce fibrotic activation of hepatic stellate cells. *Sci. Rep.* **2017**, *7*, 3710. [CrossRef] [PubMed]
33. Lua, I.; Li, Y.; Zagory, J.A.; Wang, K.S.; French, S.W.; Sevigny, J.; Asahina, K. Characterization of hepatic stellate cells, portal fibroblasts, and mesothelial cells in normal and fibrotic livers. *J. Hepatol.* **2016**, *64*, 1137–1146. [CrossRef] [PubMed]
34. Chen, L.; Brigstock, D.R. Integrins and heparan sulfate proteoglycans on hepatic stellate cells (HSC) are novel receptors for HSC-derived exosomes. *FEBS Lett.* **2016**, *590*, 4263–4274. [CrossRef]
35. Kouwaki, T.; Fukushima, Y.; Daito, T.; Sanada, T.; Yamamoto, N.; Mifsud, E.J.; Leong, C.R.; Tsukiyama-Kohara, K.; Kohara, M.; Matsumoto, M.; et al. Extracellular Vesicles Including Exosomes Regulate Innate Immune Responses to Hepatitis B Virus Infection. *Front. Immunol.* **2016**, *7*, 335. [CrossRef]
36. Verma, V.K.; Li, H.; Wang, R.; Hirsova, P.; Mushref, M.; Liu, Y.; Cao, S.; Contreras, P.C.; Malhi, H.; Kamath, P.S.; et al. Alcohol stimulates macrophage activation through caspase-dependent hepatocyte derived release of CD40L containing extracellular vesicles. *J. Hepatol.* **2016**, *64*, 651–660. [CrossRef]
37. Momen-Heravi, F.; Bala, S.; Kodys, K.; Szabo, G. Exosomes derived from alcohol-treated hepatocytes horizontally transfer liver specific miRNA-122 and sensitize monocytes to LPS. *Sci. Rep.* **2015**, *5*, 9991. [CrossRef]
38. Hirsova, P.; Ibrahim, S.H.; Krishnan, A.; Verma, V.K.; Bronk, S.F.; Werneburg, N.W.; Charlton, M.R.; Shah, V.H.; Malhi, H.; Gores, G.J. Lipid-induced Signaling Causes Release of Inflammatory Extracellular Vesicles from Hepatocytes. *Gastroenterology* **2016**. [CrossRef]
39. Kakazu, E.; Mauer, A.S.; Yin, M.; Malhi, H. Hepatocytes release ceramide-enriched pro-inflammatory extracellular vesicles in an IRE1alpha-dependent manner. *J. Lipid Res.* **2016**, *57*, 233–245. [CrossRef]

40. Povero, D.; Eguchi, A.; Niesman, I.R.; Andronikou, N.; de Mollerat du Jeu, X.; Mulya, A.; Berk, M.; Lazic, M.; Thapaliya, S.; Parola, M.; et al. Lipid-induced toxicity stimulates hepatocytes to release angiogenic microparticles that require Vanin-1 for uptake by endothelial cells. *Sci. Signal.* **2013**, *6*, ra88. [CrossRef]
41. Kim, J.H.; Lee, C.H.; Lee, S.W. Exosomal Transmission of MicroRNA from HCV Replicating Cells Stimulates Transdifferentiation in Hepatic Stellate Cells. *Mol. Nucleic Acids* **2019**, *14*, 483–497. [CrossRef] [PubMed]
42. Wang, R.; Ding, Q.; Yaqoob, U.; de Assuncao, T.M.; Verma, V.K.; Hirsova, P.; Cao, S.; Mukhopadhyay, D.; Huebert, R.C.; Shah, V.H. Exosome Adherence and Internalization by Hepatic Stellate Cells Triggers Sphingosine 1-Phosphate-dependent Migration. *J. Biol. Chem.* **2015**, *290*, 30684–30696. [CrossRef] [PubMed]
43. Li, X.; Chen, R.; Kemper, S.; Brigstock, D. Extracellular vesicles from hepatocytes are therapeutic for toxin-mediated fibrosis and gene expression in the liver. *Front. Cell Dev. Biol.* **2019**. [CrossRef] [PubMed]
44. Jiang, W.; Tan, Y.; Cai, M.; Zhao, T.; Mao, F.; Zhang, X.; Xu, W.; Yan, Z.; Qian, H.; Yan, Y. Human Umbilical Cord MSC-Derived Exosomes Suppress the Development of CCl4-Induced Liver Injury through Antioxidant Effect. *Stem Cells Int.* **2018**, *2018*, 6079642. [CrossRef] [PubMed]
45. Li, T.; Yan, Y.; Wang, B.; Qian, H.; Zhang, X.; Shen, L.; Wang, M.; Zhou, Y.; Zhu, W.; Li, W.; et al. Exosomes derived from human umbilical cord mesenchymal stem cells alleviate liver fibrosis. *Stem Cells Dev.* **2013**, *22*, 845–854. [CrossRef] [PubMed]
46. Qu, Y.; Zhang, Q.; Cai, X.; Li, F.; Ma, Z.; Xu, M.; Lu, L. Exosomes derived from miR-181-5p-modified adipose-derived mesenchymal stem cells prevent liver fibrosis via autophagy activation. *J. Cell Mol. Med.* **2017**. [CrossRef] [PubMed]
47. Mardpour, S.; Hassani, S.N.; Mardpour, S.; Sayahpour, F.; Vosough, M.; Ai, J.; Aghdami, N.; Hamidieh, A.A.; Baharvand, H. Extracellular vesicles derived from human embryonic stem cell-MSCs ameliorate cirrhosis in thioacetamide-induced chronic liver injury. *J. Cell. Physiol.* **2018**, *233*, 9330–9344. [CrossRef]
48. Ohara, M.; Ohnishi, S.; Hosono, H.; Yamamoto, K.; Yuyama, K.; Nakamura, H.; Fu, Q.; Maehara, O.; Suda, G.; Sakamoto, N. Extracellular Vesicles from Amnion-Derived Mesenchymal Stem Cells Ameliorate Hepatic Inflammation and Fibrosis in Rats. *Stem Cells Int.* **2018**, *2018*, 3212643. [CrossRef]
49. Povero, D.; Pinatel, E.M.; Leszczynska, A.; Goyal, N.P.; Nishio, T.; Kim, J.; Kneiber, D.; de Araujo Horcel, L.; Eguchi, A.; Ordonez, P.M.; et al. Human induced pluripotent stem cell-derived extracellular vesicles reduce hepatic stellate cell activation and liver fibrosis. *JCI Insight* **2019**, *5*. [CrossRef]
50. Rong, X.; Liu, J.; Yao, X.; Jiang, T.; Wang, Y.; Xie, F. Human bone marrow mesenchymal stem cells-derived exosomes alleviate liver fibrosis through the Wnt/beta-catenin pathway. *Stem Cell Res.* **2019**, *10*, 98. [CrossRef]
51. Bruno, S.; Pasquino, C.; Herrera Sanchez, M.B.; Tapparo, M.; Figliolini, F.; Grange, C.; Chiabotto, G.; Cedrino, M.; Deregibus, M.C.; Tetta, C.; et al. HLSC-Derived Extracellular Vesicles Attenuate Liver Fibrosis and Inflammation in a Murine Model of Non-alcoholic Steatohepatitis. *Mol. Ther.* **2019**. [CrossRef] [PubMed]
52. Chen, L.; Chen, R.; Kemper, S.; Cong, M.; You, H.; Brigstock, D.R. Therapeutic effects of serum extracellular vesicles in liver fibrosis. *J. Extracell. Vesicles* **2018**, *7*, 1461505. [CrossRef] [PubMed]
53. Pranitha, P.; Sudhakaran, P.R. Fibronectin dependent upregulation of matrix metalloproteinases in hepatic stellate cells. *Indian J. Biochem. Biophys.* **2003**, *40*, 409–415. [PubMed]
54. Dodig, M.; Ogunwale, B.; Dasarathy, S.; Li, M.; Wang, B.; McCullough, A.J. Differences in regulation of type I collagen synthesis in primary and passaged hepatic stellate cell cultures: The role of alpha5beta1-integrin. *Am. J. Physiol. Gastrointest Liver Physiol.* **2007**, *293*, G154–G164. [CrossRef]
55. Rodriguez-Juan, C.; de la Torre, P.; Garcia-Ruiz, I.; Diaz-Sanjuan, T.; Munoz-Yague, T.; Gomez-Izquierdo, E.; Solis-Munoz, P.; Solis-Herruzo, J.A. Fibronectin increases survival of rat hepatic stellate cells–a novel profibrogenic mechanism of fibronectin. *Cell. Physiol. Biochem.* **2009**, *24*, 271–282. [CrossRef]
56. Milliano, M.T.; Luxon, B.A. Initial signaling of the fibronectin receptor (alpha5beta1 integrin) in hepatic stellate cells is independent of tyrosine phosphorylation. *J. Hepatol.* **2003**, *39*, 32–37. [CrossRef]
57. Huang, G.; Brigstock, D.R. Integrin expression and function in the response of primary culture hepatic stellate cells to connective tissue growth factor (CCN2). *J. Cell Mol. Med.* **2011**, *15*, 1087–1095. [CrossRef]
58. Antonyak, M.A.; Li, B.; Boroughs, L.K.; Johnson, J.L.; Druso, J.E.; Bryant, K.L.; Holowka, D.A.; Cerione, R.A. Cancer cell-derived microvesicles induce transformation by transferring tissue transglutaminase and fibronectin to recipient cells. *Proc. Natl. Acad. Sci. USA* **2011**, *108*, 4852–4857. [CrossRef]

59. Yuan, O.; Lin, C.; Wagner, J.; Archard, J.A.; Deng, P.; Halmai, J.; Bauer, G.; Fink, K.D.; Fury, B.; Perotti, N.H.; et al. Exosomes Derived from Human Primed Mesenchymal Stem Cells Induce Mitosis and Potentiate Growth Factor Secretion. *Stem Cells Dev.* **2019**, *28*, 398–409. [CrossRef]
60. Gho, Y.S.; Lee, C. Emergent properties of extracellular vesicles: A holistic approach to decode the complexity of intercellular communication networks. *Mol. Biosyst.* **2017**, *13*, 1291–1296. [CrossRef]

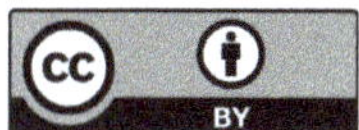

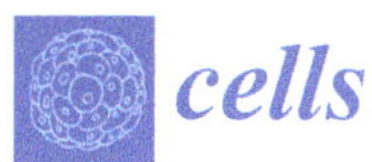
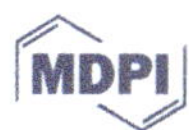
Article

Depletion of Bone Marrow-Derived Fibrocytes Attenuates TAA-Induced Liver Fibrosis in Mice

Felix Hempel [1,†], Martin Roderfeld [1,†], Rajkumar Savai [2,3], Akylbek Sydykov [3], Karuna Irungbam [1], Ralph Schermuly [3], Robert Voswinckel [4,5], Kernt Köhler [6], Yury Churin [1], Ladislau Kiss [3], Jens Bier [3], Jörn Pons-Kühnemann [7] and Elke Roeb [1,*]

1. Department of Gastroenterology, Justus Liebig University, D-35392 Giessen, Germany; felix.hempel@med.jlug.de (F.H.); martin.roderfeld@innere.med.uni-giessen.de (M.R.); kukuirungbam@gmail.com (K.I.); yury.churin@innere.med.uni-giessen.de (Y.C.)
2. Max Planck Institute for Heart and Lung Research, Member of the German Center for Lung Research (DZL), Member of the Cardio-Pulmonary Institute (CPI), D-61231 Bad Nauheim, Germany; rajkumar.savai@mpi-bn.mpg.de
3. Department of Internal Medicine, Cardio-Pulmonary Institute (CPI), Universities of Giessen and Marburg Lung Center (UGMLC), Member of the German Center for Lung Research (DZL), Justus Liebig University, D-35392 Giessen, Germany; akylbek.sydykov@innere.med.uni-giessen.de (A.S.); ralph.schermuly@innere.med.uni-giessen.de (R.S.); ladislau.kiss@innere.med.uni-giessen.de (L.K.); jens.bier@innere.med.uni-giessen.de (J.B.)
4. Department of Internal Medicine, Bürgerhospital, D-61169 Friedberg, Germany; robert.voswinckel@gz-wetterau.de
5. Department of Internal Medicine, Hochwaldkrankenhaus, D-61231 Bad Nauheim, Germany
6. Institute of Veterinary Pathology, Justus Liebig University, D-35392 Giessen, Germany; kernt.koehler@vetmed.uni-giessen.de
7. Institute of Medical Informatics, Justus Liebig University, D-35392 Giessen, Germany; joern.pons@informatik.med.uni-giessen.de

* Correspondence: elke.roeb@innere.med.uni-giessen.de; Tel.: +49-641-985-42338

† These authors contributed equally.

Received: 20 September 2019; Accepted: 5 October 2019; Published: 7 October 2019

Abstract: Bone marrow-derived fibrocytes (FC) represent a unique cell type, sharing features of both mesenchymal and hematopoietic cells. FC were shown to specifically infiltrate the injured liver and participate in fibrogenesis. Moreover, FC exert a variety of paracrine functions, thus possibly influencing the disease progression. However, the overall contribution of FC to liver fibrosis remains unclear. We aimed to study the effect of a specific FC depletion, utilizing a herpes simplex virus thymidine kinase (HSV-TK)/Valganciclovir suicide gene strategy. Fibrosis was induced by oral thioacetamide (TAA) administration in C57BL/6J mice. Hepatic hydroxyproline content was assessed for the primary readout. The HSV-TK model enabled the specific depletion of fibrocytes. Hepatic hydroxyproline content was significantly reduced as a result of the fibrocyte ablation (−7.8%; 95% CI: 0.7–14.8%; $p = 0.033$), denoting a reduced deposition of fibrillar collagens. Lower serum alanine transaminase levels (−20.9%; 95% CI: 0.4–36.9%; $p = 0.049$) indicate a mitigation of liver-specific cellular damage. A detailed mode of action, however, remains yet to be identified. The present study demonstrates a relevant functional contribution of fibrocytes to chronic toxic liver fibrosis, contradicting recent reports. Our results emphasize the need to thoroughly study the biology of fibrocytes in order to understand their importance for hepatic fibrogenesis.

Keywords: fibrocytes; liver fibrosis; bone marrow; myofibroblasts; thioacetamide (TAA); HSV-TK

1. Introduction

Liver fibrosis is denoted by the excess deposition of extracellular matrix (ECM) components in response to chronic liver injury, such as viral hepatitis, cholestatic disorders, alcoholic liver disease or non-alcoholic fatty liver disease (NAFLD). With perpetuated injury, liver fibrosis might progress to cirrhosis and facilitate hepatocellular carcinoma (HCC) formation [1]. Fibrosis accounts for severe morbidity and mortality and has been shown to determine the outcome of patients with NAFLD [2].

Bone marrow-derived fibrocytes (FC) represent a unique cell type, sharing features of both hematopoietic and mesenchymal cells. While their secretion of collagens and other ECM components resembles fibroblasts, they express various leucocyte markers (e.g., CD34, CD45, CD11b, Ly6C, and F4/80) [3,4] and are hence commonly identified by the simultaneous expression of CD45 and collagen I [5]. Fibrocytes comprise ~0.5% of peripheral blood leucocytes and rapidly enter the site of injury in physiological and pathological wound healing processes [3,6]. Since they had been explicitly described by Bucala et al. in 1994 [3], FC have been shown to participate in fibrotic diseases of the lung [7], kidney [8], heart [9], and colon [10,11]. Moreover, they are implicated in the pathogenesis of asthma [12], inflammatory bowel disease [10,13], and ocular disorders [14].

In recent years, the mechanisms of hepatic fibrogenesis have been studied extensively. Activated hepatic stellate cells (HSCs) and, to a lesser extent, portal fibroblasts were identified as the main source of contractile, α-SMA$^+$ myofibroblasts in the liver, which, being absent under healthy conditions, drive scar tissue formation during hepatic fibrogenesis [15–17]. HSCs are therefore commonly considered the key to understanding and treating liver fibrosis [15,18,19]. However, there is compelling evidence that FC, in fact, contribute to liver fibrosis. Fate-tracing studies demonstrated that fibrocytes specifically infiltrate the liver upon injury [20] and participate in fibrogenesis by the secretion of ECM components [21,22]. Furthermore, FC constitute a potential source of myofibroblasts. Although the transdifferentiation into myofibroblasts has been shown both in vitro [7,23] and in vivo [12], its relevance remains controversial.

Besides their direct contribution to fibrogenesis, FC exert a variety of paracrine functions (reviewed in references [24,25]), thus possibly influencing liver fibrosis. FC, on the one hand, express the fibrogenic mediators TGF-β and PDGF [24,26], which are essential for the activation and proliferation of myofibroblasts [1,27]. FC can acquire an inflammatory phenotype, characterized by the production of cytokines (e.g., TNF-α, IL-1β, and CCL2,-3,-4) and eicosanoids [26,28], and their capability of antigen presentation [29]. On the other hand, FC are able to promote the degradation of ECM components via the secretion of matrix metalloproteinases (MMPs) [30,31], regulate angiogenesis [32,33], and exert antimicrobial defense mechanisms [34].

Given the complex interplay of the aforementioned factors in the pathogenesis of liver fibrosis, the overall contribution of FC remains highly speculative. We therefore seek to characterize the role of FC on experimental liver fibrosis in vivo by specific depletion of these cells. Utilizing the well-established herpes simplex virus thymidine kinase (HSV-TK)/Valganciclovir (VCV) model, driven by a collagen I promotor, we depleted collagen I-expressing cells of bone marrow (BM) origin [35–38] in C57BL/6J mice. All collagen-producing cells herein co-express the HSV-TK, making them susceptible to killing by Valganciclovir. BM of such mice was transplanted into non-transgenic mice in order to limit the effect to cells of BM origin. Introducing the HSV-TK via bone marrow transplantation circumnavigates the issue of an unstable expression of the widely used markers CD34 and, as shown recently, CD45 in fibrocytes [5]. Additionally, the collagen-promotor driven expression of HSV-TK enables the killing of fibrocytes in various stages of their development or differentiation. Although a CD14$^+$ cell population, located in the bone marrow, is assumed to be the origin of fibrocytes [23], the exact differentiation pathways remain poorly understood. Thus, the results and possible side effects of an approach that interferes with alleged monocyte precursors in order to deplete fibrocytes, as reported recently [39], seem hardly predictable to us.

While different animal models of murine liver fibrosis have been described [40], with CCl_4-induced liver injury certainly being the most popular, we chose to induce fibrosis with thioacetamide (TAA).

TAA, administered via drinking water, causes a chronic-toxic, more slowly progressing fibrosis with only moderately increased serum transaminase levels, thus closely mimicking alcoholic liver fibrosis in humans [41,42]. The aim of the present study was two-fold: To determine whether the depletion of fibrocytes (1) ameliorates fibrosis, as indicated by decreased hepatic hydroxyproline content, and (2) attenuates liver cell damage, denoted by reduced serum alanine transaminase levels.

2. Materials and Methods

2.1. Animal Experiments

The present study was performed with permission of the State of Hesse, Regierungspraesidium Giessen, according to section 8 of the German Law for the protection of animals and conforms to the NIH guide for the care and use of laboratory animals. All experiments were approved by the committee on the ethics of animal experiments of the Regierungspraesidium Giessen, Germany (permit number: V54-19c 20 15c GI20/10 Nr. G21_2016 and JLU Nr. 532_M). Col-HSV-TK mice were generated at the Max Planck Institute for Heart and Lung Research animal facility (Bad Nauheim, Germany), as described previously [38]. In brief, purified Col1-HSV-TK-IRES-EGFP plasmids (Supplementary Figure S1a) were microinjected into the pronucleus of a fertilized ovum obtained from super-ovulated female mice. Subsequently, groups of injected embryos were re-implanted into the oviducts of pseudo-pregnant female mice. The litters were bred with wild-type C57BL/6J mice. Female, positively genotyped mice were paired again with wild-type mice to create a heterozygous Col-HSV-TK colony. After genotyping, offspring were used for the experiments. All mice were housed in a pathogen-free environment under a constant 12-hour light-dark cycle at 22 °C temperature and 50% humidity. The mice were fed standard chow (ALTROMIN, Lage, Germany) and water ad libitum.

5×10^6 bone marrow (BM) cells were transplanted from male Col-HSV-TK (FC-Ablation) or C57BL/6J wild-type mice (Control) into 12 weeks old lethally irradiated (11 Gy, ^{60}Co) female C57BL/6J mice via tail vein injection ($n = 16$ for each group). For FC depletion during fibrogenesis after 4 weeks of reconstitution 300 mg/l TAA (Sigma-Aldrich, Munich, Germany) and 8.3 mg/l VCV (Roche, Basel, Switzerland) were administered orally via drinking water for 18 weeks. Mice were sacrificed at the age of 34 weeks. A summary of the animal experiment is depicted schematically in Figure 1a.

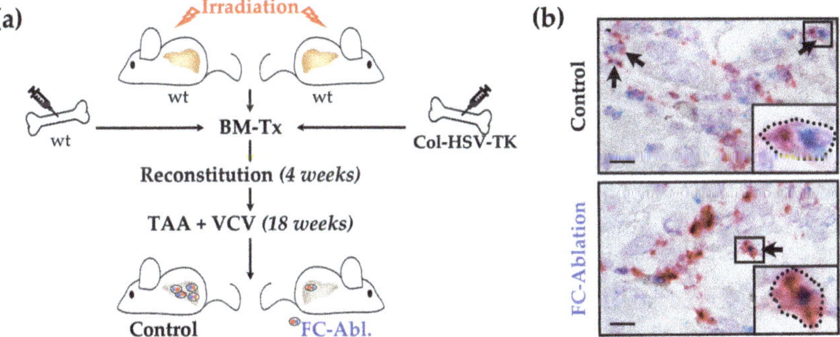

Figure 1. Suicide gene strategy enabled fibrocyte depletion. (**a**) Schematic representation of the animal experiments including lethal irradiation, bone marrow transplantation (BM-Tx), and treatment with valganciclovir (VCV) and thioacetamide (TAA). While TAA induces hepatic fibrosis, VCV is metabolized into toxic compounds by all cells expressing herpes simplex virus thymidine kinase (HSV-TK). (**b**) Successful depletion was confirmed by RNA in situ hybridization. Fibrocytes (FC, black arrows) were identified by the simultaneous expression of *Col1a1* (red) and *Ptprc* (CD45, blue) transcripts. The details in boxes were enlarged in individual panels in the lower right part of the micrograph. Note that individual and possibly *Col1a1/Ptprc* co-expressing cells were detected in the fibrocyte-ablated group. Magnification 1000×, bars 10 μm.

For FC ablation during regeneration, TAA but not VCV was given until the age of 34 weeks. Thereafter, the TAA-administration was stopped and VCV was added during a 4-week regeneration period. Untreated female C57BL/6J mice, sacrificed at the age of 34 and 38 weeks, served as supercontrols (SC). Liver samples were shock frosted and stored at −80 °C or preserved for histology as indicated below. Serum samples were stored at −80 °C until analysis of alanine aminotransferases (ALT) by routine clinical chemistry on a Reflotron Plus Analyzer (Roche, Mannheim, Germany).

2.2. RNA in Situ Hybridization Assay

Liver samples were fixed in 1% paraformaldehyde for 12 h, embedded in paraffin and cut into 5 µm sections. RNAscope® 2.5 HD Duplex RNA in situ hybridization assay (Advanced Cell Diagnostics, Newark, CA, USA) was performed according to the manufacturer's instructions, applying standard pretreatment conditions [43]. The ethanol incubation following target retrieval was performed for ten minutes and the ninth amplification step was extended to one hour. Specific probes were used for the detection of type I collagen- (*Mm-Col1a1*, #319379) and CD45- (*Mm-Ptprc*, #318651) gene expression. Positive- and negative-controls were carried out using probes specific to murine housekeeping-genes (*Mm-Ppib/Mm-Polr2a*, #321651) and a bacterial gene (*dapB*, #320751).

2.3. Histology and Immunohistochemistry

Paraffin-embedded liver samples were cut into 3–6 µm sections and routine hematoxylin/eosin and Masson's trichrome staining were performed. For Sirius Red/Fast Green staining, sections were deparaffinized, hydrated, incubated in a staining solution consisting of 0.1% Sirius Red (Polysciences, Inc., Warrington, PA, USA) and 0.1% Fast Green (Roth, Karlsruhe, Germany) in saturated picric acid (Chroma, Münster, Germany) for one hour and differentiated in 1% acetic acid for 45 seconds.

To perform immunohistochemical stainings, peroxidase activity was blocked with 3% hydrogen peroxide. Afterwards, sections were boiled for 10 minutes either in citrate buffer (pH 6.0, Collagen I), Tris-EDTA buffer (pH 9.0, CD45) or no target retrieval was performed (α-SMA). Sections were then blocked with 10% BSA (PAA, Pasching, Austria) and 2.5% normal horse serum (Vector Laboratories, Inc., Burlingame, CA, USA) and incubated with specific antibodies (Rabbit anti Collagen I polyclonal antibody, ab34710, Abcam, Cambridge, UK; Rabbit anti CD45 polyclonal antibody, 20103-1-AP, Proteintech, Rosemont, IL, USA; Mouse anti α-SMA monoclonal antibody, 61001, Progen, Heidelberg, Germany), diluted 1:200 in 10% BSA in PBS. Secondary antibodies coupled with horseradish peroxidase (MP-7401/MP-7452) or alkaline phosphatase (MP-5401) and corresponding substrates (SK-4100) were used for detection (all purchased from Vector Laboratories, Inc., Burlingame, CA, USA). Unspecific isotype IgGs were used to control the specificity of the secondary antibodies. Sections were counterstained with hematoxylin to visualize nuclei.

All sections were eventually dehydrated and mounted with Pertex® (Medite, Burgdorf, Germany). Photographs were taken using a Leica DMRB microscope (Leica, Wetzlar, Germany) equipped with a Canon EOS 600D with Canon EOS Utility 2 software, version 2.14 (Canon, Tokyo, Japan).

2.4. Pathological Staging and Grading

Hepatic staging and grading were performed by a trained pathologist (K.K.) in a blinded fashion. Hematoxylin/eosin and Masson's trichrome-stained sections were evaluated, utilizing the scoring system suggested by Ishak et al. [44].

2.5. Morphometric Analysis

As many liver lobules as possible were photographed in two Sirius Red/Fast Green-stained sections of each mouse (magnification 200×, blinded for groups). Images suitable for analysis were identified following predefined exclusions criteria and the red stained area was quantified using the color threshold tool in ImageJ, version 1.51 [45]. To quantify the stained area in CD45 immunohistochemical sections, as many non-overlapping high-power fields as possible were photographed using a Biozero

BZ-8000 microscope (magnification 200×, Keyence, Osaka, Japan). Suitable images were converted to 8-bit grey scale and the threshold tool in ImageJ was used to quantify the stained area.

2.6. Hydroxyproline Assay

Total hepatic hydroxyproline content was quantified as described previously [41].

2.7. Quantitative Real-Time PCR

RNA extraction from full liver lysates and elimination of genomic DNA was performed using the RNeasy Mini- (QIAGEN, Hilden, Germany) and TURBO DNAfree-Kit (Thermo Fisher Scientific, Waltham, MA, USA), each following the manufacturer's instructions. RNA integrity and purity were assessed by gel electrophoresis and spectrophotometry, equal amounts of RNA were then subjected to cDNA synthesis, using the iScript cDNA Synthesis-Kit (Bio-Rad, Hercules, CA, USA). qPCR was carried out, including one of the primer pairs listed in Supplementary Table S2 and SYBR-Green/ROX dye. *Hprt* was validated and used as a reference gene. Statistical tests and computation of confidence intervals were performed on ΔC_T-values, calculated as

$$\Delta C_T = C_T(\text{reference gene}) - C_T(\text{gene of interest}). \tag{1}$$

Fold-changes were calculated as

$$\text{fold-change} = 2^{\Delta C_T(\text{FC - Abl.}) - \Delta C_T(\text{Ctrl})}. \tag{2}$$

2.8. Gene Expression Array

84 fibrosis-related genes were analyzed using the RT^2 Profiler™ PCR Array Mouse Fibrosis (PAMM-120ZC, QIAGEN, Hilden, Germany) according to the manufacturer's instructions. RNA was prepared as described above and cDNA synthesis was performed with RT^2 First Strand Kit (QIAGEN, Hilden, Germany) on pooled samples (fibrocyte-ablated and control group, $n = 15$ per group). Data analysis was conducted utilizing the QIAGEN data analysis web portal.

2.9. Western Blot Analysis

Western blot experiments were performed as described previously [46] using 1:1.000 diluted antibodies against α-SMA (Mouse anti α-SMA monoclonal antibody, 61001, Progen, Heidelberg, Germany), Bax (Rabbit anti Bax polyclonal antibody, #2772), and Bcl-2 (Rabbit anti Bcl-2 polyclonal antibody, #2876). Rabbit anti α-Tubulin polyclonal antibodies (#2144, all purchased from Cell Signaling Technology, Inc., Danvers, MA, USA) or Mouse anti ß-Actin monoclonal antibodies (sc-47778, Santa Cruz Biotechnology, Inc., Dallas, TX, USA) were used for loading controls.

2.10. Multiplex ELISA

Mouse Magnetic Luminex Assay (LXSAMSM, R&D Systems, Minneapolis, MN, USA) was performed according to the manufacturer's protocol to quantify hepatic protein levels of fibrosis- and inflammation-relevant factors. Luminex® 200 flow-cytometer and xPONENT® software, version 3.1 (Luminex Corp., Austin, TX, USA), were used for measurements and data analysis.

2.11. Proteome Profiling

Mouse XL Cytokine Array Kit (ARY028, R&D Systems, Minneapolis, MN, USA) was used to test pooled samples ($n \geq 15$ per group) of native liver lysates according to the manufacturer's instructions. Regions of interest (ROIs) were defined on high resolution scans of the membranes in ImageJ and the mean grey values (OD) were retrieved. After subtraction of the lowest OD ($OD_{background}$), every pair of ROIs was assigned a relative OD-value relative to the pair of ROIs with the highest OD ($OD_{reference}$) using the equation

$$\text{Relative } OD_{ROI}\,[\%] = \frac{OD_{ROI} - OD_{background}}{OD_{reference}} \times 100. \quad (3)$$

Linear regression was performed to calculate expected values for the fibrocyte ablated group.

2.12. Eicosanoid Profiling

The concentrations of eicosanoids were assessed in pooled liver lysates (fibrocyte-ablated-, control-, and supercontrol-group, $n \geq 8$ per group) via LC-MS/MS as described before [47].

2.13. Statistical Analysis

Statistical analysis was performed using GraphPad Prism, version 8.20 for Mac (GraphPad software, La Jolla, CA, USA). Unpaired t-test (two-tailed) was applied for hypothesis testing, if normal distribution of data was not negated after evaluating histograms and QQ-plots. If normal distribution of data was rejected, then the Mann-Whitney *U* test was applied. The significance level α was set to 0.05; *p*-values < 0.05 were labeled with an asterisk (*). For explorative analyses, unpaired t-tests (two-tailed) were performed where appropriate. No correction for multiple comparisons was applied. Data are depicted as means or median ± 95% confidence intervals or SEM.

3. Results

3.1. Suicide Gene Strategy Enabled the Depletion of Bone Marrow-Derived Fibrocytes

TAA- and VCV-treatment was well tolerated during the animal experiments. After reconstitution from bone marrow transplantation, mice gained weight steadily, regardless of group affiliation. Basic observational data are provided in Supplementary Figure S1. Due to drastic weight loss, one out of the 32 mice was euthanized ahead of schedule. A subsequently performed autopsy of the euthanized mouse remained inconclusive, yet confirmed the successful reconstitution of bone marrow.

RNA in situ hybridization was performed on liver sections to visualize the suicide gene strategy's success. Bone marrow-derived fibrocytes were identified by the simultaneous expression of *Ptprc* (CD45) and *Col1a1* mRNA (collagen type I α-1 chain, Figure 1b). A considerable amount of fibrocytes, most frequently located in the periportal area and interportal septi, was detected in mice of the control group. While single cells remained, a marked reduction of the number of fibrocytes was observed in mice which received Col-HSV-TK bone marrow (Figure 1b, bottom).

3.2. Depletion of Fibrocytes Attenuated Hepatic Fibrogenesis

TAA-administration induced a marked perilobular fibrosis in mice of the control (Ctrl)- and fibrocyte-ablated group (FC-Abl., Figure 2a,b). Irregular liver architecture and regenerative nodules indicated beginning cirrhosis in some mice. Total liver hydroxyproline content was reduced by 7.8% (95% CI: 0.7%–14.8%; Figure 2c) in fibrocyte-ablated mice, denoting a reduced deposition of fibrillar collagens. The difference is considered statistically significant ($p = 0.033$). Neither the pathologist's staging depicted in Table 1, nor the morphometric analysis of histological samples (Figure 2d) showed differences between the control- and fibrocyte-ablated group.

Table 1. Staging according to Ishak et al.

Stage	0	1	2	3	4	5	6	Median
Supercontrol	3	5	0	0	0	0	0	1
Control	0	0	0	8	6	2	0	3.5 [1]
FC-Ablation	0	0	0	6	5	4	0	4 [1]

[1] $p = 0.476$; Mann-Whitney *U* test was applied.

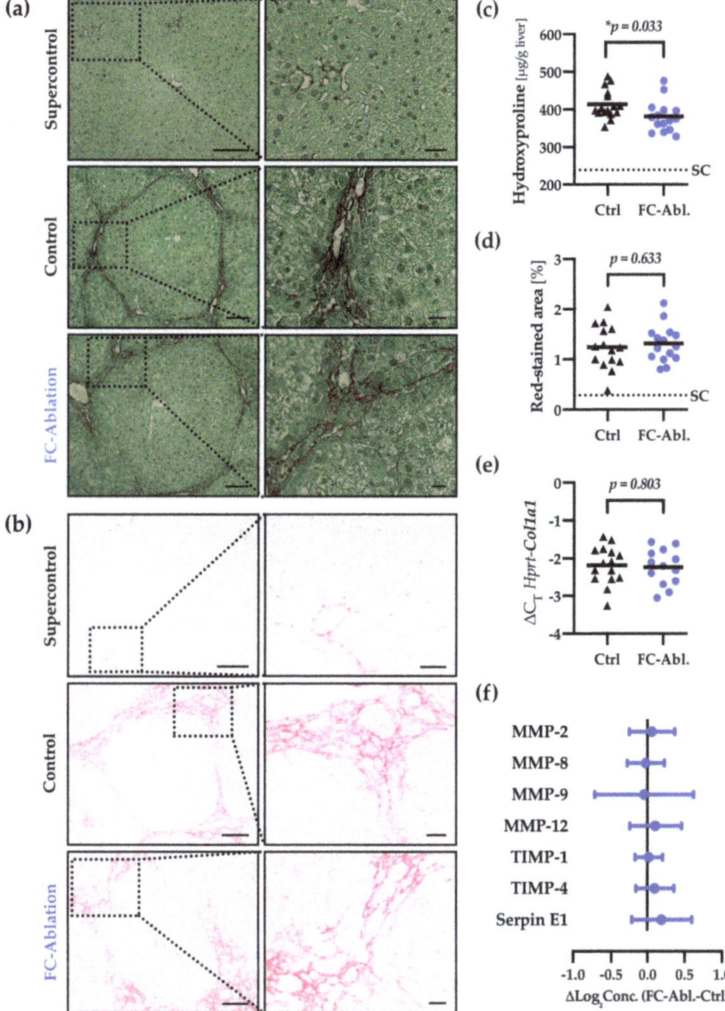

Figure 2. Fibrocyte ablation attenuated hepatic fibrogenesis. Fibrillar collagen distribution was visualized by (**a**) Sirius Red/Fast Green staining and (**b**) immunohistochemical staining of collagen I on formalin fixed, paraffin-embedded liver sections. TAA-treatment caused pronounced periportal and bridging fibrosis as well as faint chicken wire sinusoidal fibrosis in the control- and fibrocyte-ablated group. Dotted boxes are shown in enlarged panels on the right side. Magnification 200×, bars 100 and 25 µm. (**c**) Quantitative assessment of hepatic hydroxyproline content revealed a reduction of fibrillar collagens in mice lacking fibrocytes. The assay was performed three times. Mean values of each individual mouse are depicted by black triangles (control) or blue dots (fibrocyte ablation). The solid line depicts the group mean, the dotted line the mean hydroxyproline level in untreated supercontrols (SC). (**d**) Morphometric analysis of Sirius Red/Fast Green-stained sections displayed a comparable extent of red-stained areas in TAA-treated mice with and without fibrocyte ablation. A total of 1361 images were analyzed (2–134 per mouse). (**e**) The transcriptional levels of *Col1a1* were equal throughout both groups. (**f**) Relative protein levels of MMP-2, MMP-8, MMP-9, MMP-12, TIMP-1, TIMP-4, and Serpin E1 were assessed utilizing a multiplex ELISA and remained constant as a result of fibrocyte ablation. Absolute concentrations and individual *p*-values are provided in Figure S4.

Next, a high-throughput analysis of 84 fibrosis-related genes was conducted; a table of the strongest regulated genes can be found in Figure S3. The gene expression of *Col1a2* (fold-change 0.88) and *Col3a1* (fold-change 0.88) was not relevantly altered in this array. Quantitative real-time PCR, moreover, demonstrated an unchanged expression of *Col1a1* in result of the fibrocyte ablation (fold-change 0.97; 95% CI: 0.74–1.26; $p = 0.803$; Figure 2e).

The extent of fibrosis is largely influenced by the degradation of ECM components. Quantitative analysis of the protein levels of several MMPs and TIMPs showed an about equal expression throughout both groups (Figure 2f). The mean group difference of all but one analyte (MMP-9) yielded 95% confidence intervals whose border values were considered irrelevant in the context of this study. For MMP-9, the high scatter in the data, possibly due to the short half-life of MMP-9, impeded a conclusive interpretation. While there is a negligible mean difference, the 95% confidence interval ranges from a considerable increase (40.0%) to a noteworthy decrease (50.4%) in the mean concentration. Absolute concentrations and individual *p*-values are provided in Figure S4. The gene expression of selected MMPs and TIMPs was not relevantly altered in the gene expression array either.

3.3. The Antifibrotic Effect was Not Accompanied by A Reduction of Myofibroblasts

Despite interindividual differences within the control- and fibrocyte-ablated group, the overall hepatic expression of α-SMA was comparable both on protein- (Figure 3a,b) and transcriptional level (fold-change 1.08; 95% CI: 0.80–1.44; $p = 0.614$; Figure 3c). Immunohistochemical staining (Figure 3b), furthermore, revealed a similar staining intensity and distribution pattern of α-SMA. Additionally, we investigated the gene expression of the most potent myofibroblast activators TGF-β and PDGF. Both were expressed about equally in the control and the fibrocyte-ablated group (fold-change 1.16 and 0.99; $p = 0.165$ and 0.951; Figure 3c, full data in Figure S5a–c).

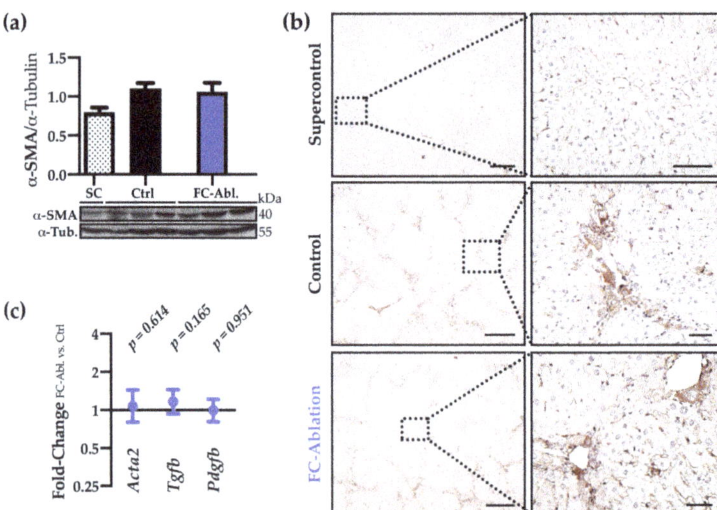

Figure 3. The antifibrotic effect was not accompanied by a reduction of myofibroblasts. (**a**) Western blot analysis and optical densitometry thereof revealed that the hepatic α-SMA levels were increased following TAA-treatment but unchanged by fibrocyte ablation. Two individual western blots were included in the analysis, a representative blot is shown. Arbitrary unit. *SC n* = 2; *Ctrl, FC-Abl. n* = 6. Mean + SEM is depicted. (**b**) Immunohistochemical staining of α-SMA (brown) demonstrated the periportal accumulation of myofibroblasts in TAA-treated animals and an unchanged expression pattern in result of the fibrocyte ablation. Representative stainings are shown. Magnification 40× and 200×, bars 400 and 50 μm. (**c**) Hepatic gene expression levels of *Acta2*, *Tgfb*, and *Pdgfb* were comparable at the end of the experiment (full data in Figure S5a–c).

3.4. Fibrocyte Ablation Lead to A Reduction of Hepatic IL-1β Levels

Next, we evaluated the hepatic infiltration and proliferation of inflammatory cells. While histological grading, performed on routine hematoxylin/eosin-staining, did not retrieve significant differences in result of fibrocyte-ablation (Table S6), immunohistochemical staining and subsequent morphometric analysis of the pan-leucocyte marker CD45 hinted at a decreased number of CD45-positive cells in the liver ($p = 0.054$; Figure 4a,b).

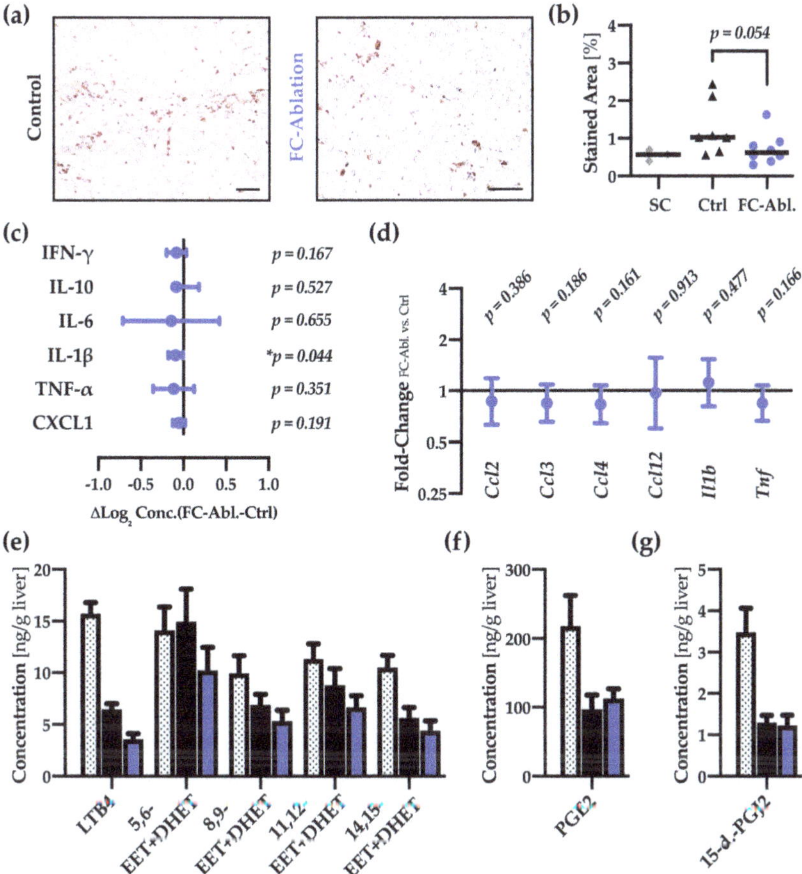

Figure 4. Fibrocyte ablation lead to a reduction of hepatic IL-1β levels. (**a**) Immunohistochemical staining of CD45 (grey) and (**b**) subsequent morphometric analysis revealed a tendentially reduced number of leukocytes in the liver of fibrocyte-ablated mice. Magnification 200×, bar 50μm. Mann-Whitney *U* test was applied. (**c**) Multiplex ELISA demonstrated a reduction of IL-1β protein levels while none of the other cytokines were significantly regulated. Absolute concentrations and individual *p*-values are provided in Figure S8. (**d**) qRT-PCR showed no regulations in a panel of inflammatory genes (full data in Figure S5d–i). (**e**–**g**) In comparison to healthy supercontrols ($n = 8$, dotted bars), absolute quantification of hepatic eicosanoids revealed a notable decrease of all but one analyte (5,6-EET + DHET) in consequence of the TAA-treatment. The level of LTB4 is considerably lower in FC-ablated mice ($n = 15$, blue), compared to controls ($n = 15$, black). Mean of three measurements + SEM are depicted.

In order to assess paracrine inflammatory functions of fibrocytes, we evaluated various cytokines on a transcriptional and protein level. Proteome Profiling of 111 cytokines was performed, yet none of the suspected mediators were strongly regulated (Figure S7). Multiplex ELISA-data of common inflammatory cytokines (Figure 4c, full data in Figure S8) revealed that the level of IL-1β was significantly decreased in fibrocyte-ablated mice (13.7 ± 0.98 vs. 12.9 ± 1.12 ng/g liver; $p = 0.044$). Moreover, genes encoding inflammatory markers (*Tnf*, *Ccl3*, and *Ccl12*) were among the strongest regulated analytes in the gene expression array (Figure S3). Significantly regulated- and further genes of interest were therefore assessed using quantitative real-time PCR (Figure 4d), yielding no significant regulations.

Since FC are known to express cysteinyl leukotrienes (CysLTs), we also sought to determine the hepatic levels of several eicosanoids (Figure 4e–g). While CysLTs were not detectable in our experimental setup, other changes in the eicosanoid profile occurred in response to the fibrogenic stimulus. The concentration of leukotriene B4 (LTB4), several isomers of epoxyeicosatrienoic acid (EETs), 15-deoxy-delta-12,14-prostaglandin J2 (15-d.-PGJ2), and prostaglandin E2 (PGE2) decreased in TAA-treated groups. FC ablation lead to a subtle attenuation of the EETs and a notable decrease of LTB4 (Figure 4e).

3.5. Liver Integrity was Ameliorated by Fibrocyte Depletion

Cell death is a key event in the pathogenesis of liver fibrosis. Significantly reduced serum levels of alanine amino transferase (ALT) demonstrated a mitigation of liver-specific cellular damage in the fibrocyte-ablated group (−20.9%; 95% CI: 0.4–36.9%; $p = 0.049$; Figure 5a). High-throughput gene expression analysis indicated a decrease of the extracellular death ligand FAS (Figure S3), providing a possible explanation in the differential regulation of apoptosis. Subsequently performed quantitative real-time PCR, however, did not support a regulation of *Fasl* (fold-change 1.04; 95% CI: 0.83–1.34; $p = 0.666$; Figure 5b). Even more, further analyses displayed a subtle downregulation of the antiapoptotic factor Bcl-2 as a consequence of the depletion of fibrocytes (Figure 5c). Neither the transcriptional analysis of *Bcl2* (fold-change 0.97; 95% CI: 0.83–1.13; $p = 0.661$; Figure 5d), nor western blotting (Figure 5e) and quantitative real-time PCR of the Bcl-2 associated factor Bax (fold-change 0.99; 95% CI: 0.86–1.15; $p = 0.921$; Figure 5f) corroborated a general regulation regarding the Bcl-2 family.

3.6. A Four-Week Period is Not Sufficient to Provoke Regression of TAA-Induced Liver Fibrosis

Lastly, we aimed to study the effects of a fibrocyte depletion on hepatic fibrolysis and regeneration. FC were depleted during a 4-week regeneration period after 18 weeks of fibrosis induction (Figure 6a). As the TAA-model induced a favorable, marked fibrosis, representing typical pathological features known from human liver fibrosis as expected (Figure 2), we anticipated a considerable regeneration after 4 weeks. Serum ALT levels, in fact, suggest an ameliorated disease state (Figure 4b). Surprisingly, fibrosis was not reduced by a 4-week regeneration period after cessation of the noxe: Total liver hydroxyproline levels remained constant in the control group after the regeneration period (409.8 ± 35.5 vs. 413.4 ± 38.2 µg/g liver; Figure 6c). FC depletion during the regeneration period did not significantly alter either hydroxyproline content (Figure 6c) or serum ALT levels (Figure 6b). We chose to not further investigate the role of FC in fibrolysis and regeneration until a protocol leading to marked liver regeneration could be established for the TAA-model.

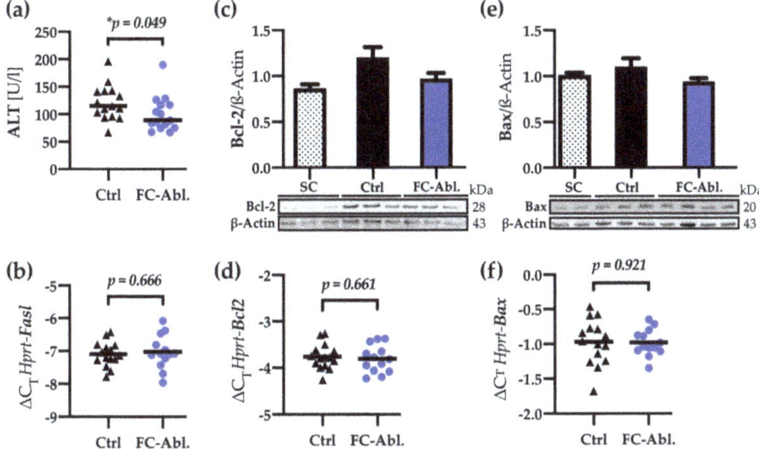

Figure 5. Liver integrity was preserved by fibrocyte ablation. (**a**) Fibrocyte ablation caused a considerable reduction in serum levels of alanine amino transferase (ALT). Median is depicted, Mann-Whitney *U* test was applied. (**b**) Quantitative real-time PCR showed an unchanged expression of *Fasl*. (**c**) Bcl-2 western blot and optical densitometry thereof hinted at a reduced expression of Bcl-2 in the fibrocyte-ablated group. Arbitrary unit. *SC n* = 5; *Ctrl, FC-Abl. n* = 6. (**d**) qPCR displayed an unchanged *Bcl2* expression. (**e**,**f**) Bax is expressed comparably on a protein and transcriptional level in the control- and fibrocyte-ablated group. Arbitrary unit; *SC n* = 4; *Ctrl n* = 10; *FC-Abl. n* = 9; All western blot experiments were performed ≥2 times, representative blots are shown. Columns and error bars depict Mean + SEM.

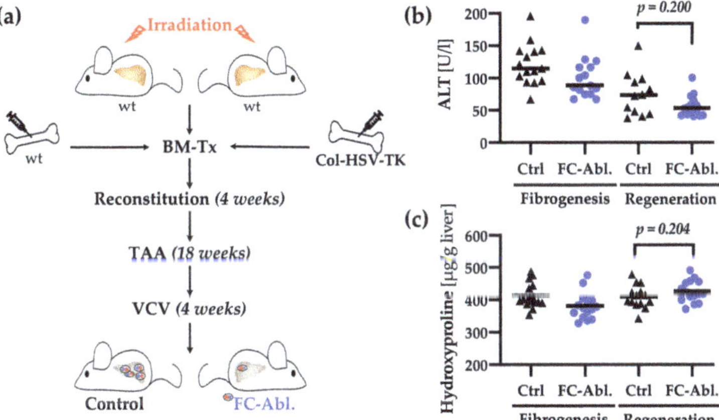

Figure 6. A four-week period was not sufficient to provoke regression of fibrosis. (**a**) Schematic representation of the animal experiments. Fibrocytes were depleted in mice of the respective group via the administration of VCV during a four-week regeneration period. (**b**) The direct comparison of serum ALT levels of mice sacrificed during fibrogenesis (see Section 3.5) and after regeneration shows an ameliorated disease state four weeks after the last TAA-administration. FC depletion during regeneration did not alter ALT levels. Median is depicted, Mann-Whitney *U* test was applied. (**c**) The direct comparison of hepatic hydroxyproline content indicates that a resolution of fibrosis cannot be observed after a regeneration period as short as four weeks. FC depletion during regeneration did not influence hydroxyproline levels. Mean is depicted, an unpaired *t*-test (two-tailed) was applied.

4. Discussion

In light of recent translational approaches in the field of liver fibrosis, a thorough understanding of fibrocyte biology is urgently needed. Bone marrow transplantation, for instance, proved beneficial in murine cholestatic fibrosis but remains controversial as a treatment option for chronic liver diseases [48]; Cenicriviroc (CVC), a dual CCR2/CCR5-inhibitor impeding the infiltration of monocytes, is a promising drug candidate for NAFLD patients with fibrosis [49,50]. Fibrocytes potentially contribute to the targeted monocyte population and are known to be recruited via CCR2, -3, -5, and -7 signaling [8,20,23,51,52]. CVC just recently provided promising results reducing fibrosis but surprisingly not reducing inflammation in NAFLD-patients, and is currently tested in a phase III trial (NCT03028740) [53].

We herein present a novel approach to investigate the role of bone marrow-derived fibrocytes in liver fibrosis. Our model enabled the specific depletion of fibrocytes, avoiding the dependence on particular surface markers or differentiation pathways. RNA in situ hybridization, however, implies that it did not entirely deplete bone marrow-derived fibrocytes (Figure 1b). This result appears in line with evidence from a study Puche et al. conducted: utilizing the HSV-TK model, about 65% of HSCs could be depleted in a CCl_4-model of hepatic fibrosis [54]. Even though our analyses suggest a superior depletion-rate, it should be a concern of future studies to closely monitor the depletion effectiveness to not underestimate the role of bone marrow-derived fibrocytes.

Our results show a functional contribution of fibrocytes to hepatic fibrogenesis. The determination of hydroxyproline content revealed a reduced deposition of fibrillar collagens as a result of the depletion of fibrocytes (Figure 2c). The present data allow a range of interpretations regarding the extent of the mitigation: While the common prediction, mainly based on fate-tracing studies and evidence from other organs, that the depletion of fibrocytes yields minor effects on hepatic fibrogenesis [15,17,55] is compatible with our data, the 95% confidence interval also spans a reduction of up to ~15%. An attenuation of that magnitude is considered highly clinically significant and would challenge our understanding of the contribution of fibrocytes. Significantly reduced serum ALT levels (Figure 5a), despite the generally moderate level of hepatocyte damage, support this notion. It appears noteworthy that (1) the reduction of hydroxyproline was not accompanied by a changed gene expression of collagen I in our study and (2) contradicting results were obtained in studies, investigating the contribution of fibrocytes to fibrosis of the liver [39] and lung [56].

The unchanged gene expression of *Col1a1*, *Col1a2*, and *Col3a1* (Figures 2e and S3) implies that a reduced secretion of collagens at the time of analysis is not the cause of the reduced hydroxyproline content. The development of fibrosis is highly dependent upon the balance of deposition and degradation of ECM-material [57]. Although fibrocytes are known to express several MMPs [30,31], the overall hepatic expression of these was unchanged in result of the fibrocyte ablation (Figure 2f), too. We therefore hypothesize that the mitigation of fibrosis is the result of a transient regulation of fibrogenesis during the disease progression. Given their properties as hematopoietic, circulating cells, fibrocytes can be found early at the site of injury [3,20]. Investigations regarding the influx of fibrocytes into the injured liver show a peak two weeks after onset of the fibrogenic stimulus [20]. It has to be considered, however, that fibrosis was induced via CCl_4 in this experiment, which provokes an accelerated disease progression, compared to the TAA model [41,42]. Taken together, these results suggest that our timepoint of analysis missed the greatest contribution of fibrocytes yet displayed a lasting effect and provide encouragement to more closely focus on the role of fibrocytes in different stages of disease progression in future research.

Ozono et al. just recently published their findings as a clodronate liposome-mediated depletion of fibrocytes »had little contribution on liver fibrosis« in a murine model of CCl_4-induced fibrosis [39]. Although the authors concluded differently, we argue that the results they present are not necessarily contradictory to ours. Morphometric analysis displays a reduction of stained fibrillar collagens by tendency (see Figure 3b in reference [39]). Smaller sample sizes (n = 8) might provide an explanation of why the level of statistical significance postulated by the authors was not reached.

Furthermore, semiquantitative means like histology with subsequent pathological evaluation (staging) or morphometric analysis perhaps lack the accuracy to detect subtle changes in the deposition of ECM components. Consistent with this claim, semiquantitative methods failed to detect the mitigation of fibrosis in our study (Table 1, Figure 2d). Solely relying on those techniques might under some circumstances therefore be inadequate to elaborate the biology of fibrocytes. Even though it will be inevitable to study the contribution of fibrocytes in different models of fibrosis, the use of distinct models and readout parameters impedes the comparability of results obtained with such.

A specific knockout of the *Col1a1* gene in fibrocytes, furthermore, yielded no significant impact on pulmonary fibrosis, even though up to 30% of collagen producing cells are assumed to be fibrocytes, suggesting a crucial role of paracrine functions [56]. We herein sought to investigate effects on the activation and proliferation of myofibroblasts, hepatic inflammation, and cell death. Since there is compelling evidence for activated HSCs being the main contributors to hepatic collagen deposition [15–17], and fibrocytes, in fact, can facilitate the activation of myofibroblast via the secretion of TGF-β and PDGF in vitro [26], a decreased activation of myofibroblasts might provide a plausible explanation for the observed attenuation of fibrosis. Even though a transient process cannot be excluded, our results, showing an unchanged expression of α-SMA, *Tgfb*, and *Pdgfb* in result of the fibrocyte depletion (Figure 3), tend to refute this hypothesis. The reduced CD45-stained area (Figure 4a,b) and the decreased hepatic concentration of IL-1β (Figure 4c) might imply an ameliorated inflammatory response in consequence of the fibrocyte depletion. Nevertheless, the evaluation of inflammatory cytokines (Figures 4c,d and S7) emphasized that bone marrow-derived fibrocytes are not a major source of inflammatory mediators at the time of analysis. These results are noteworthy, given the fact that previous research provided evidence for a participation of fibrocytes in inflammatory processes [26,34,58] and entities like scleroderma, rheumatoid diseases, and asthma are associated with fibrocytes (reviewed in reference [24]). Our findings call for careful considerations, especially regarding the interpretation of cultivation and stimulation experiments performed with fibrocytes. Lastly, the decreased levels of serum ALT (Figure 5a) can be interpreted as a result of ameliorated fibrosis. They might, however, also display an attenuation of hepatic cell death, caused by the depletion of fibrocytes, leading to reduced profibrogenic stimuli. Serum amyloid P, which is known to inhibit the differentiation of fibrocytes [59], prevented hepatic cell damage in CCl_4-induced acute liver injury [60]. While multiple forms of hepatic cell death are known [61], we found subtle regulations regarding apoptosis. Contradictory and partly not reproducible results herein forbid a conclusive interpretation.

In summary, we herein demonstrate a functional contribution of bone marrow-derived fibrocytes to hepatic fibrogenesis. However, a definitive mode of action could not be identified. It has to be considered that neither our analyses of paracrine fibrocyte functions, despite covering the crucial mediators of hepatic fibrogenesis, were exhaustive nor the previous cultivation and fate-tracing studies necessarily elucidated the entire range of fibrocyte functions in a complex in vivo setting. Since it is, due to the high plasticity and little number of cells, often troublesome to study fibrocytes in vivo, it is noteworthy that properly planned animal experiments with a rigorous statistically substantiated design according to the 3R principles enabled the generation of robust results. Fibrocytes should be considered in future research to acquire a thorough understanding of the biology of hepatic fibrosis.

Supplementary Materials: The following are available online at http://www.mdpi.com/2073-4409/8/10/1210/s1, Figure S1: Schematic gene construction and basic experimental data, Table S2: Primer sequences used in quantitative real-time PCR, Figure S3: Gene Expression Array results, Figure S4: Hepatic protein concentrations of MMPs and TIMPs, Figure S5: Detailed quantitative real-time PCR results, Table S6: Grading according to Ishak et al., Figure S7: Proteome Profiling of inflammatory cytokines, Figure S8: Hepatic protein concentrations of inflammatory cytokines.

Author Contributions: Conceptualization, M.R. and E.R.; Data curation, F.H. and M.R.; Formal analysis, F.H., M.R. and J.P.-K.; Funding acquisition, M.R.; Investigation, F.H., M.R., A.S., K.I., K.K., Y.C. and J.B.; Methodology, F.H., M.R., R.S. (Rajkumar Savai), R.V., L.K. and J.B.; Project administration, M.R. and E.R.; Resources, M.R., R.S. (Ralph Schermuly), K.K. and E.R.; Supervision, M.R.; Validation, F.H.; Visualization, F.H.; Writing—original draft, F.H. and M.R.; Writing—review & editing, F.H., M.R., K.I., L.K., J.B. and E.R.

Funding: This work was supported by grants from the German Research Foundation (RO 957/10-1 to E.R.), Max Planck Society, Cardio-Pulmonary Institute (CPI), and the German Center for Lung Research (DZL). F.H. received starting grants from the Justus Liebig University Giessen.

Acknowledgments: The authors thank Dirk Krambrich for performing irradiation experiments and Annette Tschuschner, Heike Müller, and Dagmar Leder for excellent technical assistance.

Conflicts of Interest: The authors declare no conflict of interest. The founding sponsors had no role in the design of the study; in the collection, analyses, or interpretation of data; in the writing of the manuscript, and in the decision to publish the results.

References

1. Bataller, R.; Brenner, D.A. Liver fibrosis. *J. Clin. Investig.* **2005**, *115*, 209–218. [CrossRef] [PubMed]
2. Dulai, P.S.; Singh, S.; Patel, J.; Soni, M.; Prokop, L.J.; Younossi, Z.; Sebastiani, G.; Ekstedt, M.; Hagstrom, H.; Nasr, P.; et al. Increased risk of mortality by fibrosis stage in nonalcoholic fatty liver disease: Systematic review and meta-analysis. *Hepatology* **2017**, *65*, 1557–1565. [CrossRef] [PubMed]
3. Bucala, R.; Spiegel, L.A.; Chesney, J.; Hogan, M.; Cerami, A. Circulating fibrocytes define a new leukocyte subpopulation that mediates tissue repair. *Mol. Med.* **1994**, *1*, 71–81. [CrossRef] [PubMed]
4. Pilling, D.; Fan, T.; Huang, D.; Kaul, B.; Gomer, R.H. Identification of markers that distinguish monocyte-derived fibrocytes from monocytes, macrophages, and fibroblasts. *PLoS ONE* **2009**, *4*, e7475. [CrossRef] [PubMed]
5. Suga, H.; Rennert, R.C.; Rodrigues, M.; Sorkin, M.; Glotzbach, J.P.; Januszyk, M.; Fujiwara, T.; Longaker, M.T.; Gurtner, G.C. Tracking the elusive fibrocyte: Identification and characterization of collagen-producing hematopoietic lineage cells during murine wound healing. *Stem Cells* **2014**, *32*, 1347–1360. [CrossRef] [PubMed]
6. Yang, L.; Scott, P.G.; Dodd, C.; Medina, A.; Jiao, H.; Shankowsky, H.A.; Ghahary, A.; Tredget, E.E. Identification of fibrocytes in postburn hypertrophic scar. *Wound Repair Regen.* **2005**, *13*, 398–404. [CrossRef] [PubMed]
7. Phillips, R.J.; Burdick, M.D.; Hong, K.; Lutz, M.A.; Murray, L.A.; Xue, Y.Y.; Belperio, J.A.; Keane, M.P.; Strieter, R.M. Circulating fibrocytes traffic to the lungs in response to CXCL12 and mediate fibrosis. *J. Clin. Investig.* **2004**, *114*, 438–446. [CrossRef]
8. Sakai, N.; Wada, T.; Yokoyama, H.; Lipp, M.; Ueha, S.; Matsushima, K.; Kaneko, S. Secondary lymphoid tissue chemokine (SLC/CCL21)/CCR7 signaling regulates fibrocytes in renal fibrosis. *Proc. Natl. Acad. Sci. USA* **2006**, *103*, 14098–14103. [CrossRef]
9. Haudek, S.B.; Xia, Y.; Huebener, P.; Lee, J.M.; Carlson, S.; Crawford, J.R.; Pilling, D.; Gomer, R.H.; Trial, J.; Frangogiannis, N.G.; et al. Bone marrow-derived fibroblast precursors mediate ischemic cardiomyopathy in mice. *Proc. Natl. Acad. Sci. USA* **2006**, *103*, 18284–18289. [CrossRef]
10. Sazuka, S.; Katsuno, T.; Nakagawa, T.; Saito, M.; Saito, K.; Maruoka, D.; Matsumura, T.; Arai, M.; Miyauchi, H.; Matsubara, H.; et al. Fibrocytes are involved in inflammation as well as fibrosis in the pathogenesis of crohn's disease. *Dig. Dis. Sci.* **2014**, *59*, 760–768. [CrossRef]
11. Kuroda, N.; Masuya, M.; Tawara, I.; Tsuboi, J.; Yoneda, M.; Nishikawa, K.; Kageyama, Y.; Hachiya, K.; Ohishi, K.; Miwa, H.; et al. Infiltrating CCR2(+) monocytes and their progenies, fibrocytes, contribute to colon fibrosis by inhibiting collagen degradation through the production of TIMP-1. *Sci. Rep.* **2019**, *9*, 8568. [CrossRef] [PubMed]
12. Schmidt, M.; Sun, G.; Stacey, M.A.; Mori, L.; Mattoli, S. Identification of circulating fibrocytes as precursors of bronchial myofibroblasts in asthma. *J. Immunol.* **2003**, *171*, 380–389. [CrossRef] [PubMed]
13. Uehara, H.; Nakagawa, T.; Katsuno, T.; Sato, T.; Isono, A.; Noguchi, Y.; Saito, Y. Emergence of fibrocytes showing morphological changes in the inflamed colonic mucosa. *Dig. Dis. Sci.* **2010**, *55*, 253–260. [CrossRef] [PubMed]
14. Zhang, F.; Liu, K.; Zhao, H.; He, Y. The emerging role of fibrocytes in ocular disorders. *Stem Cell Res. Ther.* **2018**, *9*, 105. [CrossRef] [PubMed]
15. Mederacke, I.; Hsu, C.C.; Troeger, J.S.; Huebener, P.; Mu, X.; Dapito, D.H.; Pradere, J.P.; Schwabe, R.F. Fate tracing reveals hepatic stellate cells as dominant contributors to liver fibrosis independent of its aetiology. *Nat. Commun.* **2013**, *4*, 2823. [CrossRef] [PubMed]

16. Iwaisako, K.; Jiang, C.; Zhang, M.; Cong, M.; Moore-Morris, T.J.; Park, T.J.; Liu, X.; Xu, J.; Wang, P.; Paik, Y.H.; et al. Origin of myofibroblasts in the fibrotic liver in mice. *Proc. Natl. Acad. Sci. USA* **2014**, *111*, E3297–E3305. [CrossRef] [PubMed]
17. Nishio, T.; Hu, R.; Koyama, Y.; Liang, S.; Rosenthal, S.B.; Yamamoto, G.; Karin, D.; Baglieri, J.; Ma, H.Y.; Xu, J.; et al. Activated hepatic stellate cells and portal fibroblasts contribute to cholestatic liver fibrosis in MDR2 knockout mice. *J. Hepatol.* **2019**, *71*, 573–585. [CrossRef] [PubMed]
18. Zhang, C.Y.; Yuan, W.G.; He, P.; Lei, J.H.; Wang, C.X. Liver fibrosis and hepatic stellate cells: Etiology, pathological hallmarks and therapeutic targets. *World J. Gastroenterol.* **2016**, *22*, 10512–10522. [CrossRef] [PubMed]
19. Higashi, T.; Friedman, S.L.; Hoshida, Y. Hepatic stellate cells as key target in liver fibrosis. *Adv. Drug Deliv. Rev.* **2017**, *121*, 27–42. [CrossRef]
20. Scholten, D.; Reichart, D.; Paik, Y.H.; Lindert, J.; Bhattacharya, J.; Glass, C.K.; Brenner, D.A.; Kisseleva, T. Migration of fibrocytes in fibrogenic liver injury. *Am. J. Pathol.* **2011**, *179*, 189–198. [CrossRef]
21. Kisseleva, T.; Uchinami, H.; Feirt, N.; Quintana-Bustamante, O.; Segovia, J.C.; Schwabe, R.F.; Brenner, D.A. Bone marrow-derived fibrocytes participate in pathogenesis of liver fibrosis. *J. Hepatol.* **2006**, *45*, 429–438. [CrossRef] [PubMed]
22. Roderfeld, M.; Rath, T.; Voswinckel, R.; Dierkes, C.; Dietrich, H.; Zahner, D.; Graf, J.; Roeb, E. Bone marrow transplantation demonstrates medullar origin of CD34+ fibrocytes and ameliorates hepatic fibrosis in Abcb4-/- mice. *Hepatology* **2010**, *51*, 267–276. [CrossRef] [PubMed]
23. Abe, R.; Donnelly, S.C.; Peng, T.; Bucala, R.; Metz, C.N. Peripheral blood fibrocytes: Differentiation pathway and migration to wound sites. *J. Immunol.* **2001**, *166*, 7556–7562. [CrossRef] [PubMed]
24. Reilkoff, R.A.; Bucala, R.; Herzog, E.L. Fibrocytes: Emerging effector cells in chronic inflammation. *Nat. Rev. Immunol.* **2011**, *11*, 427–435. [CrossRef] [PubMed]
25. Kleaveland, K.R.; Moore, B.B.; Kim, K.K. Paracrine functions of fibrocytes to promote lung fibrosis. *Expert Rev. Respir. Med.* **2014**, *8*, 163–172. [CrossRef] [PubMed]
26. Chesney, J.; Metz, C.; Stavitsky, A.B.; Bacher, M.; Bucala, R. Regulated production of type I collagen and inflammatory cytokines by peripheral blood fibrocytes. *J. Immunol.* **1998**, *160*, 419–425. [PubMed]
27. Seki, E.; Brenner, D.A. Recent advancement of molecular mechanisms of liver fibrosis. *J. Hepatobiliary Pancreat. Sci.* **2015**, *22*, 512–518. [CrossRef]
28. Vannella, K.M.; McMillan, T.R.; Charbeneau, R.P.; Wilke, C.A.; Thomas, P.E.; Toews, G.B.; Peters-Golden, M.; Moore, B.B. Cysteinyl leukotrienes are autocrine and paracrine regulators of fibrocyte function. *J. Immunol.* **2007**, *179*, 7883–7890. [CrossRef]
29. Chesney, J.; Bacher, M.; Bender, A.; Bucala, R. The peripheral blood fibrocyte is a potent antigen-presenting cell capable of priming naive T cells in situ. *Proc. Natl. Acad. Sci. USA* **1997**, *94*, 6307–6312. [CrossRef]
30. Higashiyama, R.; Inagaki, Y.; Hong, Y.Y.; Kushida, M.; Nakao, S.; Niioka, M.; Watanabe, T.; Okano, H.; Matsuzaki, Y.; Shiota, G.; et al. Bone marrow-derived cells express matrix metalloproteinases and contribute to regression of liver fibrosis in mice. *Hepatology* **2007**, *45*, 213–222. [CrossRef]
31. Garcia-de-Alba, C.; Becerril, C.; Ruiz, V.; Gonzalez, Y.; Reyes, S.; Garcia-Alvarez, J.; Selman, M.; Pardo, A. Expression of matrix metalloproteases by fibrocytes: Possible role in migration and homing. *Am. J. Respir Crit. Care Med.* **2010**, *182*, 1144–1152. [CrossRef] [PubMed]
32. Hartlapp, I.; Abe, R.; Saeed, R.W.; Peng, T.; Voelter, W.; Bucala, R.; Metz, C.N. Fibrocytes induce an angiogenic phenotype in cultured endothelial cells and promote angiogenesis in vivo. *FASEB J.* **2001**, *15*, 2215–2224. [CrossRef] [PubMed]
33. Li, J.; Tan, H.; Wang, X.; Li, Y.; Samuelson, L.; Li, X.; Cui, C.; Gerber, D.A. Circulating fibrocytes stabilize blood vessels during angiogenesis in a paracrine manner. *Am. J. Pathol.* **2014**, *184*, 556–571. [CrossRef] [PubMed]
34. Kisseleva, T.; von Kockritz-Blickwede, M.; Reichart, D.; McGillvray, S.M.; Wingender, G.; Kronenberg, M.; Glass, C.K.; Nizet, V.; Brenner, D.A. Fibrocyte-like cells recruited to the spleen support innate and adaptive immune responses to acute injury or infection. *J. Mol. Med. (Berl)* **2011**, *89*, 997–1013. [CrossRef] [PubMed]
35. Borrelli, E.; Heyman, R.; Hsi, M.; Evans, R.M. Targeting of an inducible toxic phenotype in animal cells. *Proc. Natl. Acad. Sci. USA* **1988**, *85*, 7572–7576. [CrossRef] [PubMed]
36. Borrelli, E.; Heyman, R.A.; Arias, C.; Sawchenko, P.E.; Evans, R.M. Transgenic mice with inducible dwarfism. *Nature* **1989**, *339*, 538–541. [CrossRef] [PubMed]

37. Heyman, R.A.; Borrelli, E.; Lesley, J.; Anderson, D.; Richman, D.D.; Baird, S.M.; Hyman, R.; Evans, R.M. Thymidine kinase obliteration: Creation of transgenic mice with controlled immune deficiency. *Proc. Natl. Acad. Sci. USA* **1989**, *86*, 2698–2702. [CrossRef]
38. Tian, B.; Han, L.; Kleidon, J.; Henke, C. An HSV-TK transgenic mouse model to evaluate elimination of fibroblasts for fibrosis therapy. *Am. J. Pathol.* **2003**, *163*, 789–801. [CrossRef]
39. Ozono, Y.; Shide, K.; Toyoshima, F.; Takaishi, Y.; Tsuchimochi, M.; Kamiunten, A.; Kameda, T.; Nakamura, K.; Miike, T.; Kusumoto, K.; et al. Monocyte-derived fibrocytes elimination had little contribution on liver fibrosis. *Hepatobiliary Pancreat. Dis. Int.* **2019**, *18*, 348–353. [CrossRef]
40. Mederacke, I. Liver fibrosis - mouse models and relevance in human liver diseases. *Z Gastroenterol.* **2013**, *51*, 55–62. [CrossRef]
41. Salguero Palacios, R.; Roderfeld, M.; Hemmann, S.; Rath, T.; Atanasova, S.; Tschuschner, A.; Gressner, O.A.; Weiskirchen, R.; Graf, J.; Roeb, E. Activation of hepatic stellate cells is associated with cytokine expression in thioacetamide-induced hepatic fibrosis in mice. *Lab. Investig.* **2008**, *88*, 1192–1203. [CrossRef] [PubMed]
42. Wallace, M.C.; Hamesch, K.; Lunova, M.; Kim, Y.; Weiskirchen, R.; Strnad, P.; Friedman, S.L. Standard operating procedures in experimental liver research: Thioacetamide model in mice and rats. *Lab. Anim.* **2015**, *49*, 21–29. [CrossRef] [PubMed]
43. Wang, F.; Flanagan, J.; Su, N.; Wang, L.C.; Bui, S.; Nielson, A.; Wu, X.; Vo, H.T.; Ma, X.J.; Luo, Y. RNAscope: A novel in situ RNA analysis platform for formalin-fixed, paraffin-embedded tissues. *J. Mol. Diagn.* **2012**, *14*, 22–29. [CrossRef] [PubMed]
44. Ishak, K.; Baptista, A.; Bianchi, L.; Callea, F.; De Groote, J.; Gudat, F.; Denk, H.; Desmet, V.; Korb, G.; MacSween, R.N.; et al. Histological grading and staging of chronic hepatitis. *J. Hepatol.* **1995**, *22*, 696–699. [CrossRef]
45. Schneider, C.A.; Rasband, W.S.; Eliceiri, K.W. NIH image to ImageJ: 25 years of image analysis. *Nat. Methods* **2012**, *9*, 671–675. [CrossRef] [PubMed]
46. Roderfeld, M.; Padem, S.; Lichtenberger, J.; Quack, T.; Weiskirchen, R.; Longerich, T.; Schramm, G.; Churin, Y.; Irungbam, K.; Tschuschner, A.; et al. Schistosoma mansoni egg-secreted antigens activate hepatocellular carcinoma-associated transcription factors c-Jun and STAT3 in hamster and human hepatocytes. *Hepatology* **2019**. [CrossRef]
47. Kiss, L.; Roder, Y.; Bier, J.; Weissmann, N.; Seeger, W.; Grimminger, F. Direct eicosanoid profiling of the hypoxic lung by comprehensive analysis via capillary liquid chromatography with dual online photodiode-array and tandem mass-spectrometric detection. *Anal. Bioanal. Chem.* **2008**, *390*, 697–714. [CrossRef]
48. Roderfeld, M.; Rath, T.; Pasupuleti, S.; Zimmermann, M.; Neumann, C.; Churin, Y.; Dierkes, C.; Voswinckel, R.; Barth, P.J.; Zahner, D.; et al. Bone marrow transplantation improves hepatic fibrosis in Abcb4-/- mice via Th1 response and matrix metalloproteinase activity. *Gut* **2012**, *61*, 907–916. [CrossRef]
49. Lefebvre, E.; Moyle, G.; Reshef, R.; Richman, L.P.; Thompson, M.; Hong, F.; Chou, H.L.; Hashiguchi, T.; Plato, C.; Poulin, D.; et al. Antifibrotic effects of the dual CCR2/CCR5 antagonist cenicriviroc in animal models of liver and kidney fibrosis. *PLoS ONE* **2016**, *11*, e0158156. [CrossRef]
50. Puengel, T.; Krenkel, O.; Mossanen, J.; Longerich, T.; Lefebvre, E.; Trautwein, C.; Tacke, F. The dual CCR2/CCR5 antagonist cenicriviroc ameliorates steatohepatitis and fibrosis in vivo by inhibiting the infiltration of inflammatory monocytes into injured liver. *J. Hepatol.* **2016**, *64*, S159–S182. [CrossRef]
51. Moore, B.B.; Kolodsick, J.E.; Thannickal, V.J.; Cooke, K.; Moore, T.A.; Hogaboam, C.; Wilke, C.A.; Toews, G.B. CCR2-mediated recruitment of fibrocytes to the alveolar space after fibrotic injury. *Am. J. Pathol.* **2005**, *166*, 675–684. [CrossRef]
52. Moore, B.B.; Murray, L.; Das, A.; Wilke, C.A.; Herrygers, A.B.; Toews, G.B. The role of CCL12 in the recruitment of fibrocytes and lung fibrosis. *Am. J. Respir Cell Mol. Biol.* **2006**, *35*, 175–181. [CrossRef] [PubMed]
53. Friedman, S.L.; Ratziu, V.; Harrison, S.A.; Abdelmalek, M.F.; Aithal, G.P.; Caballeria, J.; Francque, S.; Farrell, G.; Kowdley, K.V.; Craxi, A.; et al. A randomized, placebo-controlled trial of cenicriviroc for treatment of nonalcoholic steatohepatitis with fibrosis. *Hepatology* **2018**, *67*, 1754–1767. [CrossRef] [PubMed]
54. Puche, J.E.; Lee, Y.A.; Jiao, J.; Aloman, C.; Fiel, M.I.; Munoz, U.; Kraus, T.; Lee, T.; Yee, H.F., Jr.; Friedman, S.L. A novel murine model to deplete hepatic stellate cells uncovers their role in amplifying liver damage in mice. *Hepatology* **2013**, *57*, 339–350. [CrossRef] [PubMed]

55. Xu, J.; Cong, M.; Park, T.J.; Scholten, D.; Brenner, D.A.; Kisseleva, T. Contribution of bone marrow-derived fibrocytes to liver fibrosis. *Hepatobiliary Surg. Nutr.* **2015**, *4*, 34–47. [PubMed]
56. Kleaveland, K.R.; Velikoff, M.; Yang, J.; Agarwal, M.; Rippe, R.A.; Moore, B.B.; Kim, K.K. Fibrocytes are not an essential source of type I collagen during lung fibrosis. *J. Immunol.* **2014**, *193*, 5229–5239. [CrossRef]
57. Hemmann, S.; Graf, J.; Roderfeld, M.; Roeb, E. Expression of MMPs and TIMPs in liver fibrosis - a systematic review with special emphasis on anti-fibrotic strategies. *J. Hepatol.* **2007**, *46*, 955–975. [CrossRef] [PubMed]
58. Gan, Y.; Reilkoff, R.; Peng, X.; Russell, T.; Chen, Q.; Mathai, S.K.; Homer, R.; Gulati, M.; Siner, J.; Elias, J.; et al. Role of semaphorin 7a signaling in transforming growth factor beta1-induced lung fibrosis and scleroderma-related interstitial lung disease. *Arthritis Rheum* **2011**, *63*, 2484–2494. [CrossRef] [PubMed]
59. Pilling, D.; Buckley, C.D.; Salmon, M.; Gomer, R.H. Inhibition of fibrocyte differentiation by serum amyloid P. *J. Immunol.* **2003**, *171*, 5537–5546. [CrossRef]
60. Cong, M.; Zhao, W.; Liu, T.; Wang, P.; Fan, X.; Zhai, Q.; Bao, X.; Zhang, D.; You, H.; Kisseleva, T.; et al. Protective effect of human serum amyloid P on CCl4-induced acute liver injury in mice. *Int. J. Mol. Med.* **2017**, *40*, 454–464. [CrossRef]
61. Luedde, T.; Kaplowitz, N.; Schwabe, R.F. Cell death and cell death responses in liver disease: Mechanisms and clinical relevance. *Gastroenterology* **2014**, *147*, 765–783. [CrossRef] [PubMed]

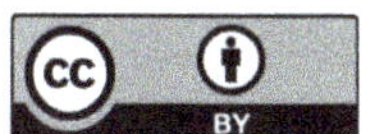

TGR5 knockout mice (TGR5 KO) have a very mild phenotype without any signs of overt liver disease [15,16]. However, TGR5 KO are more susceptible towards cholestatic and inflammatory liver injury [17–19]. While TGR5 is responsive to all human primary and secondary BAs, irrespective of conjugation state, the secondary BA taurolithocholic acid (TLC) represents the most potent TGR5 BA agonist [6,20]. Interestingly, feeding wildtype (WT) mice a diet enriched in 1% (*w/w*) LCA triggers within a few days segmental bile duct obstruction by crystal precipitation leading to the development of focal areas of necrosis (bile infarcts) with subsequent recruitment and accumulation of neutrophils, as well as to the induction of periportal fibrosis [21,22]. Using mice deficient for either the intercellular adhesion molecule-1 (ICAM-1 KO mice) or the catalytic subunit of NADPH oxidase (gp91phox KO mice), it was demonstrated that the contribution of neutrophils to liver injury following LCA feeding is negligible. Thus, the hepatotoxicity stems from LCA and its metabolites directly, and this model can be used to rapidly induce severe cholestatic liver injury, which also shows characteristics of sclerosing cholangitis [21,22].

The burden of liver diseases continues to rise in European countries and accounts for approximately 150,000 deaths per year attributed to liver disease, of which about two-thirds of patients die before the age of 65 years [23]. The most important non-malignant complication of chronic liver disease in humans is the development of portal hypertension (PH). PH results from increased intrahepatic vascular resistance, which is due to structural changes within the sinusoids during fibrosis development, to dysfunction of HSCs and LSECs as well as to microvascular thrombosis and platelet dysfunction [24,25]. Nitric oxide (NO) is an essential regulator of portal pressure. However, NO release from LSECs is decreased in cirrhotic livers, contributing to LSEC dysfunction [24]. We have previously demonstrated that TGR5 is expressed in LSECs, where activation of the receptor induced expression and activation of endothelial NO synthase (eNOS) and subsequent generation of NO [1].

While TGR5 was not expressed in quiescent HSCs in vitro and in vivo, cultivation of isolated HSCs on plastic dishes, which triggers differentiation into a myofibroblast-like phenotype (activated HSCs), led to an upregulation of TGR5 mRNA and protein levels [4,26]. These findings suggest that BA signaling via TGR5 may play a role in the regulation of hepatic vascular tone and portal pressure under physiological but also disease conditions. Since LCA feeding not only resulted in severe cholestatic liver injury and recruitment of inflammatory cells, but also rapid development of periductal fibrosis [21], we studied the impact of short-term LCA diet supplementation in TGR5 WT and KO mice.

2. Materials and Methods

2.1. Materials

Dulbecco's modified Eagle Medium (DMEM) was from Gibco (Thermo Fisher Scientific, Waltham, MA, USA). FCS was acquired from Perbio Science (Bonn, Germany). Pencillin, streptomycin, and amphotericin B were purchased from Gibco (Thermo Fisher). Taurolithocholic acid (TLC) and forskolin were purchased from Sigma-Aldrich (St. Louis, MO, USA). DMSO (Dimethyl sulfoxide) was acquired from Carl Roth (Karlsruhe, Germany). The TGR5 agonist RO5527239((R,E)-1-(4-(3-(hydroxyimino)-3-(2-methylpyridin-4-yl)-1-o-tolylpropyl)phenyl)piperi-dine-4-carboxylic acid) was kindly provided by F. Hoffmann-La Roche, (Basel, Switzerland) [27]. Pronase P and Dnase I for isolation of murine HSCs were also from F. Hoffmann-La Roche. Pronase E for isolation of HSCs was purchased from Sigma-Aldrich and collagenase type I from Worthington (Lakewood, WA, USA). Collagenase type I for isolation of LSECs was from Sigma-Aldrich.

2.2. Animal Experiments

TGR5 transgenic mice were a generous gift from K. Schoonjans and J. Auwerx and have been shown to overexpress TGR5 in different tissues, including liver [28]. TGR5 knockout (KO) mice were kept on a C57BL/6 background and were kindly provided by the Schering-Plough Research-Institute (Kenilworth, NJ, USA) [15,29]. Heterozygous animals were used for breeding to obtain littermate TGR5 knockout and wildtype animals. Mice were bred and kept in the central animal facility of Düsseldorf University (ZETT) and had access to water and food ad libitum. A 12 h light/dark cycle was maintained. TGR5 KO and WT male mice aged 8–12 weeks were fed a diet containing 1% (*w*/*w*) lithocholic acid (LCA, ssniff, Soest, Germany) for 84 h or standard chow diet ad libitum. After 84 h of feeding, mice were anesthetized by intraperitoneal injection of ketamine/sodium pentobarbital solution. Blood was collected and anesthetized animals were subjected to portal vein perfusion prior to collection of liver tissue. All animal experiments were approved by the local authorities (LANUV).

2.3. Serum Analysis

Serum samples of WT and TGR5 KO mice were taken at the end of the experiment. Serum was analyzed for AST and ALT using the Spotchem Analyzer (Axon Lab AG, Reichenbach, Germany).

2.4. Determination of Hepatic Hydroxyproline Content

Hydroxyproline content was determined from liver tissue (TGR5 KO and WT) according to I.S. Jamall [30].

2.5. Isolation of Hepatic Stellate Cells

HSCs were isolated from 4–6 month-old female WT C57BL/6 mice. Mice were kept under the same conditions as described above. Mice were anesthetized and placed under a heating lamp. After cannulation of the portal vein, the liver was perfused using HBSS buffer (37 °C). Following a perfusion with pronase E (0.2% in HBSS buffer) and collagenase type I (0.025% in HBSS buffer), that led to digestion of collagen and lysis of hepatocytes, the liver was removed and mechanically diced. The liver cell solution was filtered and resuspended in a pronase/Dnase solution (0.125%) for further digestion. After filtration through a 70 μm cell strainer, the solution was diluted in HBSS and centrifuged at 500× *g* for 7 min. The supernatant containing cell debris was removed. The cell pellet was resuspended in HBSS containing 0.25% BSA and then mixed with 28.7% Nycodenz gradient solution (Cosmo bio USA, Carlsbad, CA, USA) to obtain a final concentration of 18% Nycodenz (*w*/*v*). This preparation was covered with 8 mL 0.25% BSA/HBSS before centrifugation for 30 min at 1400× *g* without brake. After centrifugation, the layer between the two buffers was harvested and centrifuged at 450× *g* for 10 min. The supernatant was discarded and the pellet was resuspended in DMEM supplemented with 10% fetal calf serum (FCS) and 1% penicillin/streptomycin/amphotericin B. The medium was exchanged every other day. Cells were kept on cell culture plates covered with collagen type 1 in a density of 2.5–3 × 10^6 cells/well in a 6-well plate. Cells were used for experiments on the next day or after seven days for experiments with activated HSCs (Supplemental Figure S1). During experiments, cells were kept in DMEM without FCS or antibiotics.

2.6. Isolation and Cultivation of LSECs

The protocol for magnetic-activated cell isolation of LSECs was adapted from [31]. After induction of anesthesia, a cannula was inserted into the portal vein for perfusion with HBSS containing collagenase type 1, leading to removal of blood and dissociation of liver cells from connective tissue. Afterwards, livers were removed, diced, and incubated in the collagenase solution for 20 min for further digestion. The cell suspension was filtered through 100 μm cell strainers and centrifuged several times for removal of collagen and cell debris. To clear the cell suspension of CD45-positive immune cells, the cell suspension was preincubated with anti-CD45 magnetic beads for 15 min at 4 °C and transferred onto LD columns in the QuadroMACS separator (Miltenyi Biotec GmbH, Bergisch Gladbach, Germany). The flow-through was centrifuged for 10 min at 500× *g* and 4 °C. The supernatant was discarded and the pellet was resuspended in ice-cold MACS-buffer, according to the manufacturer's protocol. For positive selection of LSECs the cell suspension was incubated with anti-CD146 MicroBeads (Miltenyi Biotec). Then the cell suspension was put on cell columns in the OctoMACS separator (Miltenyi Biotec), according to protocol provided by the company. The flow-through was discarded and the columns were flushed with MACS-buffer containing 0.05% BSA after removal of columns from the magnetic field. The cell suspension was centrifuged and the pellet was resuspended in cell culture medium (DMEM, supplemented with 10% FCS and 1% antibiotics). Cells were cultured in cell culture dishes covered with collagen type I with the following densities: 24-well: 800,000–900,000 cells/well; and 6-well: 3–3.5 × 10^6 cells/well. Culture medium was removed and cells were washed in PBS after 24 h in culture. Cells were treated with serum-free medium containing DMSO, 10 µM TGR5 agonist, 25 µM taurolithocholic acid, or 10 µM forskolin for 24 h.

2.7. Gene Expression Assay

RNA from liver samples of the above-mentioned mice or of LSECs was extracted using the Maxwell 16 LEV simply RNA Tissue Kit (Promega, Madison, WI, USA) and the Maxwell 16 Instrument (Promega, Madison, WI, USA), according to the manufacturer's instructions.

A DNA microarray platform (Affymetrix) was used for global gene expression analysis.

Total RNA preparations were checked for RNA integrity by Agilent 2100 Bioanalyzer quality control. Mean RNA integrity number (RIN) was 7.3 ± 0.4 (range 6.5 to 8.1) for liver tissue from chow-fed animals and 7.8 ± 0.3 (range 6.5 to 8.8) for liver tissue from LCA-fed animals. RNA was further analyzed by photometric Nanodrop measurement and quantified by fluorometric Qubit RNA assays (Life Technologies).

Synthesis of biotin-labeled cDNA was performed according to the manufacturers' protocol (WT Plus Reagent Kit; Affymetrix, Inc., Thermo Fisher Scientific, Waltham, MA, USA). Briefly, 100 ng of total RNA was converted to cDNA. After amplification by in vitro transcription and 2nd cycle synthesis, cDNA was fragmented and biotin labeled by terminal transferase. Finally, end-labeled cDNA was hybridized to Affymetrix Mouse Gene 2.0 ST Gene Expression Microarrays for 16 h at 45 °C, stained by strepatavidin/phycoerythrin conjugate and scanned as described in the manufacturers´ protocol. Data analyses on Affymetrix CEL files are described in Section 2.14—Statistical Analysis of Expression Data. The gene expression data can be downloaded from the NCBI GEO database (https://www.ncbi.nlm.nih.gov/geo/, accession number GSE139075).

For real-time PCR, 1 µg of this RNA was used to generate cDNA utilizing the QuantiTect Reverse Transcription Kit (Qiagen, Hilden, Germany). Gene expression was quantified using Taqman Gene Expression Assays (Thermo Fisher Scientific, Waltham, MA, USA, assay order information can be obtained upon request) and the Lightcycler 480 II (Roche Diagnostics, Rotkreuz, Switzerland). Data were produced in duplicates for each gene. Mean values of cycle numbers of the target gene were subtracted from the mean of cycle numbers of the house-keeping gene succinatdehydrogenase (SDHA) for the respective sample. These values taken to the power of 2 are the mRNA expression of the target genes in relation to SDHA expression. The number of independent experiments performed are given in the text/figure legends. At least three independent experiments were performed. In order to rule out a regulation of the chosen house-keeping gene SDHA in response to LCA feeding, we initially analyzed expression of selected genes in relation to SDHA, hypoxanthine phosphoriosyltransferase-1 (HPRT-1), and glyceraldehyde-3-phosphate dehydrogenase (GAPDH). Since no difference in regulation was observed between these house-keeping genes, we continued the experiments with SDHA, as shown in Table 1 and Figure 3.

2.8. ET-1 ELISA

For analysis of ET-1 secretion from LSECs, cells were kept in culture after isolation as described for 24 h. After washing of cells with PBS, they were treated with serum-free medium containing DMSO, 10 µM TGR5 agonist, 25 µM TLC, or 10 µM forskolin for 24 h. Then, the supernatant was collected and transferred onto amicon ultra-10 centrifugal filters (Merck Millipore, Burlington, NJ, USA) to concentrate the supernatant (1:10). The concentrated supernatant was analyzed for ET-1 levels using the Quantikine kit system for murine ET-1 (Research and Diagnostic Systems Inc, Minneapolis, MN, USA), according to the provided protocol. LSECs were washed and incubated with a fixed amount of

50 µL lysis buffer for protein isolation. Measurement of protein concentration in lysate was performed in the Multiskan Spectrum (Thermo Fisher) and ET-1 concentration in the supernatant was normalized relative to protein concentration.

2.9. HSC Contraction Assay

For quantification of activated HSC contraction, 6-well plates were covered with a thick layer of 1 mL/well rat tail collagen. Rat HSCs were isolated as described before [32]. Cells were put on 6-well plates at a density of 6×10^5 cells/well. Cells were kept in DMEM supplemented with 10% FCS and 1% antibiotics for 7 days. Medium was exchanged every 48 h starting the day after isolation. At day 7 after isolation, cells were treated with serum-free medium containing DMSO, 10 µM TGR5 agonist, or 10 µM forskolin for 30 min. After detachment of collagen lattices from the 6-well surface, cells were treated with ET-1 (Sigma-Aldrich) at a concentration of 1nM to induce contraction for 2 h and 24 h. Photos of cell/collagen lattice areas were taken at the time of ET-1 addition and after 2 h and 24 h (Supplementary Figure S2). Surface area was measured using the ImageJ distribution Fiji V.2.0.0 [33,34]. The lattice area used as control treated with DMSO and vehicle for the respective time points was set to 1.0.

2.10. Measurement of Portal Pressure

TGR5 KO and WT mice on chow or LCA diet (1%, 84 h) were anesthetized and the portal vein was cannulated. Invasive blood pressure measurement was performed using the pressure transducer P75 and amplifier from Hugo Sachs Electronics (Harvard Apparatus GmbH, March, USA). Additionally, 6-week-old WT mice were anesthetized and cannulation of portal vein for blood pressure measurement was done. Mice livers were then perfused with either control HBSS solution or a solution containing 10 µM TGR5 agonist for 15 min. Subsequently, increasing concentrations of ET-1 (5, 10, and 15 nM) were added to the perfusion media for 15 min each. Perfusion pressure in the portal vein was measured constantly over the whole time course. Mean portal pressure was taken for each condition of each mouse. Portal pressure under control conditions (t = 0) of HBSS buffer perfusion supplemented with DMSO (=vehicle) were set to 1.0.

2.11. Hematoxylin Eosin- and Picro-Sirius Red Staining

Liver samples were fixed in 4% paraformaldehyde, embedded in paraffin, and sliced into sections of 5 µm. Following rehydration, liver slides were stained in hematoxylin (Hematoxylin Solution Gill No.3, Sigma Aldrich) for 1 min and in eosin for 3 min. Alternatively, slides were treated with the Picro-Sirius Red staining kit according to the manufacturer's instructions (Polysciences, Warrington, FL, USA). After dehydration, slides were mounted with VectaMount (Vectorlabs, Burlingame, CA, USA). Images were acquired on a Zeiss AxioLab A1 Microscope (Carl Zeiss, Jena, Germany) with 63×, 40×, 20×, and 10× objectives.

2.12. Immunofluorescence of Cells in Culture

HSCs were isolated and kept in culture as described above. Seven days after isolation, cells were incubated with serum-free medium containing either DMSO, 10 µM TGR5 agonist, or 10 µM forskolin. After 24 h, cells were washed with PBS and incubated with 5 µg/mL wheat germ agglutinin (WGA) (Thermo Fisher) labeled with AlexaFluor-594 in PBS for 10 min at 37 °C to stain glycoproteins or glycolipids within the outer leaflet of the plasma membrane [35]. Cells were fixed with ice-cold methanol for 3 min after removal of the WGA-solution. After washing of cells, unspecific binding was blocked using a solution of 5% FCS in PBS for 30 min. Activated HSCs were treated with either primary antibodies for Endothelin-A receptor (Abcam, Cambridge, UK) (1:500) or just blocking solution as negative control for 1 h. A secondary antibody labeled with AlexaFluor-488 (Dianova, Hamburg, Germany) (1:100) was used for detection of the primary antibody and incubated for 1 h. LSECs were fixed with methanol and incubated with antibodies directed against vascular endothelial Cadherine (Santa Cruz Biotechnology, Dallas, USA) (1:100) and TGR5 (Gpbar1 8/50, Roche) (1:20). Secondary antibodies labeled with Cyanine-3 (Dianova) (1:500) or fluorescein (Dianova) (1:100) were used at dilutions of 1:500 and 1:100, respectively. Intranuclear DNA was labeled by Hoechst 34580 (Thermo Fisher) (1:20,000). Pictures of LSECs were taken using the confocal microscope LSM 510 (Carl Zeiss, Jena, Germany). HSCs were imaged using a LSM 810 confocal laser microscope (Carl Zeiss, Jena, Germany). Colocalization analysis of murine hepatic stellate cells was carried out using Pearson's correlation coefficient calculated by the coloc2 plugin for ImageJ after selection of representative regions of interest ROIs in cell surface areas [33,34].

2.13. Statistical Evaluation

The data are presented as means and the standard error of the mean (SEM). Statistical significance was tested using the two-sided Student's *t*-test or the Wilcoxon signed-ranked test as appropriate. A *p*-value < 0.05 was considered a significant result and a *p*-value < 0.01 was considered a highly significant result.

2.14. Statistical Analysis of Expression Data

Data preprocessing and all subsequent analyses were performed using the statistical programming language R, version 3.5.0 (R Development Core Team 2018). Normalization of the raw microarray data (CEL files) was done using RMA as implemented in the R package oligo. Normalization was performed on a set of, in total, 18 CEL files. To determine differentially expressed genes, the R package limma was used [36]. Adjustment for multiple testing was conducted with the method of Benjamini and Hochberg (FDR, false discovery rate) [37]. A gene was called differentially expressed if the adjusted *p*-value was <0.05 and log2 fold change was <−1.5 (downregulated) or >1.5 (upregulated). A volcano plot was generated that plots log2 fold change on the x-axis and statistical significance on the y-axis (-log10 of the FDR-adjusted *p*-value). Heatmaps were used to visualize z-scores (expression values standardized per gene to mean 0 and standard deviation 1), ordered according to average linkage hierarchical clustering of genes and experiments, respectively. Gene ontology enrichment analysis was performed based on probe set IDs with the topGO package [38], using Fisher's exact test and the elim method. Only results from the biological process ontology were considered. The cutoff for the enrichment *p*-value was set to 0.05.

3. Results

3.1. LCA Feeding Results in a Significant Upregulation of Genes Associated with Cholestasis, Inflammation, and Extracellular Matrix Remodeling

Feeding of a chow diet supplemented with 1% LCA over 3.5 days (84 h) resulted in a severe cholestatic liver injury in wildtype (WT) mice, as described previously [21]. Liver tissue of LCA-fed WT mice was compared to chow-fed WT littermates by gene array analysis. In total, 332 and 263 genes were significantly up- or downregulated, respectively ($p < 0.05$; FDR-adjusted, and log2 fold change <−1.5 or >1.5; Supplementary Tables S1 and S2). Overrepresented Gene Ontology (GO) groups among the upregulated genes were associated with proliferation, inflammation, and extracellular matrix organization (Supplementary Tables S1 and S3, Figure 1). The four upregulated genes with the lowest *p*-values were the acute phase proteins serum amyloid A3 (Saa3) (46.2-fold up) and orosomucoid 2 (Orm2) (42.4-fold up), the bacterial siderophore binding protein lipocalin 2 (Lcn2) (32.4-fold up) that is expressed in neutrophils, and the pattern recognition receptor MARCO (macrophage receptor with collagenous structure, 17.4-fold up), which is found on macrophages and dendritic cells (Supplementary Table S1). The most significantly overrepresented GO groups among the downregulated genes were associated with oxidation-reduction processes, sodium-independent organic anion transport, and bile acid biosynthesis. The rate-limiting enzyme of bile acid synthesis, Cyp7a1 (89.0-fold down), was among the strongest downregulated genes (Supplementary Tables S2 and S4). Therefore, gene expression profiling of the livers of mice under LCA diet revealed a profile of an inflamed, cholestatic organ undergoing extracellular matrix reorganization [21,22].

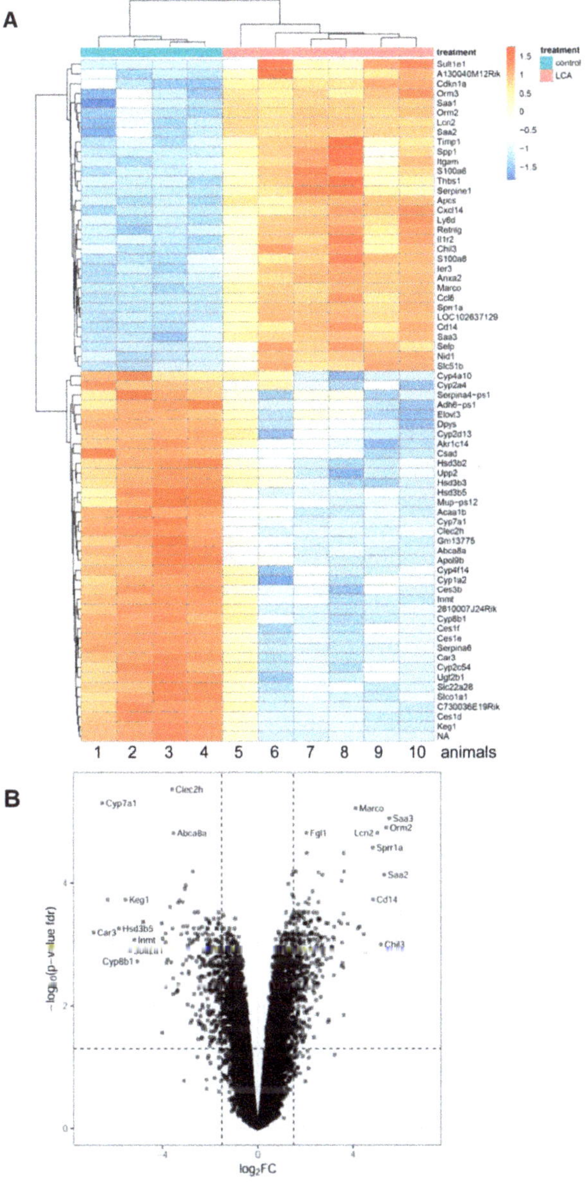

Figure 1. Influence of a chow diet supplemented with 1% lithocholic acid (LCA) over 3.5 days on gene expression in liver tissue of mice. (**A**) Heatmaps of z-scores (expression values standardized per gene to mean 0 and standard deviation 1) of the strongest differentially-regulated genes ($p < 0.05$ and log2 fold change >3 (upregulated) or <−3 (downregulated)). Each row corresponds to a gene, each column to a mouse. Rows and columns were ordered according to average linkage hierarchical clustering. (**B**) Volcano plot: On the x-axis, the $\log_2$ fold change is plotted, and on the y-axis, -log10 of the false discovery rate (FDR)-adjusted p-value is plotted.

We have previously reported that cholestatic liver injury in response to bile duct ligation is more severe in TGR5 knockout (KO) mice as compared to WT littermates [19]. Therefore, we analyzed liver damage following LCA feeding in TGR5 WT and TGR5 KO littermates.

3.2. *Liver Damage in Response to LCA Feeding is Aggravated in TGR5 KO Mice and Results in Increased Portal Pressure*

Liver damage in response to LCA feeding was more pronounced in TGR5 KO mice as compared to WT mice, as demonstrated by significantly higher serum levels of AST (WT LCA ($n = 12$) 6586 ± 898 IU/L vs. KO LCA ($n = 10$) 10,629 ± 1422 IU/L (1.6-fold increase), $p < 0.05$) and more extensive bile infarcts on liver histology (Figure 2A–C). Furthermore, a significant increase in portal venous pressure was observed in LCA-fed TGR5 KO mice as compared to LCA-fed WT or chow-fed TGR5 KO mice, respectively (WT LCA ($n = 7$) 3.9 ± 0.4 cmH_20 vs. KO LCA ($n = 6$) 5.7 ± 0.6 cmH_20 (1.4-fold increase), $p < 0.05$) (Figure 2D). There was no difference in portal pressure between chow-fed mice of both genotypes.

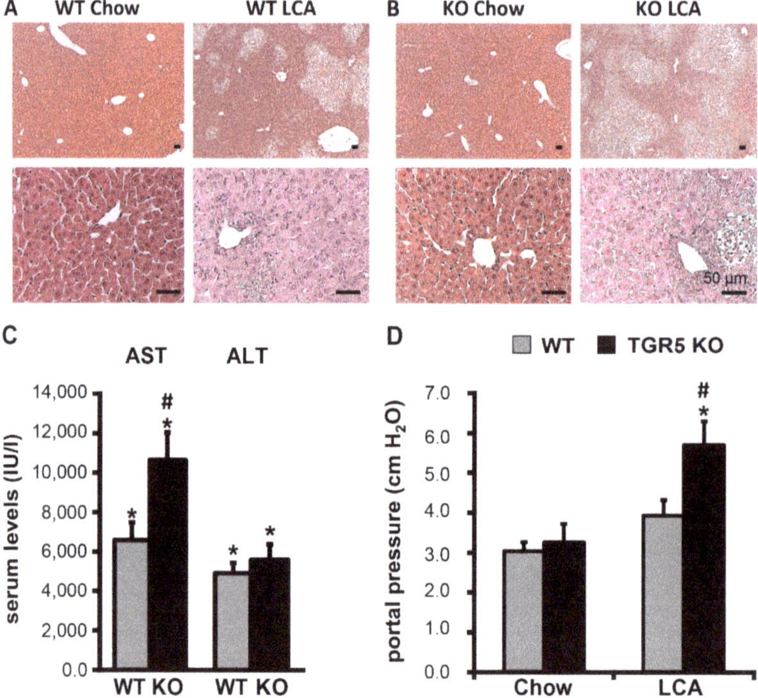

Figure 2. LCA feeding induces a more pronounced liver injury in TGR5 knockout mice as compared to littermate controls. (**A**) Hematoxylin and eosin staining of representative liver sections from wildtype mice fed with either a chow or LCA-enriched diet (1% *wt/wt*) for 84 h. (**B**) H&E staining of liver sections from TGR5 knockout (KO) mice. LCA feeding results in a more severe liver injury in TGR5 KO mice as compared to controls. Bars = 50 µm. (**C**) Serum AST and ALT-levels (in IU/l) increase significantly in mice of both genotypes following LCA feeding ($n = 10$–12 for LCA-fed and $n = 4$ for chow-fed mice of each genotype). (**D**) Measurement of portal vein perfusion pressure (in cm H_20) of wildtype (WT) and TGR5 KO mice fed with either chow or LCA diet ($n = 5$–7). All data are shown as mean ± standard error of the mean (SEM). * Statistically significant difference between the LCA- and chow-fed mice of the same genotype ($p < 0.05$); # statistically significant difference between WT and TGR5 KO mice fed the same diet ($p < 0.05$).

3.3. Genes Associated with HSC Activation are Significantly Upregulated in TGR5 KO Mice as Compared to WT Littermates

Gene expression analysis by semi-quantitative real-time PCR revealed a similar pattern of gene regulation in both genotypes after LCA feeding. As expected, induction of cholestasis by LCA feeding resulted in a significant downregulation of Cyp7a1 and Cyp8b1, the rate limiting enzymes of bile acid synthesis. In line with the increase in liver damage, a significant upregulation of the genes encoding receptor-interacting serine/threonine-protein kinases 1 and 3 (RIPK1 and RIPK3), as well as caspase-3, was observed (Table 1). Furthermore, we found a significant induction of pro-inflammatory genes such as tumor necrosis factor-α (TNF-α), CCL2, interleukin-1β (IL-1β) and pro-fibrogenic chemokine receptors CCR1, CCR5 (Table 1) [21,22,39]. Interestingly, genes related to sinusoidal endothelial dysfunction, activation of HSCs, and fibrosis development, such as platelet-derived growth factor receptor-α (PDGFRα), PDGFRβ, transforming growth factor-β1 (TGF-β1), and endothelin-1 (ET-1), were upregulated in both WT and TGR5 KO mice following LCA feeding. However, the observed increase was significantly higher in TGR5 KO mice (PDGFRα: WT LCA ($n = 7$) 3.52 ± 0.8 vs. KO LCA ($n = 10$) 7.30 ± 1.4, 2.1-fold increase in TGR5 KO, $p < 0.05$; PDGFRβ: WT LCA ($n = 12$) 4.0 ± 0.6 vs. KO LCA ($n = 12$) 6.23 ± 0.75, 1.6-fold increase, $p < 0.05$; TGF-β1: WT LCA ($n = 7$) 7.81 ± 0.8 vs. KO LCA ($n = 9$) 11.8 ± 1.4, 1.5-fold increase, $p < 0.05$; ET-1: WT LCA ($n = 14$) 8.58 ± 1.1 vs. KO LCA ($n = 11$) 13.9 ± 2.4, 1.6-fold increase, $p < 0.05$) (Figure 3A–D). Sirius red staining of liver tissue after 3.5 days of LCA feeding revealed a slight increase in periportal collagen deposition, but no overt hepatic fibrosis in both genotypes, which was in line with measurements of hydroxyproline content in liver tissue (Figure 4A,B). Expression of genes encoding collagen-1α1, collagen-1α2 were upregulated in both genotypes following LCA feeding for 3.5 days, indicating initiation of extracellular matrix synthesis, as described earlier (Figure 4B) [21,22].

Table 1. Selection of genes significantly regulated in livers of TGR5 wildtype (WT) and TGR5 knockout (KO) after LCA feeding for 84 h as compared to chow-fed animals of the same genotypes. Data were generated by real-time PCR, as described in Section 2—Materials and Methods. Gene expression is presented in relation to the house-keeping gene SDHA. Values for WT mice on chow diet were set to 1.0. * Significantly different as compared to chow-fed animals of the same genotype ($p < 0.05$); ** significantly different as compared to chow-fed animals of the same genotype ($p < 0.01$); # significantly different as compared to WT animals of the same treatment group ($p < 0.05$). All data are expressed as mean ± SEM. Green and red boxes indicate a statistically significant downregulation or upregulation, respectively, of a gene in TGR5 KO as compared to WT littermates receiving the same treatment.

	WT Chow		WT LCA		WT LCA		KO LCA	
	Mean	SEM	MW	SEM	MW	SEM	MW	SEM
Col1α1	1.00	0.57	1.71	0.81	65.77 **	18.57	68.82 **	13.78
Col1α2	1.00	0.35	1.69	0.39	25.59 **	6.53	21.67 **	3.39
PAI-1	1.00	0.27	0.92	0.31	120.21 **	24.53	160.23 **	29.05
TIMP-1	1.00	0.44	4.03	2.74	492.23 *	159.09	456.28 **	93.63
VEGF-C	1.00	0.21	2.00	0.50	5.26 *	1.69	7.23 *	1.64
eNOS	1.00	0.26	1.43	0.46	10.07 **	1.39	10.19 **	1.46
VAP-1	1.00	0.70	0.40	0.12	5.78 *	1.98	4.92 **	1.03
CD163	1.00	0.23	1.50	0.13	16.23 **	4.64	16.53 **	3.12
CCR1	1.00	0.55	1.89	0.50	134.81 **	32.27	111.67 **	21.33
CCR5	1.00	0.37	3.16 #	0.26	35.52 **	8.26	17.20 **#	3.18
CXCR3	1.00	0.20	1.57	0.42	3.11 **	0.67	5.35 **#	0.67
CXCR4	1.00	0.37	0.83	0.22	14.53 **	3.53	13.41 **	2.68
CXCR7	1.00	0.45	1.32	0.38	28.23 **	7.24	26.56 **	5.45
CCL2	1.00	0.50	1.40	0.80	293.80 **	30.39	384.99 **	71.68
CCL3	1.00	0.50	3.46	1.58	98.31 **	18.18	95.45 **	15.64
CCL4	1.00	0.76	1.26	0.37	55.92 **	12.79	38.48 **	6.40
CCL25	1.00	0.28	2.14	0.20	3.16 **	0.34	3.13 **	0.34

Table 1. *Cont.*

	WT Chow		WT LCA		WT LCA		KO LCA	
	Mean	**SEM**	**MW**	**SEM**	**MW**	**SEM**	**MW**	**SEM**
CXCL1	1.00	0.76	0.35	0.07	14.48 **	1.64	9.38 **#	1.00
CXCL10	1.00	0.17	1.22	0.42	9.69 **	1.95	5.03 **#	0.68
IL1β	1.00	0.20	1.91	0.44	16.34 **	2.91	17.07 **	2.41
IL10	1.00	0.08	1.24	0.32	26.43 **	4.13	48.14 **	12.76
TNFα	1.00	0.59	2.19	0.94	19.78 **	3.49	21.39 **	3.35
TGF-β2	1.00	0.50	1.00	0.32	16.55 **	2.86	16.95 **	2.71
TGFβR1	1.00	0.06	1.66	0.50	7.99 **	0.94	8.84 **	0.92
CyclinD1	1.00	0.31	1.36	0.35	17.57 **	2.81	8.95 **#	0.98
SOX9	1.00	0.17	1.24	0.06	16.03 **	2.89	16.02 **	1.00
Caspase3	1.00	0.20	1.65	0.20	10.92 **	1.98	10.46 **	1.38
RIPK1	1.00	0.14	1.28	0.12	4.00 **	0.49	4.32 **	0.50
RIPK3	1.00	0.27	1.89	0.45	21.74 **	2.72	28.57 **	3.27
MT-1	1.00	0.48	1.15	0.36	140.44 **	40.83	104.00 **	28.48
MT-2	1.00	0.38	1.21	0.59	293.15 *	97.95	186.38 **	46.39
CYP7A1	1.00	0.22	2.23	0.57	0.01 **	0.00	0.01 **	0.00
CYP8B1	1.00	0.28	1.20	0.26	0.01 *	0.00	0.01 *	0.00

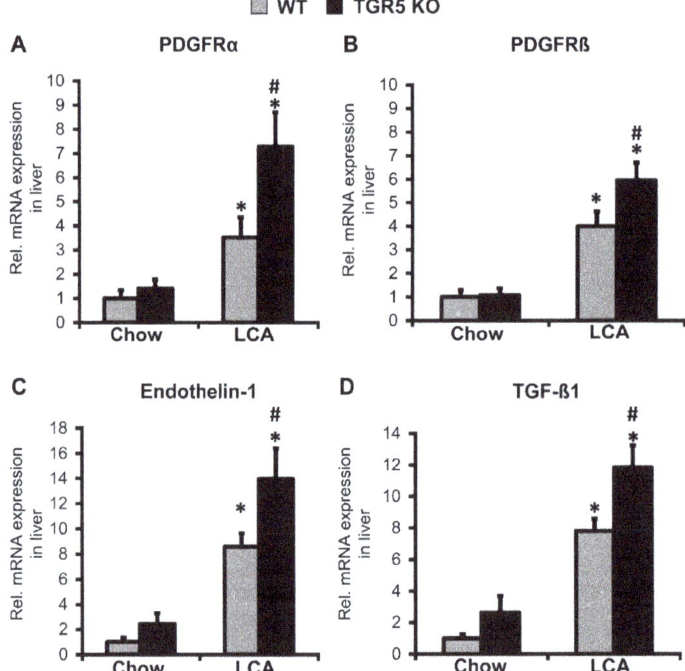

Figure 3. Expression of genes related to portal hypertension and fibrosis development are significantly higher in liver tissue of TGR5 KO mice as compared to WT littermates in response to LCA feeding. (**A–D**) Semi-quantitative real-time PCR analysis of liver tissue revealed an upregulation of mRNA expression PDGFRα, PDGRFβ, endothelin-1, and TGF-β1 following LCA feeding. The increase was more pronounced in mice deficient for TGR5. Data are presented as mean ± SEM (n = 4–12). * Statistically significant difference between the LCA- and chow-fed mice of the same genotype ($p < 0.05$); # statistically significant difference between WT and TGR5 KO mice fed the same diet ($p < 0.05$; using the two-sided Student's t-test).

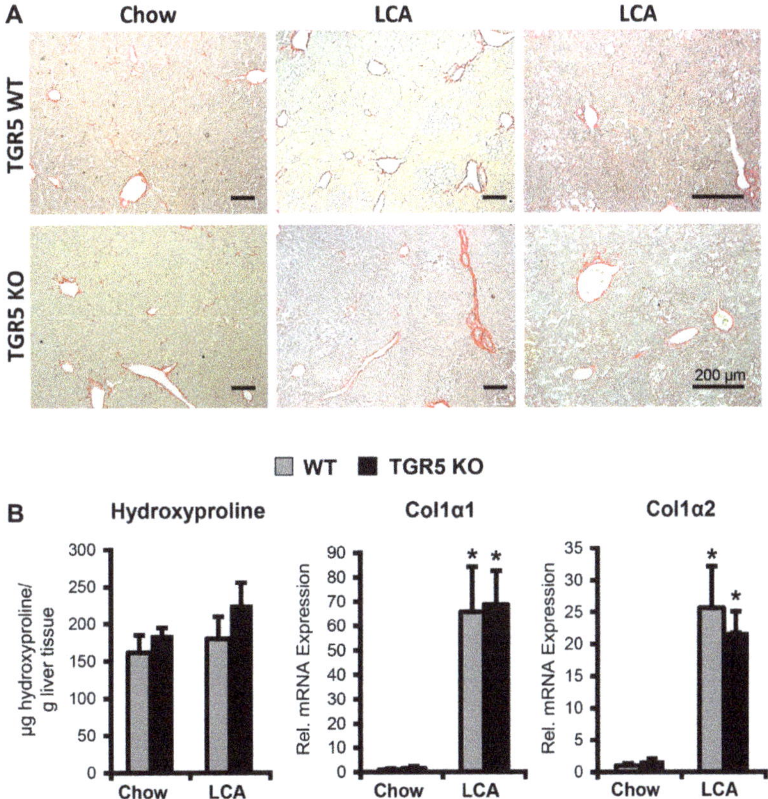

Figure 4. LCA-feeding triggers an increase in extracellular matrix production in both genotypes. (**A**) Representative Sirius red staining from one chow-fed and two LCA-fed animals of each genotype demonstrates a slight increase in fibrous tissue in both genotypes. Bars = 200 µm. (**B**) Measurement of hydroxyproline content in liver tissue showed a slight increase following LCA feeding, which did not reach significance (n = 8–10 animals per genotype LCA group, n = 3 animals per genotype for chow group). However, expression of collagen-1α1 and collagen-1α2 increased significantly after LCA feeding in both genotypes (qPCR: n = 12–14 LCA-fed animals per genotype, n = 4 chow-fed animals per genotype). Liver tissue from WT animals is shown in grey, while tissue from TGR5 KO mice is represented by black bars. All data are shown as mean ± SEM. * Statistically significant difference between the LCA- and chow-fed mice of the same genotype ($p < 0.05$) (n = 8–10).

3.4. *Activation of TGR5 in LSECs Lowers ET-1 Expression and Secretion*

ET-1 in liver is mainly secreted by LSECs under physiological conditions [24]. We have previously demonstrated that rat and human LSECs express TGR5 [1,4]. To determine whether secretion of ET-1 from LSECs was modulated by TGR5, LSECs were isolated from WT mice. Expression and localization of TGR5 in these primary cells was confirmed by immunofluorescence staining with an antibody against TGR5 and an antibody against vascular endothelial cadherin (Ve-Cad). TGR5 was localized in the plasma membrane, as well as in intracellular vesicular structures (Figure 5A). Treatment of primary murine LSECs with vehicle (DMSO), taurolithocholic acid (TLC, 25 µM), a non-bile acid TGR5 agonist (RO5527239, 10 µM) [27], and forskolin (10 µM) for 24 h resulted in a significant decrease in ET-1 mRNA expression (DMSO vs. TLC (n = 10) 1.0 vs. 0.76 ± 0.06 (1.3-fold reduction, $p < 0.01$); DMSO vs. TGR5 Ago (n = 7) 1.0 vs. 0.73 ± 0.08 (1.4-fold reduction, $p < 0.05$); DMSO vs. forskolin

(n = 6) 1.0 vs. 0.58 ± 0.12 (1.7-fold reduction, $p < 0.05$)) (Figure 5B). We have previously demonstrated that stimulation of TGR5 in LSECs through coupling to a stimulatory G protein triggered an increase in intracellular cAMP [1]. Therefore, forskolin, a direct activator of adenylate cyclase, was used as TGR5-independent positive control [1]. Furthermore, detection of ET-1 in the cell culture supernatant of these cells demonstrated a reduction in ET-1 protein levels in response to TLC, the TGR5 Ago, and forskolin (Figure 5C) (DMSO vs. TLC (n = 10) 1.0 vs. 0.80 ± 0.05 (1.3-fold reduction, $p < 0.01$); DMSO vs. TGR5 Ago (n = 9) 1.0 vs. 0.67 ± 0.12 (1.5-fold reduction, $p < 0.05$); DMSO vs. forskolin (n = 5) 1.0 vs. 0.54 ± 0.11 (1.9-fold reduction, $p < 0.05$)). Thus, stimulation of TGR5 not only reduces ET-1 mRNA expression, but also ET-1 secretion from LSECs.

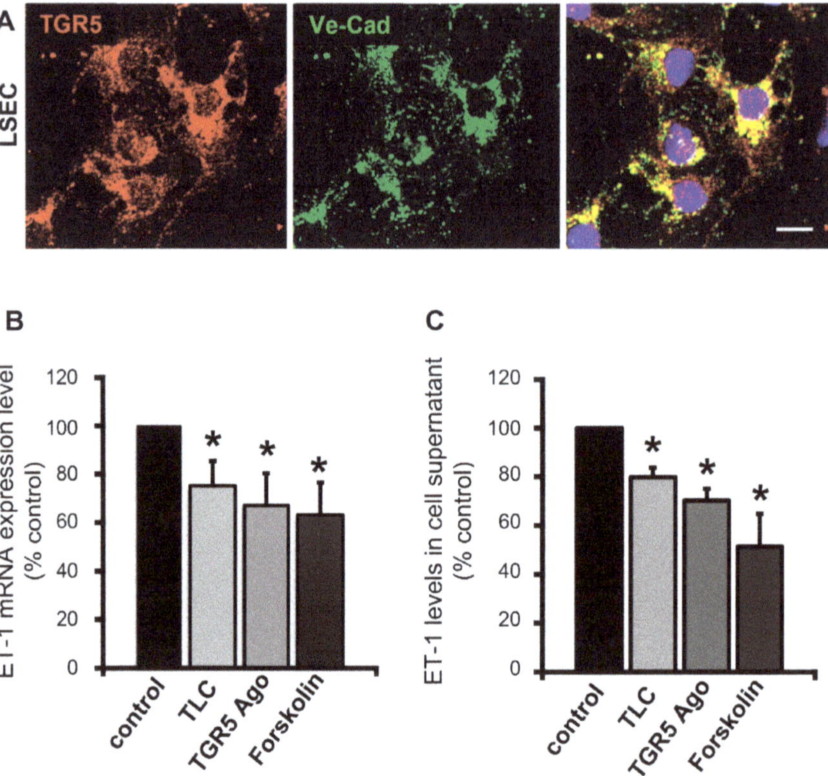

Figure 5. Stimulation of TGR5 in isolated liver sinusoidal endothelial cells (LSECs) reduces endothelin-1 (ET-1) mRNA expression and secretion. (**A**) Immunofluorescence staining of TGR5 in isolated LSECs (in red) demonstrates localization of the receptor within the plasma membrane, as well as in intracellular vesicular structures. An antibody against vascular endothelial cadherin (VE-cad, shown in green) was used to visualize cell junctions near the plasma membrane. Nuclei were stained with Hoechst (shown in blue). Bar = 10 μm. (**B**) ET-1 mRNA levels in isolated murine LSECs in response to a 24-h incubation with DMSO (=control), TLC (25 μM), a TGR5 agonist (10 μM), or forskolin (10 μM). The mRNA level after DMSO treatment was set to 100%. (**C**) Detection of ET-1 protein amounts by ELISA in the cell supernatant of LSECs incubated for 24 h with DMSO (=control), TLC (25 μM), a TGR5 agonist (10 μM), or forskolin (10 μM). ET-1 protein levels after stimulation with DMSO were set to 100%. Data are presented as mean ± SEM (n = 6–9). * Statistically significant difference as compared to DMSO-treated controls ($p < 0.05$).

3.5. Activation of TGR5 in HSCs Attenuates ET-1-Mediated Contractility

Activated HSCs are able to contract, leading to an increase in portal pressure due to their perivascular location in the space of Disse [40]. ET-1 has been identified as one of the key mediators regulating HSC contractility [24,41]. Since we observed an increase in portal pressure solely in TGR5 KO mice after LCA feeding, we hypothesized that activation and contraction of HSCs may contribute to this phenotype. To determine whether ET-1-dependent HSC contraction is modulated by TGR5, HSC contraction in response to ET-1 was analyzed. Rat HSCs were cultivated on collagen lattices for 7 days [40]. After this interval, DMSO, a TGR5 agonist (10 μM), or forskolin (10 μM) were added to the culture medium 30 min prior to stimulation with ET-1 (1 nM). Measurement of the collagen lattice surface area 2 h and 24 h after addition of ET-1 revealed a significantly smaller reduction in relative surface area in TGR5 agonist- or forskolin-treated cells, indicating an attenuation of HSC contractility (Figure 6A); 2 h: DMSO/ET-1 vs. TGR5 Ago/ET-1 1.0 vs. 1.64 ± 0.11 pixels^2; DMSO/ET-1 vs. forskolin/ET-1 1.0 vs. 2.85 ± 0.36 pixels^2, $n = 12$, $p < 0.01$; 24 h: DMSO/ET-1 vs. TGR5 Ago/ET-1 1.0 vs. 1.89 ± 0.27 pixels^2; DMSO/ET-1 vs. forskolin/ET-1 1.0 vs. 3.96 ± 0.51, $n = 12$, $p < 0.01$. It was previously shown that cAMP may desensitize the ET-1 receptor-A (ET_AR) towards its ligand on activated HSCs through internalization. Thus, the ET_AR's responsiveness is being shifted from picomolar to nanomolar concentrations [42]. Since TGR5 is coupled to a stimulatory G protein [6,8], we hypothesized that ligand binding to TGR5 could result in increased intracellular cAMP levels and internalization of the ET_AR. Immunofluorescence staining localized the ET_AR within the plasma membrane of HSCs, as demonstrated by colocalization with the plasma membrane marker wheat germ agglutinin (WGA) (Figure 6B). Treatment with the TGR5 agonist reduced the amount of ET_AR within the plasma membrane, indicating internalization of the receptor (Figure 6C) (DMSO vs. TGR5 Ago ($n = 8$–9) 0.37 ± 0.06 Pearson's correlation coefficient vs. 0.11 ± 0.04, 3.4-fold decrease, $p < 0.01$).

3.6. Activation of TGR5 Inhibits the ET-1-Mediated Increase in Portal Pressure

Perfusion of mouse livers with buffer containing only DMSO as vehicle did not cause any significant changes in portal perfusion pressure. A challenge of these mice with increasing concentrations of ET-1 led to a dose-dependent increase in portal perfusion pressure. Addition of a TGR5 agonist to the ET-1-enriched perfusion buffer significantly reduced the ET-1-mediated rise in portal pressure as compared to vehicle containing perfusion buffer, indicating that TGR5 activation rapidly reduces ET-1-mediated portal hypertension (DMSO vs. TGR5 Ago/+1 nM ET-1 2.41 ± 0.26 cmH_20 vs. 1.42 ± 0.18 cmH_20 (1.7-fold decrease); DMSO vs. TGR5 Ago/+5 nM ET-1 2.9 ± 0.18 cmH_20 vs. 1.89 ± 0.28 cmH_20 (1.5-fold decrease), DMSO vs. TGR5 Ago/+15 nM ET-1 3.14 ± 0.15 cmH_20 vs. 2.20 ± 0.3 cmH_20 (1.4-fold decrease), ($n = 5$–6), $p < 0.05$) (Figure 7A).

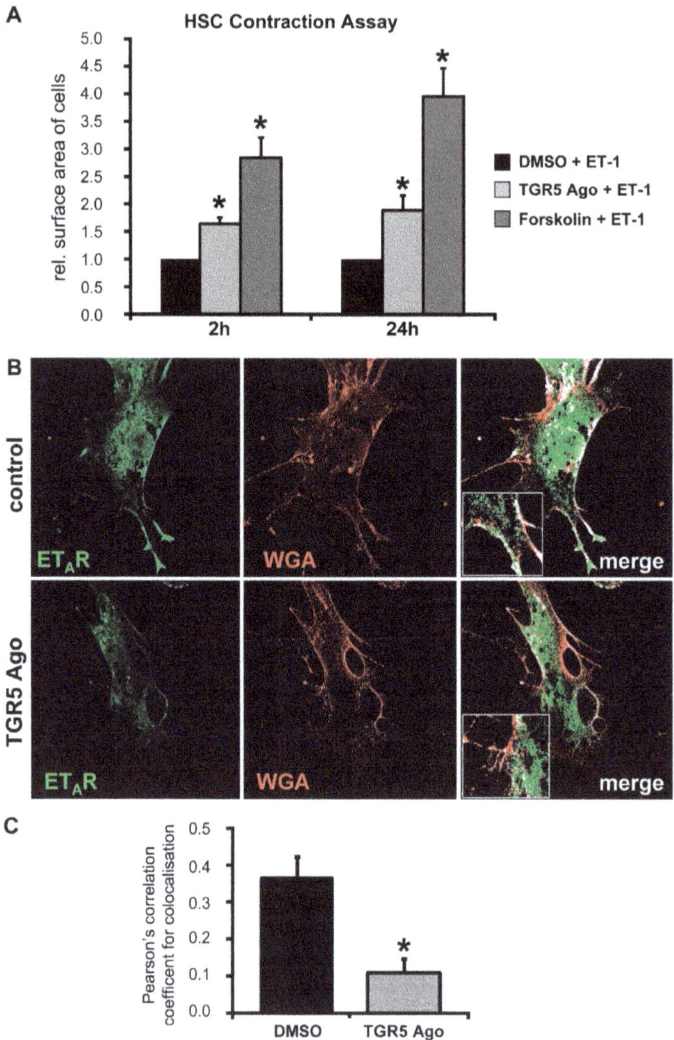

Figure 6. Stimulation of TGR5 in isolated HSCs triggers internalization of the endothelin A receptor (ET_AR), thus reducing the contractile response towards ET-1. (**A**) Contraction of rat HSCs on collagen lattices was measured in response to ET-1 after pre-incubation with DMSO, a TGR5 agonist (10 µM), or forskolin (10 µM), which was used as TGR5-independent positive control. Surface area of collagen lattices served as indirect measure of contractile activity 2 h and 24 h after ET-1 addition. Surface area of cells/collagen lattices treated with DMSO and ET-1 was set to 1.0. Data are shown as mean ± SEM ($n = 12$); * statistically significant from DMSO/ET-1-treated cells ($p < 0.01$). (**B**) Immunofluorescence staining of murine HSCs using an antibody directed against the ET_AR (in green) and Alexa-543 coupled wheat germ agglutinin (WGA, shown in red) to stain the cell surface. HSCs were incubated with either DMSO or a TGR5 agonist (10 µM) for 24 h prior to fixation and immunofluorescence staining. Colocalization of ET_AR and WGA was determined using the coloc2 plugin for ImageJ. Colocalized pixels are shown in white in the merge images. (**C**) Colocalization was quantified using Pearson's correlation coefficient for colocalization, as determined by the coloc2 plugin for ImageJ for each selected region of interest (ROI). Data are shown as mean ± SEM; * statistically significant from DMSO-treated cells ($n = 8$–9; 2–3 different ROIs per condition of three different cell isolations) ($p < 0.05$).

A

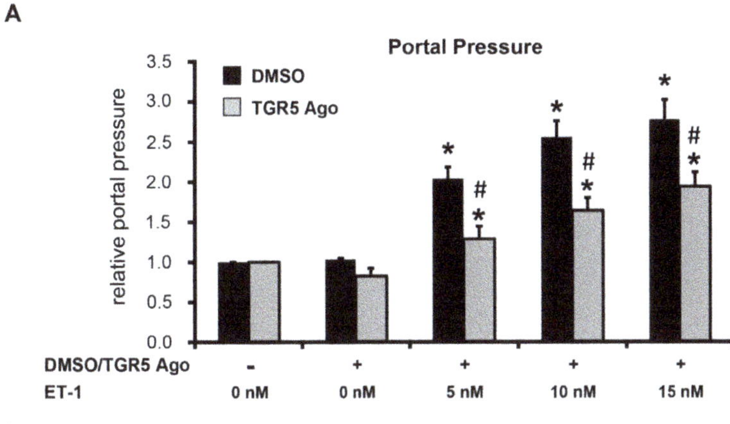

B

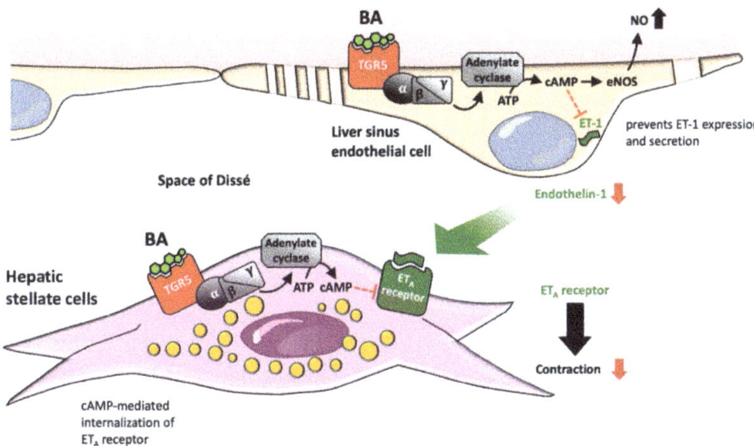

Figure 7. TGR5-dependent regulation of portal perfusion pressure. (**A**) Portal perfusion pressure of TGR5 transgenic mice (TGR5tg) was continuously measured in the presence of DMSO or a TGR5 agonist and increasing concentrations of ET-1. Perfusion was performed with either DMSO or a TGR5 agonist (10 µM) and increasing concentrations of endothelin-1 (ET-1, 5–15nM). Data are shown relative to controls, where the perfusion pressure in the presence of DMSO-containing perfusion buffer following an equilibrium phase of 15 min at the starting point was set to 1.0. All data are shown as mean ± SEM; * statistically significant from DMSO-treated cells ($p < 0.05$) (n = 6–9). (**B**) Cartoon depicting the mechanisms of TGR5-dependent inhibition of ET-1 signaling within the sinusoid. Activation of TGR5 through cAMP inhibits transcription and subsequent secretion of ET-1 from LSECs. ET-1, produced by LSECs, is known to induce contraction of activated HSCs cells by binding to the ET_AR, leading to an increase of intrahepatic vascular resistance and, hence, the development of portal hypertension. Activation of TGR5 in HSCs promotes internalization of the ET_AR, reducing ligand binding at the cell surface and thus contractile activity. In conclusion, ligand binding to TGR5 activates two mechanisms that act synergistically to reduce intrahepatic vascular resistance and, thus, portal hypertension.

4. Discussion

Liver injury of various etiologies triggers morphological and functional changes within hepatic sinusoids, resulting in development of fibrosis and portal hypertension [24,43,44]. Disturbances of the intercellular crosstalk within the sinusoids, especially between LSECs and HSCs, contribute to fibrosis development and microvascular dysfunction [24,43,44]. Multiple paracrine signals, such as NO, ET-1, TGF-β, PDGF, and VEGF, as well as various cytokines and chemokines that are being secreted not only from LSECs, hepatocytes, cholangiocytes, immune cells, but also from platelets, modulate LSEC and HSC phenotype under physiological and pathophysiological conditions [44,45]. Gene expression analysis of liver tissue following LCA feeding for 84 h revealed an enrichment in signaling pathways related to inflammation, proliferation, and matrix remodeling, which was in line with histological analysis of the livers. Interestingly, mice deficient for the G protein-coupled BA receptor TGR5 were more susceptible towards LCA-induced liver injury, resulting in elevated AST serum levels, more pronounced bile infarcts, and an elevated portal perfusion pressure. TGR5 is highly expressed in cholangiocytes, where activation of the receptor triggers formation of the bicarbonate umbrella, promotes tight junction integrity, and inhibits apoptosis, thus protecting cholangiocytes from bile acid toxicity [9,11,46,47]. Lack of TGR5 therefore renders mice more susceptible towards bile acid-induced biliary injury, as observed previously, in response to common bile duct ligation (CBDL) [19] and now in the LCA model. Furthermore, TGR5 exerts anti-inflammatory functions in monocytes and macrophages [4,6,13,14,18]. Absence of TGR5 resulted in elevated expression and secretion of chemokines and cytokines in response to lipopolysaccharide injection or common bile duct ligation [18,19]. Following LCA feeding, we observed a significant induction of hepatic mRNA expression of various cytokines, chemokines, and pro-fibrogenic chemokine receptors such as CCR1 and CCR5 [39]. Interestingly, expression of the chemokine receptor CCR5 was already induced 3-fold in TGR5 KO mice under chow-fed conditions, which has been previously reported for white adipose tissue in TGR5-deficient animals [13]. CXCL10 and its receptor CXCR3 have been implicated in fibrosis development in models of congenital hepatic fibrosis and carbon tetrachloride (CCl_4)-mediated fibrosis [48,49]. While upregulation in comparison to chow-fed WT animals of CXCL10 was 9-fold in WT and 5-fold in TGR5 KO, respectively, CXCR3 mRNA expression was induced 3-fold in WT and 5-fold in TGR5 KO following LCA feeding. Interestingly, in patients with chronic liver disease, serum CXCL10 levels, but not hepatic CXCL10 mRNA levels, were positively correlated with portal hypertension, fibrosis stage, and disease progression [50,51]. To which extent the CXCL10–CXCR3 signaling pathway contributes to the phenotypes of our LCA-fed mice is unclear. CXCL1, which is secreted from LSECs following mechanical stretching, triggers formation of sinusoidal microthrombi, thereby increasing portal pressure independent of cirrhosis [52]. Hepatic CXCL1 mRNA expression was significantly induced in LCA-fed mice. In comparison to chow-fed WT mice, CXCL1 levels were 14.5- and 9.4-fold higher in LCA-fed WT and TGR5 KO mice, respectively. However, in TGR5 KO mice, CXCL1 levels were low under chow-fed conditions and increased 27-fold in response to LCA. Thus, microthrombosis may also contribute to portal hypertension in LCA-fed TGR5 KO animals.

Moreover, expression of PDGFRα/β, TGF-β1 and ET-1, which are related to HSC activation, development of fibrosis, and portal hypertension, were upregulated in both genotypes in response to LCA. However, mRNA levels were significantly higher in livers of TGR5 KO mice as compared to liver tissue from WT littermates. While periportal fibrosis, as measured by Sirius red staining and hydroxyproline content, was not significantly increased in either genotype as early as 3.5 days after starting the LCA feeding, expression of collagen was significantly upregulated in both genotypes, suggesting initiation of fibrogenesis in line with previous data [21]. Since TGR5 is expressed both in LSECs and activated HSCs, we further explored TGR5-mediated effects in these cell types. Stimulation of TGR5 on LSECs reduced ET-1 expression, as well as its secretion, and reduced the responsiveness of activated HSCs towards ET-1 through internalization of the ET_AR. These two mechanisms may act synergistically to reduce ET-1 signaling within the sinusoid (Figure 7B). In rats, treatment with a TGR5 agonist (BAR501) for 6 days prior to cannulation of the portal vein lowered the rise in portal perfusion pressure in response to norepinephrine [53]. Furthermore, administration of the TGR5 agonist inhibited portal hypertension in mice treated for 9 weeks with CCl_4, while it did not affect fibrosis development [53], suggesting an effect on the hepatic microvasculature independent of extracellular matrix deposition. As underlying molecular mechanisms, the authors demonstrated that TGR5 activation induces expression and also non-genomically promotes activation of cystathione-γ-lyase (CSE), resulting in increased production of hydrogen sulfide (H_2S), a potent vasodilator [53,54]. Amongst others, we have previously shown that TGR5 may also trigger serine phosphorylation of eNOS, thereby promoting NO generation, which again leads to vasodilation of hepatic sinusoids [1,53]. Taken together, TGR5 agonists promote generation and secretion of vasodilatory agents (H_2S and NO) and inhibit expression and secretion of the potent vasoconstrictor ET-1 from LSECs [1,7,46,53,54]. While the function of TGR5 in LSECs has been previously studied, the role of TGR5 for HSC activation and function remained elusive. Interestingly, the rise in hepatic PDGFRα/β expression was more pronounced in TGR5 KO mice as compared to WT littermates after LCA-feeding. PDGF-β, which may be derived from either LSECs or platelets, can signal to activated HSCs through its receptor PDGFRβ and promote cell proliferation, migration, and development of a pro-angiogenic HSC phenotype [55,56]. Furthermore, it was recently demonstrated that PDGF-β plays a role in the trans-differentiation processes of HSCs into an activated phenotype, and that administration of an anti-PDGF-β antibody (MPR8457) inhibits development and progression of biliary fibrosis in Abcb4 KO mice, which serve as a chronic model for sclerosing cholangitis [56,57]. Moreover, cAMP may desensitize activated HSCs towards ET-1 through internalization of the ET_AR [42]. Using a non-BA TGR5 ligand, we could demonstrate that activation of the receptor promotes retrieval of ET_AR from the plasma membrane, explaining the reduced ET-1-dependent contractility of activated HSCs in the presence of a TGR5 agonist in vitro. In summary, TGR5 activation reduces hepatic vascular resistance through several mechanisms, both in LSECs and in HSCs, that act synergistically. Through modulation of PDGFRβ expression, it may also contribute to the response of HSCs to microvascular thrombosis and platelet-derived signals. A recent study explored the effect of the non-bile acid TGR5 ligand oleanolic acid in a rat model of liver fibrosis development [58]. Treatment with oleanolic acid significantly reduced fibrogenesis in vivo; however, a direct effect on HSCs in vitro was not observed, since the cell lines used did not express TGR5 [58]. It was previously reported that TGR5 expression, which is very low in quiescent HSCs, is upregulated during the activation of HSCs into a myofibroblast-like phenotype [4,26]. Thus, stimulation of TGR5 on activated HSCs may contribute to the beneficial effects of oleanolic acid on fibrosis development in the above model [58]. Furthermore, mice deficient in both TGR5 and the nuclear bile acid receptor FXR were generated and showed an enrichment in gene expression pathways associated with liver fibrosis and inflammation in line with our study [59]. Since FXR agonists convey beneficial effects in preclinical models of liver fibrosis and portal hypertension [60], it is highly anticipated that TGR5/FXR double-KO mice will also develop LSEC and HSC dysfunction and portal hypertension. Thus, targeting of BA signaling becomes an interesting strategy to reverse morphological changes and dysfunction of cell types residing in the hepatic sinusoids, thereby attenuating portal hypertension and fibrosis development.

Supplementary Materials: The following are available online at http://www.mdpi.com/2073-4409/8/11/1467/s1, Figure S1: Expression of TGR5 in rodent HSCs Figure S2: HSC contraction assay Table S1: Differentially upregulated genes LCA vs. chow; Table S2: Differentially downregulated genes LCA vs. chow; Table S3: Enriched GO pathways LCA vs. chow; Table S4: Downregulated GO pathways LCA vs. chow.

Author Contributions: C.K. co-designed the study, performed the experiments, interpreted the data, and wrote the manuscript. V.K. designed the study, interpreted the results, and wrote the manuscript. M.R. performed and interpreted the animal experiments. J.S. created the figures and reviewed the manuscript. K.K. performed the gene array experiments and reviewed the manuscript. B.H., J.R., and J.G.H. performed the gene array analysis, designed the figures, and reviewed the manuscript. K.S. provided the transgenic animals, supported the data analysis, and carefully reviewed the manuscript. D.H. provided the stellate cells, interpreted the data, and carefully reviewed the manuscript.

Funding: This work was funded by the German Research Foundation (DFG) through the Collaborative Research Centre 974 (SFB 974).

Acknowledgments: Expert technical assistance by Stefanie Lindner, Nichole Eichhorst, and Claudia Rupprecht is gratefully acknowledged.

Conflicts of Interest: The authors declare that there are no potential conflicts of interest.

References

1. Keitel, V.; Reinehr, R.; Gatsios, P.; Rupprecht, C.; Görg, B.; Selbach, O.; Häussinger, D.; Kubitz, R. The G-protein coupled bile salt receptor TGR5 is expressed in liver sinusoidal endothelial cells. *Hepatology* **2007**, *45*, 695–704. [CrossRef] [PubMed]
2. Pols, T.W.; Nomura, M.; Harach, T.; Lo Sasso, G.; Oosterveer, M.H.; Thomas, C.; Rizzo, G.; Gioiello, A.; Adorini, L.; Pellicciari, R.; et al. TGR5 activation inhibits atherosclerosis by reducing macrophage inflammation and lipid loading. *Cell Metab.* **2011**, *14*, 747–757. [CrossRef] [PubMed]
3. Deutschmann, K.; Reich, M.; Klindt, C.; Droge, C.; Spomer, L.; Häussinger, D.; Keitel, V. Bile acid receptors in the biliary tree: TGR5 in physiology and disease. *Biochim. Biophys. Acta Mol. Basis Dis.* **2018**, *1864*, 1319–1325. [CrossRef] [PubMed]
4. Keitel, V.; Donner, M.; Winandy, S.; Kubitz, R.; Häussinger, D. Expression and function of the bile acid receptor TGR5 in Kupffer cells. *Biochem. Biophys. Res. Commun.* **2008**, *372*, 78–84. [CrossRef] [PubMed]
5. Kordes, C.; Sawitza, I.; Götze, S.; Häussinger, D. Bile acids and stellate cells. *Dig. Dis.* **2015**, *33*, 332–337. [CrossRef] [PubMed]
6. Kawamata, Y.; Fujii, R.; Hosoya, M.; Harada, M.; Yoshida, H.; Miwa, M.; Fukusumi, S.; Habata, Y.; Itoh, T.; Shintani, Y.; et al. AG protein-coupled receptor responsive to bile acids. *J. Biol. Chem.* **2003**, *278*, 9435–9440. [CrossRef]
7. Keitel, V.; Stindt, J.; Häussinger, D. Bile Acid-Activated Receptors: GPBAR1 (TGR5) and Other G Protein-Coupled Receptors. *Handb. Exp. Pharmacol.* **2019**, *256*, 19–49.
8. Maruyama, T.; Miyamoto, Y.; Nakamura, T.; Tamai, Y.; Okada, H.; Sugiyama, E.; Nakamura, T.; Itadani, H.; Tanaka, K. Identification of membrane-type receptor for bile acids (M-BAR). *Biochem. Biophys. Res. Commun.* **2002**, *298*, 714–719. [CrossRef]
9. Keitel, V.; Cupisti, K.; Ullmer, C.; Knoefel, W.T.; Kubitz, R.; Häussinger, D. The membrane-bound bile acid receptor TGR5 is localized in the epithelium of human gallbladders. *Hepatology* **2009**, *50*, 861–870. [CrossRef]
10. Keitel, V.; Reich, M.; Häussinger, D. TGR5: Pathogenetic role and/or therapeutic target in fibrosing cholangitis? *Clin. Rev. Allergy Immunol.* **2015**, *48*, 218–225. [CrossRef]
11. Merlen, G.; Kahale, N.; Ursic-Bedoya, J.; Bidault-Jourdainne, V.; Simerabet, H.; Doignon, I.; Tanfin, Z.; Garcin, I.; Péan, N.; Gautherot, J.; et al. TGR5-dependent hepatoprotection through the regulation of biliary epithelium barrier function. *Gut* **2019**. [CrossRef] [PubMed]
12. Perino, A.; Schoonjans, K. TGR5 and Immunometabolism: Insights from Physiology and Pharmacology. *Trends Pharmacol. Sci.* **2015**, *36*, 847–857. [CrossRef] [PubMed]
13. Perino, A.; Pols, T.W.; Nomura, M.; Stein, S.; Pellicciari, R.; Schoonjans, K. TGR5 reduces macrophage migration through mTOR-induced C/EBPbeta differential translation. *J. Clin. Investig.* **2014**, *124*, 5424–5436. [CrossRef] [PubMed]
14. Guo, C.; Xie, S.; Chi, Z.; Zhang, J.; Liu, Y.; Zhang, L.; Zheng, M.; Zhang, X.; Xia, D.; Ke, Y.; et al. Bile Acids Control Inflammation and Metabolic Disorder through Inhibition of NLRP3 Inflammasome. *Immunity* **2016**, *45*, 944. [CrossRef] [PubMed]
15. Vassileva, G.; Golovko, A.; Markowitz, L.; Abbondanzo, S.J.; Zeng, M.; Yang, S.; Hoos, L.; Tetzloff, G.; Levitan, D.; Murgolo, N.J.; et al. Targeted deletion of Gpbar1 protects mice from cholesterol gallstone formation. *Biochem. J.* **2006**, *398*, 423–430. [CrossRef] [PubMed]
16. Maruyama, T.; Tanaka, K.; Suzuki, J.; Miyoshi, H.; Harada, N.; Nakamura, T.; Miyamoto, Y.; Kanatani, A.; Tamai, Y. Targeted disruption of G protein-coupled bile acid receptor 1 (Gpbar1/M-Bar) in mice. *J. Endocrinol.* **2006**, *191*, 197–205. [CrossRef]
17. Pean, N.; Doignon, I.; Garcin, I.; Besnard, A.; Julien, B.; Liu, B.; Branchereau, S.; Spraul, A.; Guettier, C.; Humbert, L.; et al. The receptor TGR5 protects the liver from bile acid overload during liver regeneration in mice. *Hepatology* **2013**, *58*, 1451–1460. [CrossRef]

18. Wang, Y.D.; Chen, W.D.; Yu, D.; Forman, B.M.; Huang, W. The G-protein-coupled bile acid receptor, Gpbar1 (TGR5), negatively regulates hepatic inflammatory response through antagonizing nuclear factor kappa light-chain enhancer of activated B cells (NF-kappaB) in mice. *Hepatology* **2011**, *54*, 1421–1432. [CrossRef]
19. Reich, M.; Deutschmann, K.; Sommerfeld, A.; Klindt, C.; Kluge, S.; Kubitz, R.; Ullmer, C.; Knoefel, W.T.; Herebian, D.; Mayatepek, E.; et al. TGR5 is essential for bile acid-dependent cholangiocyte proliferation in vivo and in vitro. *Gut* **2016**, *65*, 487–501. [CrossRef]
20. Sato, M.; Sato, K.; Furuse, M. Change in hepatic and plasma bile acid contents and its regulatory gene expression in the chicken embryo. *Comp. Biochem. Physiol. B Biochem. Mol. Biol.* **2008**, *150*, 344–347. [CrossRef]
21. Fickert, P.; Fuchsbichler, A.; Marschall, H.U.; Wagner, M.; Zollner, G.; Krause, R.; Zatloukal, K.; Jaeschke, H.; Denk, H.; Trauner, M. Lithocholic acid feeding induces segmental bile duct obstruction and destructive cholangitis in mice. *Am. J. Pathol.* **2006**, *168*, 410–422. [CrossRef] [PubMed]
22. Woolbright, B.L.; Li, F.; Xie, Y.; Farhood, A.; Fickert, P.; Trauner, M.; Jaeschke, H. Lithocholic acid feeding results in direct hepato-toxicity independent of neutrophil function in mice. *Toxicol. Lett.* **2014**, *228*, 56–66. [CrossRef] [PubMed]
23. Pimpin, L.; Cortez-Pinto, H.; Negro, F.; Corbould, E.; Lazarus, J.V.; Webber, L.; Sheron, N.; EASL HEPAHEALTH Steering Committee. Burden of liver disease in Europe: Epidemiology and analysis of risk factors to identify prevention policies. *J. Hepatol.* **2018**, *69*, 718–735. [CrossRef] [PubMed]
24. McConnell, M.; Iwakiri, Y. Biology of portal hypertension. *Hepatol. Int.* **2018**, *12* (Suppl. 1), 11–23. [CrossRef] [PubMed]
25. Iwakiri, Y.; Shah, V.; Rockey, D.C. Vascular pathobiology in chronic liver disease and cirrhosis—Current status and future directions. *J. Hepatol.* **2014**, *61*, 912–924. [CrossRef]
26. Sawitza, I.; Kordes, C.; Götze, S.; Herebian, D.; Häussinger, D. Bile acids induce hepatic differentiation of mesenchymal stem cells. *Sci. Rep.* **2015**, *5*, 13320. [CrossRef]
27. Ullmer, C.; Alvarez Sanchez, R.; Sprecher, U.; Raab, S.; Mattei, P.; Dehmlow, H.; Sewing, S.; Iglesias, A.; Beauchamp, J.; Conde-Knape, K. Systemic bile acid sensing by G protein-coupled bile acid receptor 1 (GPBAR1) promotes PYY and GLP-1 release. *Br. J. Pharmacol.* **2013**, *169*, 671–684. [CrossRef]
28. Thomas, C.; Gioiello, A.; Noriega, L.; Strehle, A.; Oury, J.; Rizzo, G.; Macchiarulo, A.; Yamamoto, H.; Mataki, C.; Pruzanski, M.; et al. TGR5-mediated bile acid sensing controls glucose homeostasis. *Cell Metab.* **2009**, *10*, 167–177. [CrossRef]
29. Vassileva, G.; Hu, W.; Hoos, L.; Tetzloff, G.; Yang, S.; Liu, L.; Kang, L.; Davis, H.R.; Hedrick, J.A.; Lan, H.; et al. Gender-dependent effect of Gpbar1 genetic deletion on the metabolic profiles of diet-induced obese mice. *J. Endocrinol.* **2010**, *205*, 225–232. [CrossRef]
30. Jamall, I.S.; Finelli, V.N.; Que Hee, S.S. A simple method to determine nanogram levels of 4-hydroxyproline in biological tissues. *Anal. Biochem.* **1981**, *112*, 70–75. [CrossRef]
31. Bartneck, M.; Topuz, F.; Tag, C.G.; Sauer-Lehnen, S.; Warzecha, K.T.; Trautwein, C.; Weiskirchen, R.; Tacke, F. Molecular response of liver sinusoidal endothelial cells on hydrogels. *Mater. Sci. Eng. C Mater. Biol. Appl.* **2015**, *51*, 64–72. [CrossRef] [PubMed]
32. Kordes, C.; Sawitza, I.; Müller-Marbach, A.; Ale-Agha, N.; Keitel, V.; Klonowski-Stumpe, H.; Häussinger, D. CD133+ hepatic stellate cells are progenitor cells. *Biochem. Biophys. Res. Commun.* **2007**, *352*, 410–417. [CrossRef] [PubMed]
33. Schneider, C.A.; Rasband, W.S.; Eliceiri, K.W. NIH Image to ImageJ: 25 years of image analysis. *Nat. Methods* **2012**, *9*, 671–675. [CrossRef] [PubMed]
34. Schindelin, J.; Arganda-Carreras, I.; Frise, E.; Kaynig, V.; Longair, M.; Pietzsch, T.; Preibisch, S.; Rueden, C.; Saalfeld, S.; Schmid, B.; et al. Fiji: An open-source platform for biological-image analysis. *Nat. Methods* **2012**, *9*, 676–682. [CrossRef] [PubMed]
35. Chazotte, B. Labeling membrane glycoproteins or glycolipids with fluorescent wheat germ agglutinin. *Cold Spring Harb. Protoc.* **2011**, *2011*. [CrossRef]
36. Smyth, G.K. Limma: Linear Models for Microarray Data. In *Bioinformatics and Computational Biology Solutions Using R and Bioconductor*; Springer: New York, NY, USA, 2005.
37. Benjamini, Y.; Hochberg, Y. Controlling the False Discovery Rate: A Practical and Powerful Approach to Multiple Testing. *J. R. Stat. Soc. Ser. B Methodol.* **1995**, *57*, 289–300. [CrossRef]

38. Alexa, A.; Rahnenführer, J.; Lengauer, T. Improved scoring of functional groups from gene expression data by decorrelating GO graph structure. *Bioinformatics* **2006**, *22*, 1600–1607. [CrossRef]
39. Seki, E.; De Minicis, S.; Gwak, G.Y.; Kluwe, J.; Inokuchi, S.; Bursill, C.A.; Llovet, J.M.; Brenner, D.A.; Schwabe, R.F. CCR1 and CCR5 promote hepatic fibrosis in mice. *J. Clin. Investig.* **2009**, *119*, 1858–1870. [CrossRef]
40. Rockey, D.C.; Housset, C.N.; Friedman, S.L. Activation-dependent contractility of rat hepatic lipocytes in culture and in vivo. *J. Clin. Investig.* **1993**, *92*, 1795–1804. [CrossRef]
41. Iwakiri, Y. Endothelial dysfunction in the regulation of cirrhosis and portal hypertension. *Liver Int.* **2012**, *32*, 199–213. [CrossRef]
42. Reinehr, R.; Fischer, R.; Häussinger, D. Regulation of endothelin-A receptor sensitivity by cyclic adenosine monophosphate in rat hepatic stellate cells. *Hepatology* **2002**, *36*, 861–873. [CrossRef] [PubMed]
43. Greuter, T.; Shah, V.H. Hepatic sinusoids in liver injury, inflammation, and fibrosis: New pathophysiological insights. *J. Gastroenterol.* **2016**, *51*, 511–519. [CrossRef] [PubMed]
44. Marrone, G.; Shah, V.H.; Gracia-Sancho, J. Sinusoidal communication in liver fibrosis and regeneration. *J. Hepatol.* **2016**, *65*, 608–617. [CrossRef] [PubMed]
45. Lee, Y.A.; Wallace, M.C.; Friedman, S.L. Pathobiology of liver fibrosis: A translational success story. *Gut* **2015**, *64*, 830–841. [CrossRef] [PubMed]
46. Keitel, V.; Häussinger, D. Role of TGR5 (GPBAR1) in Liver Disease. *Semin. Liver Dis.* **2018**, *38*, 333–339. [PubMed]
47. Beuers, U.; Hohenester, S.; de Buy Wenniger, L.J.; Kremer, A.E.; Jansen, P.L.; Elferink, R.P. The biliary HCO(3)(-) umbrella: A unifying hypothesis on pathogenetic and therapeutic aspects of fibrosing cholangiopathies. *Hepatology* **2010**, *52*, 1489–1496. [CrossRef]
48. Hintermann, E.; Bayer, M.; Pfeilschifter, J.M.; Luster, A.D.; Christen, U. CXCL10 promotes liver fibrosis by prevention of NK cell mediated hepatic stellate cell inactivation. *J. Autoimmun.* **2010**, *35*, 424–435. [CrossRef]
49. Kaffe, E.; Fiorotto, R.; Pellegrino, F.; Mariotti, V.; Amenduni, M.; Cadamuro, M.; Fabris, L.; Strazzabosco, M.; Spirli, C. beta-Catenin and interleukin-1beta-dependent chemokine (C-X-C motif) ligand 10 production drives progression of disease in a mouse model of congenital hepatic fibrosis. *Hepatology* **2018**, *67*, 1903–1919. [CrossRef]
50. Lehmann, J.M.; Claus, K.; Jansen, C.; Pohlmann, A.; Schierwagen, R.; Meyer, C.; Thomas, D.; Manekeller, S.; Claria, J.; Strassburg, C.P.; et al. Circulating CXCL10 in cirrhotic portal hypertension might reflect systemic inflammation and predict ACLF and mortality. *Liver Int.* **2018**, *38*, 875–884. [CrossRef]
51. Tacke, F.; Zimmermann, H.W.; Berres, M.L.; Trautwein, C.; Wasmuth, H.E. Serum chemokine receptor CXCR3 ligands are associated with progression, organ dysfunction and complications of chronic liver diseases. *Liver Int.* **2011**, *31*, 840–849. [CrossRef]
52. Hilscher, M.B.; Sehrawat, T.; Arab, J.P.; Zeng, Z.; Gao, J.; Liu, M.; Kostallari, E.; Gao, Y.; Simonetto, D.A.; Yaqoob, U.; et al. Mechanical Stretch Increases Expression of CXCL1 in Liver Sinusoidal Endothelial Cells to Recruit Neutrophils, Generate Sinusoidal Microthombi, and Promote Portal Hypertension. *Gastroenterology* **2019**, *157*, 193–209. [CrossRef] [PubMed]
53. Renga, B.; Cipriani, S.; Carino, A.; Simonetti, M.; Zampella, A.; Fiorucci, S. Reversal of Endothelial Dysfunction by GPBAR1 Agonism in Portal Hypertension Involves a AKT/FOXOA1 Dependent Regulation of H2S Generation and Endothelin-1. *PLoS ONE* **2015**, *10*, e0141082. [CrossRef] [PubMed]
54. Renga, B.; Bucci, M.; Cipriani, S.; Carino, A.; Monti, M.C.; Zampella, A.; Gargiulo, A.; d'Emmanuele di Villa Bianca, R.; Distrutti, E.; Fiorucci, S. Cystathionine gamma-lyase, a H2S-generating enzyme, is a GPBAR1-regulated gene and contributes to vasodilation caused by secondary bile acids. *Am. J. Physiol. Heart Circ. Physiol.* **2015**, *309*, H114–H126. [CrossRef] [PubMed]
55. Semela, D.; Das, A.; Langer, D.; Kang, N.; Leof, E.; Shah, V. Platelet-derived growth factor signaling through ephrin-b2 regulates hepatic vascular structure and function. *Gastroenterology* **2008**, *135*, 671–679. [CrossRef]
56. Yoshida, S.; Ikenaga, N.; Liu, S.B.; Peng, Z.W.; Chung, J.; Sverdlov, D.Y.; Miyamoto, M.; Kim, Y.O.; Ogawa, S.; Arch, R.H.; et al. Extrahepatic platelet-derived growth factor-beta, delivered by platelets, promotes activation of hepatic stellate cells and biliary fibrosis in mice. *Gastroenterology* **2014**, *147*, 1378–1392. [CrossRef] [PubMed]

57. Fickert, P.; Pollheimer, M.J.; Beuers, U.; Lackner, C.; Hirschfield, G.; Housset, C.; Keitel, V.; Schramm, C.; Marschall, H.U.; Karlsen, T.H.; et al. Characterization of animal models for primary sclerosing cholangitis (PSC). *J. Hepatol.* **2014**, *60*, 1290–1303. [CrossRef]
58. Kaya, D.; Kaji, K.; Tsuji, Y.; Yamashita, S.; Kitagawa, K.; Ozutsumi, T.; Fujinaga, Y.; Takaya, H.; Kawaratani, H.; Moriya, K.; et al. TGR5 Activation Modulates an Inhibitory Effect on Liver Fibrosis Development Mediated by Anagliptin in Diabetic Rats. *Cells* **2019**, *8*, 1153. [CrossRef]
59. Ferrell, J.M.; Pathak, P.; Boehme, S.; Gilliland, T.; Chiang, J.Y.L. Deficiency of Both Farnesoid X Receptor and Takeda G Protein-Coupled Receptor 5 Exacerbated Liver Fibrosis in Mice. *Hepatology* **2019**, *70*, 955–970. [CrossRef]
60. Schwabl, P.; Hambruch, E.; Seeland, B.A.; Hayden, H.; Wagner, M.; Garnys, L.; Strobel, B.; Schubert, T.L.; Riedl, F.; Mitteregger, D.; et al. The FXR agonist PX20606 ameliorates portal hypertension by targeting vascular remodelling and sinusoidal dysfunction. *J. Hepatol.* **2017**, *66*, 724–733. [CrossRef]

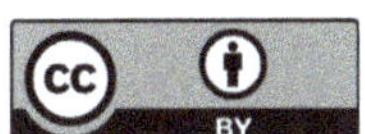

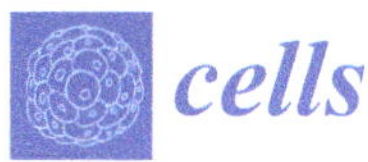

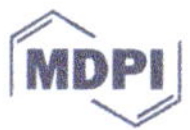

Article

Single Cell RNA Sequencing Identifies Subsets of Hepatic Stellate Cells and Myofibroblasts in Liver Fibrosis

Oliver Krenkel [1,2], Jana Hundertmark [1,3], Thomas P. Ritz [1], Ralf Weiskirchen [4] and Frank Tacke [3,*]

1 Department of Medicine III, University Hospital Aachen, D-52074 Aachen, Germany; okrenkel@ukaachen.de (O.K.); jhundertmark@ukaachen.de (J.H.); tritz@ukaachen.de (T.P.R.)
2 Boehringer-Ingelheim Pharma GmbH & Co. KG, D-88397 Biberach an der Riss, Germany
3 Department of Hepatology/Gastroenterology, Charité University Medical Center, D-13353 Berlin, Germany
4 Institute of Molecular Pathobiochemistry, Experimental Gene Therapy and Clinical Chemistry (IFMPEGKC), University Hospital Aachen, D-52074 Aachen, Germany; rweiskirchen@ukaachen.de
* Correspondence: frank.tacke@charite.de; Tel.: +49-30-450-553022

Received: 1 May 2019; Accepted: 22 May 2019; Published: 24 May 2019

Abstract: Activation of hepatic stellate cells (HSCs) and their trans-differentiation towards collagen-secreting myofibroblasts (MFB) promote liver fibrosis progression. During chronic liver disease, resting HSCs become activated by inflammatory and injury signals. However, HSCs/MFB not only produce collagen, but also secrete cytokines, participate in metabolism, and have biomechanical properties. We herein aimed to characterize the heterogeneity of these liver mesenchymal cells by single cell RNA sequencing. In vivo resting HSCs or activated MFB were isolated from C57BL6/J mice challenged by carbon tetrachloride (CCl_4) intraperitoneally for 3 weeks to induce liver fibrosis and compared to in vitro cultivated MFB. While resting HSCs formed a homogenous population characterized by high platelet derived growth factor receptor β (PDGFRβ) expression, in vivo and in vitro activated MFB split into heterogeneous populations, characterized by α-smooth muscle actin (α-SMA), collagens, or immunological markers. S100 calcium binding protein A6 (S100A6) was a universal marker of activated MFB on both the gene and protein expression level. Compared to the heterogeneity of in vivo MFB, MFB in vitro sequentially and only transiently expressed marker genes, such as chemokines, during culture activation. Taken together, our data demonstrate the heterogeneity of HSCs and MFB, indicating the existence of functionally relevant subsets in hepatic fibrosis.

Keywords: hepatic stellate cells; myofibroblasts; liver fibrosis; scRNASeq

1. Introduction

Hepatic stellate cell (HSC) activation and their trans-differentiation to myofibroblasts (MFB) due to chronic hepatic inflammation is a major hallmark feature of liver fibrosis [1]. Preventing or reversing excessive hepatic scarring is a major therapeutic target in treating chronic liver diseases, such as viral hepatitis and alcoholic and non-alcoholic steatohepatitis [2]. Resting HSC store lipids, such as retinol, can become activated following triggering signals released by damaged hepatocytes or activated local immune cells, such as e.g., Kupffer cells. Activating signals include transforming growth factor-β (TGF-β), platelet derived growth factors as well as various cytokines, such as interleukin-1β (IL-1β), and tumor necrosis factor-α (TNF-α) [3]. Activated MFB alter the composition and density of the extracellular matrix, by secreting collagens, and release inflammatory mediators, including chemokines and cytokines, thereby aggravating local inflammation. Interestingly, a variety of different functions have been assigned to HSCs and/or MFB, ranging from extracellular matrix production, mechanical properties (e.g., contraction and vascular resistance regulation in the liver), and lipid metabolism to immune regulation [4], raising the question about yet unrecognized, functionally diverse subsets of HSCs/MFB. The aim of this study was therefore the evaluation of the heterogeneity of resting HSCs and activated MFB, both in vivo and in vitro, by single cell RNA sequencing (scRNASeq) analysis. We found that resting platelet derived growth factor receptor β- (PDGFR-β) positive HSCs show a high homogeneity, while activated α-smooth muscle actin- (α-SMA) positive MFB split into four different subpopulations, characterized by uniquely expressed gene patterns related to collagen synthesis or immunologic functions. We could identify S100 calcium binding protein A6 (S100A6) as a key marker of activated MFB. Furthermore, we found that in vitro activated MFB lack key functions of in vivo activated MFB as the production of various chemokines, such as CC-chemokine ligand 2 (CCL2) and CXC-chemokine ligand 1 (*CCL1*).

Taken together, our data demonstrate the heterogeneity of activated MFB in vivo and highlight the differences of in vivo and in vitro activated MFB, leading to a better understanding of HSCs to MFB trans0differentation during liver fibrosis.

2. Materials and Methods

2.1. *Animal Models and Induction of Liver Fibrosis*

C57Bl6/J mice were housed under specific pathogen free conditions in the animal facility of the University Hospital, Aachen. All experiments that are described were approved by the corresponding legal authorities (Landesamt für Natur, Umwelt und Verbraucherschutz NRW, LANUV NRW). To induce hepatic fibrosis, mice received intraperitoneal injections of 0.5 mL per kg bodyweight carbon tetrachloride (CCl_4) three times per week for a total of three weeks. Controls received an equivalent amount of oil. After three weeks, mice were euthanized and analyzed as detailed below.

2.2. *Isolation of Ultrapure Hepatic Stellate Cells by Flow Cytometric Sorting*

Ultrapure HSCs were isolated from the liver of healthy C57Bl6/J mice by collagenase digestion and differential gradient centrifugation, followed by fluorescence activated cell sorting (FACS) purification for UV autofluorescence as described before [5]. In detail, the liver was perfused via the *Vena portae* with a prewarmed perfusion HEPES buffer to remove remaining blood from the tissue. the liver was then perfused with 0.5 mg/mL pronase E (Merck, Darmstadt, Germany) and 0.75 U/mL collagenase P (Roche, Basel, Switzerland) for 4.5 min each. The liver was then removed and additionally digested at 37 °C in a water bath for another 20 min. After filtering via a 40 μm cell strainer, HSCs were purified by ultraviolet autofluorescence by using a BD FACS Aria II SORP Cell Sorter (BD Biosciences, Franklin Lakes, NJ, USA).

2.3. *Cultivation of Hepatic Stellate Cells*

4×10^5 purified HSCs were seeded on an uncoated 6 well plate in Dulbecco's Modified Eagle Medium (DMEM) with 10% heat inactivated fetal calf serum (FCS) and 1% penicillin/streptomycin. After one, three, seven, or nine days, cells were then detached by accutase treatment for 10 min. Afterwards, the detached cells were washed once with cold phosphate-buffered saline (PBS) and pelleted by centrifugation at 570 rcf for 5 min in a cold centrifuge. Cells were then resuspended at 500 cells per μl in cold PBS with 0.1% bovine serum albumin (BSA) and directly subjected to the single cell RNA sequencing analysis, according to the manufacturers protocol.

2.4. *Isolation of Liver Non-Parenchymal Cells*

Livers were perfused with cold PBS, followed by digestion for 40 min at 37 °C with 100 μg/mL Collagenase D and 50 μg/mL DNase I (Worthington Biochemicals, Lakewood, NJ, USA). Digestion was stopped by adding cold HBSS with 0.1 mM EDTA. Single cell suspension was obtained by using a 40 μm cell strainer. After washing once with cold PBS, liver non-parenchymal cells were purified by 18% Nycodenz gradient centrifugation. Obtained cells were then stained with CD31-FITC and CD45-APC-Cy7 (BD Biosciences, Heidelberg, Germany). Retinol droplets were measured as autofluorescence by UV-laser excitation. Dead cells were excluded by Hoechst 33342 staining (Sigma-Aldrich, Taufkirchen, Germany).

2.5. Single-Cell RNA Sequencing

Freshly isolated cells, or in vitro cultivated MFB, were analyzed by using the Chromium Single Cell 5′ kit (10× Genomics, Pleasanton, CA, USA), according to manufacturer's protocol. In detail, cells were resuspended at 500 cells per μL in sterile filtered cold PBS containing 0.1% BSA. The experiment was conducted for 5000 recovered cells. After, library generation sequencing was performed by Illumina sequencing on a NextSeq 550 (IZKF genomics facility of the RWTH Aachen University, Aachen, Germany) as detailed before [6]. Primary analysis was done by using an in-house pipeline based on "cellranger" (10× Genomics). Additional analysis was then performed by using the "Seurat" (v2.3.2) [7] package for R (v3.5) (https://www.r-project.org/). Cluster identification was based on the 50 most significant principal components.

2.6. Immunohistochemistry

Immunohistochemistry was performed on formalin-fixed and paraffin-embedded (FFPE) liver sections for α-smooth muscle actin (α-SMA) (clone ASM-1/1A4; Sigma-Aldrich, Taufkirchen, Germany), platelet derived growth factor-β (PDGFR-β) (clone 42G12; Abcam, Cambridge, UK), and S100 calcium binding protein A6 (S100A6) (clone EPNCIR121; Abcam). All primary antibodies were diluted 1:100. For immunofluorescence, secondary goat anti-mouse Cy5 (Abcam) and goat anti-rabbit Al488 (Abcam) were used at a dilution of 1:200. Nuclei were stained with DAPI (Sigma-Aldrich, Taufkirchen, Germany). Micrographs were taken using an Axio Observer Z1 equipped with an Axio Cam MR (Zeiss, Oberkochen, Germany)

3. Results

3.1. Single Cell RNA Sequencing Identifies Four Different Clusters of Myofibroblasts

Chronic liver injury involves the activation of HSCs and their subsequent transformation towards collagen secreting MFB. To assess the heterogeneity of activated MFB, we isolated liver non-leukocytes non-parenchymal cells from three weeks-CCl_4-treated mice and rested HSCs from untreated control mice. The presence of liver fibrosis after three weeks of CCl_4 treatment was confirmed by a hematoxylin and eosin (H&E) stain as well as α smooth muscle actin (α-SMA) immunohistochemistry on FFPE tissue sections (Figure 1A). To capture all potential hepatic MFB from fibrotic livers, we excluded CD31 positive endothelial cells as well as CD45 positive leukocytes, but subjected all remaining double negative cells to scRNASeq analysis. FACS purified retinol positive HSCs, isolated from livers of untreated mice, served as a control (Figure 1B). Both HSCs and MFB were identified by their expression of platelet derived growth factor receptor-β (*Pdgfrb*), while the expression of alpha smooth muscle actin (*Acta2*), collagen, type III, alpha 1 (*Col3a1*), and transforming growth factor, beta induced (*Tgfbi*) allowed the distinction of differently activated states of HSCs and MFB (Figure 1C).

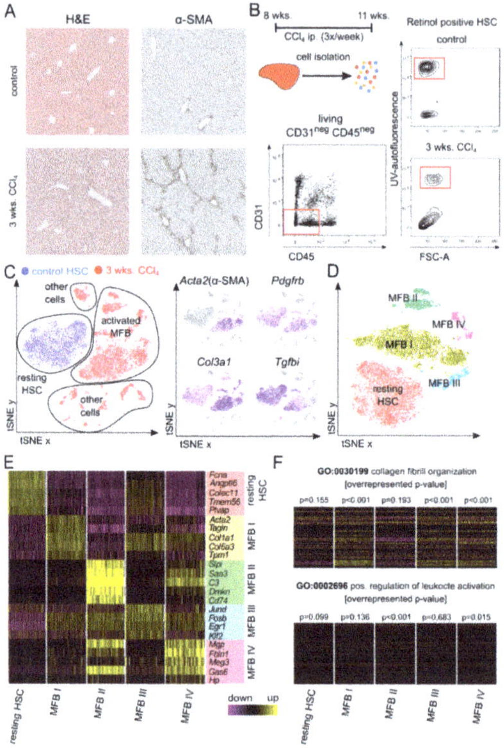

Figure 1. Identification of four sub-populations of activated myofibroblasts (MFB) by single cell RNA sequencing (scRNASeq). (**A**) Representative images of formalin fixed and paraffin-embedded hematoxylin and eosin (H&E) or anti-α-smooth muscle (α-SMA) stained liver sections of control mice and mice subjected to repetitive carbon tetrachloride (CCl_4) injections for 3 weeks. (**B**) Treatment scheme of mice during CCl_4 treatment. Gating strategy for the isolation of resting hepatic stellate cells (HSCs) from healthy mice and activated MFB from CCl_4 treated mice by FACS. (**C**) t-distributed stochastic neighbor embedding (t-SNE) plots mapping the identity of cells to resting HSCs (blue) and MFB from CCl_4 treated liver (red), and the expression of marker genes used for identifying HSCs and MFB. (**D**) Definitive subset clustering of resting HSCs and activated MFB after exclusion of contaminating cells from scRNASeq data sets. (**E**) Log fold change (avg-logFC) gene expression of the top five marker genes for each cluster. For a better comparability, the number of cells in each cluster is aligned. (**F**) Avg-logFC gene expression of genes in the corresponding Gene Ontology (GO) categories, with overrepresented p-value in each cluster. $n = 4$ with an average of 5000 cells per condition and ~60,000 reads per cell.

In the next step, we excluded contaminating endothelial cells, leukocytes, and hepatocytes from our dataset to identify clusters of resting HSCs and activated MFB. We found that the HSCs form a highly homogenous cluster, while the MFB separated into four different sub-clusters, which we termed MFB I to IV (Figure 1D). Analysis of the most significantly expressed marker genes for each cluster allowed the further functional differentiation of these subtypes (Figure 1E). Besides common markers, such as PDGFR-β or various collagens, resting HSCs were uniquely characterized by a high expression of ficolin A (*Fcna*), which has been described to trim extracellular collagen as well as being an activator of a lectin complement pathway, and the hepatokine (*Angptl6*), an inducer of energy expenditure and regulator of the expression of fibroblast derived growth factor 21 (*Fgf21*) in white adipose tissue [8,9].

The major population of activated MFB, termed MFB I, was defined by a high expression of *Acta2*, the smooth muscle cell specific cytoskeletal protein, transgelin (*Tglna*), as well as various types of collagens, such as *Col1a1*, *Col3a1*, or *Col6a3*. The second cluster, MFB II, expressed less extracellular matrix associated genes, but did express the inflammation associated serum leukocyte protease inhibitor (*Slpi*), complement factor C3 (*C3*), serum amyloid A3 (*Saa3*), and cluster of differentiation 74 (*Cd74*). These data indicate towards the existence of a distinct subset of immunoregulatory MFB, characterized by a reduced capacity of modulating the extracellular matrix. The subset, MFB III, comprised proliferating fibroblasts, indicated by an expression of components of the activator protein 1 (*Ap1*) transcription factor, such as anti-apoptotic jun D (*Jund*) and its dimer forming partner *FBJ osteosarcoma oncogene B* (*FosB*). The smallest subset, MFB IV, displayed a mixed phenotype with a high expression of extracellular matrix modulators, such as the matrix gla protein (*Mgp*) and fibulin 1 (*Fbln1*), as well as growth arrest specific 6 (*Gas6*). Some of these marker genes have been described for portal fibroblasts [10]. While clusters MFB I, III, and IV showed a high expression of genes associated with the Gene Ontology (GO) category collagen fibril organization and extracellular matrix buildup (Figure 1F), cluster MFB II expressed less matrix associated genes, and more genes associated with the GO category positive regulation of leukocytes and immune regulation (Figure 1F). Due to the combination of characteristics of myeloid leukocytes, as well as of myofibroblasts, cluster MFB II most likely includes trans-differentiated myeloid myofibroblasts, which have been described before [11].

3.2. S100A6 Represents a Marker for Activated Myofibroblasts

At present, α-SMA is largely accepted as a marker of activated MFB [12]. However, in our scRNASeq analysis, this marker only recognized a subset of activated MFB (see Figure 1C). We therefore wanted to identify markers that are uniquely and uniformly upregulated on all subsets of activated MFB in vivo (Figure 2A). We found that the S100 calcium binding protein A 6 (*S100a6*) is highly upregulated on activated MFB but not on resting HSCs (Figure 2A,B). We first confirmed the presence of S100A6 positive cells in the periportal (i.e., fibrotic) areas of CCl_4-treated livers by immunohistochemistry (Figure 2C). By using immunofluorescence co-staining for PDGFR-β (red) and S100A6 (green) we could then confirm the presence of double positive cells, corroborating the MFB phenotypes observed by our scRNASeq analysis (Figure 2D).

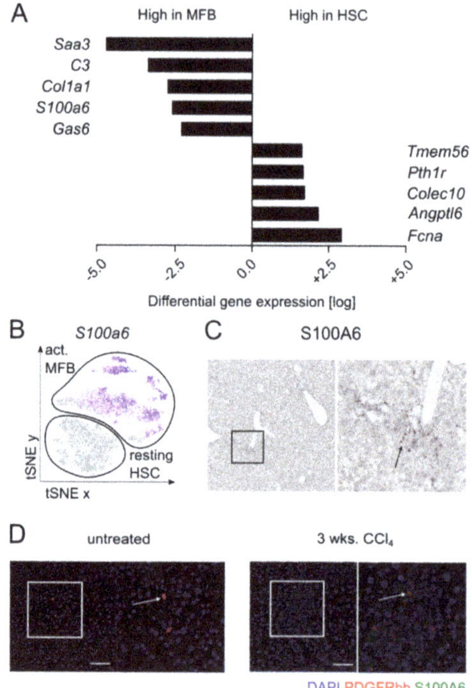

Figure 2. The S100 calcium binding protein A 6 (S100A6) expression marks activated myofibroblasts. (**A**) Differential gene expression analysis of HSCs versus MFB, showing the top five genes upregulated in both groups. (**B**) t-SNE plot of relative gene expression of S100A6, based on scRNASeq analyses from normal and fibrotic mouse livers. (**C**) Representative image of immunohistochemistry staining for S100A6 in CCl_4-treated fibrotic liver. (**D**) Representative images of immunofluorescence co-staining for PDGFR-β (red) and S100A6 (green) on untreated and CCl_4-treated fibrotic liver. Nuclei are stained with DAPI (4′,6-diamidino-2-phenylindole, blue). Scale bar represents 100 μm.

3.3. *Differential Expression of Chemokines and Collagens by Activated Myofibroblast Subsets*

Upregulated expression of chemokines, such as CCL2, CXCL1, or CXCL12, and collagens, particularly COL1A2, COL3A1, or COL5A2, are often named attributes for activated MFB [13]. We herein wanted to analyze whether different subsets of either chemokine or collagen-producing MFB sub-clusters exist in fibrotic livers in vivo (Figure 3A). By scRNASeq analysis, the expression of collagens is homogenously upregulated in activated MFB, while chemokines show a more restricted pattern. While the monocyte recruiting chemokine *Ccl2* is expressed by both resting HSCs and MFB, neutrophil recruiting *Cxcl1* is strongly associated with activated MFB only. *Cxcl12,* on the other hand, is highly expressed by both HSCs and MFB, except for cluster MFB II, representing myeloid myofibroblasts (Figure 3A,B and Supplementary Table S1). By correlating the expression of the chemokine *Ccl2* with *Col3a1* on a single-cell level, resting HSCs comprised cells that express only *Col3a1*, cells co-expressing *Col3a1*, or cells that only express *Ccl2*. Interestingly, activated MFB could be differentiated by their expression of *Ccl2*, while all cells highly expressed *Col3a1* (Figure 3C). These data confirm the universal importance of an upregulated collagen expression during the activation of HSCs to MFB, while resting HSCs and selected MFB clusters demonstrate the capacity to secrete chemokines and thereby modulate the inflammatory environment in their surroundings.

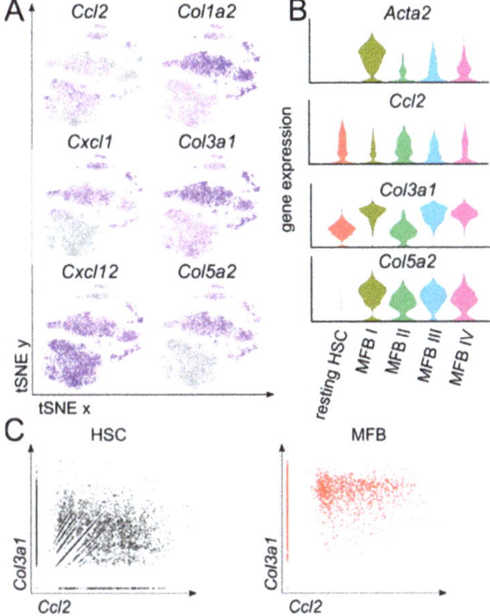

Figure 3. Differential chemokine and collagen gene expression patterns in hepatic stellate cells and myofibroblasts. (**A**) Feature plots showing the relative gene expression strength of selected marker genes. (**B**) Violin plots showing the relative gene expression of activation markers. (**C**) Gene plots for the normalized gene expression of *Col3a1* and *Ccl2*. $n = 4$ with an average of 5000 cells per condition and ~60,000 reads per cell.

3.4. *In Vitro Activated MFB Share Key Characteristics of In Vivo MFB*

Our scRNASeq analyses revealed a striking heterogeneity of MFB in vivo compared to resting HSCs, indicating a functional diversity of these cells during fibrogenesis in vivo. This prompted us to investigate to which extent in vitro activated MFB would reflect this heterogeneity as well. Ultrapure FACS-sorted mouse HSCs were therefore cultivated for up to 9 days on uncoated plastic dishes, the standard model of HSCs to MFB trans-differentiation in vitro [14]. HSCs and MFB were harvested at baseline, day 1, day 3, and days 7 and 9 for scRNASeq analysis (Figure 4A). On the one hand, scRNASeq analysis revealed that in vitro activated MFB clustered dependent on the time of cultivation and could be differentiated into early (day 1), intermediate (day 3), and late (day 7 and day 9) MFB (Figure 4B,C). On the other hand, in vitro activation induced a remarkable MFB heterogeneity over time, which became apparent at the intermediate (day 3) and the late (days 7 and 9) time-point. A more granular analysis of the scRNASeq data generated from the culture-activated HSCs/MFB revealed sub-clusters at all time-points (Figure 4C), for which the marker gene expression patterns varied (Figure 4D and Supplementary Table S2).

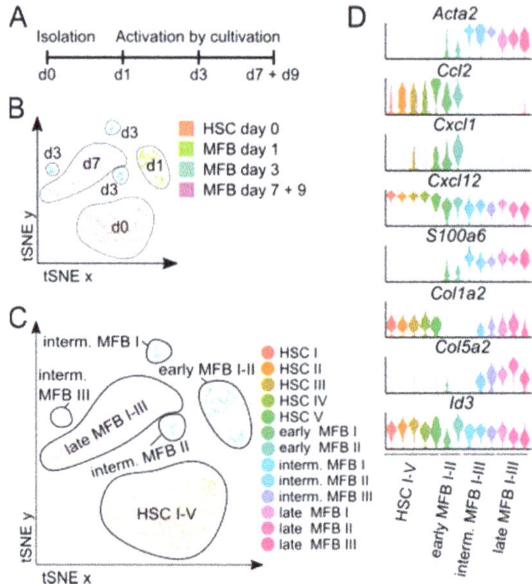

Figure 4. Single-cell RNA sequencing analysis of in vitro activated myofibroblasts. (**A**) Schematic overview of the experimental setup. (**B**) t-SNE plot showing all in vitro activated MFB and resting HSCs dependent on their origin. (**C**) t-SNE plot showing all in vitro activated MFB and resting HSCs dependent on cluster. (**D**) Violin plots showing the relative expression of selected marker genes for each cluster. $n = 4$ with an average of 1000 cells per condition.

We then particularly looked at some markers that we had identified from the in vivo data sets (compare to Figures 2 and 3). The expression of α-SMA (*Acta2*) and *S100a6* was found to be upregulated from early to late MFB in vitro, indicating the relevance of *S100a6* expression as a marker of activated MFB and revealing a high concordance with the in vivo data. For collagens, we observed a clear upregulation of *Col1a2* or *Col5a2* over time during MFB maturation in vitro (Figure 4D). On the contrary, chemokine expression tended to decrease in sequential samples during culture-induced MFB activation. The production of the chemokines *Ccl2* and *Cxcl1* was only found in early MFB, while late MFB populations from day 3 to day 9 did not show any expression of these chemokines. *Cxcl12* displayed the highest expression in resting HSCs and early MFB (Figure 4D). While in vivo, MFB from fibrotic livers consisting of heterogeneous subsets, in which either collagens or chemokines were highly expressed, in vitro activated MFB only expressed these marker genes in a time-dependent manner and not simultaneously, indicating in vitro activation reflected important aspects of MFB biology only transiently during cultivation.

4. Discussion

HSCs trans-differentiation to MFB is a key event in the progression from chronic liver injury to liver fibrosis, which occurs as a consequence of chronic hepatic inflammation e.g., following alcoholic or non-alcoholic steatohepatitis. Liver fibrosis is also considered as a cornerstone event in the progression toward liver cirrhosis or hepatocellular carcinoma [15]. Given the wide range of functional contributions of HSCs and MFB for liver physiology and for fibrogenesis [4], a better understanding of the heterogeneity and subpopulations of HSC and MFB may help to identify novel therapeutic targets to treat liver fibrosis. The upregulation of collagens and α-SMA in MFB is a well-established finding [16] and was confirmed by our single-cell based data for MFB in vivo as well as in vitro. While almost all was MFB upregulated collagen production, only half of the cells expressed chemokines. This was even more striking in vitro, in which chemokine expression appeared early after HSC activation and was down-regulated during later maturation. Activated MFB secrete chemokines capable of recruiting myeloid cells from the circulation, such as e.g., neutrophils via CXCL1 and monocytes via CCL2, which has been linked to exacerbated hepatic inflammation [3]. In fact, HSCs had been reported to induce monocyte chemotaxis via CCL2 upon recognizing danger signals via toll-like receptor 4 [17]. Our scRNASeq data support that this is a feature of HSCs and early activated MFB in vitro, while the existence of MFB sub-populations in fibrotic livers in vivo allows to maintain the production of inflammatory chemokines and cytokines during fibrogenesis. On the other hand, as this feature was missing in our in vitro MFB dataset for the late MFB, we conclude that the use of plastic adherence cultivated MFB may not be a useful tool for analyzing chemokine production by MFB when the cells are being studied after 7 days of culture. However, it needs to be noted that we did not further evaluate other stimuli or cultivation methods as TGF-β or platelet derived growth factor subunit beta (PDGF-β) for the in vitro culture, which could potentially give different results regarding collagen and chemokine expression.

The scRNASeq data sets generated in this work may help to guide future studies on the functional relevance and interactions of HSC/MFB subsets. For instance, we identified S100A6 as a novel marker of activated MFB, following liver fibrosis, which could be confirmed in vitro. The functional involvement of S100A6 for HSCs/MFB signaling, however, requires further evaluation. Data from mouse models of fibrosis indicated that recombinant S100A6 would aggravate fibrogenesis via inducing HSCs proliferation [18]. While S100A6 was consistently found across HSCs/MFB in vivo and in vitro, some MFB properties appear restricted to distinct clusters and/or differentiation states. Cluster MFB II showed characteristics of both leukocytes by expressing CD74, C3 or SLPI but also expressed various collagens. These cells might represent macrophages that have trans-differentiated into myofibroblasts, which has been described for renal fibrosis previously [11] and could potentially explain parts of the immunologic properties that have often been assigned to HSCs and/or trans-differentiated MFB [4].

Importantly, more work is needed to get a better spatial resolution on the MFB populations in fibrosis. The cluster MFB IV showed some features that had been previously reported for portal fibroblasts [19]. It will be important to confirm the scRNASeq data in other models of liver fibrosis, such as bile duct ligation leading to a preferential expansion of the portal fibroblasts, and to define the exact localization of the MFB sub-clusters in fibrotic livers in vivo. Last, but not least, it will be important to identify HSC and MFB populations in human liver. scRNASeq data from healthy human liver already indicated the existence of HSC clusters [20], and similar analyses from cirrhotic human livers are currently ongoing.

Taken together, our scRNASeq analyses from healthy and fibrotic mouse livers demonstrated a yet unrecognized heterogeneity of HSCs and MFB in vivo, suggesting a concerted interplay of functionally diverse MFB subsets during liver fibrogenesis.

Supplementary Materials: The following are available online at http://www.mdpi.com/2073-4409/8/5/503/s1, Table S1: Mean gene expression of HSC and MFB I-IV, Table S2: Mean gene expression of HSC I-V and early, intermediate and late MFB.

Author Contributions: F.T. guided the research. O.K., T.P.R., and R.W. designed and performed the experiments. O.K. and J.H. performed the RNA sequencing analysis. F.T., R.W., and O.K. wrote the manuscript. All authors reviewed and approved the manuscript.

Funding: This work was supported by the German Research Foundation (DFG; Ta434/5-1 and SFB/TRR57). The study sponsor had no role in the study design or in the collection, analysis, or interpretation of data.

Conflicts of Interest: The authors declare no conflict of interest.

References

1. Alegre, F.; Pelegrin, P.; Feldstein, A.E. Inflammasomes in Liver Fibrosis. *Semin. Liver Dis.* **2017**, *37*, 119–127. [CrossRef] [PubMed]

2. Higashi, T.; Friedman, S.L.; Hoshida, Y. Hepatic stellate cells as key target in liver fibrosis. *Adv. Drug Deliv. Rev.* **2017**, *121*, 27–42. [CrossRef] [PubMed]
3. Weiskirchen, R.; Tacke, F. Liver Fibrosis: From Pathogenesis to Novel Therapies. *Digest. Dis.* **2016**, *34*, 410–422. [CrossRef] [PubMed]
4. Weiskirchen, R.; Tacke, F. Cellular and molecular functions of hepatic stellate cells in inflammatory responses and liver immunology. *Hepatobiliary Surg. Nutr.* **2014**, *3*, 344–363. [PubMed]
5. Bartneck, M.; Warzecha, K.T.; Tag, C.G.; Sauer-Lehnen, S.; Heymann, F.; Trautwein, C.; Weiskirchen, R.; Tackeet, F. Isolation and time lapse microscopy of highly pure hepatic stellate cells. *Anal. Cell Pathol.* **2015**, *2015*. [CrossRef] [PubMed]
6. Krenkel, O.; Hundertmark, J.; Abdallah, A.T.; Kohlhepp, M.; Puengel, T.; Roth, T.; Branco, D.P.P.; Mossanen, J.C.; Luedde, T.; Trautwein, C.; et al. Myeloid cells in liver and bone marrow acquire a functionally distinct inflammatory phenotype during obesity-related steatohepatitis. *Gut* **2019**. [CrossRef] [PubMed]
7. Butler, A.; Hoffman, P.; Smibert, P.; Papalexi, E.; Satija, R. Integrating single-cell transcriptomic data across different conditions, technologies, and species. *Nat. Biotechnol.* **2018**, *36*, 411–420. [CrossRef] [PubMed]
8. Kang, S.G.; Yi, H.S.; Choi, M.J.; Ryu, M.J.; Jung, S.; Chung, H.K.; Chang, J.Y.; Kim, Y.K.; Lee, S.E.; Kim, H.W.; et al. ANGPTL6 expression is coupled with mitochondrial OXPHOS function to regulate adipose FGF21. *J. Endocrinol.* **2017**, *233*, 105–118. [CrossRef] [PubMed]
9. Kim, M.J.; Namkung, J.; Chang, J.S.; Kim, S.J.; Park, K.S.; Kong, I.D. Leptin regulates the expression of angiopoietin-like 6. *Biochem. Biophys. Res. Commun.* **2018**, *502*, 397–402. [CrossRef] [PubMed]
10. Koyama, Y.; Wang, P.; Liang, S.; Iwaisako, K.; Liu, X.; Xu, J.; Zhang, M.; Sun, M.; Cong, M.; Karin, D.; et al. Mesothelin/mucin 16 signaling in activated portal fibroblasts regulates cholestatic liver fibrosis. *J. Clin. Invest.* **2017**, *127*, 1254–1270. [CrossRef] [PubMed]
11. Meng, X.M.; Wang, S.; Huang, X.R.; Yang, C.; Xiao, J.; Zhang, Y.; To, K.F.; Nikolic-Paterson, D.J.; Lan, H.Y. Inflammatory macrophages can transdifferentiate into myofibroblasts during renal fibrosis. *Cell Death. Dis.* **2016**, *7*. [CrossRef] [PubMed]
12. Weiskirchen, R.; Weiskirchen, S.; Tacke, F. Organ and tissue fibrosis: Molecular signals, cellular mechanisms and translational implications. *Mol. Aspects Med.* **2019**, *65*, 2–15. [CrossRef] [PubMed]
13. Tsuchida, T.; Friedman, S.L. Mechanisms of hepatic stellate cell activation. *Nat. Rev. Gastroenterol. Hepatol.* **2017**, *14*, 397–411. [CrossRef] [PubMed]
14. Tacke, F.; Weiskirchen, R. Update on hepatic stellate cells: Pathogenic role in liver fibrosis and novel isolation techniques. *Expert Rev. Gastroenterol. Hepatol.* **2012**, *6*, 67–80. [CrossRef] [PubMed]
15. Dulai, P.S.; Singh, S.; Patel, J.; Soni, M.; Prokop, L.J.; Younossi, Z.; Sebastiani, G.; Ekstedt, M.; Hagstrom, H.; Nasr, P.; et al. Increased risk of mortality by fibrosis stage in nonalcoholic fatty liver disease: Systematic review and meta-analysis. *Hepatology* **2017**, *65*, 1557–1565. [CrossRef] [PubMed]
16. Lee, Y.A.; Wallace, M.C.; Friedman, S.L. Pathobiology of liver fibrosis: A translational success story. *Gut* **2015**, *64*, 830–841. [CrossRef] [PubMed]
17. Seki, E.; De Minicis, S.; Osterreicher, C.H.; Kluwe, J.; Osawa, Y.; Brenner, D.A.; Schwabe, R.F. TLR4 enhances TGF-beta signaling and hepatic fibrosis. *Nat. Med.* **2007**, *13*, 1324–1332. [CrossRef] [PubMed]
18. Xia, P.; He, H.; Kristine, M.S.; Guan, W.; Gao, J.; Wang, Z.; Hu, J.; Han, L.; Li, J.; Han, W.; et al. Therapeutic effects of recombinant human S100A6 and soluble receptor for advanced glycation end products(sRAGE) on CCl4-induced liver fibrosis in mice. *Eur. J. Pharmacol.* **2018**, *833*, 86–93. [CrossRef] [PubMed]
19. Karin, D.; Koyama, Y.; Brenner, D.; Kisseleva, T. The characteristics of activated portal fibroblasts/myofibroblasts in liver fibrosis. *Differentiation* **2016**, *92*, 84–92. [CrossRef] [PubMed]
20. MacParland, S.A.; Liu, J.C.; Ma, X.Z.; Innes, B.T.; Bartczak, A.M.; Gage, B.K.; Manuel, J.; Khuu, N.; Echeverri, J.; Linares, I.; et al. Single cell RNA sequencing of human liver reveals distinct intrahepatic macrophage populations. *Nat. Commun.* **2018**, *9*. [CrossRef] [PubMed]

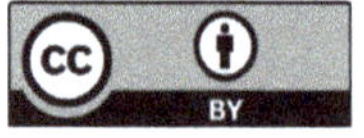

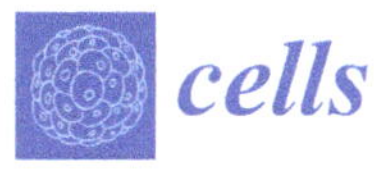

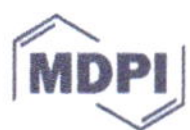

Article

Influence of Liver Fibrosis on Lobular Zonation

Ahmed Ghallab [1,2,*], Maiju Myllys [1], Christian H. Holland [3,4], Ayham Zaza [1], Walaa Murad [5], Reham Hassan [1,2], Yasser A. Ahmed [6], Tahany Abbas [5], Eman A. Abdelrahim [5], Kai Markus Schneider [7], Madlen Matz-Soja [8], Jörg Reinders [1], Rolf Gebhardt [8], Marie-Luise Berres [7], Maximilian Hatting [7], Dirk Drasdo [1,9], Julio Saez-Rodriguez [3,4], Christian Trautwein [7] and Jan G. Hengstler [1,*]

1 Leibniz Research Centre for Working Environment and Human Factors at the Technical University Dortmund, 44139 Dortmund, Germany; Myllys@ifado.de (M.M.), zaza@ifado.de (A.Z.); Hassan@ifado.de (R.H.), Reinders@ifado.de (J.R.); dirk.dras@gmail.com (D.D.)

2 Department of Forensic Medicine and Toxicology, Faculty of Veterinary Medicine, South Valley University, Qena 83523, Egypt

3 Faculty of Medicine, Institute of Computational Biomedicine, Heidelberg University, Bioquant—Im Neuenheimer Feld 267, 69120 Heidelberg, Germany; christian.holland@bioquant.uni-heidelberg.de (C.H.H.); julio.saez@bioquant.uni-heidelberg.de (J.S.-R.)

4 Faculty of Medicine, Joint Research Centre for Computational Biomedicine (JRC-COMBINE), RWTH Aachen University, Pauwelsstrasse 19, 52074 Aachen, Germany

5 Histology Department, Faculty of Medicine, South Valley University, Qena 83523, Egypt; walaamurad1991@yahoo.com (W.M.); tahany_abbass@yahoo.com (T.A.); emaneweda@yahoo.com (E.A.A.)

6 Department of Histology, Faculty of Veterinary Medicine, South Valley University, Qena 83523, Egypt; yasser.ali@vet.svu.edu.eg

7 Department of Medicine III, University Hospital RWTH Aachen, Aachen University, 52074 Aachen, Germany; Kai.Markus.Schneider@gmail.com (K.M.S.); mberres@ukaachen.de (M.-L.B.); mhatting@ukaachen.de (M.H.); ctrautwein@ukaachen.de (C.T.)

8 Faculty of Medicine, Rudolf-Schönheimer-Institute of Biochemistry, Leipzig University, 04103 Leipzig, Germany; Madlen.Matz@medizin.uni-leipzig.de (M.M.-S.); Rolf.Gebhardt@medizin.uni-leipzig.de (R.G.)

9 Modelling and Analysis for Medical and Biological Applications (MAMBA), Inria Paris & Sorbonne Université LJLL, 2 Rue Simone IFF, 75012 Paris, France

* Correspondence: Ghallab@ifado.de (A.G.); Hengstler@ifado.de (J.G.H); Tel.: +49-02311084356 (A.G.); +49-02311084348 (J.G.H.)

Received: 5 November 2019; Accepted: 28 November 2019; Published: 2 December 2019

Abstract: Little is known about how liver fibrosis influences lobular zonation. To address this question, we used three mouse models of liver fibrosis, repeated CCl_4 administration for 2, 6 and 12 months to induce pericentral damage, as well as bile duct ligation (21 days) and mdr2$^{-/-}$ mice to study periportal fibrosis. Analyses were performed by RNA-sequencing, immunostaining of zonated proteins and image analysis. RNA-sequencing demonstrated a significant enrichment of pericentral genes among genes downregulated by CCl_4; vice versa, periportal genes were enriched among the upregulated genes. Immunostaining showed an almost complete loss of pericentral proteins, such as cytochrome P450 enzymes and glutamine synthetase, while periportal proteins, such as arginase 1 and CPS1 became expressed also in pericentral hepatocytes. This pattern of fibrosis-associated 'periportalization' was consistently observed in all three mouse models and led to complete resistance to hepatotoxic doses of acetaminophen (200 mg/kg). Characterization of the expression response identified the inflammatory pathways TGFβ, NFκB, TNFα, and transcription factors NFKb1, Stat1, Hif1a, Trp53, and Atf1 among those activated, while estrogen-associated pathways, Hnf4a and Hnf1a, were decreased. In conclusion, liver fibrosis leads to strong alterations of lobular zonation, where the pericentral region adopts periportal features. Beside adverse consequences, periportalization supports adaptation to repeated doses of hepatotoxic compounds.

Keywords: zonation; liver lobule; chronic liver disease; cytochrome P450; inflammation; bile duct ligation; acetaminophen

1. Introduction

Prevalence and mortality of liver diseases, including fibrosis and cirrhosis, continue to grow in Europe [1]. The increase in alcohol consumption and obesity-associated non-alcoholic fatty liver disease (NAFLD) in recent years has contributed to this development. Liver fibrosis is a complex wound-healing process that leads to inflammation and scarring [2,3]. It occurs as a consequence of chronic liver damage, caused by different etiologies, including chronic intoxication, viral infections, genetic diseases, or metabolic disorders due to super-nutrition [2]. Liver fibrosis requires the interaction of several cell types, myofibroblasts, macrophages, hepatocytes and immune cells that are orchestrated by a spectrum of cytokines, chemokines and mediators such as lipids, hormones and reactive oxygen species [3–5]. Progressive fibrosis is characterized by the excessive accumulation of the extracellular matrix which compromises the functional architecture of the organ [3,6].

Liver zonation is the spatial separation of a large spectrum of different metabolic pathways along the porto-central axis of the liver lobule, which is essential for liver function [7,8]. For example, xenobiotic metabolism by cytochrome P450 enzymes (CYP) is located in the approximately 50% of hepatocytes in the center of the liver lobule [9,10]. This serves to detoxify xenobiotics before they are drained into the central vein [2,11]. However, for compounds metabolically activated by CYPs, such as CCl_4 or acetaminophen, the zonated expression causes a pericentral pattern of necrosis [12,13]. A zonated metabolic pattern is also known for ammonia metabolism [14]. While urea-cycle enzymes detoxify ammonia by high capacity and low affinity mechanism in the periportal and midzonal regions, low remaining ammonia concentrations are removed from the sinusoidal blood by a pericentral ring of glutamine synthetase positive hepatocytes that act by a low capacity, high affinity mechanism [15–17]. Further zonated functions include glycolysis, gluconeogenesis, glycogenesis, the TCA-cycle, glutamine metabolism and lipogenesis [2,7].

While liver fibrosis and the mechanisms of zonation have already been intensively studied [18–21], little is known about how liver fibrosis influences lobular zonation. In the present study, we used three different mouse models of liver fibrosis, chronic CCl_4 intoxication, bile duct ligation (BDL) and the knockout of mdr2. For all three fibrosis models, we observed a loss of pericentral factors, while the entire lobule adapts periportal features. Besides of several adverse consequences, 'periportalization' is responsible for adaptation to toxic stress during the pathogenesis of liver fibrosis and leads to resistance to the hepatotoxic compound acetaminophen (APAP).

2. Materials and Methods

2.1. Experimental Animals

Eight to 10 week-old male C57BL/6N mice (Janvier Labs, France) and 8- to 64-week-old $Mdr2^{-/-}$ mice and age-matched controls were used. The mice were housed under 12 h light/dark cycles at a controlled ambient temperature of 25 °C and fed ad libitum on a standard diet (Ssniff, Soest, Germany) with free access to water. Three to 5 mice were used for each time point and condition given in the result section. All experiments were approved by the local animal protection authorities (application number: 84-02.04.2017.A177).

2.2. Induction of Chronic Liver Injury by CCl_4 and Bile Duct Ligation (BDL)

For induction of progressive pericentral fibrosis, carbon tetrachloride (CCl_4, 1 g/kg b.w. in olive oil) was repeatedly injected intraperitoneally (i.p.) twice a week for 2, 6 and 12 months. The vehicle controls received only olive oil in the same way as the CCl_4 groups. Samples were collected on day 6 after the last CCl_4 or oil injection. In order to induce periportal fibrosis, the extrahepatic common bile duct was ligated under anaesthesia as previously described [22]. Liver tissue samples were collected on day 21 post-BDL or sham operation.

2.3. Induction of Acute Liver Injury by Acetaminophen (APAP)

In order to induce acute liver injury, a dose of 200 mg/kg b.w. APAP was dissolved in warm phosphate-buffered saline (PBS) and i.p. injected. The mice were fasted overnight before APAP injection.

2.4. Sample Collection

At the time points indicated in the result section, the mice were anaesthetised by an i.p. injection of ketamine (100 mg/kg b.w.) and xylazine (10 mg/kg b.w.). After the loss of reflexes, blood as well as liver tissue samples were collected. The blood samples were collected from the portal vein, the hepatic vein, and the right heart chamber in EDTA-coated syringes as previously described [15]. The samples were centrifuged at 13,000 rpm for 10 min in order to separate plasma. The collected plasma was stored at −80 °C until used for analyses. After blood collection, the remaining blood was removed by perfusion trans-cardially with 40 mL PBS. Subsequently, the whole liver was excised and specimens were collected from defined anatomical positions as follow: (i) a specimen of approximately 1 cm size was taken from the left liver lobe, fixed in 4% paraformaldehyde (PFA) for 2 days and then embedded in paraffin for 2D staining; (ii) a specimen of approximately 0.5 cm size was taken from the left liver lobe and immediately embedded in Tissue-Tek®cryomold in Neg-50 media (ThermoFisher Scientific, Oberhausen, Germany), frozen in 2-methylbutane and stored at −80 °C until used for cryosection preparation; (iii) a specimen of approximately 0.5 cm size was taken from the median liver lobe, fixed in 4% PFA for 2 days, incubated in 30% sucrose for 2 days, and then embedded in Tissue-Tek®cryomold in Neg-50 media, frozen in 2-methylbutane and stored at −80 °C until used for preparation of liver slices; (iv) a specimen of approximately 20 mg weight was taken from the left liver lobe, snap-frozen in liquid nitrogen and stored at −80 °C until used for RNA isolation.

2.5. Histopathology

Haematoxylin and eosin staining was performed in 5 µm-thick paraffin embedded tissue sections using a standard protocol. In order to visualize collagen accumulation during chronic liver disease progression, picrosirius red staining was performed in 5 µm-thick paraffin embedded tissue sections using a commercially available kit (Polyscience Europe GmbH, Eppelheim, Germany), according to the manufacturer's instructions.

2.6. Gene Expression Analyses

Quantitative real time polymerase chain reaction (qRT-PCR). Total RNA was isolated from frozen liver tissue using QIAzol Lysis Reagent (Qiagen, Hilden, Germany). cDNA synthesis was performed from 2 µg of isolated RNA using a commercially available kit (High-Capacity cDNA Reverse Transcription Kit, Applied Biosystems, Schwerte, Germany). qRT-PCR analyses were performed using TaqMan 7500 Real-Time PCR, TaqMan universal PCR Master Mix (Applied Biosystems, Schwerte, Germany), and TaqMan gene expression assays (ThermoFisher Scientifics, Oberhausen, Germany). Gene expression values were normalized to GAPDH, calculated using the ΔΔCt method, and are expressed as fold changes over untreated control samples.

2.7. RNA-Seq Analysis

Pre-processing and normalization. The count matrix was derived from FASTQ files of wild-type, CCl_4 plus olive oil and pure olive oil samples using the web application BioJupies [23]. The samples were normalized using the R package edgeR (version 3.25.8) [24].

Differential gene expression analysis. Differential gene expression analysis was performed with the R package limma (version 3.39.18) [25]. To extract the effect of chronic CCl_4 intoxication, we computed contrasts comparing the treated samples (CCl_4 plus olive oil) versus matched olive oil samples. While there are matched oil samples for month 2 and 12, there were no oil samples for month 6 available. As the oil effect was relatively constant across time we imputed oil expression values for month 6 by taking the arithmetic mean of month 2 and month 12. A gene was considered as differentially expressed with abs(logFC) $\geq$ 1.5 and FDR $\leq$ 0.05.

2.8. Functional Genomics Analysis of the CCl_4 Signature

Pathway analysis with PROGENy. Pathway activity scores were calculated with the functional genomics tools PROGENy [26,27]. While classical pathway analysis methods (e.g., Kyoto Encyclopedia of Genes and Genomes (KEGG) pathway analysis) rely on gene sets containing genes of pathway members PROGENy exploits so called "footprint gene sets" containing not the pathway members but the most responsive genes upon corresponding pathway perturbation. PROGENy was applied on contrast using the moderated t-value as a gene-level statistic.

Transcription factor (TF) analysis with DoRothEA. DoRothEA is a high-quality data resource of TF-target interactions (regulons) [26,28]. Coupling DoRothEA regulons with a statistical method allows to infer TF activity from the expression of its transcriptional targets. We used as statistical method the function viper from the R package viper (version: 1.17.0) [29] that computes for each TF a normalized enrichment score that we consider as TF activity. DoRothEA in combination with viper was applied on contrasts using moderated t-values as a gene-level statistic.

Gene Ontology (GO) term enrichment. We used the R package msigdf (https://github.com/ToledoEM/msigdf) to query GO terms (biological process and molecular functions) from MsigDB. Gene set enrichment analysis was performed on contrasts using the R package fgsea (version 1.10.0) [30] with 100,000 permutations. The moderated t-value was used as a gene-level statistic.

Construction of consensus pericentral and periportal gene sets. Consensus pericentral and periportal gene sets were constructed by integrating pericentral and periportal gene sets from three independent studies [31–33]. Gene sets reported by Braeuning et al. [31] were extracted from their corresponding Supplementary Table S1. Saito et al. [33] made their data available for both male and female mice. Since only male mice were used in the here presented work we focused on common (with respect to male and female mice) and male specific pericentral and periportal genes. Halpern et al. [32] do not provide explicit pericentral and periportal gene sets in their supplement; therefore, we generated them systematically starting from their Supplementary Tables S1 and S2. Supplementary Table S1 contains the UMI counts of 1415 hepatocytes/cells. Supplementary Table S2 reports information about the spatial organization of the 1415 cells across the 9 lobule layer (layer 1 is the most pericentral and layer 9 is the most periportal layer). For each cell and lobule layer combination a probability is given that indicates the likelihood that a cell was originally located in the respective layer. We started our analysis pipeline by removing genes that were expressed in less than 15 cells (out of 1415). Subsequently, we normalized the sub-setted count matrix using the R package scran (version 1.11.27) [34]. To assign cells to a specific lobule layer we selected for each cell the layer with the highest probability yielding in a zonation table reporting the spatial distribution of all cells across the lobule. Given this zonation table we identified genes with significant monotonic expression changes across the lobule layer by applying the exact version of the Jonckheere–Terpstra test from the R package clinfun (version 1.0.15, https://cran.r-project.org/web/packages/clinfun/index.html). Monotonically increasing genes (from layer 1–9) were considered as potential periportal and monotonic decreasing as potential pericentral genes. Only genes with an FDR $\leq$ 0.001 were considered as pericentral and periportal gene set members. As the three independent studies were published within more than a decade we updated all MGI gene symbols to their current alias using the function alias2SymbolTable from the limma package (version: 3.39.18) [25]. The consensus pericentral and periportal gene sets contain only those genes that are reported in at least two studies.

Characterization of the overlap of pericentral/periportal genes and the most responsive genes of CCl_4 treatment. In this analysis, the overlap of pericentral and periportal genes with the differentially expressed genes after CCl_4 treatment is characterized with over-representation analysis (ORA). To ensure a reasonable overlap size we relaxed the condition of differentially expressed genes to abs(logFC) ≥ 0.8 and FDR ≤ 0.2. We identified the final overlap gene set (for both zonations: pericentral and periportal) independently of time by taking the union of overlapping genes across all time points (months 2–12). ORA was performed using Fisher's exact test. The number of background genes has been set to 20,000 as this reflects a typical number of genes in a mouse transcriptome experiment. We tested the following gene sets: GO terms (molecular functions and biological processes), DoRothEA regulon's, PROGENy's footprint gene sets, KEGG gene sets. *P*-values were corrected using Benjamini Hochberg correction (false discovery rate, FDR) [35].

2.9. Immunohistochemistry

Immunohistochemistry analysis was performed in five µm-thick frozen or formalin-fixed paraffin-embedded liver tissue sections using antibodies against CYP3A (Biotrend, Cologne, Germany), CYP1A, CYP2C (a gift from Dr. R. Wolf, Biochemical Research Centre, University of Dundee, Dundee, UK), CYP2E1, Arginase1 (Sigma-Aldrich Corp., St. Louis, MO, USA), GS (BD Bioscience, Heidelberg, Germany), and CPS1 (Abcam, Cambridge, UK) (Table 1). The following horseradish peroxidase-conjugated secondary antibodies were used: anti-rabbit IgG (Agilent, Santa Clara, CA, USA), anti-mouse IgG (Sigma-Aldrich Corp., St. Louis, MO, USA), and anti-rat IgG (Linaris GmbH, Heidelberg, Germany) (Table 1). In order to visualize the target signal, the tissues were stained with either 3,3′-diaminobenzidine solution (Vector Laboratories, Peterborough, UK) or AEC+ high sensitivity substrate chromogen (Agilent, Santa Clara, CA, USA). The nuclei were visualized by counter-staining with Mayer's haematoxylin.

Table 1. Antibodies and staining conditions.

Target	Tissue Section	Primary Antibody		Secondary Antibody	
		Antibody	Dilution	Antibody	Dilution
CYP3A	Frozen	Rabbit anti-CYP3A1	1:250	Swine anti-rabbit	1:20
CYP1A	Frozen	Rat anti-CYP1A2	1:500	Rabbit anti-rat IgG	1:1000
CYP2C	Frozen	Rat anti-CYP2C6	1:250	Rabbit anti-rat IgG	1:1000
CYP2E1	Frozen/ FFPE	Rabbit anti-CYP2E1	1:100	Swine anti-rabbit	1:20
GS	FFPE	Mouse anti-GS	1:1000	anti-mouse	1:500
Arginase1	FFPE	Anti-arginase-1 antibody, rabbit monoclonal	1:500	Swine anti-rabbit	1:20
CPS1	FFPE	Anti-CPS1 antibody—liver mitochondrial marker	1:500	Swine anti-rabbit	1:20

2.10. Immunostaining of Liver Slices

CYP2E1 immunostaining was done in 200 µm-thick liver slices prepared using a cryostat microtome. After washing, permeabilization and blocking steps the slices were incubated for 3 days with a primary antibody against CYP2E1 (Sigma-Aldrich Corp., St. Louis, MO, USA, 1:50). Subsequently, the slices were incubated for 2 days with CyTM3-conjugated AffiniPure; F(ab′)2 fragment donkey anti-rabbit secondary antibody (Dianova, Hamburg, Germany, 1:100). The nuclei were visualized by counterstaining with 4,6-diamidino-2-phenylindole. In order to allow 3D imaging of the thick slices, the tissue was cleared by successive immersion in 50% (*v*/*v*), 75% (*v*/*v*) and 100% (*v*/*v*) tetrahydrofuran, 15 min each, followed by immersion in di-benzyl ether (Sigma-Aldrich Corp., St. Louis, MO, USA) for at least 10 min. Subsequently, Z-stacks of approximately 120 µm-depth were acquired using a custom-modified inverted LSM MP7 (Zeiss, Jena, Germany) with an LD C-Apochromat 40 × 1.1 water immersion objective.

2.11. Image Analyses and 3D Reconstructions

In order to provide an unbiased and quantitative description of histological slices, a problem-specific image analysis pipeline was developed. Depending on the utilized staining and after performing necessary preprocessing, various related features were segmented. These segmentations were verified by domain knowledge experts, serving as a gold standard. Subsequent measurements were then performed before producing the final summary statistic. Both ImageJ [36] and Matlab R2019a were utilized throughout the quantification process. The former was used for exploration and the later for developing dedicated programs. In the case of bright field scans and after obtaining satisfactory segmentation of a CYP-positive area as well as the associated corresponding background, a ratio was recorded. For the 3D reconstruction, individual structures (nuclei, CYP-positive area and the vessels) were also first segmented and verified. The final reconstruction and visualization were prepared using Imaris 9.3 software.

2.12. Ammonia Assay

Ammonia concentrations were measured from 20 μL whole blood samples directly after collection. The analysis was done using the Blood Ammonia Meter PocketChem BA PA-4140 (Arkray.inc, Amstelveen, The Netherlands).

2.13. Transaminase Activity Assay

Alanine transaminase (ALT) and aspartate transaminase (AST) activities were measured from plasma samples after dilution 1:10 in PBS. The analysis was done at the Central Laboratory Facility at University Hospital RWTH Aachen (Aachen, Germany).

2.14. Statistical Analysis

Statistical analysis of the data other than the RNA-seq was done using SPSS software, version 26. An independent samples *t*-test was used. $p < 0.05$ was considered statistically significant.

3. Results

3.1. RNA-Seq Demonstrates Downregulation of Pericentral and Upregulation of Periportal Genes in Fibrosis

Genome-wide expression response caused by CCl_4. To study the influence of fibrosis on liver zonation, we established a mouse model with two intraperitoneal injections of 1 g/kg CCl_4 per week over 12 months (Figure 1A). Only a relatively mild fibrosis was observed up to six months (Figure 1B). However, between months 6 and 12, the mice progressed into severe fibrosis characterized by wide Sirius red positive fibrotic streets, regenerative nodules and fibrosis-associated macroscopically visible tumor nodules (Figure 1B).

For RNA-seq analysis CCl_4-treated mice were processed after 0, 2, 6 and 12 months; olive oil controls were included after 2 and 12 months. Liver tissues of six mice per condition were analyzed (Figure 2A). A principal component analysis (PCA) of the RNA-seq data showed a good clustering of each group of six mice (Figure 2B). Treatment with CCl_4 caused a shift in the inverse direction of principal component 1 (PC1) that explains ~30% of the variance in the data (Figure 2B). PC2 represents the combined effects of olive oil, the solvent of CCl_4, and aging (Figure 2B). Differential gene expression analysis revealed that 80/85, 95/89 and 261/902 genes were significantly [abs(logFC) $\geq$ 1.5 and FDR $\leq$ 0.05] up/downregulated after 2, 6 and 12 months of CCl_4 treatment compared to olive oil controls, respectively, with partially very strong, more than 1000-fold expression changes (Figure 2C; lists of differential genes: Table S1). Strongly and consistently upregulated genes (Figure 2D) comprise extracellular matrix-associated genes, such as *Col28a1*, whose role in liver fibrosis is well-known; the variable domains of immunoglobulin heavy chains, suggesting infiltration of B cells/plasma cells [37], e.g., Ighv10-3, Ighv1-9, Ighv4-57-1, Ighv1-22, Ighv4-57-1; the liver-derived peptide hormone hepcidin-2 which supports iron homeostasis [38]; and some factors that so far have not been considered as primary genes affected by liver damage, such as gliomedin (*Gldn*), a protein expressed by myelinating Schwann cells [39] and the leucine-rich repeat and transmembrane domain-containing protein 2 (Lrtm2). Among the strongest downregulated genes (Figure 2D) are several major urinary proteins (Mups), also known as $\alpha_2\mu$-globulins, such as Mup19, Mup21, Mup15, Mup17, Mup-ps16, Mup-ps14 and Mup12. Expression of Mup proteins is known to be induced by androgens and they are physiologically relevant, because they bind small hydrophobic molecules, such as steroid hormones, lipids and retinoids in plasma [40]; several cytochrome P450 enzymes; the sushi domain-containing protein 4 (SUSD4) which inhibits complement factors [41]; calpains (e.g., capn11, Capn8) that act as calcium-dependent cysteine proteases, fatty acid elongase 3 (Elovl3); and roquois homeobox protein 1 (lrx1-6) that is known as a cardiac transcription factor [42]. The role of many of these differential genes in liver fibrosis remains unknown. Characterization of the CCl_4-induced expression response by pathway analysis using the functional genomics tools PROGENy identified the inflammatory pathways TGFβ, NFκB, TNFα and hypoxia-induced signaling as most active (Figure 2E; Table S2), which is in agreement with previous studies [43]. Estrogen and androgen associated pathways were among the most decreased in the CCl_4-exposed livers for all time points compared to corresponding oil samples. Transcription factor (TF) activities were inferred with DoRothEA and were dominated by TF with an increased activity that mediate inflammation (e.g., NFKb1, Stat1) cell stress as well as hypoxia response (Hif1a, Trp53, Atf1) and support proliferation (e.g., E2f1, Ef3, Egr1). TFs with reduced activities are known to mediate mature liver functions, such as Hnf4a, Hnf1a, Esr2 and the Fox genes (Figure 2F; Table S3). Enriched GO-terms such as actin-binding, angiogenesis, cell cycle, death and immune response further round out the picture of an inflamed, regenerating tissue (Figure 2G; Table S4).

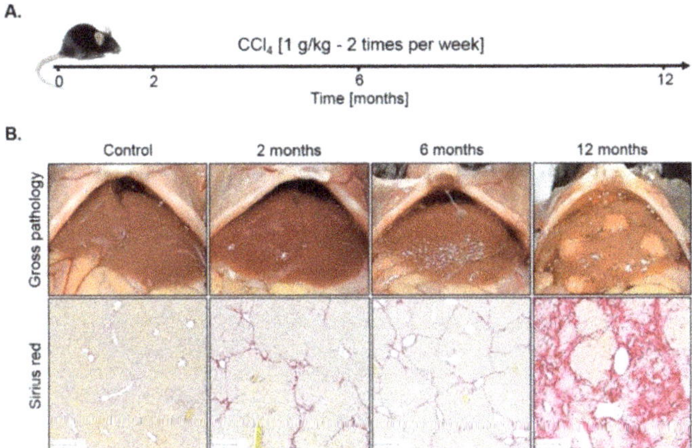

Figure 1. Mouse model of liver fibrosis induced by CCl_4 administration. (**A**) Treatment schedule. (**B**) Macroscopical alterations and visualization of fibrosis by Sirius red staining. Scale bars: 200 μm.

The solvent controls with olive oil alone showed expression changes after 2 and 12 months, respectively, compared to untreated mice at time zero (Table S5). No age-matched untreated controls were included, because the study was designed to identify CCl_4 induced expression changes. Administration of CCl_4 in oil and comparison to oil controls represents a frequently used protocol.

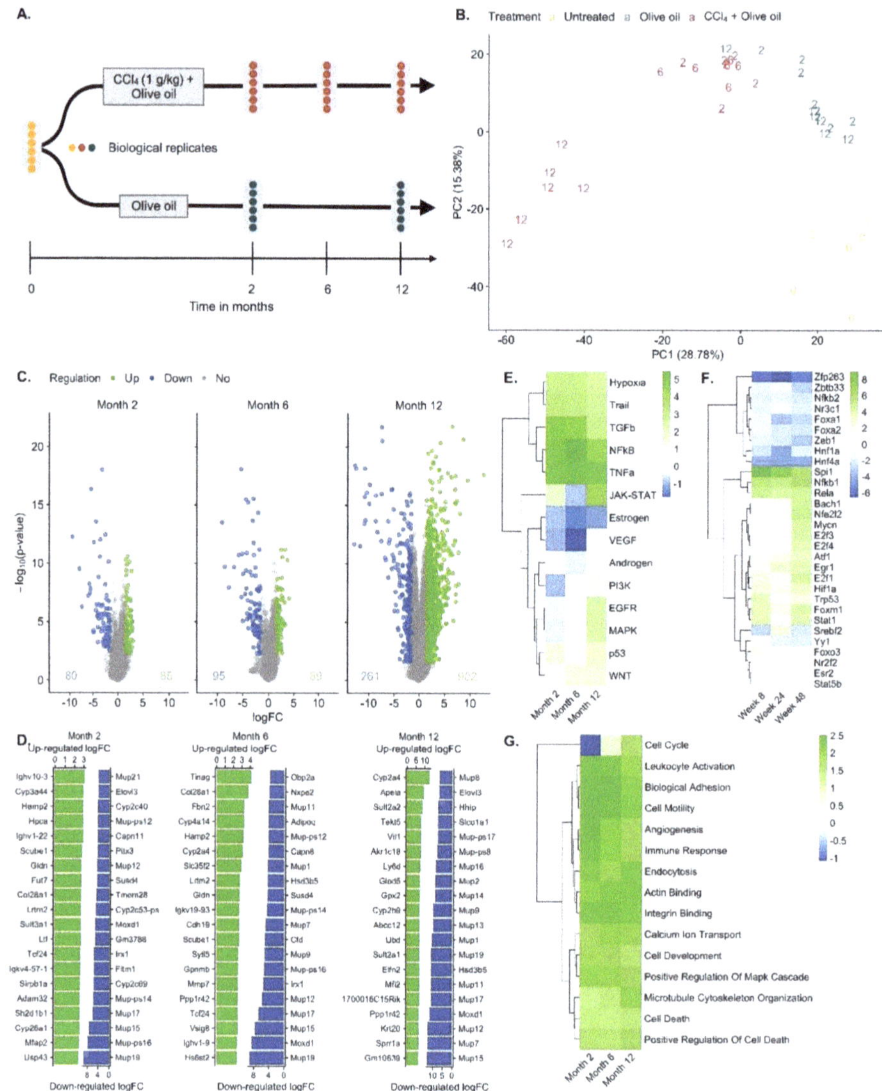

Figure 2. Bioinformatics of RNA-seq data of mouse liver tissue after exposure to CCl_4 for up to one year. **A**. Analysis schedule; **B**. Principal component analysis (PCA). Untreated mice at the time point zero (0), the day of onset of exposure for the other mouse groups, period of olive oil exposure in blue (2 and 12 months) and period of CCl_4 (solved in olive oil) exposure (2, 6 and 12 months) in red. **C**. Visualization of significantly up (green) and downregulated (blue) genes after 2, 6 and 12 months of CCl_4 exposure. **D**. The 20 most up- and downregulated genes after 2, 6 and 12 months exposure to CCl_4. **E**. Up- and downregulated pathways via PROGENy. The color legend indicates pathway activity (z-score). **F**. Transcription factor (TF) activities computed with DoRothEA. The color legend indicates TF activity (normalized enrichment score, NES). **G**. Enriched Gene Ontology (GO) groups. The color legend indicates the degree of enrichment (NES).

CCl_4-induced expression response in relation to zonated genes. To study a possible zonation of genes up- or downregulated in CCl_4-induced fibrosis, a consensus list of pericentral and periportal genes was established, containing 136 and 83 genes, respectively (Table S6). To our knowledge, three previous studies identified genes with zonated expression [31–33], whose overlap was relatively low (Table S6; Figure S5). Hence, genes were included in the consensus list, when they were identified as pericentral or periportal by at least two of the three published studies (Table S6). Genes were ranked by a gene-level statistic (here moderated t-value provided by limma) indicating the strength of their deregulation in response to CCl_4 treatment with upregulated genes at the top ranks (left side of the x-axis) and downregulated at the bottom of the list (right) (Figure 3A). Each vertical line on top of the x-axis represents a member of the pericentral or periportal gene set. The y-axis represents the enrichment score (ES), where values higher than zero indicate enrichment of zonated genes among upregulated and values smaller than zero among downregulated genes. Pericentral genes were significantly enriched among downregulated genes at all time points of CCl_4 treatment (Gene Set Enrichment Analysis (GSEA), p-values of 3.99×10^{-4} for month 2, 3.73×10^{-4} for month 6 and 2.77×10^{-4} for month 12). Periportal genes were significantly enriched among upregulated genes only after two and six but not after 12 months of CCl_4 treatment (GSEA, p-values of 1.42×10^{-4} for month 2, 0.013 for month 6). (Figure 3B). P-values were not adjusted for multiple hypothesis testing as we tested only 2 gene sets per signature. Leading edge analysis identified a set of downregulated pericentral and upregulated periportal genes across all time points that are mainly driving the significant GSEA results (Figure 3C, Table S7). We also characterized the overlap of pericentral/periportal genes and the most responsive genes of CCl_4 treatment across all time points using over-representation analysis. Analyzing the downregulated pericentral genes, biological processes such as monocarboxylic acid metabolism, epoxygenase P450, and glutamine family catabolic process and the KEGG pathways primary bile acid biosynthesis as well as arginine and proline metabolism were enriched; the transcription factor small heterodimer partner (SHP; synonym: Nr0b2), an interaction partner of HNF4α and LXRα, showed increased activity (Figure 3D). Among the periportal upregulated genes' GO groups associated with lipid metabolism, triglyceride lipase, and phospholipid transport were enriched. Some hits are listed in Figure 3D and the complete list is available in Table S8. Thus, during CCl_4-induced liver fibrosis, a complex conglomerate of inflammatory pathways orchestrate downregulation of pericentral and upregulation of periportal genes that further will be referred to as 'periportalized' lobular zonation.

Expression of several genes with a zonated expression pattern was validated by quantitative real-time polymerase chain reaction (qRT-PCR, Figure 4). Analysis of pericentrally expressed genes, solute carrier family 1 member 2 (GLT1), glutamine synthetase (GS), ornithine amino-transferase (Oat), and the vascular/hepatic-type arginine vasopressin receptor (Avpr1a), confirmed a strong downregulation during CCl_4 treatment, particularly between months 6 and 12 (Figure 4A). In contrast, the periportal genes glutaminase 2 (Gls2), the urea cycle enzyme carbamoyl phosphate synthetase 1 (CPS1) and the gluconeogenesis enzyme phosphoenolpyruvate carboxykinase 1 (PCK1) showed an increase until month 6, followed by a decrease at month 12 (Figure 4B). The urea cycle enzyme arginase 1 (Arg1) showed little change until month six followed by a moderate decrease at month twelve (Figure 4B). Thus, qRT-PCR of selected genes confirmed a strong decrease of the pericentral genes, while the changes of periportal genes are weaker and more complex, characterized by an increase until month 6 and a decrease between months 6 and 12, an observation that will be interpreted in the context of the immunostaining data described below.

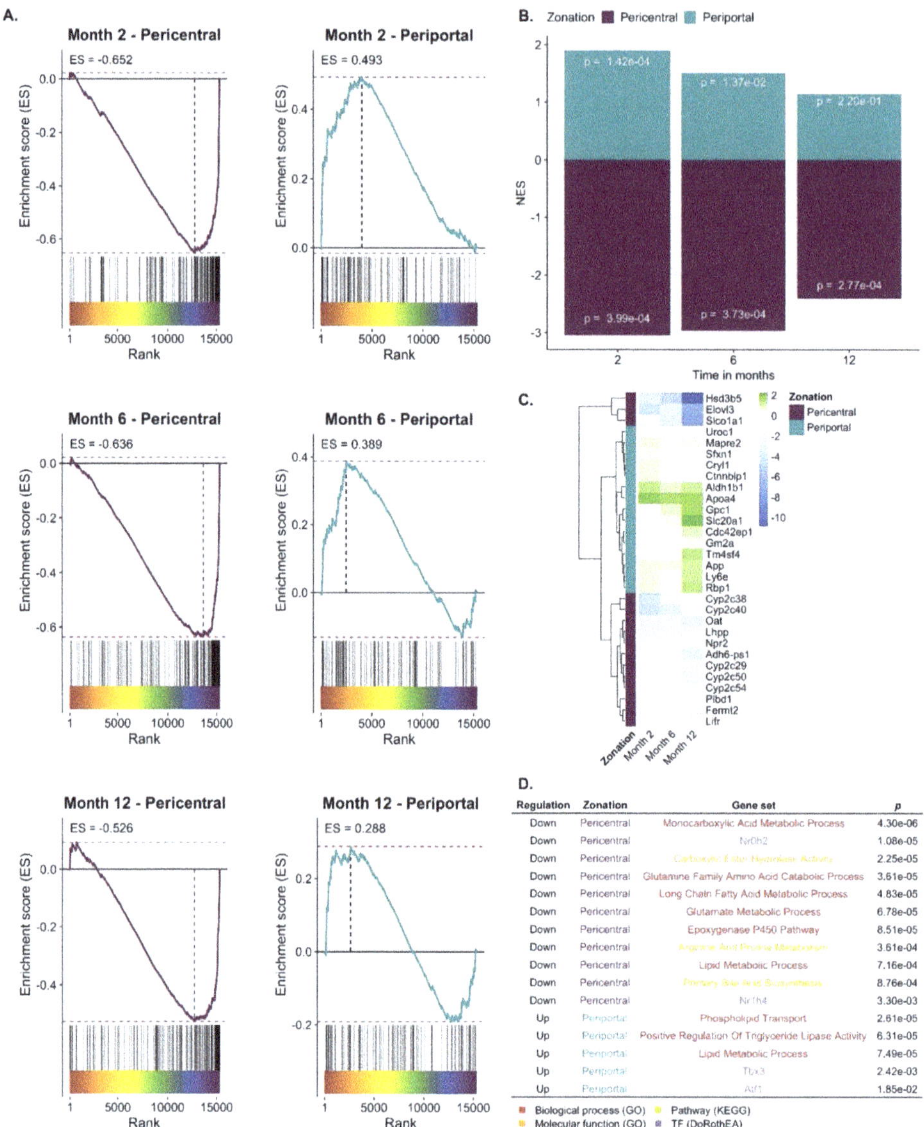

Figure 3. Periportalization of CCl_4 exposed liver tissue. **A**. Enrichment of pericentral and periportal genes among genes up or downregulated by CCl_4 exposure. **B**. Summarized results of Gene Set Enrichment Analysis (GSEA) showing normalized enrichment score (NES) and *p*-values. **C**. Leading edge of periportal and pericentral gene set that mainly accounts for the enrichment score of the gene set. The color scheme indicates the logFC. **D**. Selection of GO-terms and TFs that characterize the overlap of CCl_4 signature and pericentral/periportal gene sets.

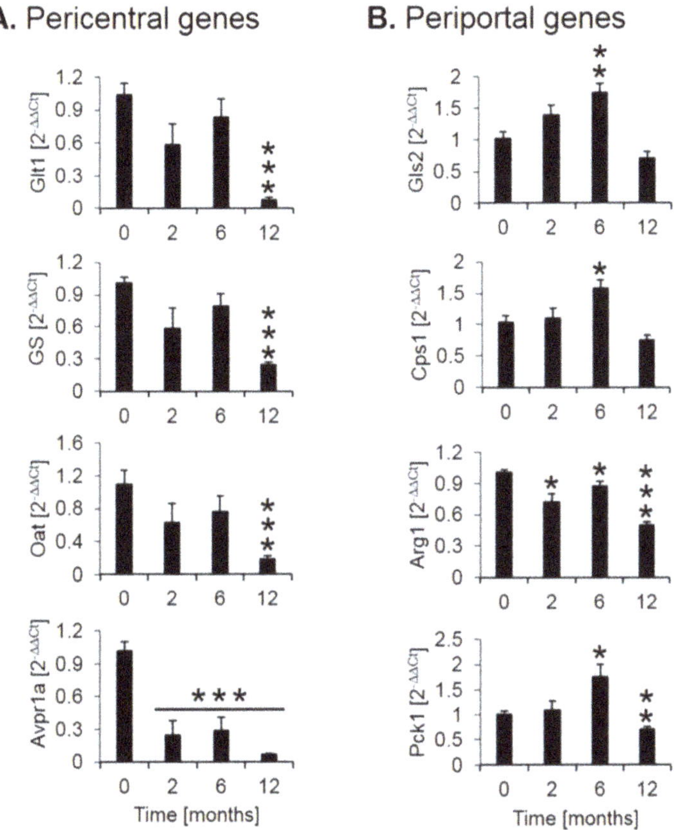

Figure 4. Quantitative real-time polymerase chain reaction (qRT-PCR) confirmation of selected pericentral (**A**) and (**B**) periportal genes. The x-axis represents the time of CCl_4 treatment, while the y-axis depicts relative RNA expression normalized to controls (0 months). Glt1: glutamate transporter 1; GS: glutamine synthetase; Oat: ornithine aminotransferase; Avpr1a: arginine vasopressin receptor 1A; Gls2: glutaminase 2; Cps1: carbamoyl phosphate synthetase I; Arg1: arginase 1; Pck1: phosphoenolpyruvate carboxykinase 1. The data are means ± standard errors of 6 mice per time point. * $p < 0.05$; ** $p < 0.01$; *** $p < 0.001$ compared to the untreated controls (0).

Spatio-temporal analysis of periportalization. Further insight into spatio-temporal changes of zonation was obtained by immunostaining. Similar results were observed for the pericentrally expressed enzymes, cytochrome P450 (CYP) 3A, 1A, 2C, 2E1 and GS (Figure 5A). Compared to controls, the CYP positive areas around central veins became narrower after 2 and 6 months of CCl_4 administration. However, contacts between CYP2E1 positive areas present in controls (Figure 5B, control; Supplementary Video 1) were maintained even after 6 months of repeated CCl_4 treatment, giving the impression of central-to-central bridging (Figure 5B, CCl_4; Supplementary Video 2). Until month 12, CYP immunostaining decreased massively. Similarly, GS showed central-to-central bridging at month two and six, followed by an almost complete loss of expression at month 12 (Figure 5A). Image analysis confirmed the decrease of the immunostained CYP1A1-positive area (Figure 5C). In controls, the periportally expressed urea cycle enzymes, arginase 1 and CPS1 showed a periportal to midzonal staining pattern with a relatively narrow negative pericentral zone (Figure 5A). The vessels in the center of arginase 1 or CPS1 positive regions are portal veins, while the vessels in negative regions represent central veins. During the one-year-period of CCl_4 administration, fibrotic streets formed between the central veins, which were particularly obvious between months 6 and 12 (Figure 5A). No expression of arginase 1 or CPS1 occurred in the fibrotic streets, while these enzymes were expressed in hepatocytes at similar levels as in control mice, even in the regenerative nodules at month 12. Whole slide scans immunostained for CYP1A and arginase 1 illustrated the narrowing of the pericentral region expressing CYP1A (months 2 and 4), followed by an almost complete loss at month 12 (Figure 5D). Vice versa, arginase1 expression extended into the pericentral region at months 2, 6 and 12 (Figure 5D).

3.2. *Confirmation of Periportalization in Further Mouse Models of Liver Fibrosis*

Bile duct ligation (BDL). This mouse model was investigated because it represents a periportal fibrosis model, in contrast to the CCl_4 model described above, where pericentral fibrosis is induced. Ligation of the common bile duct leads to the formation of bile infarcts due to the rupture of the apical hepatocyte membrane in the acute phase up to day three [22]. In the chronic phase after approximately seven days, the liver adapts to the obstruction of the bile duct, bile infarcts do no longer occur and the infarct regions regenerate. However, a slowly progressing periportal fibrosis occurs in the chronic phase. In the present study, mice at day 21 after BDL were compared to sham-operated controls (Figure 6A). Macroscopically, BDL mice showed a strongly distended gallbladder with transparent, so-called 'white bile' (Figure 6B). Histologically, a strong ductular response was observed accompanied by periportal fibrosis (Figure 6B).

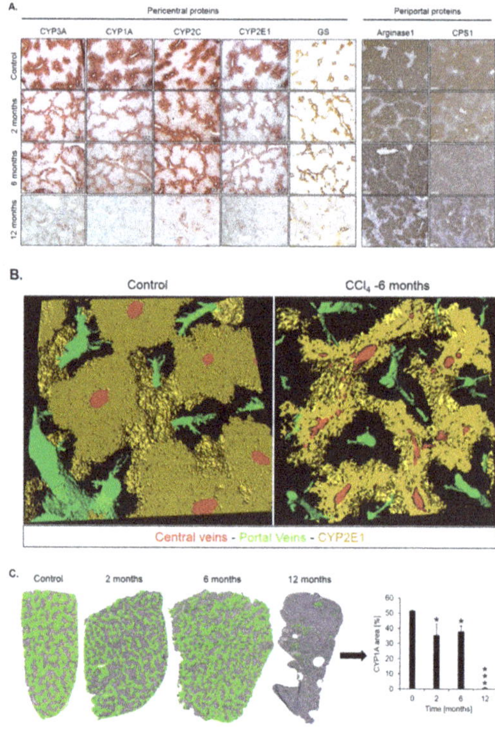

Figure 5. *Cont.*

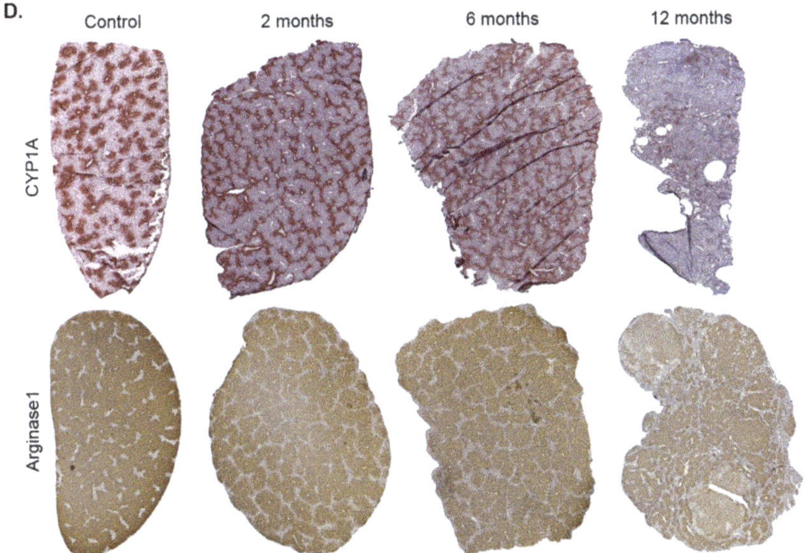

Figure 5. Spatio-temporal analysis of periportalization of selected pericentral and periportal enzymes. (**A**) Immunostaining of the pericentral proteins cytochrome P450 3A, 1A, 2C, 2E and glutamine synthetase (GS) as well as the periportal proteins arginase 1 and carbamoyl phosphate synthetase 1 (CPS1). The left margin indicates the time of treatment with CCl_4. Scale bars: 200 µm. (**B**) 3D-Reconstructions of CYP1A immunostained liver tissue showing normal pericentral zonation in control (left), and central-to-central bridging at month six of CCl_4 intoxication. (**C**) Whole slide scans of CYP1A-immunostained liver lobules at 2, 6 and 12 months after CCl_4 treatment with segmentation (green) and quantification of the fraction of the CYP1A positive area. The data are means ± standard errors of 3 mice per time point. * $p < 0.05$; *** $p < 0.001$ compared to the untreated controls (0). (**D**) Whole slide scans of CYP1A and arginase1 positive liver tissue.

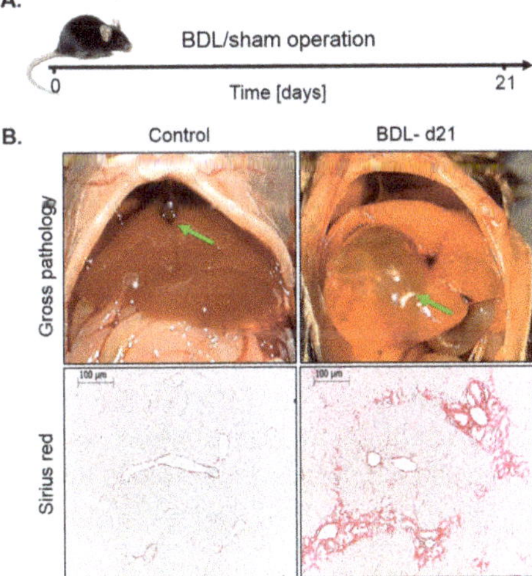

Figure 6. Periportal fibrosis after bile duct ligation (BDL). (**A**) Experimental schedule. (**B**) Macroscopic appearance and visualization of fibrosis by Sirius red staining. Scale bars: 100 µm.

Immunostaining for CYP2E1 and GS showed a massive decrease 21 days after BDL (Figure 7A). While the CYP2E1 positive area amounted to approximately 50% of the total tissue area in controls, this value fell to only approximately 14% after BDL (Figure 7C,D). Corresponding analysis of the periportal enzymes arginase 1 and CPS1 showed that the negative pericentral regions in controls become positive ('periportalized') after BDL (Figure 7B). Whole slide scans immunostained for CYP2E1 and CPS1 confirmed the results shown in Figure 7 (Figure S1). Therefore, BDL associated fibrosis was accompanied by similar changes in zonation as fibrosis induced by chronic administration of CCl_4. $Mdr2^{-/-}$ mice represent a further model of periportal fibrosis. Similar to the CCl_4 model and BDL, also eight- and 64-week-old knockout mice showed reduced expression of CYP2E1 (Figure S2).

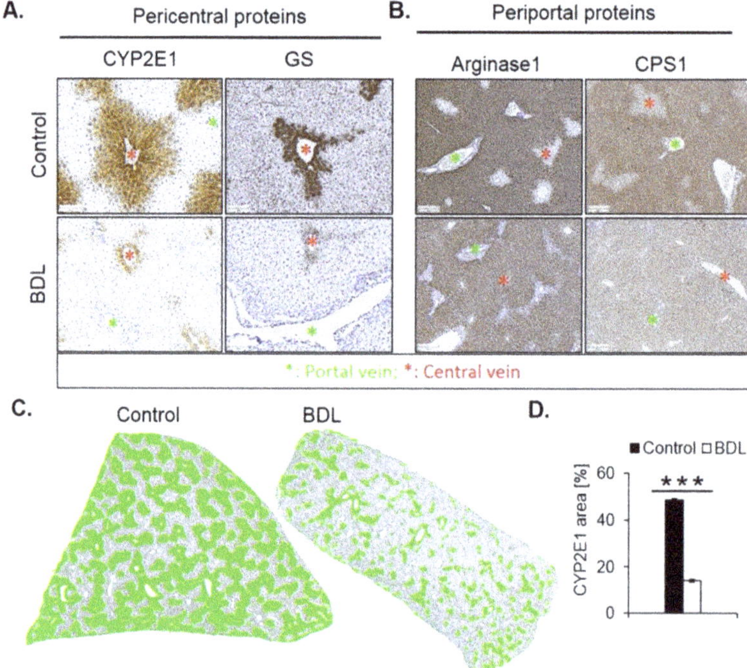

Figure 7. Periportalization of lobular zonation after BDL. (**A**) Immunostaining of the pericentral proteins CYP2E1 and GS. Scale bars: 100 µm. (**B**) Immunostaining of the periportal proteins arginase1 and CPS1. Scale bars: 200 µm. (**C**) CYP2E1-immunostained whole slide scans of liver lobules of BDL mice, and segmentation of the positive area (green). (**D**) Quantification of the fraction of CYP2E1 positive tissue 21 days after BDL and in controls. The data are means ± standard errors of 3 mice per group. *** $p < 0.001$ compared to the sham controls (0).

3.3. *Functional Consequences of Compromised Zonation: Adaptation to Hepatotoxicants*

Fibrosis associated disturbed lobular zonation causes several adverse functional consequences. An example is compromised ammonia detoxification. The loss of the fine-tuned interaction of the periportal high capacity (urea cycle) and the pericentral high-affinity (GS) compartments leads to increased ammonia blood concentrations. We compared ammonia concentrations in the portal vein, liver vein and heart blood of mice after 1 year of treatment with CCl_4 and untreated controls. The much higher concentrations in the hepatic vein of CCl_4 mice demonstrate the loss of the capacity of the fibrotic liver to reduce ammonia to very low concentrations of <30 µg/dL (Figure 8).

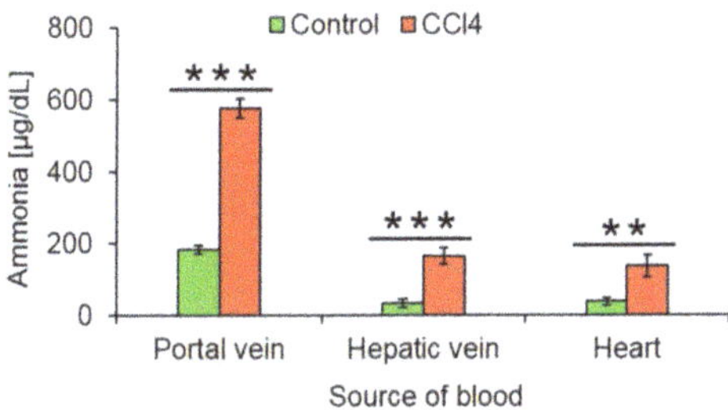

Figure 8. Increased ammonia blood concentrations after 1 year CCl_4 treatment. The data are means ± standard errors of 6 mice per group. ** $p < 0.01$; *** $p < 0.001$ compared to the corresponding controls (0).

Moreover, we wondered if the loss of the pericentrally located cytochrome P450 enzymes may lead to resistance against hepatotoxicants that require metabolic activation by these enzymes. To test this hypothesis, we exposed one year CCl_4-treated fibrotic mice and olive oil controls to a hepatotoxic dose of APAP (200 mg/kg) (Figure 9A). In oil controls, APAP macroscopically caused the characteristic dotted pattern, indicating pericentral necrosis (Figure 9B) that was confirmed histologically (Figure 9D). Interestingly, APAP-induced no visible necrosis in the fibrotic livers after one year of chronic CCl_4 intoxication (Figure 9B,D, Figure S4). These results were confirmed by analysis of the liver enzymes ALT and AST that increased after APAP administration in oil controls but not in fibrotic livers (Figure 9C). Immunostaining for CYP2E1 illustrated that the CYP2E1 positive pericentral regions were destroyed by APAP (Figure 9E). In contrast, the periportalized fibrotic livers without detectable CYP2E1 expression did not show any necrotic hepatocytes around central veins (Figure 9E). The corresponding H&E-stained whole slide scans are available in Figure S4).

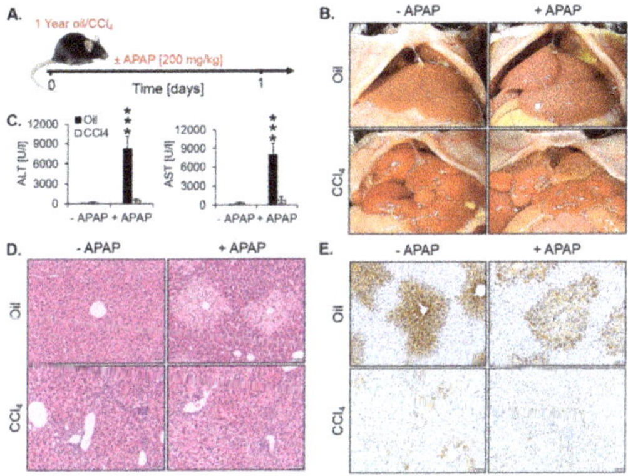

Figure 9. Acetaminophen (APAP) resistance of mice after one year of treatment with CCl_4. (**A**) Experimental schedule. (**B**) Macroscopic appearance. (**C**) The concentration of liver enzymes in the blood. The data are means ± standard errors of 5 mice per time point. *** $p < 0.001$ compared to the corresponding controls without APAP intoxication. (**D**) H&E-stained tissue. Scale bars: 100 µm. (**E**) CYP2E1 immunostaining. Scale bars: 100 µm.

To analyze whether fibrosis-associated resistance to APAP is a generalizable phenomenon, a similar experiment was performed in mice with BDL-associated fibrosis. For this purpose, BDL mice and sham controls were overnight fasted from the evening of day 20 after surgery and 200 mg/kg APAP were administered on the morning of day 21 to be analyzed 24 h later (Figure 10A). Interestingly, BDL mice were resistant to APAP (Figure 10C,D; Figure S5), similar to the observation made in CCl_4-induced fibrosis.

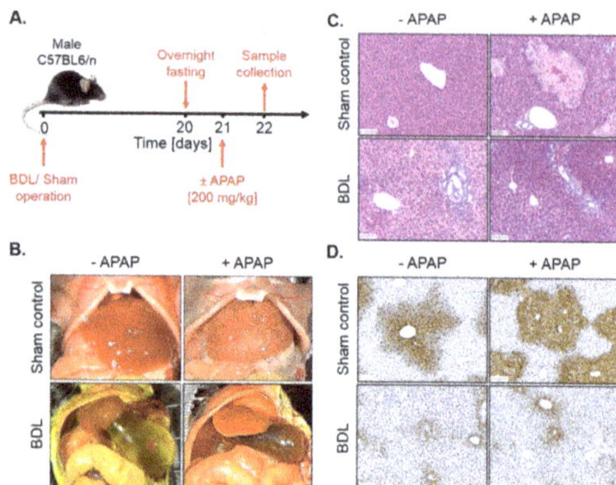

Figure 10. APAP resistance of mice 21 days after BDL. (**A**) Experimental schedule. (**B**) Macroscopic appearance. (**C**) H&E staining. Scale bars: 100 µm. (**D**) CYP2E1 immunostaining. Scale bars: 100 µm.

4. Discussion

Little is known about how liver fibrosis influences hepatic zonation. Here, we show that fibrosis of different etiologies causes 'periportalization', which means that the entire liver lobule including the pericentral region adopts a periportal pattern of gene expression (graphical abstract). We first observed this phenomenon in the mouse model of CCl_4 established here, where severe fibrosis was induced by repeated induction of pericentral liver necrosis over a period of one year. Recently, several genome-wide studies have identified genes that show a preferentially pericentral or periportal expression pattern [31–33]. We established a consensus list of periportal and pericentral genes that overlapped in at least two of the three studies. The genome-wide analysis showed that pericentral genes are enriched among the genes downregulated by CCl_4, while the periportal genes are enriched among the upregulated genes. This phenomenon occurred already at the earliest analyzed time point of two months.

Analysis of selected pericentral genes by immunostaining and qRT-PCR showed that the downregulation of pericentral genes occurred in two phases. Phase 1 until month 6 is characterized by 'central-to-central bridging'. In this period, the pericentral area with positive immunostaining of e.g., cytochrome P450 enzymes becomes narrower but areas of contact between neighboring pericentral regions are maintained. In this first phase, RNA levels of the analyzed pericentral genes show a statistically significant but moderate, less than 2-fold decrease. Phase 2 occurs between months six and twelve and is characterized by a massive formation of fibrotic streets. In this period, immunostaining of cytochrome P450s and glutamine synthetase is almost completely lost and RNA levels decrease by more than 10-fold.

Immunostaining of the periportal genes arginase 1 and CPS1 shows that they begin to be newly expressed in the pericentral region during CCl_4 treatment. In controls, they are expressed in periportal and midzonal hepatocytes but not in a narrow region around the central vein. While pericentral proteins retreat, arginase 1 and CPS1 advance towards the central vein until finally all hepatocytes express these periportal genes. The extension of periportal enzymes into the pericentral region is accompanied by a moderate but statistically significant increase in RNA levels (e.g., of CPS1) at months 2 and 6. However, between months 6 and 12, expression of several periportal genes decreases again. This is most likely explained by the massive formation of fibrotic streets that contain myofibroblasts, macrophages and further inflammation-associated cells that do not express (periportal) liver genes. Therefore, periportal liver genes will be diluted by the RNA of the cells forming fibrotic streets. Nevertheless, immunostaining suggests that expression levels, e.g., of arginase 1 and CPS1, do not decrease in the remaining hepatocytes of the regenerative nodules at month 12. Rather, the hepatocyte fraction of total liver mass decreases.

The loss of pericentrally expressed metabolizing enzymes has different consequences. One of them is an increase of ammonia concentrations in the liver vein blood and the systemic circulation. During the passage through the fibrotic, 1-year CCl_4-treated liver, ammonia concentrations still decrease from ~600 μg/dL concentrations in the portal vein to ~180 μg/dL in the liver vein. However, the destruction of the pericentral high affinity detoxification system by glutamine synthetase [15,16] prevents further reduction of ammonia concentrations to normal levels (<30 μg/dL). The reason for the strongly increased ammonia concentrations in portal vein blood (~600 μg/dL) may be due to increased intestinal ammonia production from urea. Because of chronic liver damage mice develop secondary kidney damage [22] with increased blood concentrations of urea. Because of the leaky gut-blood barrier in chronic liver damage, urea reaches bacterial ureases in the intestinal lumen that generate ammonia, which is absorbed into intestinal capillaries and drains into the portal vein [44–46]. However, the latter mechanism still requires experimental validation. The data clearly show that 'periportalization' of liver lobules causes loss of detoxifying functions. The increase in ammonia or urea concentrations to the observed levels will lead to long-term consequences but is not immediately life-threatening. This is in contrast to acute intoxication by hepatotoxicants that may be lethal. In this context, the loss of pericentrally expressed metabolizing enzymes can be interpreted as an adaptive response to chronic CCl_4 exposure. CCl_4 is metabolically activated by cytochrome P450 2E1 and further CYPs to form the reactive trichloromethyl free radical and the trichloromethyl peroxyl radical [2]. Therefore, the downregulation of cytochrome P450 enzymes is an efficient strategy to survive repeated exposure to toxins that require metabolic activation. This leads to the question as to why also mouse models of periportal fibrosis cause downregulation of pericentral genes. In the present study, we used BDL that is known to preferentially cause periportal liver damage and fibrosis [47,48]. Also, $mdr2^{-/-}$ mice are a model of periportal fibrosis [49]. At first glance, it may be difficult to understand why the downregulation of pericentral genes should offer a survival advantage to BDL and $mdr2^{-/-}$ mice. In this context, co-evolution between plants and herbivores should be considered [50]. Plants responded to herbivory by formation of plant toxins, many of them metabolically activated by pericentral liver enzymes, such as pyrrolizidine alkaloids and mycotoxins [51]. Herbivores responded by several evolutionary strategies, particularly by novel detoxifying enzymes. Also the periportalization of liver lobules under toxic stress could be interpreted as an adaptive process in animal–plant warfare. Periportalization seems to represent a stereotypical response to different types of inflammatory stress, possibly because the liver lacks the ability to activate distinct adaptive zonation programs for pericentral and periportal damage. This corresponds to previous studies, demonstrating that different types of acute and chronic inflammatory stimuli activate the same gene regulatory networks, whereby upregulation of inflammatory genes occurs simultaneously to the downregulation of metabolic genes [52]; interestingly, both inflammatory and metabolic genes are controlled by the same upstream mechanisms [52]. A strength of the present study is that six individual mice were included for each condition of the time-resolved analysis. This allowed sufficient statistical power to demonstrate the significance of the process of periportalization identified here.

In conclusion, liver fibrosis leads to periportalization of liver lobules. Periportalization occurs as a common response to pericentral and also periportal damage. It allows the liver to adapt to the repeated exposure to hepatotoxic compounds that require metabolic activation by pericentrally expressed enzymes.

Supplementary Materials: The following are available online at http://www.mdpi.com/2073-4409/8/12/1556/s1: **Supplemental figures.** Figure S1. Immunostaining of CYP2E1 and CPS1 in whole slide scans after BDL. Figure S2. Sirius red and CYP2E1 staining of 8 and 64 week-old $mdr2^{-/-}$ mice and 64 week-old wild type (WT) mice. Figure S3. H&E staining of livers (whole slide scans) after 1-year exposure to olive oil and CCl_4. Figure S4. H&E staining of livers (whole slide scans) 21 days after BDL compared to sham-operated controls. Figure S5. Overlap of pericentral and periportal genes between three different studies. **Supplemental tables.** Table S1. Significantly (abs(logFC) $\geq$ 1.5 and FDR $\leq$ 0.05) up and downregulated genes after 2, 6 and 12 months of treatment of the mice with 1 g/kg CCl_4. Table S2. Characterization of CCl_4 induced expression response by PROGENy pathway analysis. Table S3. Transcription factor activities of genes differentially expressed after CCl_4 exposure. The column confidence is an empirical classification indicating how confident we are about the TF activity prediction based on the confidence of its regulon. The confidence class range from A–E with being A the highest confident class. Table S4. Analysis of GO group enrichment based on genes differentially expressed after CCl_4 exposure. Only those GO terms are shown that were significantly enriched (FDR $\leq$ 0.05) in at least one-time point. Table S5. Significantly (abs(logFC) $\geq$ 1.5 and FDR $\leq$ 0.05) up and downregulated genes after 2, 6 and 12 months of treatment of the mice with olive oil. Table S6. List of zonated pericentral and periportal genes. A. Consensus list including genes that were identified as zonated in at least two of the three studies Braeuning et al., 2006; Saito et al., 2013; Halpern et al., 2017. B. Zonated genes in Braeuning et al., 2006; C. Zonated genes in Saito et al., 2013; D. Zonated genes in Halpern et al., 2017. Table S7. Table of leading-edge genes for pericentral and periportal gene set members that mainly account for the corresponding gene set enrichment score. Table S8. Significantly over-represented gene sets (p-value $\leq$ 0.05) that characterize the overlap of the CCl_4 signature and pericentral/periportal gene set, respectively. **Supplemental Videos.** Supplemental video 1. 3D reconstructions of control mouse liver immunostained for CYP2E1. Supplemental video 2. 3D reconstructions of fibrotic mouse liver on month 6 of repeated CCl_4 intoxication immunostained for CYP2E1.

Author Contributions: A.G.; J.G.H.: Study concept and design; acquisition of data; analysis and interpretation of data; drafting of the manuscript; critical revision of the manuscript; obtained funding; study supervision. M.M.; W.M.; R.H.; Y.A.A.; T.A.; E.A.A.; K.M.S.; J.R.; M.-L.B.; M.H.: acquisition of data; analysis and interpretation of data; drafting of the manuscript; critical revision of the manuscript. C.H.H.; J.S.-R.: Biostatistical analyses of the RNA-seq. data; analysis and interpretation of data; drafting of the manuscript; critical revision of the manuscript. M.M.-S.; R.G.: critical revision of the manuscript. A.Z.; D.D.: Image analysis; 3D reconstructions; drafting of the manuscript; critical revision of the manuscript. C.T.: Drafting of the manuscript; critical revision of the manuscript; obtained funding.

Funding: This study was supported by the BMBF (Germany) funded project LiSyM (FKZ 031L0052; 031L0045; 031L0049).

Acknowledgments: We thank Zaynab Hobloss and Brigitte Begher-Tibbe -Leibniz Research Centre for Working Environment and Human Factors, Technical University Dortmund, Dortmund, Germany, for competent technical assistance.

Availability of Data and Material: The code to perform the presented RNA-seq study is written in R and is freely available on GitHub: https://github.com/saezlab/LiverPeriportalization [53].

Conflicts of Interest: The authors declare no conflicts of interest.

Abbreviations

APAP	acetaminophen
ALT	alanine transaminase
AST	aspartate transaminase
i.p.	intraperitoneal
BDL	bile duct ligation
PBS	phosphate-buffered saline
CCl4	carbon tetrachloride
CYP450	cytochrome P450
CPS1	carbamoyl phosphate synthase
FFPE	formalin-fixed paraffin embedded
GS	glutamine synthetase
Mdr2	multidrug resistance gene 2
RNA-seq	RNA sequencing
TGFβ	Transforming growth factor beta
NFκB	nuclear factor kappa-light-chain-enhancer of activated B cells
TNFα	Tumor necrosis factor alpha
TCA-cycle	tricarboxylic acid cycle
GAPDH	Glyceraldehyde-3-phosphate dehydrogenase
UMI	unique molecular identifier
GSEA	Gene Set Enrichment Analysis
MGI	Mouse Genome Informatics

References

1. Pimpin, L.; Cortez-Pinto, H.; Negro, F.; Corbould, E.; Lazarus, J.V.; Webber, L.; Sheron, N.; Committee, E.H.S. Burden of liver disease in Europe: Epidemiology and analysis of risk factors to identify prevention policies. *J. Hepatol.* **2018**, *69*, 718–735. [CrossRef] [PubMed]
2. Godoy, P.; Hewitt, N.J.; Albrecht, U.; Andersen, M.E.; Ansari, N.; Bhattacharya, S.; Bode, J.G.; Bolleyn, J.; Borner, C.; Bottger, J.; et al. Recent advances in 2D and 3D in vitro systems using primary hepatocytes, alternative hepatocyte sources and non-parenchymal liver cells and their use in investigating mechanisms of hepatotoxicity, cell signaling and ADME. *Arch. Toxicol.* **2013**, *87*, 1315–1530. [CrossRef] [PubMed]
3. Weiskirchen, R.; Tacke, F. Liver fibrosis: Which mechanisms matter? *Clin. Liver Dis.* **2016**, *8*, 94–99. [CrossRef] [PubMed]
4. Gressner, A.M.; Weiskirchen, R. Modern pathogenetic concepts of liver fibrosis suggest stellate cells and TGF-beta as major players and therapeutic targets. *J. Cell Mol. Med.* **2006**, *10*, 76–99. [CrossRef]
5. Leist, M.; Ghallab, A.; Graepel, R.; Marchan, R.; Hassan, R.; Bennekou, S.H.; Limonciel, A.; Vinken, M.; Schildknecht, S.; Waldmann, T.; et al. Adverse outcome pathways: Opportunities, limitations and open questions. *Arch. Toxicol.* **2017**, *91*, 3477–3505. [CrossRef]
6. Hoehme, S.; Brulport, M.; Bauer, A.; Bedawy, E.; Schormann, W.; Hermes, M.; Puppe, V.; Gebhardt, R.; Zellmer, S.; Schwarz, M.; et al. Prediction and validation of cell alignment along microvessels as order principle to restore tissue architecture in liver regeneration. *Proc. Natl. Acad. Sci. USA* **2010**, *107*, 10371–10376. [CrossRef]
7. Gebhardt, R.; Matz-Soja, M. Liver zonation: Novel aspects of its regulation and its impact on homeostasis. *World J. Gastroenterol.* **2014**, *20*, 8491–8504. [CrossRef]
8. Kietzmann, T. Liver Zonation in Health and Disease: Hypoxia and Hypoxia-Inducible Transcription Factors as Concert Masters. *Int J. Mol. Sci.* **2019**, *20*. [CrossRef]
9. Schenk, A.; Ghallab, A.; Hofmann, U.; Hassan, R.; Schwarz, M.; Schuppert, A.; Schwen, L.O.; Braeuning, A.; Teutonico, D.; Hengstler, J.G.; et al. Physiologically-based modelling in mice suggests an aggravated loss of clearance capacity after toxic liver damage. *Sci. Rep.* **2017**, *7*, 6224. [CrossRef]
10. Sezgin, S.; Hassan, R.; Zuhlke, S.; Kuepfer, L.; Hengstler, J.G.; Spiteller, M.; Ghallab, A. Spatio-temporal visualization of the distribution of acetaminophen as well as its metabolites and adducts in mouse livers by MALDI MSI. *Arch. Toxicol.* **2018**, *92*, 2963–2977. [CrossRef]
11. Hewitt, N.J.; Lechon, M.J.; Houston, J.B.; Hallifax, D.; Brown, H.S.; Maurel, P.; Kenna, J.G.; Gustavsson, L.; Lohmann, C.; Skonberg, C.; et al. Primary hepatocytes: Current understanding of the regulation of metabolic enzymes and transporter proteins, and pharmaceutical practice for the use of hepatocytes in metabolism, enzyme induction, transporter, clearance, and hepatotoxicity studies. *Drug Metab. Rev.* **2007**, *39*, 159–234. [CrossRef] [PubMed]
12. Hammad, S.; Braeuning, A.; Meyer, C.; Mohamed, F.; Hengstler, J.G.; Dooley, S. A frequent misinterpretation in current research on liver fibrosis: The vessel in the center of CCl4-induced pseudolobules is a portal vein. *Arch. Toxicol.* **2017**, *91*, 3689–3692. [CrossRef] [PubMed]
13. Hoehme, S.; Hengstler, J.G.; Brulport, M.; Schafer, M.; Bauer, A.; Gebhardt, R.; Drasdo, D. Mathematical modelling of liver regeneration after intoxication with CCl(4). *Chem. Biol. Interact.* **2007**, *168*, 74–93. [CrossRef] [PubMed]
14. Bartl, M.; Pfaff, M.; Ghallab, A.; Driesch, D.; Henkel, S.G.; Hengstler, J.G.; Schuster, S.; Kaleta, C.; Gebhardt, R.; Zellmer, S.; et al. Optimality in the zonation of ammonia detoxification in rodent liver. *Arch. Toxicol.* **2015**, *89*, 2069–2078. [CrossRef] [PubMed]
15. Ghallab, A.; Celliere, G.; Henkel, S.G.; Driesch, D.; Hoehme, S.; Hofmann, U.; Zellmer, S.; Godoy, P.; Sachinidis, A.; Blaszkewicz, M.; et al. Model-guided identification of a therapeutic strategy to reduce hyperammonemia in liver diseases. *J. Hepatol.* **2016**, *64*, 860–871. [CrossRef] [PubMed]
16. Schliess, F.; Hoehme, S.; Henkel, S.G.; Ghallab, A.; Driesch, D.; Bottger, J.; Guthke, R.; Pfaff, M.; Hengstler, J.G.; Gebhardt, R.; et al. Integrated metabolic spatial-temporal model for the prediction of ammonia detoxification during liver damage and regeneration. *Hepatology* **2014**, *60*, 2040–2051. [CrossRef]
17. Van Straten, G.; van Steenbeek, F.G.; Grinwis, G.C.; Favier, R.P.; Kummeling, A.; van Gils, I.H.; Fieten, H.; Groot Koerkamp, M.J.; Holstege, F.C.; Rothuizen, J.; et al. Aberrant expression and distribution of enzymes of the urea cycle and other ammonia metabolizing pathways in dogs with congenital portosystemic shunts. *PLoS ONE* **2014**, *9*, e100077. [CrossRef]

18. Hernandez-Gea, V.; Friedman, S.L. Pathogenesis of liver fibrosis. *Annu. Rev. Pathol.* **2011**, *6*, 425–456. [CrossRef]
19. Luedde, T.; Schwabe, R.F. NF-kappaB in the liver—Linking injury, fibrosis and hepatocellular carcinoma. *Nat. Rev. Gastroenterol. Hepatol.* **2011**, *8*, 108–118. [CrossRef]
20. Tacke, F.; Weiskirchen, R. Update on hepatic stellate cells: Pathogenic role in liver fibrosis and novel isolation techniques. *Expert Rev. Gastroenterol. Hepatol.* **2012**, *6*, 67–80. [CrossRef]
21. Zimmermann, H.W.; Seidler, S.; Nattermann, J.; Gassler, N.; Hellerbrand, C.; Zernecke, A.; Tischendorf, J.J.; Luedde, T.; Weiskirchen, R.; Trautwein, C.; et al. Functional contribution of elevated circulating and hepatic non-classical CD14CD16 monocytes to inflammation and human liver fibrosis. *PLoS ONE* **2010**, *5*, e11049. [CrossRef] [PubMed]
22. Ghallab, A.; Hofmann, U.; Sezgin, S.; Vartak, N.; Hassan, R.; Zaza, A.; Godoy, P.; Schneider, K.M.; Guenther, G.; Ahmed, Y.A.; et al. Bile Microinfarcts in Cholestasis Are Initiated by Rupture of the Apical Hepatocyte Membrane and Cause Shunting of Bile to Sinusoidal Blood. *Hepatology* **2019**, *69*, 666–683. [CrossRef]
23. Torre, D.; Lachmann, A.; Ma'ayan, A. BioJupies: Automated Generation of Interactive Notebooks for RNA-Seq Data Analysis in the Cloud. *Cell Syst.* **2018**, *7*, 556.e3–561.e3. [CrossRef]
24. Robinson, M.D.; McCarthy, D.J.; Smyth, G.K. edgeR: A Bioconductor package for differential expression analysis of digital gene expression data. *Bioinformatics* **2010**, *26*, 139–140. [CrossRef] [PubMed]
25. Ritchie, M.E.; Phipson, B.; Wu, D.; Hu, Y.; Law, C.W.; Shi, W.; Smyth, G.K. limma powers differential expression analyses for RNA-sequencing and microarray studies. *Nucl. Acids Res.* **2015**, *43*, e47. [CrossRef]
26. Holland, C.H.; Szalai, B.; Saez-Rodriguez, J. Transfer of regulatory knowledge from human to mouse for functional genomic analysis. *Biochim. Biophys. Acta Gene Regul. Mech.* **2019**. [CrossRef]
27. Schubert, M.; Klinger, B.; Klunemann, M.; Sieber, A.; Uhlitz, F.; Sauer, S.; Garnett, M.J.; Bluthgen, N.; Saez-Rodriguez, J. Perturbation-response genes reveal signaling footprints in cancer gene expression. *Nat. Commun.* **2018**, *9*, 20. [CrossRef]
28. Garcia-Alonso, L.; Holland, C.H.; Ibrahim, M.M.; Turei, D.; Saez-Rodriguez, J. Benchmark and integration of resources for the estimation of human transcription factor activities. *Genome Res.* **2019**, *29*, 1363–1375. [CrossRef]
29. Alvarez, M.J.; Shen, Y.; Giorgi, F.M.; Lachmann, A.; Ding, B.B.; Ye, B.H.; Califano, A. Functional characterization of somatic mutations in cancer using network-based inference of protein activity. *Nat. Genet.* **2016**, *48*, 838–847. [CrossRef]
30. Korotkevich, G.; Sukhov, V.; Sergushichev, A. Fast gene set enrichment analysis. *bioRxiv* **2019**. [CrossRef]
31. Braeuning, A.; Ittrich, C.; Kohle, C.; Hailfinger, S.; Bonin, M.; Buchmann, A.; Schwarz, M. Differential gene expression in periportal and perivenous mouse hepatocytes. *FEBS J.* **2006**, *273*, 5051–5061. [CrossRef]
32. Halpern, K.B.; Shenhav, R.; Matcovitch-Natan, O.; Toth, B.; Lemze, D.; Golan, M.; Massasa, E.E.; Baydatch, S.; Landen, S.; Moor, A.E.; et al. Single-cell spatial reconstruction reveals global division of labour in the mammalian liver. *Nature* **2017**, *542*, 352–356. [CrossRef] [PubMed]
33. Saito, K.; Negishi, M.; James Squires, E. Sexual dimorphisms in zonal gene expression in mouse liver. *Biochem. Biophys. Res. Commun.* **2013**, *436*, 730–735. [CrossRef]
34. Lun, A.T.; McCarthy, D.J.; Marioni, J.C. A step-by-step workflow for low-level analysis of single-cell RNA-seq data with Bioconductor. *F1000Res* **2016**, *5*, 2122. [CrossRef] [PubMed]
35. Benjamini Y, Y.D. The control of the false discovery rate in multiple testing under dependency. *Ann. Statist.* **2001**, *29*, 1165–1188.
36. Goto, M. Immediate CT image processing-Dynamic range compression processing. *Nihon Hoshasen Gijutsu Gakkai Zasshi* **2019**, *75*, 688–692. [CrossRef]
37. Watson, C.T.; Breden, F. The immunoglobulin heavy chain locus: Genetic variation, missing data, and implications for human disease. *Genes Immun.* **2012**, *13*, 363–373. [CrossRef]
38. Poli, M.; Anower, E.K.F.; Asperti, M.; Ruzzenenti, P.; Gryzik, M.; Denardo, A.; Gordts, P.; Arosio, P.; Esko, J.D. Hepatic heparan sulfate is a master regulator of hepcidin expression and iron homeostasis in human hepatocytes and mice. *J. Biol. Chem.* **2019**, *294*, 13292–13303. [CrossRef]
39. Han, H.; Kursula, P. The olfactomedin domain from gliomedin is a beta-propeller with unique structural properties. *J. Biol. Chem.* **2015**, *290*, 3612–3621. [CrossRef]
40. Charkoftaki, G.; Wang, Y.; McAndrews, M.; Bruford, E.A.; Thompson, D.C.; Vasiliou, V.; Nebert, D.W. Update on the human and mouse lipocalin (LCN) gene family, including evidence the mouse Mup cluster is result of an "evolutionary bloom". *Hum. Genom.* **2019**, *13*, 11. [CrossRef]

41. Holmquist, E.; Okroj, M.; Nodin, B.; Jirstrom, K.; Blom, A.M. Sushi domain-containing protein 4 (SUSD4) inhibits complement by disrupting the formation of the classical C3 convertase. *FASEB J.* **2013**, *27*, 2355–2366. [CrossRef] [PubMed]
42. Hu, W.; Xin, Y.; Zhang, L.; Hu, J.; Sun, Y.; Zhao, Y. Iroquois Homeodomain transcription factors in ventricular conduction system and arrhythmia. *Int. J. Med. Sci.* **2018**, *15*, 808–815. [CrossRef] [PubMed]
43. Godoy, P.; Widera, A.; Schmidt-Heck, W.; Campos, G.; Meyer, C.; Cadenas, C.; Reif, R.; Stober, R.; Hammad, S.; Putter, L.; et al. Gene network activity in cultivated primary hepatocytes is highly similar to diseased mammalian liver tissue. *Arch. Toxicol.* **2016**, *90*, 2513–2529. [CrossRef] [PubMed]
44. Häussinger, D. Ammonia, urea production and pH regulation. In *Textbook of Hepatology*; Rodes, J., Benhamou, J.P., Blei, A.T., Eds.; Blackwell Publishing: Malden, MA, USA, 2007; Volume 181, p. 192.
45. Hawkins, R.A.; Jessy, J.; Mans, A.M.; De Joseph, M.R. Effect of reducing brain glutamine synthesis on metabolic symptoms of hepatic encephalopathy. *J. Neurochem.* **1993**, *60*, 1000–1006. [CrossRef]
46. Jones, E.A.; Smallwood, R.A.; Craigie, A.; Rosenoer, V.M. The enterohepatic circulation of urea nitrogen. *Clin. Sci.* **1969**, *37*, 825–836.
47. Jansen, P.L.; Ghallab, A.; Vartak, N.; Reif, R.; Schaap, F.G.; Hampe, J.; Hengstler, J.G. The ascending pathophysiology of cholestatic liver disease. *Hepatology* **2017**, *65*, 722–738. [CrossRef]
48. Vartak, N.; Damle-Vartak, A.; Richter, B.; Dirsch, O.; Dahmen, U.; Hammad, S.; Hengstler, J.G. Cholestasis-induced adaptive remodeling of interlobular bile ducts. *Hepatology* **2016**, *63*, 951–964. [CrossRef]
49. Lammert, F.; Wang, D.Q.; Hillebrandt, S.; Geier, A.; Fickert, P.; Trauner, M.; Matern, S.; Paigen, B.; Carey, M.C. Spontaneous cholecysto- and hepatolithiasis in Mdr2-/- mice: A model for low phospholipid-associated cholelithiasis. *Hepatology* **2004**, *39*, 117–128. [CrossRef]
50. Wöll, S.; Kim, S.H.; Greten, H.J.; Efferth, T. Animal plant warfare and secondary metabolite evolution. *Nat. Prod. Bioprospect.* **2013**, *3*, 1–7. [CrossRef]
51. Hessel-Pras, S.; Braeuning, A.; Guenther, G.; Adawy, A.; Enge, A.M.; Ebmeyer, J.; Henderson, C.J.; Hengstler, J.G.; Lampen, A.; Reif, R. The pyrrolizidine alkaloid senecionine induces CYP-dependent destruction of sinusoidal endothelial cells and cholestasis in mice. *Arch. Toxicol.* **2019**. [CrossRef]
52. Campos, G.; Schmidt-Heck, W.; De Smedt, J.; Widera, A.; Ghallab, A.; Pütter, L.; González, D.; Edlund, K.; Cadenas, C.; Marchan, R.; et al. In-flammation-associated suppression of metabolic gene networks in acute and chron-ic liver disease. *Arch. Toxicol.* **2019**. (Accepted).
53. R Core Team. R: A language and Environment for Statistical Computing. R Foundation for Statistical Computing. Available online: https://www.R-project.org/ (accessed on 7 November 2019).

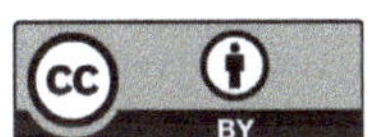

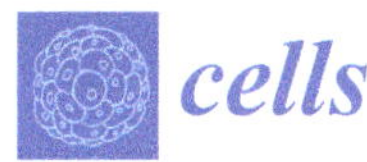

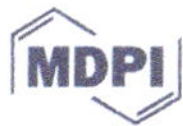

Review

Ubiquitin-Like Post-Translational Modifications (Ubl-PTMs): Small Peptides with Huge Impact in Liver Fibrosis

Sofia Lachiondo-Ortega [1], Maria Mercado-Gómez [1,†], Marina Serrano-Maciá [1,†], Fernando Lopitz-Otsoa [2], Tanya B Salas-Villalobos [3], Marta Varela-Rey [1], Teresa C. Delgado [1,*] and María Luz Martínez-Chantar [1]

1 Liver Disease Lab, CIC bioGUNE, Centro de Investigación Biomédica en Red de Enfermedades Hepáticas y Digestivas (CIBERehd), 48160 Derio, Spain; slachiondo@cicbiogune.es (S.L.-O.); mmercado@cicbiogune.es (M.M.-G.); mserrano@cicbiogune.es (M.S.-M.); mvarela.ciberehd@cicbiogune.es (M.V.-R.); mlmartinez@cicbiogune.es (M.L.M.-C.)

2 Liver Metabolism Lab, CIC bioGUNE, 48160 Derio, Spain; flopitz@cicbiogune.es

3 Department of Biochemistry and Molecular Medicine, School of Medicine, Autonomous University of Nuevo León, Monterrey, Nuevo León 66450, Mexico; bernardette.salas@gmail.com

* Correspondence: tcardoso@cicbiogune.es; Tel.: +34-944-061318; Fax: +34-944-061301

† These authors contributed equally to this work.

Received: 6 November 2019; Accepted: 1 December 2019; Published: 4 December 2019

Abstract: Liver fibrosis is characterized by the excessive deposition of extracellular matrix proteins including collagen that occurs in most types of chronic liver disease. Even though our knowledge of the cellular and molecular mechanisms of liver fibrosis has deeply improved in the last years, therapeutic approaches for liver fibrosis remain limited. Profiling and characterization of the post-translational modifications (PTMs) of proteins, and more specifically NEDDylation and SUMOylation ubiquitin-like (Ubls) modifications, can provide a better understanding of the liver fibrosis pathology as well as novel and more effective therapeutic approaches. On this basis, in the last years, several studies have described how changes in the intermediates of the Ubl cascades are altered during liver fibrosis and how specific targeting of particular enzymes mediating these ubiquitin-like modifications can improve liver fibrosis, mainly in in vitro models of hepatic stellate cells, the main fibrogenic cell type, and in pre-clinical mouse models of liver fibrosis. The development of novel inhibitors of the Ubl modifications as well as novel strategies to assess the modified proteome can provide new insights into the overall role of Ubl modifications in liver fibrosis.

Keywords: Ubiquitination; NEDDylation; SUMOylation; HCC; chronic liver disease; NAFLD; NASH

1. Chronic Liver Disease (CLD)

Liver injury induces inflammation, necrosis of hepatocytes, angiogenesis, the wound-healing response and the accumulation of extracellular matrix (ECM) proteins; followed by a process of hepatocyte regeneration to replace dead hepatocytes and restore the physiological liver mass [1,2]. Liver fibrosis typically reverts after elimination of the causative injury. However, if the damage persists and a chronic response is established, liver fibrosis can progress to cirrhosis, which is characterized by the distortion of the hepatic parenchyma and vascular structures that can eventually lead to hepatic loss of function and potential loss of reversibility [3]. At this stage, if the injury is not withdrawn, patients are at risk of end-stage liver disease and complications such as portal hypertension, hepatocellular carcinoma (HCC), and liver failure [3,4].

1.1. Etiology and Pathophysiology of Chronic Liver Disease (CLD)

Chronic liver disease (CLD) affects 800 million people worldwide and accounts for approximately 2 million deaths worldwide annually, representing a global major public health issue [4–6]. Alcohol abuse and associated alcoholic liver disease (ALD), viral hepatitis, and non-alcoholic fatty liver disease (NAFLD) are the most common causes of CLD. However, inherited disorders (such as alpha antitrypsin deficiency, hemochromatosis, and cystic fibrosis), drugs, cholestatic disease (such as primary biliary cholangitis (PBC), and primary sclerosing cholangitis (PSC)), and immune disorders also contribute to this common pathology [4].

Alcoholic liver disease (ALD) and NAFLD share a similar pathological progression, ranging from simple steatosis to alcoholic steatohepatitis (ASH) or non-alcoholic steatohepatitis (NASH). fibrosis, cirrhosis, and HCC [7]. Whereas excessive alcohol consumption is the main cause of ALD, the pathogenesis of NAFLD is related with obesity, insulin resistance and/or the metabolic syndrome, gut microbiota dysbiosis, environmental or nutritional factors, and genetic and epigenetic factors (reviewed by [8]). On the other hand, cholestatic disease [such as primary biliary cholangitis (PBC) and primary sclerosing cholangitis (PSC)] are associated with chronic damage to the cholangiocytes of the biliary tree, leading to reductions in the bile flow, persistent injury to the biliary epithelium and hepatocytes, inflammation, fibrogenesis and potentially carcinogenesis [4,9].

1.2. Liver Fibrosis and Cell Types

Liver damage leads to death of hepatocytes and cholangiocytes, which induces the release of pro-inflammatory mediators and stimulates phagocytosis of dead cell bodies by liver macrophages, mainly Kupffer cells and bone marrow-derived recruited monocytes [10]. Macrophages in the liver can also produce pro-inflammatory factors, such as reactive oxygen species (ROS), CC-chemokine ligand 2 (CCL2), tumor necrosis factor (TNF), interleukin-6 (IL-6), and 1β (IL-1β), thus triggering the wound-healing response, and stimulating the production of extracellular matrix components by myofibroblasts [11].

In ALD, the hepatocyte injury is mainly related to the oxidative metabolism of ethanol, whereas in NAFLD it depends on the lipotoxicity that induces cell death and lipo-apoptosis. When liver fibrosis is developed in an onset of ALD or NAFLD, the excessive deposition of ECM proteins is principally observed around the sinusoids (peri-sinusoidal fibrosis) and around groups of hepatocytes (peri-cellular fibrosis), and is mainly due to hepatic stellate cells (HSC) [4,12]. When fibrosis is developed in an onset of cholestasis, in addition to chronic damage to cholangiocytes, bile acids elicit hepatocyte injury and death [4,13,14]. In chronic diseases of the biliary tract, the excessive deposition of ECM proteins is principally observed around the injured bile ducts (biliary fibrosis pattern) and is mainly characterized by the proliferation of reactive ductular cells and myofibroblasts originated from portal fibroblast and HSC [4,15,16]. However, the contribution of portal fibroblasts to the development of fibrosis after cholestatic damage, compared to that of the HSC, is controversial [17].

As mentioned before, despite other minor cell sources (reviewed by [4]), HSC are the main sources of myofibroblasts in response to toxic liver injury [18,19]. In a healthy liver, HSC are in a quiescent state in which they accumulate retinoids. In response to toxic liver injury, HSC suffer a transdifferentiation process from a quiescent into an activated phenotype known as myofibroblasts [20]. These activated HSCs have a higher degree of proliferation and migration, hence repopulating the damaged liver, acquiring contractility by expressing alpha smooth muscle actin (α-SMA), expressing pro-inflammatory [(monocyte chemoattractant protein-1 (MCP-1), platelet-derived growth factor (PDGF), mouse stem cell factor (mSCF), CCL2, and CCL21, as well as IL-1β) and pro-fibrogenic markers (TGF-β)], and as well as increasing the synthesis of ECM proteins [collagen I (COL1A1) and III (COL1A3), fibronectin and tissue inhibitor of metalloproteinase (TIMP)], and of pro-angiogenic mediators [like vascular endothelial growth factor A (VEGFA), angiopoietin-1 or -2, and the homodimer (PDGF-BB)] [21,22]. One of the principal factors involved in HSC-induced proliferation is PDGF, which is upregulated in the fibrotic liver, whereas transforming growth factor (TGF-β) is the main profibrogenic factor and contributes positively to the transdifferentiation process of HSCs into myofibroblasts. Briefly, TGF-β binds and activates TGF-β receptors (TβR), of which there are three different forms (TβRI, TβRII, and TβRIII). Smads are the effector proteins of the TGF superfamily ligands. There are 8 Smad proteins which include: receptor-regulated R-Smads (Smads 1, 2, 3, 5, and 8), common-mediator Co-Smads (Smad4), and inhibitory I-Smads (Smads 6, 7). When TβRI is activated, Smads are recruited to the receptor and phosphorylated, resulting in their activation and increased affinity for Smad4. Then the Smad2/3/4 heteromeric complex translocates to the nucleus, where it has an immediate effect on the gene expression of several hundred of genes. TGF-β signaling is terminated when the activated Smads are either dephosphorylated or degraded [23,24].

1.3. *Overview of the Current Treatment Options for Chronic Liver Disease and Liver Fibrosis*

Current therapeutic interventions targeting CLD are etiology-dependent. Whereas in the last years, a quantum leap has been made in the therapy of hepatitis-induced CLD thanks to the development of novel and effective anti-viral drugs [25,26], therapeutic interventions in the case of ALD remain abstinence, treating the alcohol withdrawal syndrome, nutritional support, glucocorticosteroids or Pentoxifylline, anti-TNF therapy, antioxidants, or liver transplantation. On the other hand, treatment options for NAFLD and NASH are mainly directed toward lifestyle changes and weight loss, in combination with drugs such as insulin sensitizers, lipid lowering agents, hepatoprotective agents, antioxidants, incretin analogues, and anti-inflammatory agents (reviewed by [7]). First-line treatment for PBC involves the ursodeoxycholic acid (UDCA), which is able to prevent the progression of the disease in approximately two thirds of the patients [27–29]. For those PBC patients with insufficient response or intolerance to UDCA, second-line therapy is obeticholic acid [30,31]. There is currently no effective pharmacological therapy for PSC being liver transplantation the most definitive treatment [32].

Importantly, current clinical guidelines reinforce that, independently of the etiology of CLD, liver fibrosis should be the pharmaceutical target stage, once liver fibrosis reversibility is a reality. Taking into consideration that liver fibrosis is a multi-step disease characterized by pan-cellular and pan-pathway mechanisms, post-translational modifications (PTMs) of proteins can provide a better understanding of the liver fibrosis pathology as well as novel and more effective therapeutic approaches.

2. Post-Translational Modifications (PTMs) by Ubiquitin-Like (Ubl) Proteins

Post-translational modifications (PTMs) of proteins play a relevant role in the functional diversity of the proteome. In most eukaryotes, PTMs refer to the covalent and reversible addition of small chemical entities into target proteins following protein biosynthesis in order to exert a dynamic control over protein function in diverse cell biological contexts. The recent advances in the fields of systems biology and proteomics, have pushed forward the interest in deciphering protein modifications and their impact on the cellular microenvironment and disease pathophysiology. The most common PTMs include phosphorylation, acetylation, glycosylation, ubiquitination, acetylation, and hydroxylation, among others.

Ubiquitination is implicated in the pathogenesis of certain human diseases, including liver fibrosis. Ubiquitin has shown to be a marker of non-alcoholic liver fibrosis and it is frequently detected at the border or within the fibrous matrix [33,34]. Under these circumstances, overall changes in the ubiquitinated proteome may reflect either modifications in the ubiquitination cascade or in the proteasomal activity. For example, Cai et al. detected, in a rat model of liver fibrosis, a reduced SMAD specific E3 ubiquitin protein ligase 2 (Smurf-2) mRNA expression, which is a HECT domain E3 Ub ligase that ubiquitinates nuclear Smads and targets them for proteasomal degradation, resulting in an increased Smad2 expression [35]. Gp78, an endoplasmic reticulum (ER)-associated E3 Ub ligase, is also a key player in the ER-associated degradation (ERAD) and responsible for ubiquitination of lipid metabolism mediators, among others. Loss of Gp78 in aged mice caused NASH with fibrosis as a result of spontaneous and random ER stress [36]. On the other hand, Wilson and colleagues have shown that the Ub C-terminal hydrolase L1 (UCHL1) is an absent DUB in quiescent HSCs but its expression is increased and positively correlates with HSC transdifferentiation, in pre-clinical mouse models and in human livers from NASH and ALD patients. Pharmacological inhibition of UCHL1 in CCl_4 and bile-duct ligated (BDL) mice or ablation of UCHL1 in vitro in cultured HSC cells reduces liver fibrogenesis [37]. Likewise, an increase in mRNA expression and immunoreactivity of synoviolin which is an E3 Ub ligase has been observed in myofibroblasts. Fibrotic human livers also showed co-localization of synoviolin and the main fibrotic marker, α-SMA [38]. This compelling evidence implicating ubiquitination in liver fibrosis led several authors to evaluate the impact of ubiquitin-like proteins (Ubls)-mediated PTMs in liver fibrosis, the topic of this Review.

Ubiquitin-like proteins (Ubls) are a family of small proteins involved in PTMs, whose name is derived from ubiquitin, the first discovered member of the family. Besides ubiquitin, the human genome encodes at least eight families of Ubls, that are considered type I Ubls: (SUMO) small ubiquitin-related modifier, NEDD8 (neural precursor cell expressed developmentally downregulated protein 8), ATG8 (autophagy-related protein 8), ATG12 (autophagy-related protein 8), URM1 (ubiquitin-related modifier 1), UFM1 (ubiquitin-fold modifier 1), FAT10 (human leukocyte antigen-F adjacent transcript 10 or ubiquitin D), and ISG15 (interferon-stimulated gene 15) [39]. Even though, sparse studies have shown alteration of the levels of some Ubls in liver fibrosis, namely ATG12 related to autophagy [40], Fat10 and UFM1 [41], and ISG15 specifically in hepatitis C [42], in this Review, we will specially focus on the relevance of NEDD8 and SUMO proteins in liver fibrosis, whose therapeutic role has been addressed in liver fibrosis. The main characteristics of these proteins in comparison to ubiquitin can be found in Table 1.

Table 1. Characterization of the structure, homology with ubiquitin, size, amino acid, and conservation between species (See Supplementary Materials for species disclosure) of ubiquitin [43] and the ubiquitin-like (Ubl) proteins, neural precursor cell expressed developmentally downregulated protein 8 (NEDD8) [44] and small ubiquitin-related modifier (SUMO) [45,46].

Ubls	Structure	Identity with Ubiquitin	Size (kDa)	Amino Acid	Highly Conserved between Species
Ubiquitin		100	8.6	76	[illegible]
NEDD8		59	8	81	[illegible]
SUMO	SUMO 1	18	≈12	≈100	[illegible]
	SUMO 2				[illegible]

2.1. NEDDylation in Liver Fibrosis

NEDDylation is a reversible ubiquitin-like PTM, characterized by the covalent conjugation of NEDD8. The pathway of the NEDDylation process involves NEDD8 specific enzymes, such as E1 activating enzymes (NAE1 and UBA3); E2 conjugating enzymes (UBE2M/UBC12 and UBE2F); E3 ligase enzymes, which catalyze NEDD8 transference to the target protein (MDM2, RBX1, FBXO11, RNF7, CBL, DCUN1D1, and DECUN1D2); and deneddylase enzymes (SENP8/NEDP1, ATXN3, USP21, CPS5, UCHL1, and UCHL3) [47,48]. Noteworthy, NEDD8 is synthetized as a precursor and must be activated at the C-terminal Gly76 mainly by NEDP1 [49] in order to be integrated inside the NEDDylation cycle and conjugated to the lysine residue of target proteins [50]. The conjugation of NEDD8 can modify its target protein in different ways, such as inducing conformational changes, changing its subcellular localization, enzymatic activation, or inhibition, competing with other Ubls or inducing its stability [51,52].

The mechanisms that trigger the deregulation of NEDDylation are not well understood, but it has been reported that the levels of NEDD8 are increased under stress conditions in vitro [53]. In fact, alterations in the NEDDylated protein levels have been described in different pathological conditions, such as neurodegenerative disorders [54] and cancer [48,55,56]. Focusing on the liver context, patients with HCC and intrahepatic cholangiocarcinoma, as well as mouse models of HCC, showed a significant increase in the global NEDDylation proteome and NEDDylation intermediates [55–59]. In addition, under diverse stress conditions, the canonical pathway of NEDDylation via NAE1 changes, being NEDD8 conjugation predominantly mediated by the Ube1 E1 ubiquitin enzyme [53]. Likewise, in HCC, where NEDDylation levels are enriched, NEDP1 protein levels disappear promoting the inhibition of ATPase activity of HSP70 and, thus the apoptosis resistance of cancer cells. Hence, these result shows how the tight regulation of the NEDD8 cycle can modulate vital cellular functions like apoptosis [60].

Regarding liver fibrosis and NEDDylation, Zubiete-Franco et al. described for the first time an increase in the global NEDDylated proteome in patients with liver fibrosis as well as in mouse models of CCl_4- and BDL-induced liver fibrosis [61]. Importantly, NAE1-specific inhibition in these mouse models showed a reduction in the liver damage associated with decreased apoptosis, inflammation, and fibrosis. These results were explained by the effect of NEDDylation inhibition in the different hepatic cell subtypes. The decrease in inflammation after NEDDylation inhibition can be explained in part by the incapacity of Cullin-1 and $SCF^{\beta TrCP}$ (E3 Ligase) to ubiquitinate and degrade IKBα, promoting NF-kB stabilization in the cytoplasm [47,48]. Interestingly, in this work the authors describe how NEDD8 levels increase in activated HSCs, and consequently neddylation inhibition could directly block its activation. Indeed, after NAE1 inhibition, HSCs show an increase of cell death partly mediated by c-Jun accumulation, a target of cullin degradation. On the other hand, it has been described that Casitas B-lineage lymphoma (c-Cbl) acts as a NEDD8 Ligase promoting TGF-β signaling and stabilization of the type II receptor (TβRII) in blood cells [62]. In agreement with this line of evidence, other authors have shown very recently that the in vivo inhibition of the transcription factor SRSF3 NEDDylation, associated with its prevention of degradation, protects mice from fibrosis [63].

In conclusion, the NEDDylation inhibition is a key mechanism to down-regulating the inflammatory response, further reducing cell damage and subsequent liver fibrosis, in addition to specifically targeting HSC death.

2.2. SUMOylation in Liver Fibrosis

SUMOylation is another ubiquitin-like PTM that consists in the covalent addition of one or multiple SUMO subunits to Lys residues usually located on the SUMO consensus motifs of target proteins. SUMOylation occurs as a hierarchically organized process catalyzed by the E1 activating enzyme, the E2 conjugating enzyme, and an E3 SUMO ligase [64]. The extension of the SUMO chain is possible thanks to a specialized type of E3 ligase family of enzymes known as E4 SUMO elongases [65].

To date, five SUMO isoforms have been described in humans, being SUMO 1, 2, and 3 the most ubiquitous. SUMO modifiers are similar in size and structure to ubiquitin, but show little sequence homology compared to ubiquitin. SUMO 2 and 3 share approximately 97% identity, whereas SUMO 1 is only 50% identical in sequence. SUMO isoforms differ in several aspects, such as in the E3 ligase preference or the ability to form SUMO chains on the substrate proteins. Moreover, different functions and mechanisms of regulation within the cell would be expected since SUMO2/3 conjugation becomes more relevant under stress conditions [64]. The SUMO E1 activating enzyme is composed by the SAE1 and UBA2 heterodimer, while Ubc9 is the only E2 SUMO conjugating enzyme recognized. Conversely, a huge range of E3 SUMO ligases exist, which are grouped in the canonical PIAS family and non-canonical E3 ligases such as RanBP2 or Cbx4, thus conferring specificity to the process [64]. SUMO-mediated modification can be reversed by the action of deSUMOylating enzymes, which are also involved in the maturation of the SUMO precursor protein. SENPs belong to the most common family of protein deSUMOylases but, unrelated DESI1, DESI2, and USPL1 SUMO proteases exist as well [66]. Since SUMOylation is mostly restricted to the nucleus, it is not a surprising fact that SUMO is involved in many nuclear processes such as DNA damage response, genome integrity, transcription regulation, as well as preservation of protein stability and modulation of subcellular localization of the substrate proteins [67,68].

SUMOylation is a highly dynamic process enabling fast global changes in the SUMO status of the proteome in response to internal and external stimuli, often stress such as heat shock, nutrient depletion, genotoxic or oxidative stress [69–72]. This rapid adaptation is possible thanks to several mechanisms of regulation that can control SUMOylation levels. In addition to deSUMOylases, the SUMO-targeted ubiquitin ligase (STUbl) enzymes can modify global SUMOylation levels by binding to SUMO chains on proteins and poly-ubiquitinating them, eventually leading to their proteasome-mediated degradation. Moreover, a crosstalk between SUMOylation and other PTMs, such as ubiquitination or phosphorylation, has also been reported to affect the SUMOylation status [73,74]. The localization of the SUMO enzymatic machinery constitutes an additional critical factor for the modulation of the SUMOylation levels [64].

Hence, controlled SUMOylation is required for normal cell behavior. According to proteomics studies, between 1000 and 3000 human proteins are modified by SUMO. The identified SUMOylated proteins are implicated in almost all cellular processes [66]. A deregulation in SUMOylation dynamics has been associated with fibrotic disorders occurring in the heart, lung, and kidney, amongst other diseases [75–77]. And there is increasing evidence that SUMOylation might play a regulatory role in liver fibrosis too [78–80].

A recent study referred to Ubc9, the only existing SUMO E2 conjugating enzyme, as a potential therapeutic target for the prevention and treatment of liver fibrosis. Protein and mRNA expression levels of Ubc9 were described to be significantly upregulated in the LX-2 liver fibrosis in vitro model, and in the HepG2 and SMMC-7721 HCC cell lines. Interestingly, shRNA-mediated silencing of Ubc9 expression in activated LX-2 cells resulted in a decreased expression of α-SMA and type I collagen fibrosis markers, as well as a diminished secretion of IL-6 and TNF profibrotic cytokines. Additionally, downregulation of Ubc9 blocked cell cycle progression and promoted activated LX-2 cell cycle arrest in G_2 phase. Importantly, an induction of apoptosis in activated LX-2 cells was detected after Ubc9 expression knockdown, mainly attributed to the abrogation of the canonical NF-κB signaling pathway, which is also a known target of SUMOylation [78].

Another piece of work placed the deSUMOylating enzyme SENP2 as a critical protein to attenuate CCl_4-induced liver fibrosis in mice by inducing activated HSC apoptosis via suppression of Wnt/β-catenin signaling program. SENP2 protein and mRNA expression levels were found to be decreased both in vitro and in vivo in activated hepatic stellate cells (HSCs) during the CCl_4-induced liver fibrosis mouse model, being those levels restored after removal of the damage stimulus. On the one hand, in vitro SENP2 overexpression resulted in a decreased α-SMA and COL1A1 protein expression in a TGF-β-activated hepatic stellate cell line. Moreover, increased expression of SENP2 reduced cell viability, favored cell cycle arrest in G_0/G_1 phase and induced apoptosis of the in vitro TGF-β-activated HSCs. On the other hand, siRNA-mediated silencing of SENP2 in TGF-β-activated HSCs induced α-SMA and COL1A1 protein expression, stimulated cell proliferation, and reduced apoptosis. Finally, the expression of the Wnt/β-catenin pathway members was downregulated upon SENP2 overexpression in TGF-β-activated HSCs, thus suggesting a therapeutic role of SENP2 in liver fibrosis [79].

Although it has not been specifically studied in the context of liver, various members of the TGF-β/Smad canonical pathway, which is common to fibrotic processes, have been found to be SUMOylated [66]. TGF-β type I receptor (TRβI/ALK5), whose phosphorylation and activation are mediated by TGF-β, is SUMOylated further enhancing the activation and modulation of the downstream Smad signaling cascade [73]. Furthermore, TGF-β signal transducers Smad proteins are also postranslationally modified by SUMOylation. For example, Smad4 SUMOylation protects it from its ubiquitination and subsequent proteasomal degradation [81]. Interestingly, Smad nuclear interacting protein 1 (SNIP1), a transcription repressor for both TGF-β and NF-κB signaling pathways, is a SUMO substrate. SNIP1 inhibits the TGF-β signaling by hampering the recruitment of p300 coactivator to the Smad complex, whereas SNIP1 SUMOylation attenuates its inhibitory effect on the TGF-β response further facilitating the expression of PAI-1 and MMP2 [82]. In summary, it is suggested that interfering in the SUMOylation of these proteins could be a potential strategy for the treatment of diseases induced by aberrant TGF-β signaling, which not only includes liver fibrosis but also HCC. Nevertheless, more focused research is needed regarding the impact of the TGF-β/Smad pathway SUMOylation in the particular context of liver fibrosis.

Conversely, a study highlights the importance of SUMOylation for liver fibrosis regression. Reduced glutathione (GSH) is implicated in many cellular processes including fibrogenesis. GSH protects against oxidative stress, which activates HSCs. Thus, high levels of GSH would maintain HSC in a quiescent state, and this requires SUMOylation of Nrf2 and MafG, which facilitate heterodimerization and activation of the antioxidant response element (ARE) located in the promoter region of many genes involved in the antioxidant defense, such as the GSH synthetic enzymes [80].

Finally, it has also been demonstrated that SUMO 1 and SUMO2/3 could play a role as autoantigens during PBC, since autoantibodies to these proteins have been detected in the sera of patients suffering from this autoimmune disease. Nonetheless, further research is needed in order to understand how the development of SUMO autoantibodies can lead to autoimmunity in PBC [83].

Overall, SUMOylation is a highly dynamic process which can have both beneficial and pathological consequences in the cellular physiology depending on the protein substrate, cell type, or context. Therefore, inhibition of global SUMOylation might not always be an ideal therapeutic strategy due to potential unforeseeable secondary effects. Alternatively, a more realistic rationale would involve the discovery and development of small molecules or peptidomimetics that block the protein–protein interactions between specific E3 SUMO ligases or SENPs and their substrates that are known to be altered in a diseased state.

2.3. *Therapeutic Strategies Targeting Ubls Modifications in Liver Fibrosis*

As a result of several studies in the last decades about the role of PTMs, specifically Ubl-mediated protein modifications, and their implication in disease, many therapeutic agents targeting these modifications have been developed lately (see Reviews [84–87]). Nevertheless, only a small fraction of these agents was tested in liver fibrosis.

Regarding ubiquitination, the role of the pharmacological inhibitor LDN 57444, an inhibitor of the deubiquitinase ubiquitin C-terminal hydrolase1 (UCHL1), was also evaluated and shown to block the progression of established fibrosis in the carbon tetrachloride (CCl_4) injured mice [37]. In addition, Indole-3-carbinol (I3C), a naturally occurring compound generated from the hydrolysis of glucobrassicin and found in high concentrations in *Brassica* vegetables, was shown to induce apoptosis of HSC through RIP1 K63 de-ubiquitination by upregulating deubiquitinase CYLD [88].

Therapeutic strategies targeting NEDDylation in liver fibrosis have also been evaluated. As it was previously mentioned, pre-clinical studies in mouse models have shown that the small pharmacological inhibitor of NEDDylation, Pevonedistat, or MLN4924 [89], is able to revert liver fibrosis [61].

Pevonedistat (MLN4924) is a potent and selective NAE1 inhibitor that is currently undergoing several clinical trials to treat some leukemias and some types of solid organ cancer pathologies. Taking this into account, translation of Pevonedistat from pre-clinical mouse models to clinical trials for liver fibrosis treatment should be a fast process. Finally, to our knowledge, the role of the inhibition of the SUMOylation pathway or specific enzymes of this pathway in liver fibrosis has not been assessed to date.

3. Concluding Remarks

In the last years, a big effort has been made on the study of the role of PTMs mediated by Ubl in liver fibrosis (Figure 1). In spite of the improved knowledge obtained on this highly dynamic and pan-cellular process of liver fibrosis and its regulation by Ubl PTMs, it is clear that novel tools need to be developed. As an example, in the last years, both tandem ubiquitin-binding entities (TUBEs) and SUMO-binding entities (SUBEs), were developed [90,91]. Briefly, TUBEs and SUBEs are recombinant proteins that comprise tandem repeats of either ubiquitin-associated (UBA) domains or SUMO-interacting motifs (SIMs) thereby recognizing with high affinity ubiquitin and SUMO molecules on modified proteins, respectively. In the liver context, the use of SUBEs has been used very recently to demonstrate the relevance of Liver Kinase B1 (LKB1) SUMOylation during the progression to Hepatocellular Carcinoma (HCC) highlighting its potential for the assessment of ubiquitinated and SUMOylated proteins in liver fibrosis [92]. Other option is to combine the use of transgenic mice with tagged Ubl PTMs where fibrosis is experimentally induced followed by isolation of the different hepatic populations playing a role on the progression of liver fibrosis. For instance, transgenic mouse models, specially dedicated to the study of the ubiquitin-proteasome system have been developed. This is the case of the mouse strains transgenic for a green fluorescent protein (GFP) reporter carrying a constitutively active degradation signal [93]. Moreover, Mayor and colleagues have developed a transgenic mouse expressing biotinylated ubiquitin and demonstrated its use for the isolation of ubiquitinated proteins from the liver by taking advantage of the specificity and strength of the biotin-avidin interaction [94]. Even though similar approaches for other Ubl modifications, such as NEDD8 and SUMO, have been used in cultured cells [95], novel in vivo approaches should be investigated. Importantly, studies to analyze the intermediates on the multiple types of hepatic cells participating in liver fibrosis and not only on HSC, as occurs in the majority of the studies found in literature, should be performed. And the reason for that is that to cure fibrosis is important not only to promote the apoptosis and the reversal of the activation of HSCs, but also to take out the injury insult mainly acting on liver hepatocytes, that is in fact driving the liver fibrosis cascade. Finally, regarding potential therapeutic approaches targeting Ubl PTMs, compelling evidence indicates that whereas NEDDylation inhibition provides a global mechanism for reversing liver fibrosis, with respect to ubiquitination and SUMOylation, we believe that potential therapeutic approaches in liver fibrosis should be more specific aiming at specific ligases with targets playing an important role in the fibrosis pathogenic processes.

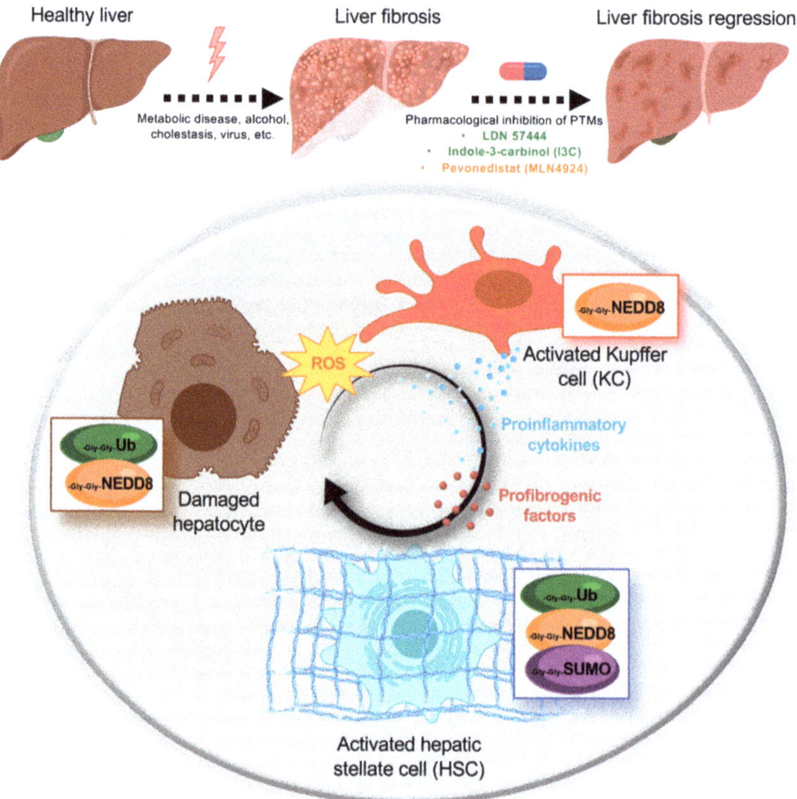

Figure 1. Schematic representation of the post-translational modifications (PTMs) described to date occurring in the main hepatic cell types involved during liver fibrosis, hepatocytes, Kupffer cells (KCs), and hepatic stellate cells (HSCs). Damage causing the transition from a normal healthy liver to a fibrotic liver are also referred, as well as the small-molecule inhibitors of PTMs that have resulted effective in the reversion of liver fibrosis.

Supplementary Materials: The following are available online at http://www.mdpi.com/2073-4409/8/12/1575/s1, Table S1: UNIPROT entry of the different species where homology of the Ubls was compared.

Author Contributions: Writing—original draft preparation, All; writing—review and editing, All.

Funding: This research was funded by Gobierno Vasco-Departamento de Salud 2013111114 (to M.L.M.-C.), ELKARTEK 2016, Departamento de Industria del Gobierno Vasco (to M.L.M.-C.), Ministerio de Ciencia, Innovación y Universidades MICINN: SAF2017-87301-R and RTI2018-096759-1-100 integrado en el Plan Estatal de Investigación Cientifica y Técnica y Innovación, cofinanciado con Fondos FEDER (to M.L.M.-C. and T.C.D. respectively), BIOEF (Basque Foundation for Innovation and Health Research): EITB Maratoia BIO15/CA/014; Asociación Española contra el Cáncer (M.S.-M., T.C.D. and M.L.M.-C.), Daniel Alagille Award from EASL (to T.C.D.), Fundación Científica de la Asociación Española Contra el Cancer (AECC Scientific Foundation) Rare Tumor Calls 2017 (to M.L.M.-C.), La Caixa Foundation Program (to M.L.M.-C.). Gilead Sciences International Research Scholars Program in Liver Disease (to M.V.-R.). Ciberehd_ISCIII_MINECO is funded by the Instituto de Salud Carlos III. We thank MINECO for the Severo Ochoa Excellence Accreditation to CIC bioGUNE (SEV-2016-0644).

Conflicts of Interest: Martínez-Chantar advises for Mitotherapeutix LLC.

References

1. Pellicoro, A.; Ramachandran, P.; Iredale, J.P.; Fallowfield, J.A. Liver fibrosis and repair: Immune regulation of wound healing in a solid organ. *Nat. Rev. Immunol.* **2014**, *14*, 181–194. [CrossRef] [PubMed]
2. Campana, L.; Iredale, J.P. Regression of Liver Fibrosis. *Semin. Liver Dis.* **2017**, *37*, 1–10. [PubMed]
3. Yoon, Y.J.; Friedman, S.L.; Lee, Y.A. Antifibrotic Therapies: Where Are We Now? *Semin. Liver Dis.* **2016**, *36*, 87–98. [CrossRef] [PubMed]
4. Parola, M.; Pinzani, M. Liver fibrosis: Pathophysiology, pathogenetic targets and clinical issues. *Mol. Asp. Med.* **2019**, *65*, 37–55. [CrossRef]
5. Byass, P. The global burden of liver disease: A challenge for methods and for public health. *BMC Med.* **2014**, *12*, 159. [CrossRef]
6. Marcellin, P.; Kutala, B.K. Liver diseases: A major, neglected global public health problem requiring urgent actions and large-scale screening. *Liver Int.* **2018**, *38* (Suppl. 1), 2–6. [CrossRef]
7. Singh, S.; Osna, N.A.; Kharbanda, K.K. Treatment options for alcoholic and non-alcoholic fatty liver disease: A review. *World J. Gastroenterol.* **2017**, *23*, 6549–6570. [CrossRef]
8. Arab, J.P.; Arrese, M.; Trauner, M. Recent Insights into the Pathogenesis of Nonalcoholic Fatty Liver Disease. *Annu. Rev. Pathol.* **2018**, *13*, 321–350. [CrossRef]
9. Fabris, L.; Spirli, C.; Cadamuro, M.; Fiorotto, R.; Strazzabosco, M. Emerging concepts in biliary repair and fibrosis. *Am. J. Physiol. Gastrointest. Liver Physiol.* **2017**, *313*, G102–G116. [CrossRef]
10. Guillot, A.; Tacke, F. Liver Macrophages: Old Dogmas and New Insights. *Hepatol. Commun.* **2019**, *3*, 730–743. [CrossRef]
11. An, L.; Wang, X.; Cederbaum, A.I. Cytokines in alcoholic liver disease. *Arch. Toxicol.* **2012**, *86*, 1337–1348. [CrossRef] [PubMed]
12. Pinzani, M.; Rombouts, K. Liver fibrosis: From the bench to clinical targets. *Dig. Liver Dis.* **2004**, *36*, 231–242. [CrossRef] [PubMed]
13. Hofmann, A.F.; Hagey, L.R. Bile acids: Chemistry, pathochemistry, biology, pathobiology, and therapeutics. *Cell Mol. Life Sci.* **2008**, *65*, 2461–2483. [CrossRef] [PubMed]
14. Arndtz, K.; Hirschfield, G.M. The Pathogenesis of Autoimmune Liver Disease. *Dig. Dis.* **2016**, *34*, 327–333. [CrossRef]
15. Iwaisako, K.; Haimerl, M.; Paik, Y.H.; Taura, K.; Kodama, Y.; Sirlin, C.; Yu, E.; Yu, R.T.; Downes, M.; Evans, R.M.; et al. Protection from liver fibrosis by a peroxisome proliferator-activated receptor delta agonist. *Proc. Natl. Acad. Sci. USA* **2012**, *109*, E1369–E1376. [CrossRef]
16. Wells, R.G.; Schwabe, R.F. Origin and function of myofibroblasts in the liver. *Semin. Liver Dis.* **2015**, *35*, e1. [CrossRef]
17. Karin, D.; Koyama, Y.; Brenner, D.; Kisseleva, T. The characteristics of activated portal fibroblasts/myofibroblasts in liver fibrosis. *Differentiation* **2016**, *92*, 84–92. [CrossRef]
18. Friedman, S.L. Hepatic stellate cells: Protean, multifunctional, and enigmatic cells of the liver. *Physiol. Rev.* **2008**, *88*, 125–172. [CrossRef]
19. Tsuchida, T.; Friedman, S.L. Mechanisms of hepatic stellate cell activation. *Nat. Rev. Gastroenterol. Hepatol.* **2017**, *14*, 397–411. [CrossRef]
20. Zhang, D.Y.; Friedman, S.L. Fibrosis-dependent mechanisms of hepatocarcinogenesis. *Hepatology* **2012**, *56*, 769–775. [CrossRef]
21. Arriazu, E.; Ruiz de Galarreta, M.; Cubero, F.J.; Varela-Rey, M.; Perez de Obanos, M.P.; Leung, T.M.; Lopategi, A.; Benedicto, A.; Abraham-Enachescu, I.; Nieto, N. Extracellular matrix and liver disease. *Antioxid. Redox Signal.* **2014**, *21*, 1078–1097. [CrossRef] [PubMed]
22. Bataller, R.; Brenner, D.A. Liver fibrosis. *J. Clin. Investig.* **2005**, *115*, 209–218. [CrossRef] [PubMed]
23. Weiss, A.; Attisano, L. The TGFbeta superfamily signaling pathway. *Wiley Interdiscip. Rev. Dev. Biol.* **2013**, *2*, 47–63. [CrossRef] [PubMed]
24. Kang, Y.; Chen, C.R.; Massague, J. A self-enabling TGFbeta response coupled to stress signaling: Smad engages stress response factor ATF3 for Id1 repression in epithelial cells. *Mol. Cell* **2003**, *11*, 915–926. [CrossRef]
25. Okada, M.; Enomoto, M.; Kawada, N.; Nguyen, M.H. Effects of antiviral therapy in patients with chronic hepatitis B and cirrhosis. *Expert Rev. Gastroenterol. Hepatol.* **2017**, *11*, 1095–1104. [CrossRef]

26. Navasa, M.; Forns, X. Antiviral therapy in HCV decompensated cirrhosis: To treat or not to treat? *J. Hepatol.* **2007**, *46*, 185–188. [CrossRef]
27. Terziroli Beretta-Piccoli, B.; Mieli-Vergani, G.; Vergani, D.; Vierling, J.M.; Adams, D.; Alpini, G.; Banales, J.M.; Beuers, U.; Bjornsson, E.; Bowlus, C.; et al. The challenges of primary biliary cholangitis: What is new and what needs to be done. *J. Autoimmun.* **2019**, 102328. [CrossRef]
28. European Association for the Study of the Liver. EASL Clinical Practice Guidelines: The diagnosis and management of patients with primary biliary cholangitis. *J. Hepatol.* **2017**, *67*, 145–172. [CrossRef]
29. Lindor, K.D.; Bowlus, C.L.; Boyer, J.; Levy, C.; Mayo, M. Primary Biliary Cholangitis: 2018 Practice Guidance from the American Association for the Study of Liver Diseases. *Hepatology* **2019**, *69*, 394–419. [CrossRef]
30. Nevens, F.; Andreone, P.; Mazzella, G.; Strasser, S.I.; Bowlus, C.; Invernizzi, P.; Drenth, J.P.; Pockros, P.J.; Regula, J.; Beuers, U.; et al. A Placebo-Controlled Trial of Obeticholic Acid in Primary Biliary Cholangitis. *N. Engl. J. Med.* **2016**, *375*, 631–643. [CrossRef]
31. Trauner, M.; Nevens, F.; Shiffman, M.L.; Drenth, J.P.H.; Bowlus, C.L.; Vargas, V.; Andreone, P.; Hirschfield, G.M.; Pencek, R.; Malecha, E.S.; et al. Long-term efficacy and safety of obeticholic acid for patients with primary biliary cholangitis: 3-year results of an international open-label extension study. *Lancet Gastroenterol. Hepatol.* **2019**, *4*, 445–453. [CrossRef]
32. Karlsen, T.H.; Folseraas, T.; Thorburn, D.; Vesterhus, M. Primary sclerosing cholangitis—A comprehensive review. *J. Hepatol.* **2017**, *67*, 1298–1323. [CrossRef] [PubMed]
33. Banner, B.F.; Savas, L.; Zivny, J.; Tortorelli, K.; Bonkovsky, H.L. Ubiquitin as a marker of cell injury in nonalcoholic steatohepatitis. *Am. J. Clin. Pathol.* **2000**, *114*, 860–866. [CrossRef] [PubMed]
34. Guy, C.D.; Suzuki, A.; Burchette, J.L.; Brunt, E.M.; Abdelmalek, M.F.; Cardona, D.; McCall, S.J.; Unalp, A.; Belt, P.; Ferrell, L.D.; et al. Costaining for keratins 8/18 plus ubiquitin improves detection of hepatocyte injury in nonalcoholic fatty liver disease. *Hum. Pathol.* **2012**, *43*, 790–800. [CrossRef] [PubMed]
35. Cai, Y.; Shen, X.Z.; Zhou, C.H.; Wang, J.Y. Abnormal expression of Smurf2 during the process of rat liver fibrosis. *Chin. J. Dig. Dis.* **2006**, *7*, 237–245. [CrossRef] [PubMed]
36. Zhang, T.; Kho, D.H.; Wang, Y.; Harazono, Y.; Nakajima, K.; Xie, Y.; Raz, A. Gp78, an E3 ubiquitin ligase acts as a gatekeeper suppressing nonalcoholic steatohepatitis (NASH) and liver cancer. *PLoS ONE* **2015**, *10*, e0118448. [CrossRef] [PubMed]
37. Wilson, C.L.; Murphy, L.B.; Leslie, J.; Kendrick, S.; French, J.; Fox, C.R.; Sheerin, N.S.; Fisher, A.; Robinson, J.H.; Tiniakos, D.G.; et al. Ubiquitin C-terminal hydrolase 1: A novel functional marker for liver myofibroblasts and a therapeutic target in chronic liver disease. *J. Hepatol.* **2015**, *63*, 1421–1428. [CrossRef]
38. Hasegawa, D.; Fujii, R.; Yagishita, N.; Matsumoto, N.; Aratani, S.; Izumi, T.; Azakami, K.; Nakazawa, M.; Fujita, H.; Sato, T.; et al. E3 ubiquitin ligase synoviolin is involved in liver fibrogenesis. *PLoS ONE* **2010**, *5*, e13590. [CrossRef]
39. Cappadocia, L.; Lima, C.D. Ubiquitin-like Protein Conjugation: Structures, Chemistry, and Mechanism. *Chem. Rev.* **2018**, *118*, 889–918. [CrossRef]
40. Kim, K.M.; Han, C.Y.; Kim, J.Y.; Cho, S.S.; Kim, Y.S.; Koo, J.H.; Lee, J.M.; Lim, S.C.; Kang, K.W.; Kim, J.S.; et al. Galpha12 overexpression induced by miR-16 dysregulation contributes to liver fibrosis by promoting autophagy in hepatic stellate cells. *J. Hepatol.* **2018**, *68*, 493–504. [CrossRef]
41. Liu, H.; Li, J.; Tillman, B.; French, B.A.; French, S.W. Ufmylation and FATylation pathways are downregulated in human alcoholic and nonalcoholic steatohepatitis, and mice fed DDC, where Mallory-Denk bodies (MDBs) form. *Exp. Mol. Pathol.* **2014**, *97*, 81–88. [CrossRef] [PubMed]
42. Lebosse, F.; Testoni, B.; Fresquet, J.; Facchetti, F.; Galmozzi, E.; Fournier, M.; Hervieu, V.; Berthillon, P.; Berby, F.; Bordes, I.; et al. Intrahepatic innate immune response pathways are downregulated in untreated chronic hepatitis B. *J. Hepatol.* **2017**, *66*, 897–909. [CrossRef] [PubMed]
43. Goldstein, G.; Scheid, M.; Hammerling, U.; Schlesinger, D.H.; Niall, H.D.; Boyse, E.A. Isolation of a polypeptide that has lymphocyte-differentiating properties and is probably represented universally in living cells. *Proc. Natl. Acad. Sci. USA* **1975**, *72*, 11–15. [CrossRef] [PubMed]
44. Kumar, S.; Tomooka, Y.; Noda, M. Identification of a set of genes with developmentally down-regulated expression in the mouse brain. *Biochem. Biophys. Res. Commun.* **1992**, *185*, 1155–1161. [CrossRef]
45. Mahajan, R.; Delphin, C.; Guan, T.; Gerace, L.; Melchior, F. A small ubiquitin-related polypeptide involved in targeting RanGAP1 to nuclear pore complex protein RanBP2. *Cell* **1997**, *88*, 97–107. [CrossRef]

46. Matunis, M.J.; Coutavas, E.; Blobel, G. A novel ubiquitin-like modification modulates the partitioning of the Ran-GTPase-activating protein RanGAP1 between the cytosol and the nuclear pore complex. *J. Cell Biol.* **1996**, *135*, 1457–1470. [CrossRef]
47. Enchev, R.I.; Schulman, B.A.; Peter, M. Protein neddylation: Beyond cullin-RING ligases. *Nat. Rev. Mol. Cell Biol.* **2015**, *16*, 30–44. [CrossRef]
48. Abidi, N.; Xirodimas, D.P. Regulation of cancer-related pathways by protein NEDDylation and strategies for the use of NEDD8 inhibitors in the clinic. *Endocr. Relat. Cancer* **2015**, *22*, T55–T70. [CrossRef]
49. Mendoza, H.M.; Shen, L.N.; Botting, C.; Lewis, A.; Chen, J.; Ink, B.; Hay, R.T. NEDP1, a highly conserved cysteine protease that deNEDDylates Cullins. *J. Biol. Chem.* **2003**, *278*, 25637–25643. [CrossRef]
50. Sundqvist, A.; Liu, G.; Mirsaliotis, A.; Xirodimas, D.P. Regulation of nucleolar signalling to p53 through NEDDylation of L11. *EMBO Rep.* **2009**, *10*, 1132–1139. [CrossRef]
51. Rabut, G.; Peter, M. Function and regulation of protein neddylation. 'Protein modifications: Beyond the usual suspects' review series. *EMBO Rep.* **2008**, *9*, 969–976. [CrossRef] [PubMed]
52. Dye, B.T.; Schulman, B.A. Structural mechanisms underlying posttranslational modification by ubiquitin-like proteins. *Annu Rev. Biophys. Biomol. Struct.* **2007**, *36*, 131–150. [CrossRef] [PubMed]
53. Leidecker, O.; Matic, I.; Mahata, B.; Pion, E.; Xirodimas, D.P. The ubiquitin E1 enzyme Ube1 mediates NEDD8 activation under diverse stress conditions. *Cell Cycle* **2012**, *11*, 1142–1150. [CrossRef] [PubMed]
54. Chen, Y.; Neve, R.L.; Liu, H. Neddylation dysfunction in Alzheimer's disease. *J. Cell Mol. Med.* **2012**, *16*, 2583–2591. [CrossRef] [PubMed]
55. Barbier-Torres, L.; Delgado, T.C.; Garcia-Rodriguez, J.L.; Zubiete-Franco, I.; Fernandez-Ramos, D.; Buque, X.; Cano, A.; Gutierrez-de Juan, V.; Fernandez-Dominguez, I.; Lopitz-Otsoa, F.; et al. Stabilization of LKB1 and Akt by neddylation regulates energy metabolism in liver cancer. *Oncotarget* **2015**, *6*, 2509–2523. [CrossRef]
56. Yu, J.; Huang, W.L.; Xu, Q.G.; Zhang, L.; Sun, S.H.; Zhou, W.P.; Yang, F. Overactivated neddylation pathway in human hepatocellular carcinoma. *Cancer Med.* **2018**, *7*, 3363–3372. [CrossRef]
57. Delgado, T.C.; Barbier-Torres, L.; Zubiete-Franco, I.; Lopitz-Otsoa, F.; Varela-Rey, M.; Fernandez-Ramos, D.; Martinez-Chantar, M.L. Neddylation, a novel paradigm in liver cancer. *Transl. Gastroenterol. Hepatol.* **2018**, *3*, 37. [CrossRef]
58. Gao, Q.; Yu, G.Y.; Shi, J.Y.; Li, L.H.; Zhang, W.J.; Wang, Z.C.; Yang, L.X.; Duan, M.; Zhao, H.; Wang, X.Y.; et al. Neddylation pathway is up-regulated in human intrahepatic cholangiocarcinoma and serves as a potential therapeutic target. *Oncotarget* **2014**, *5*, 7820–7832. [CrossRef]
59. Embade, N.; Fernandez-Ramos, D.; Varela-Rey, M.; Beraza, N.; Sini, M.; Gutierrez de Juan, V.; Woodhoo, A.; Martinez-Lopez, N.; Rodriguez-Iruretagoyena, B.; Bustamante, F.J.; et al. Murine double minute 2 regulates Hu antigen R stability in human liver and colon cancer through NEDDylation. *Hepatology* **2012**, *55*, 1237–1248. [CrossRef]
60. Bailly, A.P.; Perrin, A.; Serrano-Macia, M.; Maghames, C.; Leidecker, O.; Trauchessec, H.; Martinez-Chantar, M.L.; Gartner, A.; Xirodimas, D.P. The Balance between Mono- and NEDD8-Chains Controlled by NEDP1 upon DNA Damage Is a Regulatory Module of the HSP70 ATPase Activity. *Cell Rep.* **2019**, *29*, 212–224. [CrossRef]
61. Zubiete-Franco, I.; Fernandez-Tussy, P.; Barbier-Torres, L.; Simon, J.; Fernandez-Ramos, D.; Lopitz-Otsoa, F.; Gutierrez-de Juan, V.; de Davalillo, S.L.; Duce, A.M.; Iruzubieta, P.; et al. Deregulated neddylation in liver fibrosis. *Hepatology* **2017**, *65*, 694–709. [CrossRef] [PubMed]
62. Zuo, W.; Huang, F.; Chiang, Y.J.; Li, M.; Du, J.; Ding, Y.; Zhang, T.; Lee, H.W.; Jeong, L.S.; Chen, Y.; et al. c-Cbl-mediated neddylation antagonizes ubiquitination and degradation of the TGF-beta type II receptor. *Mol. Cell* **2013**, *49*, 499–510. [CrossRef] [PubMed]
63. Kumar, D.; Das, M.; Sauceda, C.; Ellies, L.G.; Kuo, K.; Parwal, P.; Kaur, M.; Jih, L.; Bandyopadhyay, G.K.; Burton, D.; et al. Degradation of splicing factor SRSF3 contributes to progressive liver disease. *J. Clin. Investig.* **2019**, *130*, 4477–4491. [CrossRef] [PubMed]
64. Zhao, X. SUMO-Mediated Regulation of Nuclear Functions and Signaling Processes. *Mol. Cell* **2018**, *71*, 409–418. [CrossRef]
65. Eisenhardt, N.; Chaugule, V.K.; Koidl, S.; Droescher, M.; Dogan, E.; Rettich, J.; Sutinen, P.; Imanishi, S.Y.; Hofmann, K.; Palvimo, J.J.; et al. A new vertebrate SUMO enzyme family reveals insights into SUMO-chain assembly. *Nat. Struct. Mol. Biol.* **2015**, *22*, 959–967. [CrossRef]

66. Hendriks, I.A.; Vertegaal, A.C. A comprehensive compilation of SUMO proteomics. *Nat. Rev. Mol. Cell Biol.* **2016**, *17*, 581–595. [CrossRef]
67. Muller, S.; Ledl, A.; Schmidt, D. SUMO: A regulator of gene expression and genome integrity. *Oncogene* **2004**, *23*, 1998–2008. [CrossRef]
68. Jackson, S.P.; Durocher, D. Regulation of DNA damage responses by ubiquitin and SUMO. *Mol. Cell* **2013**, *49*, 795–807. [CrossRef]
69. Golebiowski, F.; Matic, I.; Tatham, M.H.; Cole, C.; Yin, Y.; Nakamura, A.; Cox, J.; Barton, G.J.; Mann, M.; Hay, R.T. System-wide changes to SUMO modifications in response to heat shock. *Sci. Signal.* **2009**, *2*, ra24. [CrossRef]
70. Yang, W.; Thompson, J.W.; Wang, Z.; Wang, L.; Sheng, H.; Foster, M.W.; Moseley, M.A.; Paschen, W. Analysis of oxygen/glucose-deprivation-induced changes in SUMO3 conjugation using SILAC-based quantitative proteomics. *J. Proteome Res.* **2012**, *11*, 1108–1117. [CrossRef]
71. Psakhye, I.; Jentsch, S. Protein group modification and synergy in the SUMO pathway as exemplified in DNA repair. *Cell* **2012**, *151*, 807–820. [CrossRef] [PubMed]
72. Bossis, G.; Melchior, F. Regulation of SUMOylation by reversible oxidation of SUMO conjugating enzymes. *Mol. Cell* **2006**, *21*, 349–357. [CrossRef] [PubMed]
73. Kang, J.S.; Saunier, E.F.; Akhurst, R.J.; Derynck, R. The type I TGF-beta receptor is covalently modified and regulated by sumoylation. *Nat. Cell Biol.* **2008**, *10*, 654–664. [CrossRef] [PubMed]
74. Desterro, J.M.; Rodriguez, M.S.; Hay, R.T. SUMO-1 modification of IkappaBalpha inhibits NF-kappaB activation. *Mol. Cell* **1998**, *2*, 233–239. [CrossRef]
75. Liu, Y.; Zhao, D.; Qiu, F.; Zhang, L.L.; Liu, S.K.; Li, Y.Y.; Liu, M.T.; Wu, D.; Wang, J.X.; Ding, X.Q.; et al. Manipulating PML SUMOylation via Silencing UBC9 and RNF4 Regulates Cardiac Fibrosis. *Mol. Ther.* **2017**, *25*, 666–678. [CrossRef]
76. Ahner, A.; Gong, X.; Frizzell, R.A. Divergent signaling via SUMO modification: Potential for CFTR modulation. *Am. J. Physiol. Cell Physiol.* **2016**, *310*, C175–C180. [CrossRef]
77. Arvaniti, E.; Vakrakou, A.; Kaltezioti, V.; Stergiopoulos, A.; Prakoura, N.; Politis, P.K.; Charonis, A. Nuclear receptor NR5A2 is involved in the calreticulin gene regulation during renal fibrosis. *Biochim. Biophys. Acta* **2016**, *1862*, 1774–1785. [CrossRef]
78. Fang, S.; Yuan, J.; Shi, Q.; Xu, T.; Fu, Y.; Wu, Z.; Guo, W. Downregulation of UBC9 promotes apoptosis of activated human LX-2 hepatic stellate cells by suppressing the canonical NF-kappaB signaling pathway. *PLoS ONE* **2017**, *12*, e0174374.
79. Bu, F.T.; Chen, Y.; Yu, H.X.; Chen, X.; Yang, Y.; Pan, X.Y.; Wang, Q.; Wu, Y.T.; Huang, C.; Meng, X.M.; et al. SENP2 alleviates CCl4-induced liver fibrosis by promoting activated hepatic stellate cell apoptosis and reversion. *Toxicol. Lett.* **2018**, *289*, 86–98. [CrossRef]
80. Ramani, K.; Tomasi, M.L.; Yang, H.; Ko, K.; Lu, S.C. Mechanism and significance of changes in glutamate-cysteine ligase expression during hepatic fibrogenesis. *J. Biol. Chem.* **2012**, *287*, 36341–36355. [CrossRef]
81. Lin, X.; Liang, M.; Liang, Y.Y.; Brunicardi, F.C.; Feng, X.H. SUMO-1/Ubc9 promotes nuclear accumulation and metabolic stability of tumor suppressor Smad4. *J. Biol. Chem.* **2003**, *278*, 31043–31048. [CrossRef] [PubMed]
82. Liu, S.; Long, J.; Yuan, B.; Zheng, M.; Xiao, M.; Xu, J.; Lin, X.; Feng, X.H. SUMO Modification Reverses Inhibitory Effects of Smad Nuclear Interacting Protein-1 in TGF-beta Responses. *J. Biol. Chem.* **2016**, *291*, 24418–24430. [CrossRef] [PubMed]
83. Janka, C.; Selmi, C.; Gershwin, M.E.; Will, H.; Sternsdorf, T. Small ubiquitin-related modifiers: A novel and independent class of autoantigens in primary biliary cirrhosis. *Hepatology* **2005**, *41*, 609–616. [CrossRef] [PubMed]
84. Veggiani, G.; Gerpe, M.C.R.; Sidhu, S.S.; Zhang, W. Emerging drug development technologies targeting ubiquitination for cancer therapeutics. *Pharmacol. Ther.* **2019**, *199*, 139–154. [CrossRef]
85. Wertz, I.E.; Murray, J.M. Structurally-defined deubiquitinase inhibitors provide opportunities to investigate disease mechanisms. *Drug Discov. Today Technol.* **2019**, *31*, 109–123. [CrossRef]
86. Liu, J.; Shaik, S.; Dai, X.; Wu, Q.; Zhou, X.; Wang, Z.; Wei, W. Targeting the ubiquitin pathway for cancer treatment. *Biochim. Biophys. Acta* **2015**, *1855*, 50–60. [CrossRef]
87. Zhou, Y.; Ji, C.; Cao, M.; Guo, M.; Huang, W.; Ni, W.; Meng, L.; Yang, H.; Wei, J.F. Inhibitors targeting the SUMOylation pathway: A patent review 20122015 (Review). *Int. J. Mol. Med.* **2018**, *41*, 3–12. [CrossRef]

88. Li, B.; Cong, M.; Zhu, Y.; Xiong, Y.; Jin, W.; Wan, Y.; Zhou, Y.; Ao, Y.; Wang, H. Indole-3-Carbinol Induces Apoptosis of Hepatic Stellate Cells through K63 De-Ubiquitination of RIP1 in Rats. *Cell Physiol. Biochem.* **2017**, *41*, 1481–1490. [CrossRef]
89. Soucy, T.A.; Smith, P.G.; Milhollen, M.A.; Berger, A.J.; Gavin, J.M.; Adhikari, S.; Brownell, J.E.; Burke, K.E.; Cardin, D.P.; Critchley, S.; et al. An inhibitor of NEDD8-activating enzyme as a new approach to treat cancer. *Nature* **2009**, *458*, 732–736. [CrossRef]
90. Hjerpe, R.; Aillet, F.; Lopitz-Otsoa, F.; Lang, V.; England, P.; Rodriguez, M.S. Efficient protection and isolation of ubiquitylated proteins using tandem ubiquitin-binding entities. *EMBO Rep.* **2009**, *10*, 1250–1258. [CrossRef]
91. Da Silva-Ferrada, E.; Xolalpa, W.; Lang, V.; Aillet, F.; Martin-Ruiz, I.; de la Cruz-Herrera, C.F.; Lopitz-Otsoa, F.; Carracedo, A.; Goldenberg, S.J.; Rivas, C.; et al. Analysis of SUMOylated proteins using SUMO-traps. *Sci. Rep.* **2013**, *3*, 1690. [CrossRef] [PubMed]
92. Zubiete-Franco, I.; Garcia-Rodriguez, J.L.; Lopitz-Otsoa, F.; Serrano-Macia, M.; Simon, J.; Fernandez-Tussy, P.; Barbier-Torres, L.; Fernandez-Ramos, D.; Gutierrez-de-Juan, V.; Lopez de Davalillo, S.; et al. SUMOylation regulates LKB1 localization and its oncogenic activity in liver cancer. *EBioMedicine* **2019**, *40*, 406–421. [CrossRef] [PubMed]
93. Lindsten, K.; Menendez-Benito, V.; Masucci, M.G.; Dantuma, N.P. A transgenic mouse model of the ubiquitin/proteasome system. *Nat. Biotechnol.* **2003**, *21*, 897–902. [CrossRef] [PubMed]
94. Lectez, B.; Migotti, R.; Lee, S.Y.; Ramirez, J.; Beraza, N.; Mansfield, B.; Sutherland, J.D.; Martinez-Chantar, M.L.; Dittmar, G.; Mayor, U. Ubiquitin profiling in liver using a transgenic mouse with biotinylated ubiquitin. *J. Proteome Res.* **2014**, *13*, 3016–3026. [CrossRef]
95. Pirone, L.; Xolalpa, W.; Mayor, U.; Barrio, R.; Sutherland, J.D. Analysis of SUMOylated Proteins in Cells and In Vivo Using the bioSUMO Strategy. *Methods Mol. Biol.* **2016**, *1475*, 161–169. [CrossRef]

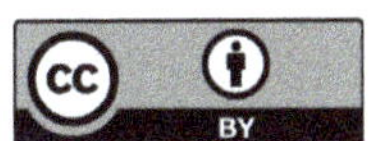

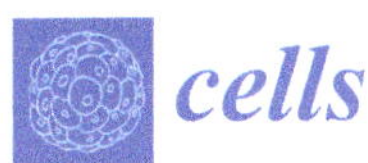
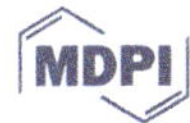

Review

Mast Cells in Liver Fibrogenesis

Ralf Weiskirchen [1,*], Steffen K. Meurer [1], Christian Liedtke [2] and Michael Huber [3,*]

1 Institute of Molecular Pathobiochemistry, Experimental Gene Therapy and Clinical Chemistry (IFMPEGKC), University Hospital, RWTH Aachen University, D-52074 Aachen, Germany; smeurer@ukaachen.de
2 Department of Internal Medicine III, University Hospital, RWTH Aachen University, D-52074 Aachen, Germany; cliedtke@ukaachen.de
3 Institute of Biochemistry and Molecular Immunology, Medical Faculty, RWTH Aachen University, D-52074 Aachen, Germany
* Correspondence: rweiskirchen@ukaachen.de (R.W.) mhuber@ukaachen.de (M.H.)

Received: 14 October 2019; Accepted: 10 November 2019; Published: 13 November 2019

Abstract: Mast cells (MCs) are immune cells of the myeloid lineage that are present in the connective tissue throughout the body and in mucosa tissue. They originate from hematopoietic stem cells in the bone marrow and circulate as MC progenitors in the blood. After migration to various tissues, they differentiate into their mature form, which is characterized by a phenotype containing large granules enriched in a variety of bioactive compounds, including histamine and heparin. These cells can be activated in a receptor-dependent and -independent manner. Particularly, the activation of the high-affinity immunoglobulin E (IgE) receptor, also known as FcεRI, that is expressed on the surface of MCs provoke specific signaling cascades that leads to intracellular calcium influx, activation of different transcription factors, degranulation, and cytokine production. Therefore, MCs modulate many aspects in physiological and pathological conditions, including wound healing, defense against pathogens, immune tolerance, allergy, anaphylaxis, autoimmune defects, inflammation, and infectious and other disorders. In the liver, MCs are mainly associated with connective tissue located in the surrounding of the hepatic arteries, veins, and bile ducts. Recent work has demonstrated a significant increase in MC number during hepatic injury, suggesting an important role of these cells in liver disease and progression. In the present review, we summarize aspects of MC function and mediators in experimental liver injury, their interaction with other hepatic cell types, and their contribution to the pathogenesis of fibrosis.

Keywords: liver; inflammation; fibrosis; mast cell; degranulation; TGF-β; animal models; translational medicine; chymase; tryptase

1. Introduction

1.1. Mast Cell Development

Mast cells (MCs) are hematopoietic cells of the myeloid lineage [1]. They can be found particularly in tissues with close contact to the environment, such as skin, gastrointestinal tract, upper airways, and lung [2]. However, MCs are also located in other vascularized organs (e.g., liver and kidney [3,4]). Correlating with their presence in various locations, MCs present as a highly heterogeneous cell population with subtype-dependent differences in cell morphology, histochemical properties, expression of granular proteases, and function, amongst others [5]. This intriguing plasticity and heterogeneity also have their origin in the differentiation process of MCs [6].

MCs originate from hematopoietic stem cells, which differentiate into MC precursors (MCps) in the bone marrow. MCps then leave the bone marrow and distribute via the blood and transendothelial migration into target tissues, where they eventually phenotypically mature in the presence of tissue-specific factors, such as cytokines, growth factors, and extracellular matrix (ECM) components.

Different maturation conditions lead to functionally diverse MCs, which can be subdivided in mice in chymase-expressing mucosa-type MCs (MMCs) and tryptase/chymase-expressing connective tissue-type MCs (CTMCs).

From a signaling perspective, MC development in vivo is strictly dependent on the expression of the receptor tyrosine kinase KIT, also known as CD117 [7]. Likewise, expression of the KIT ligand stem cell factor (SCF) is mandatory for MC development in vivo [8]. Another prominent MC receptor is the high-affinity receptor for IgE (FcεRI) [9], which is important, amongst other factors, for defense against helminths, but also for the induction of allergic reactions. The co-expression of both KIT and FcεRI, in addition to distinct cytoplasmic metachromatic granules (also termed secretory lysosomes), characterizes mature MCs [2].

With respect to the distribution of MCps through the blood to respective target tissues, productive interactions between surface molecules of MCps and endothelial cells are required for transendothelial migration [10]. As an example, the homing of MCps to the small intestine is dependent on the α4β7 integrin on the MCps, and MAdCAM-1 and VCAM1 as counterligands on the endothelial cells [11]. For α4β7 integrin activation by inside-out signaling, ligand-induced activation of CXCR2 on MCps is required [12]. After migration to the different tissues, MCps differentiate into tissue-specific mature MCs, which can belong to either of the two major subclasses of MCs, MMCs or CTMCs. In addition to the subtype- and tissue-specific changes in secretory potential (e.g., differential content of secretory lysosomes and configuration of signaling systems), mature MCs downregulate cell-surface adhesion molecules and chemokine receptors [13,14]. Intriguingly, by using a new fate mapping mouse model, Gentek et al. recently demonstrated that MCs have dual developmental origins [15]. Whereas most skin MCs are of primitive origin during embryogenesis (i.e., yolk sac derived), adult definitive MCs originate from definitive hematopoietic stem cells of the aorta-gonad-mesonephros vascular endothelium. Moreover, in this study it was demonstrated that replenishment of adult tissue MCs predominantly occurs via the proliferation/differentiation of long-lived tissue-resident precursors [15]. These data were in principle verified by Li et al. [16]. However, by applying two different fate mapping mouse models, they could demonstrate that most CTMCs even derive from late erythro-myeloid progenitors generated at the hemogenic endothelium of the yolk sac.

1.2. Different Roles of Mast Cells in Physiology and Pathophysiology

MCs take part in processes of innate and adaptive immunity, alerting the body to invasion by bacteria and parasites, and regulating lymphocyte reactions [17,18]. Moreover, through the release of different proteases, MCs are able to attenuate snake-venom-induced and honeybee-venom-induced pathology by degrading the proteinaceous venom components [19]. They also promote homeostasis by limiting endothelin-1-induced toxicity in a carboxypeptidase-A3-dependent manner [20,21]. Also, on the beneficial side, MCs have a positive impact on bone repair, most likely by recruiting vascular endothelial cells during the inflammatory phase, and by coordinating anabolic and catabolic activities during tissue remodeling [22]. Moreover, myocardial MCs regulate heart function after a myocardial infarction [23], and mucosal MCs in the intestinal epithelium execute anti-helminth immunity [24].

In addition to these beneficial functions, MCs play detrimental roles as well, e.g., as central effector cells in acute allergic disorders (such as rhinitis, asthma, and anaphylactic reactions) [25]. Moreover, MCs promote T cell-driven collagen-induced arthritis. However, they are dispensable for antibody-induced arthritis in which T cells are bypassed [26]. MCs are also known to modulate the growth/metastasis of certain solid tumors [27] and can contribute to the development of various fibrotic diseases [28]. In septic peritonitis, MCs have been demonstrated to suppress the phagocytosis of bacteria by peritoneal macrophages in an IL-4-dependent manner. Thus, MCs can aggravate the outcome of severe bacterial infections [29]. Neither the number of positive nor the number of negative functions of MCs mentioned above are exhaustive; nevertheless, they provide an idea about the variety of the biological functions of MCs.

In addition, detrimental outcomes are known for patients suffering from mastocytosis, which is a rare and heterogeneous disease characterized by the expansion and accumulation of clonal (neoplastic) tissue MCs in one or more organ systems [30,31]. Mastocytosis can be divided into subvariants of cutaneous mastocytosis, different types of systemic mastocytosis (SM), and localized MC tumors. SM is further divided into several subtypes (i.e., indolent SM, smoldering SM, SM with an associated hematologic neoplasm, aggressive SM, and MC leukemia [30,31]). The different subtypes of mastocytosis exert highly variable clinical courses, ranging from asymptomatic with a normal life expectancy to fatal with high mortality within months or weeks [30,31]. Additionally, clinical conditions related to MC activation, where symptoms are recurrent, are accompanied by an increase in MC-derived mediators in biological fluids, and are responsive to treatment with MC-stabilizing or mediator-targeting drugs, can/might be diagnosed as MC activation syndrome (MCAS) [32] (for a proposed diagnostic algorithm for MCAS we refer to Valent et al. [33]). In conclusion, MCs can be regarded as a versatile cell type with differential functions in physiological and pathophysiological settings, and hence, MCs are very attractive drug targets.

1.3. Mast Cell Mediators

The most eye-catching feature of MCs visualized using electron microscopy is the multitude of electron-dense vesicles/granula. These organelles are secretory lysosomes that store preformed pro-inflammatory mediators (e.g., histamine; proteoglycans, such as heparin and chondroitin-sulfate; various proteases, such as tryptase, chymase, carboxypeptidase A3, granzyme B, and active caspase-3; and certain cytokines) that are released immediately upon antigen-triggered activation of the IgE-bound FcεRI in a process called degranulation [34–37]. Another important MC-selective receptor able to induce the process of degranulation upon recognition of its ligand(s) is the Mas-related G protein-coupled receptor X2 (MRGPRX2; in mice: MRGPRB2), which can trigger the secretory response upon binding to antimicrobial peptides, neuropeptides, eosinophil peroxidase, and various peptidergic drugs, amongst others [38]. Before the identification of this receptor, many detrimental reactions in patients were referred to as "drug-induced pseudoallergies" without having the notion that it is only one receptor that recognizes this variety of different molecules [39].

A further immediate response of MCs is the generation and release of arachidonic acid metabolites, particularly the leukotrienes LTB_4 and LTC_4, and prostaglandin PGD_2. These mediators, in a situation-dependent context, are able to initiate, amplify, or attenuate inflammatory responses. Furthermore, they can influence the magnitude, duration, and nature of subsequent immune responses [40]. In addition, MCs are capable of producing and secreting numerous cytokines, chemokines, growth factors, and angiogenic factors mediating multiple pro-inflammatory, anti-inflammatory, and/or immunoregulatory effects in a situation-dependent manner [2,41]. Amongst others, MCs are able to synthesize and secrete TNF-α, IL-1β, IL-3, IL-5, IL-6, IL-8, IL-9, IL-13, CCL5, TGF-β1, and FGF.

The composition of MC responses is largely dependent on the activated receptor(s). In response to an antigen, MCs degranulate and produce arachidonic acid metabolites, as well as cytokines and chemokines. In contrast, the stimulation of MCs via cytokines or pattern recognition receptors (e.g., toll-like receptors (TLRs)) only induces the generation of arachidonic acid metabolites and cytokines/chemokines. With respect to TLR4 activation by lipopolysaccharide (LPS), MCs are markedly different compared to macrophages concerning their receptor composition and organization of signaling pathways. MCs do not express the GPI-anchored protein mCD14, which affects the chemotype of recognized LPS molecules (R-LPS >> S-LPS) [42]. Moreover, upon LPS recognition, MCs do not activate the TRIF pathway, and thus, MCs do not produce IFN-β [43,44].

1.4. Murine Models to Study Mast Cell Involvement

To study the role of MCs in different disease situations, mostly mouse models are used, though models in rats, hamsters, dogs, and rabbits have also been used for the investigation of certain diseases. Most mouse studies have made use of animals that do not express KIT and thus are devoid, though not completely, of MCs ("*Kit* mutant MC-deficient mice"). Different mutant mice carrying mutations in the *Kit* gene/locus have been frequently used (e.g., WBB6F$_1$-*Kit*$^{W/W\text{-}v}$ and C57BL/6-*Kit*$^{W\text{-}sh/W\text{-}sh}$ mice [7,45]) to study disease development in the absence of MCs. Moreover, in vitro differentiated bone-marrow-derived MCs (BMMCs) have been used to engraft an MC population in these genetically MC-deficient mice ("MC knock-in mice") and disease development has been studied [46]. If changes in MC-deficient mice, compared to the respective wild-type mice, could be reverted via the re-establishment of MC populations, then this was taken as a proof of MC involvement in the particular disease process. However, it should be noted that KIT is also expressed on hematopoietic stem cells and almost all myeloid progenitor cells, allowing for altered adaptive and innate immune reactions in KIT-deficient mice, which cannot only be attributed to missing MCs. Not unexpected, using a *Kit*-independent mouse model of MC deficiency (Cpa3$^{Cre/+}$ mice (Cre-Master mice) carrying a targeted insertion of Cre recombinase in the carboxypeptidase A3 locus), Feyerabend et al. could not verify all results from studies that used *Kit*-dependent MC-deficient mouse models [47]. Examples of such MC-independent diseases were antibody-induced autoimmune arthritis and experimental autoimmune encephalomyelitis. Additional mutant mice with constitutive MC deficiency unrelated to *Kit* abnormalities are the *Mcpt5-Cre; R-DTA* mice and the *Cpa3-Cre; Mcl1*$^{fl/fl}$ mice. For the generation of *Mcpt5-Cre; R-DTA* mice, *Mcpt5-Cre* transgenic mice [48] were crossed with *R-DTA*$^{fl/fl}$ mice [49] to yield a mouse strain in which CTMCs are ablated by the expression of the diphtheria toxin α chain [50]. For the generation of transgenic *Cpa3-Cre; Mcl1*$^{fl/fl}$ mice (also known as "Hello Kitty" mice), mice expressing *Cre* under the control of a *Cpa3* promoter fragment were crossed with *Mcl1*$^{fl/fl}$ mice [51], allowing for the deletion of the gene of the anti-apoptotic factor MCL1 [52]. The different mouse models of MC deficiency have been comprehensively reviewed by Galli et al. [53].

2. Fibrosis: Some General Aspects

The term fibrosis describes a pathological situation defined by the overgrowth, hardening, and excessive scarring that can affect nearly all tissues [54]. The scarring process is mainly characterized by the replacement of normal parenchymal tissue by connective tissue. The process is initiated by neutrophilic inflammation, which can result from various stimuli, such as mechanical injury, infections, autoimmune attacks, toxins, or radiation. Mechanistically, this process aims to eliminate the initial cause of injury and preserve the function of the affected organ [55].

The primary inflammatory response is well-orchestrated and requires engagement of the local vascular system and components of the immune system, as well as the systemic coordination of endocrine and neurological mediators [54]. This interconnection is driven by a variety of soluble factors (chemokines, cytokines). During acute inflammation, resident immune cells (e.g., macrophages, dendritic cells, MCs) are the most important in the initial phase. These cells are equipped with pattern recognition receptors (PRRs) playing a crucial role in the detection of pathogen-associated molecular patterns (PAMPs) and damage-associated molecular patterns (DAMPs) [54,55]. These receptors differ in their ligand recognition and defined subsets can identify a broad range of proteins, nucleic acids, or glycans [56,57]. After ligand recognition, these receptors induce various cellular responses resulting in the release of different inflammatory mediators that in turn provoke the typical five cardinal clinical signs of inflammation, namely *rubor* (redness), *calor* (heat), *tumor* (swelling), *dolor* (pain), and *functio laesa* (loss of function).

If this first-line defense is insufficient to eliminate the disease-causing agent and inflammation persists, various immune cells, such as macrophages and T-lymphocytes, are triggered to produce high quantities of cytokines and enzymes, which subsequently provoke more lasting damage. As a consequence, parenchymal cell death occurs, which is associated with an uncontrolled release of pro-fibrogenic mediators that in turn lead to activation of a pro-fibrogenic cell population with the capacity to synthesize large quantities of ECM components [58]. In this regard, members of the TGF-β family of cytokines are of fundamental importance, acting as a common master switch. TGF-β strongly promotes the synthesis of collagen and fibronectin in both epithelial and mesenchymal cells and further suppresses the process of inflammation [58]. Other important soluble mediators triggering the process of fibrogenesis are members of the platelet-derived growth factor (PDGF) family and connective tissue growth factor (CTGF). While PDGFs are highly competent mitogens and chemoattractants for fibrogenic cells, CTGF contains structural features serving as TGF-β binding domains, thereby enhancing its biological activity or sequestering other members of the TGF-β gene family, such as bone-morphogenetic proteins (BMPs), which usually act as opposing factors for TGF-β [59]. In concert with TGF-β, these mediators increase the number and activity of myofibroblasts (MFBs) and their progenitors, thereby promoting fibrogenesis in a variety of organs including skin, heart, kidney, pancreas, lung, liver, and others. Strikingly, the population of cells capable of synthesizing ECM consists of resident pro-fibrogenic cells, such as hepatic stellate cells (HSCs) and portal myofibroblasts, progenitors invading the inflamed tissue, and cells that become activated and acquire fibrogenic features [55]. These cells are preserved between different organs. The final ECM-producing cell type, the myofibroblast, can originate from cellular subsets including resident fibroblasts, mesothelial cells, circulating fibrocytes, epithelial cells, endothelial cells, pericytes, vascular smooth muscle cells, Gli1^{+} perivascular mesenchymal stem cell-like cells, and other more specialized cells that are present within different organs or tissue. In kidney, these are, for example, podocytes found in the lining of the Bowman's capsules in the nephrons or tubular epithelial cells that might also acquire migratory properties and transit into a myofibroblast-like phenotype capable of synthesizing ECM components [55].

2.1. Common Mediators in Inflammation and Fibrogenesis

Both inflammation and fibrogenesis are complex processes in which numerous pro-inflammatory and pro-fibrogenic mediators can be involved. On one hand, there are chemokines considered to regulate immune cell entry into the inflamed tissue. On the other hand, there is a convolute of cytokines that modulate important functions in the inflammatory response and in the progression of inflammation to fibrosis. In addition, enhanced production of non-peptidic factors, such as reactive oxygen species (ROS), oxidized lipid mediators, and acetaldehyde, contribute to endothelial dysfunction and tissue injury during inflammation [60].

Chemokines are a group of small, mostly basic, structurally-related molecules that modulate the trafficking of leukocytes and have critical immunological functions [61]. In the last few decades, different chemokines have emerged as important molecules whose importance extends far beyond their most famous function as inflammatory mediators [61]. For several chemokines, the exact functions in different organs were identified, while others can act in an organ-independent manner [55]. Prototypically, the C-C motif chemokine 2 (CCL2), also known as monocyte chemoattractant protein-1 (MCP-1), can activate tissue macrophages and fibroblasts during the inflammatory response in many organs. Chemokines are produced by a broad range of cells and can act in an autocrine and paracrine manner. They bind to surface-exposed receptors and transmit their signals via specific intracellular signaling pathways that modulate the expression or activity of downstream targets. Besides TGF-β and PDGF that were already discussed above, different interleukins (ILs) possessing pleiotropic activities in the innate and adaptive immune response critically contribute to the onset and progression of inflammatory responses. However, their biological activity and impact in different disease settings is more variable than the effects mediated by TGF-β and PDGF. In addition, individual members of the IL family can have overlapping, but also distinct, biological activities and may exert pro- or anti-inflammatory activities [62]. Another important cytokine in the process of inflammation and fibrosis is the tumor necrosis factor-α (TNF-α), which belongs to the TNF family composed of about 20 different proteins and is produced by macrophages, amongst others [63]. The activation of its cognate receptors (TNFR1 and TNFR2) stimulates two different signaling pathways. While TNFR1 activates NF-κB and is associated with apoptosis, TNFR2 mainly triggers cell survival pathways [64]. Therefore, it is obvious that this dual activity makes TNF-α one of the key switches that determines the outcome of an inflammatory response.

Some of the biological activities of ROS are directly linked to its potential to induce TGF-β expression and activity [65]. Under physiological conditions, NADPH oxidase-derived ROS are essential modulators of signal transduction pathways that control cell growth, proliferation, migration, differentiation, apoptosis, diverse biochemical pathways, and immune responses [66]. However, elevated ROS quantities cause direct irreversible oxidative damage of all kinds of biomolecules, thereby contributing to various pathological alterations, including inflammation [66]. In particular, ROS is known to induce parenchymal cell necrosis and apoptosis and stimulate the production and release of pro-fibrogenic signaling molecules [55].

Similarly, oxidized (phospho-)lipids, such as oxidized phosphatidylcholine, can be formed and accumulate in macrophages during fibrogenesis [67]. The oxidized products promote M2 polarization of macrophages and the enhanced production of TGF-β, thereby critically contributing to fibrogenic signaling cascades. A direct effect of acetaldehyde on type I collagen expression in HSCs is mediated through acetaldehyde-responsive elements (AcRE), which are co-localized with the TGF-β-responsive element [68]. Although the mechanisms leading to an increase of collagen expression by TGF-β and acetaldehyde rely on the formation of H_2O_2, the kinetics of these mediators in triggering collagen expression are different. Therefore, it was assumed that early acetaldehyde-dependent events induce TGF-β expression and create an H_2O_2-dependent autocrine loop that amplifies the fibrogenic process [68].

More recently, it was realized that parenchymal cells under inflammatory conditions can form extracellular membranous vesicles (exosomes) that are generated by inward budding of the plasma membrane into early endosomes and multivesicular endosomes [69]. The cargo of these particles can contain diverse molecules (proteins, mRNA, microRNA, DNA, lipids), which can be transferred to distant recipient cells. Although their precise function in the transmission of signals between the different cells is not fully understood, first reports have demonstrated that in alcoholic hepatitis, hepatocyte-derived exosomes contain different microRNAs that induce a hyperinflammatory phenotype in monocytes/macrophages [70]. Similarly, a high-fat diet in rats increased the number of circulating extracellular vesicles that promote inflammation [71]. These pilot studies confirm the assumption that exosomes can mediate the communication between donor and target cells and reprogram the cells involved in inflammation. Intriguingly, recent data by Metcalfe et al. [72] showed the generation of extracellular vesicles (EVs) with an MC signature in patients with SM, which could transfer KIT to an HSC line eliciting proliferation, cytokine production, and differentiation.

2.2. *Liver Fibrogenesis: A Number of Different Cell Types Contributing to the Initiation and Progression of Fibrosis*

In the liver, viral infections (hepatitis), metabolic diseases, cholestasis, parasites, drugs, alcohol, genetic determinants, and a variety of environmental factors can lead to the initiation and progression of fibrogenesis. Like in many other organs, the pathogenic sequence begins with parenchymal cell destruction and inflammation. Hepatocytes, building 70–85% of the main parenchymal tissue, can metabolize, detoxify, and inactivate exogenous compounds. However, if the acute or chronic exposure to a toxicant is too high, the cellular phenotype of these cells becomes detrimentally altered. Cell necrosis occurs, causing many factors to leak out of injured cells, resulting in the activation of liver-resident macrophages, designated as Kupffer cells. In addition, the damaged tissue is infiltrated by various kinds of lymphocytes, which further increase the concentration of pro-inflammatory and pro-fibrotic mediators. In particular, the concentrations of TGF-β and PDGF increase. This, in turn, leads to the activation and propagation of HSCs that lose their quiescent phenotype and transdifferentiate into proliferative and extracellular matrix-producing MFBs [73]. In addition, portal fibroblasts, comprising a small population of the fibroblast cell lineage surrounding the portal vein to maintain the integrity of the portal tract, acquire a myofibroblast-like phenotype, start to proliferate, and synthesize extracellular matrix. Moreover, mesenchymal progenitor cells and fibrocytes recruited from the bone marrow are other sources of cells contributing to the generation of excessive scar formation [73]. Also, liver sinusoidal endothelial cells (LSEC) forming the wall of the hepatic sinusoids lose their fenestrae during hepatic fibrosis and form a basement membrane, preventing the physiological bidirectional exchange of molecules between hepatocytes and hepatic blood sinusoids. This corroborates with a significant synthesis and release of soluble factors, such as TGF-β and PDGF, again triggering the fibrogenic response.

However, it should be mentioned that fibrogenesis is not a unidirectional path. Regression or even full resolution can be achieved by the withdrawal of the injurious agent and is regularly seen in patients undergoing successful causative treatment of their underlying disease [74].

2.3. Mouse Models of Liver Fibrosis: What Can be Learned for Human Disease?

In hepatology research, preclinical mouse models are still essential for analyzing complex disease-associated changes to unravel cellular reactions, signaling pathways, and networks, as well as for the preclinical testing of novel therapeutic useful anti-inflammatory or anti-fibrotic drugs [62]. The usage of mice is majorly attributable to the fact that mice are inexpensive, can be bred in large quantities on an inbred genetic background helping to establish reproducible results, and having general features in anatomy and biology that are similar to humans [62]. Nowadays, a large number of well-established injury models are commonly used in experimental and molecular hepatology. For most of these models, we have recently published standard operating protocols (SOPs) that provide information about the scientific background, treatment, duration, and burden [75–84].

In Table 1, we exclusively list relevant experimental models that have been the focus of liver-related MC research.

Table 1. Established mouse injury models that have been the focus of liver-related mast cell research.

Model	Procedure and Typical Time of Sacrifice	Outcome	Model for Human Liver Disease	Reference
CCl_4	Single or repeated i.p. application (1 h–6 wks), regular inhalation or application by gavage (11–15 wks)	Early: inflammation; late: centrilobular liver damage, fibrosis/cirrhosis induced by forming radicals	Intoxication, acute liver damage, fibrosis	[75]
LPS LPS/D-GalN LPS/BCG	I.p. injection or application of LPS in drinking water alone or in combination with D-GalN; i.p. injection of LPS/BCG (2–8 h)	Inflammation (LPS), acute hepatic failure (LPS/D-GalN), lethal hepatitis (LPS/BCG)	Acute systemic and hepatic inflammation; lethal hepatitis	[79]
DEN DMN	I.p., oral (drinking water, diet, gavage), inhalation, intratracheal, or intragastric instillation (6–50 wks)	Time-dependent liver damage (neutrophilic infiltration, extensive centrilobular hemorrhagic necrosis, bile duct proliferation, fibrosis, and bridging necrosis ending in hepatocarcinogenesis)	Early: intoxication, late: fibrosis, cirrhosis, HCC	[81]
BDL	Surgical ligation of the common biliary duct (5 days–4 wks)	Early: liver cell injury, severe inflammation; late: advanced hepatic fibrosis	Early: liver injury and jaundice, late: cholestatic liver diseases	[82,83]
Mdr2$^{-/-}$	Homozygous disruption of the multidrug resistance 2 gene	Significant increase of bilirubin, alkaline phosphatase, aspartate aminotransferase already at age of 6–14 wks	Cholestatic liver injury	[85]

Abbreviations used are: BCG: bacillus Calmette–Guérin, BDL: bile duct ligation, CCl_4: carbon tetrachloride D-GalN: D-galactosamine, DEN: diethylnitrosamine, DMN: dimethylnitrosamine, h: hour(s), HCC: hepatocellular carcinoma; i.p.: intraperitoneal, LPS: lipopolysaccharide, wks: weeks.

in SM. In this setting, MC numbers are highly increased in the liver [89,90]. It is a common feature that MC numbers increase in tissues during the process of fibrogenesis and the expansion of the MC pool in the liver is a common characteristic of liver fibrosis in humans and animal models due to damage by chemical toxins, viral infections, and cholestasis [91–94]. In fact, the physiological number of MCs in the liver is sparse and MC numbers strongly increase upon different pathological conditions [4,95–97]. According to Gentek et al., such an increase in MC numbers might occur via proliferation/differentiation of long-lived tissue-resident precursors [15].

The localization of MCs in the liver is mostly restricted to portal tracts and MCs are recruited to these areas under pathological conditions [98]. They are most likely absent from sinusoids and liver parenchyma [95,96]. However, in human liver, ≈10% of MCs have a perisinusoidal location [92]. Because of the prominent appearance in the portal tracts, most studies have been performed in the setting of cholangiopathies [99]. In those models, the inflammatory and fibrotic responses emanate from the portal fields based on a biliary reaction [82,83]. Due to this, the focus has been put on the interaction of MCs with cholangiocytes and to the pathways driving fibrogenic responses in HSCs/portal (myo)fibroblasts (see below). Nevertheless, there are a few reports addressing the crosstalk of MCs with other immune cells, i.e., Kupffer cells (see below) and the main cell type in the liver, i.e., the hepatocytes. For the latter, it was shown in vitro that syngenic BMMCs co-cultured with primary hepatocytes increases hepatocyte proliferation [100].

The infiltration (of myeloid lineage-derived cells from the bone marrow) and accumulation (differentiation of liver resident precursor cells, which can be differentiated in the presence of SCF) of MCs in the insulted liver has been shown in several studies and is unquestionable [101]. Even more, the isolation of MCs from liver of BDL-treated animals has been established [102]. It should be noted that not only the presence of MCs itself is of vital importance, but also the type of MCs within the liver (i.e., CTMCs or MMCs), when the functional interplay of cells is considered. General responses regulated by FcεRI or KIT are common to all MCs, whereas the contribution of effector enzymes for crosstalk with other cells varies in between different MC types [103]. A study in human liver tissue demonstrated that the amount of tryptase/chymase-positive MCs is higher than tryptase-positive cells in healthy and chronically diseased livers [104]. The cells isolated from BDL rats were chymase- and tryptase-positive, reflecting that these cells most likely represent CTMCs [102].

3.1. SCF–KIT Axis as Chemotactic Guidance

Initial work aimed to identify the factor(s) governing MC infiltration (chemotaxis). There have been several factors identified that govern MC migration [105]. Those include two key factors that act as a chemoattractant for MCs and that are important in the process of liver fibrosis. The first one and the most potent is TGF-β1, which is increasingly expressed in the liver under fibrogenic conditions [106,107]. However, aside migration/chemotaxis, TGF-β1 has an impact on several critical functions of MC biology, including proliferation, apoptosis, effector synthesis, and degranulation (see below). In the second line, stem cell factor (SCF), which is an essential factor for MC proliferation, survival, and differentiation is also a potent chemoattractant for MCs and circulating MC progenitors [108–110]. The SCF transcript can be differentially spliced, resulting in alternative transcripts, which differ in the presence or absence of exon 6. Both encoded proteins are membrane-bound but the longer one, including exon 6, can be more easily proteolytically cleaved to generate soluble SCF [111]. SCF is produced by fibroblasts and endothelial cells, and both the membrane-bound and soluble SCF bind to the surface tyrosine kinase membrane receptor KIT (CD117), which leads to the recruitment of MC progenitors and activation of MCs in the tissue.

Recruitment of MCs to the liver requires the liberation of progenitors into the circulation and entry into the tissue at the destination site. In this scenario, extravasation of circulating MC progenitors is facilitated by the interaction of MC progenitors with endothelial cells [11]. This contact can be mediated by the α4β7 integrin, as has been shown for murine MC homing/recruitment to the small intestine [11]. For human MCs, attachment to endothelial cells was shown to rely on the α4β1 integrin subunits [112]. As mentioned above, endothelial cells express the MC chemoattractant SCF.

In order to substantiate SCF as the basis for MC recruitment during liver disease, the expression of SCF in normal as well as diseased livers from patients suffering from PBC or PSC was analyzed using RT-qPCR and ELISA showing that SCF was increased. The corresponding SCF mRNA could be detected in human and rat primary HSCs. The expression of SCF increased during the culture, activation, and transdifferentiation of primary rat HSCs. In turn, isolated human skin MCs adhered in co-culture to HSC monolayer cells, most likely via membrane-bound SCF, since this interaction could be blocked by anti-SCF antibodies [110]. HSCs do not constitutively express SCF, but it can be induced by MCs in a TNF-α-dependent fashion [113]. In addition to HSCs, SCF is produced by keratinocytes, airway epithelial cells, and endothelial cells. In a recent paper, another critical player in fibrosis, i.e., cholangiocytes, have been shown to express and secrete SCF, in contrast to hepatocytes, which do not express SCF [114]. Inhibition of SCF expression in *Mdr2*$^{-/-}$ mice decreases MC recruitment in vivo. In vitro deprivation of SCF in cholangiocytes reduces MC migration and HSC activation. As a consequence, histamine levels, biliary reaction, and fibrosis were reduced in *Mdr2*$^{-/-}$ mice [115]. Moreover, it has been shown that the SCF-mediated migration of MCs depends on the activity of the sheddase/metallproteinase ADAM10 [115].

In addition to migration/recruitment, recombinant human SCF, as well as NIH3T3 fibroblasts (in co-culture), have the capability to induce the differentiation of MC precursors isolated from human fetal liver [116–118]. Indeed, mouse NIH3T3 fibroblast cells express SCF constitutively [119]. Analysis of glucocorticoids (dexamethasone) on a co-culture of MCs with NIH3T3 fibroblasts or HSCs showed that dexamethasone blocks NIH3T3-mediated MC proliferation, while it has no effect on HSC-mediated MC proliferation, because the latter induces SCF expression in HSC at a post-translational level [119].

In a recent work, Kim and colleagues analyzed extracellular vesicles (EVs) of patients suffering from SM. They found that EVs show an MC signature, including the proteins tryptase, FcεRI, and KIT [72]. Incubation of HSCs in vitro with these purified EVs led to the transfer of functional KIT to stellate cells. This transfer caused an increase in HSC proliferation, cytokine production, and differentiation. These effects were blocked by KIT inhibition, while in in vivo experiments, the application of EVs to mice increased α-smooth muscle actin (α-SMA) production and the presence of human KIT in mouse HSCs. These results suggest that KIT expression/presence on HSCs causes activation of these cells [72]. A mutual involvement of Kupffer cells in the recruitment of MCs to the liver was demonstrated in an endotoxin liver injury model that causes hepatocyte damage, an inflammatory reaction, and MC infiltration. Treatment of those animals with an agonist for the liver X receptor (LXR; GW3965), highly expressed in Kupffer cells, leads to reduced liver affection and reduction in MC count [120]. If this effect is mediated by Kupffer cells, or if the agonist has a direct impact on MCs is questionable since the LXR agonist GW3965 directly blocks at least inflammatory cytokine production of BMMC [121].

3.2. *Impact of Mast Cells and Mediators on Liver Disease and Individual Cells*

Once MCs have infiltrated into the interstitial tissue of the portal tracts, MCs most likely get activated by environmental factors. Through the process of hyperplasia and degranulation (Figure 2), effector molecules are liberated, which in turn act on surrounding cells, including bile duct epithelial cells, HSCs, portal fibroblasts, and resident Kupffer cells. In addition, these mediators are further triggers that recruit circulating immune cells to the site of injury. On the other hand, it has been described that the contents liberated after degranulation of MCs can act in an endocrine fashion via the bile ductules/bile showing long-range effects [122]. In addition to the "classical" degranulation, a cell-to-cell interaction has been described and termed transgranulation. This interaction occurs with MCs and fibroblasts/vascular endothelial cells and describes the direct transfer of granules from MCs via pseudopodia to the communicating cell. This process has been observed in vitro as well as in vivo [123].

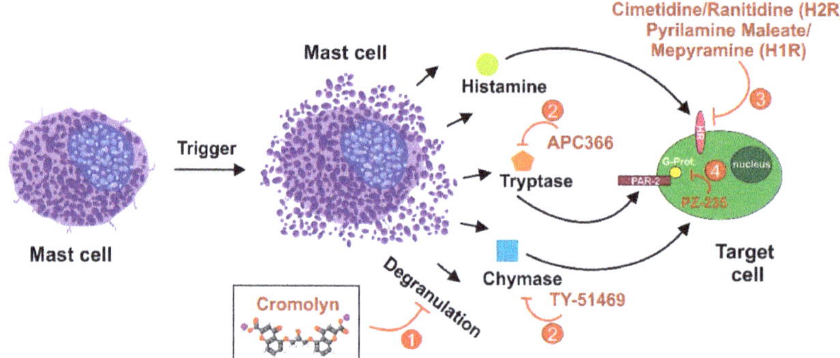

Figure 2. Regulation of mast cell (MC) effector functions. Upon liver damage, MCs increase in the liver tissue and degranulation is triggered by environmental factors. The released MC effectors modulate target cell functions in receptive cells, such as hepatic stellate cells, portal myofibroblasts, and cholangiocytes. There are several possible ways to interfere with MC effector functions: (1) MC stabilizers like cromolyn block the general release of MC granula, and inhibitors can inactivate liberated (2) proteases, (3) block different types of histamine receptors, or (4) can modulate downstream signaling in target cells. Abbreviations used are: APC366, *N*-(1-hydroxy-2-naphthoyl)-L-arginyl-L-prolinamide; G-Prot., G protein; HR, histamine receptor; H1R, histamine receptor H1; H2R, histamine receptor H2; PAR-2, protease-activator receptor-2; PZ-235, P2pal-18S cell-penetrating pepducin targeting the intracellular i3 loop of PAR-2; TY-51469, 2-[4-[(5-fluoro-3-methyl-1-benzothiophen-2-yl)sulfonylamino]-3-methylsulfonylphenyl]-1,3-thiazole-4-carboxylic acid.

In kinetic experiments using CCl_4 intoxication, MC infiltration was associated with individual stages of fibrosis. At the time points with significant MC infiltration, HSCs were not yet activated. Therefore, the authors concluded that MCs are indicators of acute inflammation [124]. Work contributed by Takeshita [125] implied that after BDL surgery in rats, MC amounts increase in the liver but not that much in the portal fields. In contrast, there is a strong but transient increase in MC number after recanalization of the bile duct [125]. The authors concluded that MCs are not involved in the early phase of fibrosis, but rather in the apoptosis of biliary epithelial cells and removal of bile ductules after recanalization [125]. However, further data from the time-resolved analysis of BDL or DMN-treated rats imply that MCs do play a role in the fibrotic phase of liver disease [95,126]. Results from CCl_4-treated rats revealed that myofibroblasts and macrophages increase in number during the first ten weeks, whereas MCs increase constantly over the period peeking in number at week 14 [127]. Nevertheless, although the function of MCs in the process of fibrosis is not completely resolved, it is common sense that most of the studies performed so far showed that MCs fulfill profibrogenic functions in diseased liver (see below).

Only one of the early works performed by Sugihara et al. implied that MCs have no consequence in the development of liver fibrosis in wild-type or MC-deprived $Kit^{Ws/Ws}$ rats and in wild-type or MC-deprived $Kit^{W/Wv}$ mice [128]. The animals were subjected to BDL and treated with CCl_4 or porcine serum (rats) and CCl_4 or BDL (mice) to induce portal tract (BDL, serum) or parenchymal fibrosis (CCl_4). The treatments lasted 21 days and were evaluated using a hydroxyproline measurement for collagen deposition and Alcian blue stain to detect MCs. Since the early time points (less than 21 days) were not taken into account, the reaction of the biliary tree and infiltration of MCs during the early events of fibrosis were not evaluated. All treatments caused fibrosis and increased quantities of MCs. However, although the overall MC quantities were approximately 20-fold higher in wild-type than in $Kit^{Ws/Ws}$ animals, the degree of fibrosis was equal in both groups. Therefore, the authors concluded that MCs have no role in fibrosis [128]. On the other hand, a recent paper analyzing the influence of MCs on fibrosis in a direct co-culture system or an indirect co-culture system composed of a human MC line and primary MCs with the human HSC line LX2 showed that soluble factor(s) derived from MCs caused a decrease in ECM/collagen I abundance in the presence or absence of TGF-β, IFN-α, or IL-10 [129]. They could show by using the APC366 tryptase inhibitor and the broad range inhibitor Chymostatin, that the key MC proteases tryptase and chymase are most likely involved in collagen I degradation. In addition, the human leukocyte antigen G (HLA-G), representing a histocompatibility antigen, is increasingly expressed in MCs when co-cultured with HSCs. This is accompanied by a significant decrease in collagen production, irrespectively of whether cells were stimulated with TGF-β, IL-10, or IFN-α, or left untreated [129]. In their study, the authors proposed MC proteases as critical mediators of collagen degradation. HLA-G has been studied by the same authors before in the setting of chronic HCV infection. They could show that HLA-G in situ is produced by MCs and is up-regulated upon stimulation with IL-10 and IFN-α, leading to the recruitment of T-lymphocytes and NK cells [130].

Nevertheless, taking into account data of MC involvement in fibrosis in lung, kidney and heart, there is a great body of evidence that MCs play a pro-fibrogenic role in liver fibrosis [131–135].

3.3. BDL-Induced Cholestasis in Mast Cell-Depleted $Kit^{W\text{-}sh/W\text{-}sh}$ Mice

In order to delineate pro-fibrogenic effects of MCs in more detail, the crosstalk of MCs with other liver resident and infiltrating cells has been analyzed in murine models of cholestatic liver injury. Due to the localization of MCs in the portal tracts of the liver, different animal models and human biopsies have been analyzed (BDL, $Mdr2^{-/-}$ mice, porcine serum injection, PBC and PSC samples) [97,136]. The animal models develop portal fibrosis and a bile duct reaction encompassing bile duct proliferation (cholangiocyte proliferation), bile duct hyperplasia, and angiogenesis as critical features [137].

In order to delineate the effects of MC absence in vivo on processes induced by cholestasis, wild-type and MC-depleted mice ($Kit^{W\text{-}sh/W\text{-}sh}$) underwent BDL surgery. Wild-type mice subjected to BDL displayed increased focal necrosis (infarct) and portal inflammatory changes that are consistent with obstruction. In BDL $Kit^{W\text{-}sh/W\text{-}sh}$ mice, the degree of focal necrosis (infarct) was reduced. Liver enzymes were significantly upregulated in wild-type mice after BDL, but this was completely ablated in BDL $Kit^{W\text{-}sh/W\text{-}sh}$ mice, suggesting diminished hepatocyte damage in the absence of MCs. Biliary and cholangiocyte proliferation was reduced in BDL $Kit^{W\text{-}sh/W\text{-}sh}$ mice. With respect to HSC function, the collagen deposition was dramatically reduced in BDL $Kit^{W\text{-}sh/W\text{-}sh}$ mice, as monitored by Fast Green/Sirius Red staining. In agreement, the expression of α-SMA, fibronectin-1, collagen I type 1α, and SYP-9 as activation markers of HSCs were decreased in BDL $Kit^{W\text{-}sh/W\text{-}sh}$ mice. In addition, there was a significant reduction in both TGF-β1 expression and secretion in BDL $Kit^{W\text{-}sh/W\text{-}sh}$ mice, while TGF-β1 levels were increased in $Kit^{W\text{-}sh/W\text{-}sh}$ mice injected with cultured MCs, supporting the concept that MCs are an important source of TGF-β1 during fibrosis progression [138]. TGF-β1 expression and secretion by antigen-stimulated MCs has been shown to induce proliferation, collagen Iα1, and monocyte chemoattractant protein-1 (MCP-1) expression in fibroblasts [139–141].

As a confirmation of the aforementioned findings, HSCs were cultured in vitro with conditioned supernatants derived from cholangiocytes isolated from BDL treated $Kit^{W\text{-}sh/W\text{-}sh}$ animals. Only when the cholangiocytes were isolated from $Kit^{W\text{-}sh/W\text{-}sh}$ animals supplemented with MCs, the corresponding supernatants have the potential to activate HSCs, as displayed by higher α-SMA expression. Those results imply that the presence of MCs triggers cholangiocytes to secrete factors that are able to cause HSC activation in vitro [138].

3.4. Tryptase/Protease-Activated Receptor-2 Axis

One of the prominent effectors secreted by MCs upon degranulation is the protease tryptase. In contrast to chymase, tryptase is found in both human MCs (MC_{TC} and MC_T) [142]. On the other hand, in the mouse, tryptase is only expressed in CTMCs but not in MMCs [143]. Tryptase, in addition to trypsin and coagulation factors, activates the protease-activated receptor (PAR)-2 via limited proteolysis of its N-terminus. Protease-activator receptor-2 (PAR-2) is expressed in hepatic endothelial cells, Kupffer cells, hepatocytes, bile duct epithelial cells, and HSCs. The expression of

PAR-2 in HSCs is increased during liver fibrosis [144]. In agreement, the analysis of PAR-1 and PAR-2 expression in isolated rat HSCs showed that mRNA expression increases during the transdifferentiation of HSCs to MFBs in culture [145].

In vivo, a PAR-2 knockout had no impact on initial liver fibrosis after 5 weeks of CCl_4 treatment but prevented the progression of fibrosis with sustained CCl_4 treatment after 8 weeks, as reflected by lower hydroxyproline content. A similar behavior was seen in the expression of α-SMA, TGF-β1, matrix metalloproteinase (MMP)-2 (gelatinase A), and tissue inhibitor of metalloproteinase (TIMP)-1. The expression of PAR-1 compensates for PAR-2 deficiency, but only in the early phase (5 weeks) and not in the late phase (8 weeks). Since activation of PAR-2 leads to the recruitment and activation of macrophages, their presence at the different time points were quantified. F4/80$^+$ macrophages are reduced after 5 and 8 weeks of treatment, whereas CD68$^+$ macrophages were only reduced at 8 weeks. These observations are consistent with a role for PAR-2 in the recruitment and later activation of macrophages in CCl_4-induced hepatic fibrosis. Therefore, these in vivo data implicate that PAR-2 is involved in the activation of HSCs, TGF-β1 synthesis, and ECM deposition, as well as macrophage recruitment.

To substantiate these findings with in vitro data, human HSC LX2 cells were induced for 48 h with the peptidic PAR-2 agonist SLIGKV. This stimulation induced proliferation of HSCs similar to that of PDGF, representing the most potent inducer of HSC proliferation. The PAR-2 agonist also led to an increase in collagen I and TGF-β1 production. Those effects were also observed when using a PAR-1 agonist, but the induction achieved with the PAR-1 and PAR-2 agonists on collagen I and TGF-β1 protein content were not additive [144]. Agonists for PAR-1, such as thrombin and SFFLRN, or agonists for PAR-2, such as tryptase and SLIGRL, induced a proliferative response in rat HSCs. Due to the sensitivity of this response to PD98059, it is most likely that the observed effects are mediated by ERK1/2 activation. In addition, tryptase and SLIGRL increased the collagen I secretion by HSCs [145]. In a more recent study, MC tryptase induced the activity of PAR-2 and increased HSC activation and proliferation, thus promoting hepatic fibrosis and implying that MCs interact directly with HSCs to drive fibrosis. The application of the MC tryptase inhibitor APC366 in BDL-induced hepatic fibrosis in rats showed that APC366 reduced hepatic fibrosis scores, collagen content, and serum biochemical parameters. Moreover, the reduced fibrosis was associated with a decreased expression of PAR-2 and α-SMA. Therefore, it was suggested that MC tryptase induces PAR-2 activation to augment HSC proliferation and promote hepatic fibrosis in rats [146].

3.5. *Chymase as an Interface for the Activation of Several Pro-fibrogenic Pathways*

The MC chymase activity is increased in the livers of patients with fibrosis or cirrhosis and there is a significant correlation between the chymase level and the degree of fibrosis [147]. Chymase can cleave the Phe8–His9 bond of the non-bioactive peptide angiotensin I (Ang I), forming its bioactive peptide angiotensin II (Ang II) in mammalian tissues including humans [148]. Ang II also induced hepatic fibrosis via the induction of α-SMA in HSCs [149]. Ang II and its angiotensin receptor 1 (AT1) are involved in the fibrotic process. In human fibrosis, MC chymase expression is increased, which is coupled with an increased expression of myofibroblast Ang II receptor, AT1. The receptor is expressed on vascular smooth muscle cells, HSCs, portal myofibroblasts, and hepatocytes. During cirrhosis, the expression of AT1 is increased in fibrotic septa and vessels. Ang II and chymase can bind to AT1 on HSCs and MFBs in fibrotic septa and promote fibrosis [150]. The effect of chymase on isolated HSCs reveals that the protease enhances HSC proliferation, TGF-β1/α-SMA protein expression, and collagen I formation [151]. In addition to the activation of Ang II, chymase was shown to enzymatically cleave the precursors of MMP-9 (pro-gelatinase B), TGF-β, and collagen I, leading to their biologically active forms [152–154]. Furthermore, the enzymatic function of MC-released chymase can produce soluble SCF via enzymatic cleavage of the membrane-bound form of SCF on stromal cells, which induces the formation of mature MCs from immature MCs via the stimulation of KIT [155]. Due to the multiple roles of chymase, which may promote organ fibrosis, this enzyme is a promising target for anti-fibrotic agents [156].

3.6. The Histamine/Histamin Receptor Axis

In the setting of cholangiocarcinoma (CCA), MCs within the tumor environment release histamine, which increases CCA progression and angiogenesis. Conversely, cholangiocytes secrete SCF, which binds and activates the MC growth factor receptor KIT. Cholangiocytes express histidine decarboxylase and its inhibition reduces CCA growth [157]. In the study by Johnson et al., MCs were detected in human CCA biopsies and their recruitment is mediated via SCF in the tumor microenvironment stimulating CCA growth. In xenograft tumor mice treated with the MC stabilizer cromolyn sodium, MC infiltration and tumor growth decreased. Inhibition of SCF in CCA blocked MC migration and MC/EMT/ECM in CCA [157]. MCs migrate into the CCA tumor microenvironment via KIT/SCF and increase tumor progression, angiogenesis, and ECM degradation [157]. In a further study analyzing histamine function, *Mdr2*$^{-/-}$ mice (PSC model) were treated with cromolyn. This treatment reduced MC protease mMCPT-1, as well as serum histamine. In agreement, human PSC samples also showed a robust expression of MC markers. Necrosis, lobular damage, and bile duct reactions, such as intrahepatic biliary mass and cholangiocyte proliferation, were also reduced via MC silencing using cromolyn in *Mdr2*$^{-/-}$ mice.

As a confirmation of the in vivo analysis, co-culture experiments of cholangiocytes with MCs induced cholangiocyte proliferation, α-SMA, fibronectin-1, and TGF-β1 production, functions that are blocked in MC depleted using an siRNA approach targeting histidine decarboxylase. In a similar experiment, MCs induced PCNA, α-SMA, and fibronectin-1 in human HSC, and these effects were also blocked by the knockdown of HDC in MCs. These in vitro results imply that cholangiocyte and HSC responses to MCs are dependent on the histamine secreted by MCs [158]. Nevertheless, the in vivo results using cromolyn have to be handled with caution because this substance directly affects HSCs and hepatocytes. Cromolyn was originally developed as an MC stabilizer. However, the activation and collagen accumulation for the HSC cell lines LX2 and HSC-T6 were reduced by 50% after cromolyn treatment at a low concentration without signs of apoptosis. Furthermore, cromolyn treatment compromised the TGF-β-induced epithelial to mesenchymal transition and replicative senescence rate of hepatocytes, which are generally associated with fibrogenesis. Taken together, cromolyn may be the basis for an effective cure for fibrosis and cirrhosis because it targets both HSCs and hepatocytes [159].

In a more reliable/specific setting to analyze the function of MC histamine, Kennedy et al. used histamine receptor antagonists. These reduced the lobular damage, necrosis, and inflammation in *Mdr2*$^{-/-}$ mice. The histamine receptors H1 (H1R) and H2 (H2HR) are upregulated in cholangiocytes of *Mdr2*$^{-/-}$ mice, as well as in human PSC and CCA. Blocking of the histamine receptor leads to decreased activation of MCs as evaluated via the detection of MC markers in *Mdr2*$^{-/-}$ mice and in the CCA model [160]. Histamine serum levels decrease in *Mdr2*$^{-/-}$ and CCA mice in the presence of respective blockers. Bile duct reaction, i.e., biliary proliferation and intrahepatic bile duct mass, were reduced. Treated *Mdr2*$^{-/-}$ mice had a lower collagen deposition and lower expression of the HSC activation marker synaptophysin-9 (Syp-9). Histamine receptor blockers do not affect activation of HSCs directly [160]. The tumor growth is blocked in the CCA model and Ki67-positive proliferating cholangiocytes were reduced. In a co-culture/conditioned medium model, MCs increased the proliferation of cholangiocytes and progression of CCA, and this effect was reduced in the presence of inhibitors. In summary, histamine receptor blockers reduce PSC and CCA progression [160]. As a general feature, MCs stimulate fibroblast proliferation [161,162] and collagen synthesis [163,164] via histamine secretion. Moreover, it has been shown that MCs themselves are competent at expressing basement membrane components, including collagen IV and laminin [165].

An early study by Akiyoshi et al. reported that MCs, portal myofibroblasts, and cholinergic nerve terminals work synergistically to promote liver fibrosis [137], demonstrating that the paracrine influence from MCs is not limited to altered HSCs and cholangiocyte function.

3.7. TGF-β1

It has been stressed before that one of the main drivers of fibrosis is TGF-β1, which is strongly upregulated in the process of fibrosis and leads to activation and ECM production by HSCs and portal fibroblasts [166]. In addition to liver resident cells, e.g., HSCs and Kupffer cells, MCs also express and secrete TGF-β1 to promote fibrosis (see above). The pro-fibrogenic master cytokine, TGF-β1, regulates the expression of proteases and their release [167]. In contrast, MC-specific receptors controlling cellular degranulation, including KIT (ligand SCF) and FcεRI (ligand IgE), are down-regulated in vitro and in vivo by TGF-β1 in a SMAD-dependent fashion [168]. In addition, TGF-β1 suppresses IL-33-induced cytokine production and MC activation by interfering with MAP kinase phosphorylation [169]. Aside from the expression and liberation of effectors, a broad spectrum of MC functions is modulated by TGF-β1, including proliferation, cell cycle control, and apoptosis [170]. Another vital function of MC biology modulated by TGF-β is migration/chemotaxis. Interestingly, chemotaxis is not mediated by the classical SMAD pathway, but by MEK1/2 signaling [171]. Moreover, the SRC family kinase FYN plays a critical role in TGF-β1-mediated MC migration in vitro and in vivo [172]. Those observations show that in the environment of fibrosis MCs may contribute to the progression of the disease by releasing TGF-β1, affecting HSCs and portal fibroblasts. In turn, MCs also express TGF-β receptors and are targets for this ligand [107]. Nevertheless, the effects are somewhat counterbalanced, leading on one hand to chemotaxis and increased effector synthesis [107,173], and on the other hand apoptosis, blocking late stage maturation and sensor suppression [173–175]. Therefore, the TGF-β1 response in MCs is a double-edged sword, which largely depends on the molecular context.

In summary, there are many mediators released by activated MCs that contribute to liver disease by directly interfering with the recruitment and activation of inflammatory blood cells, stimulating proliferation of pro-fibrogenic cells, promoting ECM synthesis, or inhibiting its degradation (Figure 3).

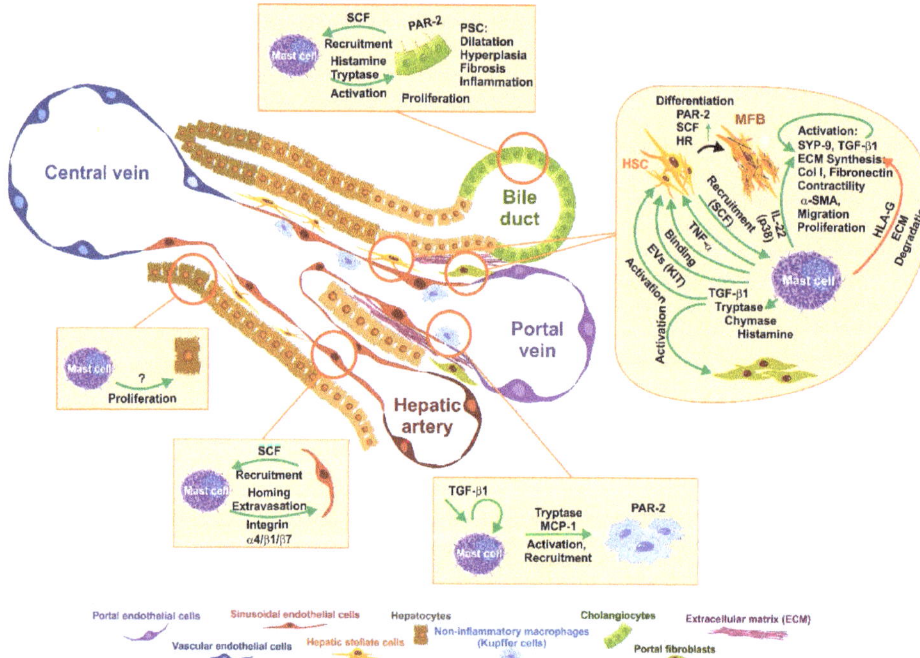

Figure 3. Schematic overview of known functional interactions between mast cells and liver cells in hepatic fibrogenesis. Mast cells (MCs) activation and degranulation leads to a production/release of many biological active compounds including TGF-β1, tryptase, chymase, histamine, TNF-α, and human leukocyte antigen G (HLA-G). These soluble mediators trigger the recruitment/activation of

inflammatory blood cells and synthesis of an extracellular matrix (ECM) by stimulating the propagation of pro-fibrogenic cells (hepatic stellate cells, portal myofibroblasts) and inhibiting its ECM degradation. Furthermore, the compounds lead to the activation of liver-resident Kupffer cells and cholangiocyte proliferation. It is further discussed that MCs modulate parenchymal cell proliferation and biological features of endothelial cells. In addition, the cargos present in extracellular vesicles (EV) that are released from MCs into the extracellular milieu facilitate pro-fibrogenic signaling pathways in recipient cells. Abbreviations used are: α-SMA, α-smooth muscle actin; Col I, collagen type I; HLA-G, human leukocyte antigen G; HR, histamine receptor; HSC, hepatic stellate cell; IL-22, interleukin 22; MCP-1, monocyte chemoattractant protein-1; MFB, myofibroblast; PAR-2, Protease-activator receptor-2; PSC, primary sclerosing cholangitis; SCF, stem cell factor; SYP-9, synaptophysin-9; TGF-β1, transforming growth factor-β1; TNF-α, tumor necrosis factor-α.

4. Mast Cells in Human Liver Disease

Today, there is first evidence demonstrating that MCs are important cellular regulators in human liver disease. In a normal human liver, MCs are associated with the connective tissue and are mainly found along the portal tracts [98]. The number of MCs in human liver is significantly increased during the pathogenesis of PBC, PSC, bile duct obstruction, hepatitis, alcohol-induced liver injury, steatosis, steatohepatitis, congenital and non-congenital liver fibrosis, liver cancer, liver rejection upon liver transplant, and liver aging [98,176,177]. Although the cellular and sub-cellular linkages of MCs to all these diseases remain unresolved, it is most likely that these cells are critically involved in the liver's fibrotic response to chronic inflammation. On the other side, MCs can exert immunomodulatory effects on other immune cells, thereby enhancing or suppressing the initiation, magnitude, and/or duration of immune cells within the liver, preventing diminished hepatobiliary functions during disease progression, or by acting as a first effector cell in an innate response to encounter antigens [176,177]. However, the knowledge of MC function in the human liver is still very limited and further fundamental studies are urgently needed to understand the full biological repertoire and activities mediated by these important immune cells in human liver homeostasis and disease.

5. Therapeutic Options

5.1. Selective Targeting of Mast Cells in Liver Fibrosis

"Personalized medicine" and "precision medicine" are keywords when it comes to discussions about successful patient-tailored treatment of diseases; such an endeavor first requires thorough and sophisticated diagnostic tools. On a different level, this also concerns pharmacological regulation of cellular activation states depending on the (patho-)physiological tissue niches, as well as patient comorbidities. The more sensitive cells are to environmental conditions, the more complicated the choice of beneficial pharmacological substances might be. This applies in particular to MCs, whose task is to recognize changes in micro-environmental conditions and occurrence of biological mediators and/or chemical substances. As already indicated in Section 1.2., MCs are endued with enormous heterogeneity, as well as fascinating plasticity; thus, depending on their localization and prevailing conditions, MCs as a whole express hundreds of mediators and surface receptors, complicating the choice of pharmacological treatment in a given pathophysiological setting. Hence, returning to the keyword of personalized medicine, deciphering the complexity of MC phenotypes in a given (patho-)physiological situation might enhance the ability to use MCs as "drug targets."

Two different pharmacological approaches, not necessarily mutually exclusive, could be followed to address and inhibit MC activity in pathophysiological situations like liver fibrosis: i) MC stabilizers, such as disodium cromoglycate (cromolyn sodium), Tranilast, ketotifen, or many others (Figure 4); and/or ii) inhibitors of MC-selective enzymes (e.g., tryptase and chymase), and antagonists for receptors of typical MC mediators, such as histamine (receptors). These mediators importantly add to the pleiotropic inflammatory functions of MCs (cf. Figure 2).

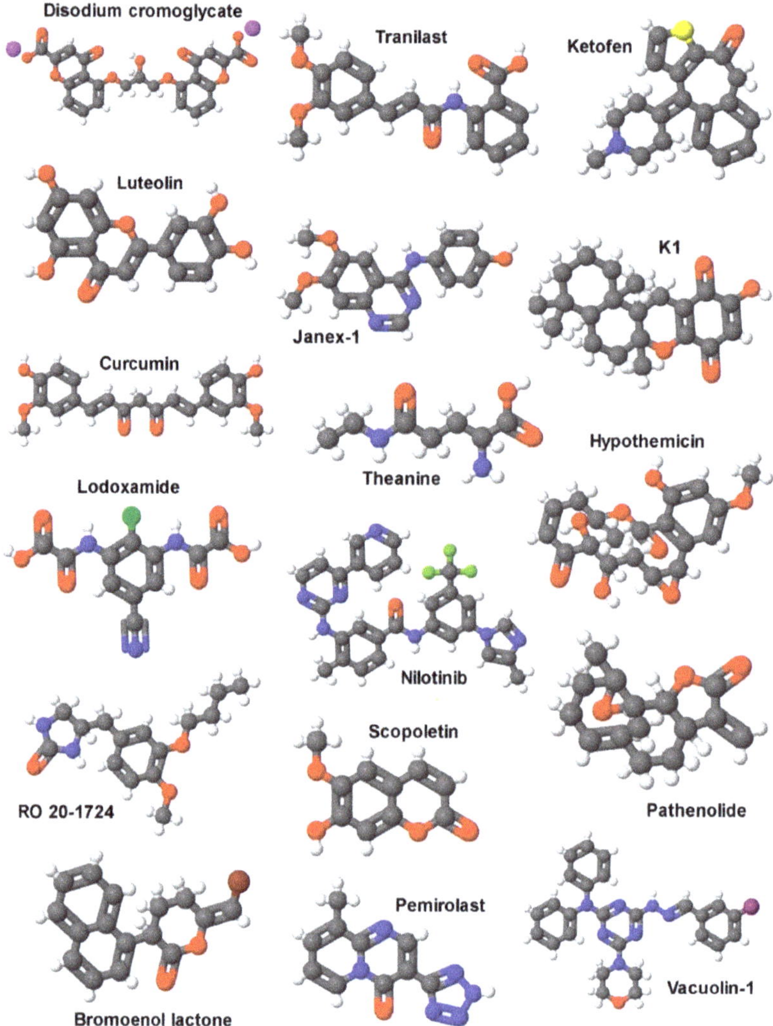

Figure 4. Naturally occurring and synthetic mast cell stabilizers with highly variant structures. Interestingly, some of these drugs, such as Tranilast, Luteolin, Curcumin, Theanine, Nilotinib, and others showed highly beneficial effects in experimental hepatic fibrosis [62]. Most of their activities are attributed to their antioxidant activity, capacity to prevent hepatic infiltration with circulating blood cells, potential to target pro-inflammatory and/or pro-fibrotic signaling pathways, or to influence extracellular matrix generation or turnover. However, none of these substances have been tested systematically regarding the modulation of mast cell stability in models of hepatic fibrogenesis. All structure images were prepared with Jmol (http://jmol.sourceforge.net/) using the following PubChem Compound Identification (CID) numbers: Bromoenol lactone (5940264), Curcumin (969516), disodium cromoglycate (27503), Hypothemicin (9929643), Janex-1 (3794), K1 (25211416), Ketofen (3827), Lodoxamide (44564), Luteolin (5280445), Nilotinib (644241), Pathenolide (7251185), Pemirolast (57697), RO 20-1724 (5087), Scopoletin (5280460), Theanine (439378), Tranilast (5282230), Vacuolin-1 (9661141). More details about the structure and functions of representative MC stabilizers can be found elsewhere [178].

Already in 1972, results from a controlled study of cromolyn sodium in patients with asthma came to the conclusion that this drug is a useful adjunct to the pharmacological treatment of asthma [179]. Since it was shown in rat peritoneal MCs that cromolyn sodium is able to attenuate IgE-mediated histamine release [180], MCs were seen as the cellular targets of this drug, fitting to their well-known detrimental role in anaphylaxis and asthma. In addition to using cromolyn sodium in patients and experimental rat models, researchers were increasingly using this drug in mouse models to prove the contributions of MCs. However, in a previous study by Galli and coworkers, in which MC-related effects of cromolyn sodium in vitro and in vivo were thoroughly compared in rat and mouse models, the authors came to the conclusion that cromolyn sodium's effectiveness and selectivity as a MC stabilizer in mice is questionable [159,181]. Nevertheless, in an in vitro model, they could demonstrate the positive effect of histamine secreted from MCs on the proliferation and activation of cholangiocytes, as well as HSCs [181]. In a model of bleomycin-induced pulmonary fibrosis, another MC stabilizer, Tranilast, was shown to be effective in suppressing fibrosis in genetically MC-deficient mice [182], raising doubt about the MC selectivity of this drug, at least in mice.

Nowadays, there are many reports testing mast cell stabilizers, such as luteolin and curcumin in vivo for their efficacy at protecting against inflammation, disease-associated apoptosis, tumorigenesis, and overshooting oxidative stress in the liver [183–187]. Unfortunately, in all these studies, the impact of these stabilizers on mast cell activity was not analyzed systematically. With respect to the mitigation of liver fibrosis, convincing studies have been published with respect to the role of MC proteases, tryptase and chymase. Tryptase β forms non-covalent ring-like tetramers and has trypsin-like activity [188,189]. Tetramerization appears to be required for proper activity and selectivity. The central pore containing the active sites of the four tryptase β molecules prohibits the access of large substrates and also suppresses inhibition by most protease inhibitors [190]. In a model of BDL-induced hepatic fibrosis in rats, treatment with the tryptase inhibitor APC366 resulted in a reduced hepatic fibrosis score, attenuated HSC proliferation, collagen content, and serum biochemical parameters [146]. In contrast to tryptase β, tryptase α is proteolytically inactive; nevertheless, it is conserved throughout evolution and significantly expressed in MCs. Very recently, Le et al. have reported the in vivo existence of biologically functional α/β tryptase heterotetramers; however, their contribution to fibrotic diseases has not been investigated yet [191].

In addition to certain soluble substrates, the G-protein-coupled receptor PAR-2 is cleaved by tryptase and appears to be its main substrate [192]. The tryptase-mediated, N-terminal cleavage of PAR-2 generates an intramolecular ligand activating PAR-2. PAR-2 has been shown to be expressed, amongst others, on fibroblasts and HSCs, and thus, in addition to tryptase inhibitors, PAR-2 antagonists might be beneficial in the treatment of liver fibrosis. Concerning liver fibrosis, rat HSCs express PAR-2 and the expression increases with the transition of stellate cells to myofibroblasts. The PAR-2 agonists, tryptase and the peptide SLIGRL, induced proliferation and collagen secretion [145], suggesting that tryptase as a PAR-2 agonist could sustain liver fibrosis. Indeed, analyzing CCl_4-induced liver fibrosis in PAR-2-deficient compared to wild-type mice, Knight et al. found a reduced progression of liver fibrosis, hepatic collagen gene expression, hydroxyproline content, TGF-β expression, and matrix metalloproteinase 2 gene expression in the absence of PAR-2. Additionally, PAR-2 activation stimulated proliferation, collagen production, and TGF-β production by human HSCs [144]. This indicated the pro-fibrogenic action of hepatic PAR-2 activation and strongly proposed a role for hepatic MCs in liver fibrosis. Interestingly, the recently identified α/β tryptase heterotetramer was also shown to cleave and activate PAR-2 [191].

Pepducins are cell-penetrating peptides acting as intracellular modulators of signal propagation from receptors of the G-protein-coupled receptor family to the associated G proteins [193]. Intriguingly, the PAR-2 pepducin PZ-235 significantly suppressed hepatic steatosis and inflammation in the experimental methionine-choline-deficient diet model in mice [194]. Moreover, PZ-235 repressed CCl_4-induced liver fibrosis, even with delayed treatment. PZ-235 also inhibited production of reactive oxygen species and hence, enhanced viability of hepatocytes in vitro [194], which might imply a reduction of necrosis-driven sterile inflammation in the course of liver fibrosis. Thus, PAR-2 pepducin inhibitors have the potential to be efficient in the treatment of liver fibrosis.

Whereas tryptase forms heparin-stabilized ring-like tetramers, which restrict the access of substrates to the active centers of the protease monomers, chymase is active as a monomeric protein, though in a macromolecular complex with heparin [195]. Accordingly, its structure sterically allows for activity against a bigger number of substrates. For instance, chymase can generate angiotensin II by cleaving the non-bioactive peptide angiotensin I [148], and cleave/activate MMP-9 [196] and TGF-β [197], all of which are associated with liver inflammation and/or fibrosis. Furthermore, human chymase was found to cleave type I pro-collagen and hence initiate collagen fibril formation [152]. Isolated rat HSCs were treated with chymase and it was shown that the proliferation and expression of α-smooth muscle actin and TGF-β1 protein were significantly enhanced in a dose-dependent manner. This implied a potential role of chymase in the development of liver fibrosis [151]. Moreover, the effect of the chymase inhibitor TY-51469 in hamsters fed a methionine- and choline-deficient (MCD) diet, which developed a marked hepatic steatosis and fibrosis, was analyzed. Both non-alcoholic steatohepatitis (NASH) and fibrosis were significantly attenuated by chymase inhibition [198,199]. Likewise, in rats fed a high-fat and high-cholesterol diet, the chymase inhibitor TY-51469 significantly attenuated all parameters associated with NASH and fibrosis [200]. Furthermore, CCl_4-induced liver fibrosis in hamsters was significantly reduced in TY-51469-treated compared to placebo-treated animals [201]. Finally, immunohistochemical analysis, as well as enzymatic activity measurements, of liver biopsies from 49 patients with chronic hepatitis revealed increased chymase levels and activity correlating with the severity of the disease. This suggested that hepatic chymase is implicated in liver fibrosis [202]. A correlative investigation of 77 patients with the aim to elucidate the function of chymase as an angiotensin-converting enzyme for the progression of liver fibrosis suggested an important role of this MC protease in the hepatic fibrosis of patients with cirrhosis [147].

5.2. *Signaling Pathways as Targets for Potential Future Therapies in Liver Fibrosis*

Another critical inflammatory mediator within the fibrotic process in the liver is the cytokine IL-1β [203]. IL-1β is a peculiar cytokine in that it is not translated by ER membrane-bound ribosomes and not secreted via the classical ER–Golgi route [204]. In contrast, pro-IL-1β is synthesized by cytoplasmic ribosomes, and for maturation and secretion, the inflammasome, a multiprotein complex (e.g., the NLRP3 inflammasome), is required for caspase-1 activation and the subsequent cleavage of pro-IL-1β to yield mature IL-1β, which then is released by the process of pyroptosis [204]. Human chymase has been demonstrated to convert the 31 kDa pro-form of IL-1β to an 18 kDa biologically active molecule [205]. This cleavage product differs from the caspase-1-processed molecule in three amino acids; however, the activity of both cytokines is comparable. Since pro-IL-1β can be released, amongst others, from necrotic cells in an alarmin-like fashion, MC chymase could contribute to the generation of IL-1β and hence to the promotion of fibrosis.

So far, the described functions of the MC proteases, tryptase and chymase, for the development of liver fibrosis and associated hepatic alterations indicated a promoting role for these diseases. However, chymase was also reported to degrade two alarmins, IL-33 and HMGB1 [206], which have been shown to play detrimental pro-fibrotic roles in liver disease. An overproduction of the mRNAs for IL-33 and its receptor ST2 was observed in mouse and human fibrotic livers, and activated HSCs were identified as the major source of IL-33 [207]. IL-33 expression in liver was sufficient for severe hepatic fibrosis in vivo by the activation and expansion of liver-resident innate lymphoid cells (ILC2), which then contribute to fibrosis by producing IL-13 [208–210]. With respect to the second alarmin, HMGB1, which is produced and released by hepatocytes and Kupffer cells, and signals via the receptor for advanced glycation end-products (RAGE) in HSCs, activation of MAPK pathways and the induction of the increased deposition of collagen has been described [211,212]. In conclusion, chymase is a double-edged sword with regard to the development of liver fibrosis; on the one hand, it cleaves/activates pro-fibrotic proteins, such as angiotensin I, MMP-9, TGF-β, and type I pro-collagen, and on the other hand, it can degrade pro-fibrotic IL-33 and HMGB1. Thus, a thorough analysis of the respective disease development and regulators involved has to be performed before chymase inhibition can be recommended.

Another central MC mediator is the biogenic amine, histamine, which also has been reported to be involved in the regulation of fibrotic diseases. Histamine is synthesized by decarboxylation of the amino acid histidine via the enzyme L-histidine decarboxylase (HDC) [213]. Degradation of histamine is catalyzed by the enzyme monoamine oxidase B (MAOB) [213]. As with tryptase and chymase, histamine as a preformed mediator is stored in secretory lysosomes and is released by the process of degranulation. The effect(s) of histamine on target cells is dependent on the type of histamine receptor(s) expressed by these cells. Histamine receptors (H1R, H2R, H3R, and H4R) belong to the family of G-protein-coupled receptors and exert their differential functions by coupling to different G proteins, which again regulate differential signaling enzymes/pathways. Whereas H1R via G_q proteins activates PLC-γ, and thus induces Ca^{2+}- and PKC-regulated signaling enzymes and transcription factors, H2R via G_s proteins positively couples to adenylyl cyclase, and thus regulates cellular processes by means of cAMP/PKA-dependent signal transduction and gene transcription. In an opposite fashion, H3R and H4R via G_i proteins inhibit adenylyl cyclase [214]. Thus, although histamine is only a single substance, it can trigger multiple cellular reactions and affect diseases in various ways.

In the livers of infants suffering from biliary atresia, histamine levels were significantly increased and positively correlated with the severity of fibrosis. Infants with severe fibrosis showed an elevated and reduced expression of HDC and DIO, respectively [213]. The *Abcb4* gene (aka *Mdr2*) encodes for the multidrug-resistant protein MDR2, and $Mdr2^{-/-}$ mice spontaneously develop severe biliary fibrosis via gross dysregulation of pro- and anti-fibrotic genes [215]. Interestingly, using H1R and H2R antagonists (mepyramine and ranitidine, respectively) alone or in combination, liver and biliary damage, as well as fibrosis in $Mdr2^{-/-}$ mice, was attenuated [160]. Moreover, these H1R and H2R antagonists also decreased the growth of CCA, angiogenesis, and epithelial–mesenchymal transition [160], clearly demonstrating the detrimental role for histamine in liver pathology.

Though so far not studied in liver, histamine was shown to affect the biology of fibroblasts in several ways. Stimulation of normal adult human lung fibroblasts with histamine enhanced the proliferation of these cells in a dose-dependent manner, mediated through the histamine receptor H2R and not H1R, which indicated a role for cAMP/PKA signaling [216]. These data were obtained using the H2R antagonist cimetidine and the H1R antagonist pyrilamine maleate. In normal human dermal fibroblasts, histamine treatment caused a clear enhancement in α-SMA expression, suggesting a role for histamine in fibroblast–myofibroblast progression [217]. Moreover, in human skin fibroblasts, histamine was found to increase proliferation and collagen production [218]. The action of histamine; however, is not only dependent on the histamine receptor(s) expressed, but also on the microenvironment of the respective cells. Hence, Lin et al. demonstrated that TGF-β1-induced expression of α-SMA in human skin fibroblasts was suppressed by histamine. In this situation, H1R activation, but not H2R or H4R activation, was responsible for the suppressive effect by histamine [219]. These few examples already clearly indicate that thorough knowledge about histamine receptor expressing cells in tissues of interest, and in addition, about the type(s) of histamine receptors expressed in these cells, must be obtained to take advantage of the substantial tool-box of various histamine receptor antagonists.

6. Conclusions

MCs are important immune cells of the myeloid lineage present in healthy liver, and to a larger degree in diseased liver. In particular, experimental models of hepatic fibrosis have shown that the overall quantities of MCs significantly increase in all kinds of liver insults. In humans, first evidence has connected elevated numbers of MCs to the pathogenesis of PBC, PSC, bile duct obstruction, hepatitis, alcohol-induced liver injury, steatosis, steatohepatitis, congenital and non-congenital liver fibrosis, liver cancer, liver rejection upon liver transplant, and liver aging. Although the impact of MCs in the initiation or progression of these disease entities is still poorly understood, it was suggested that they contribute to the liver's fibrotic response to chronic inflammation. However, MCs possess favorable immunomodulatory properties on other immune cells and act as a first effector cell in the innate response when encountering antigens. In this regard, the role of MCs in hepatic fibrosis is unclear and merits particular interest. Potential therapeutic MC-targeted strategies are the blockade of MC activity by MC stabilizers, inhibition of MC-selective enzymes, and the application of antagonists binding to receptors associated with an MC function. However, none of these approaches has been systematically tested in appropriate models and further experimental, translational, and clinical studies are urgently needed to explore whether the different compounds are beneficial in the therapy of hepatic fibrosis or its progression to cirrhosis or hepatocellular carcinoma.

Author Contributions: Writing-original draft preparation, R.W., S.K.M., C.L., and M.H.; writing-review and editing, R.W., S.K.M., C.L., and M.H.; funding acquisition, R.W., C.L., and M.H.; visualization, R.W., and S.K.M.

Funding: R.W., C.L., and M.H. are supported by the German Research Foundation (DFG, SFB/TRR57, Projects P04, P13, and Q3; HU794/12-1) and by the Interdisciplinary Centre for Clinical Research (IZKF) within the Faculty of Medicine at the RWTH Aachen University (Projects O3-1, O3-4, and O3-5). None of the funding sources exerted influence on content or decision to submit this review for publication. This research received no external funding.

Acknowledgments: The authors are grateful to Sabine Weiskirchen (Institute of Molecular Pathobiochemistry, Experimental Gene Therapy and Clinical Chemistry, University Hospital Aachen, Aachen) for kindly preparing the figures and the graphical abstract for this review.

Conflicts of Interest: The authors declare no conflict of interest.

References

1. Ribatti, D.; Crivellato, E. Mast cell ontogeny: An historical overview. *Immunol. Lett.* **2014**, *159*, 11–14. [CrossRef] [PubMed]
2. Metz, M.; Maurer, M. Mast cells–key effector cells in immune responses. *Trends Immunol.* **2007**, *28*, 234–241. [CrossRef] [PubMed]
3. Ehara, T.; Shigematsu, H. Mast cells in the kidney. *Nephrology (Carlton)* **2003**, *8*, 130–138. [CrossRef] [PubMed]
4. Farrell, D.J.; Hines, J.E.; Walls, A.F.; Kelly, P.J.; Bennett, M.K.; Burt, A.D. Intrahepatic mast cells in chronic liver diseases. *Hepatology* **1995**, *22*, 1175–1181. [CrossRef]
5. Welle, M. Development, significance, and heterogeneity of mast cells with particular regard to the mast cell-specific proteases chymase and tryptase. *J. Leukoc. Biol.* **1997**, *61*, 233–245. [CrossRef]
6. Galli, S.J.; Borregaard, N.; Wynn, T.A. Phenotypic and functional plasticity of cells of innate immunity: Macrophages, mast cells and neutrophils. *Nat. Immunol.* **2011**, *12*, 1035–1044. [CrossRef]
7. Kitamura, Y.; Go, S.; Hatanaka, K. Decrease of mast cells in W/Wv mice and their increase by bone marrow transplantation. *Blood* **1978**, *52*, 447–452. [CrossRef]
8. Nocka, K.; Buck, J.; Levi, E.; Besmer, P. Candidate ligand for the c-kit transmembrane kinase receptor: KL, a fibroblast derived growth factor stimulates mast cells and erythroid progenitors. *EMBO J.* **1990**, *9*, 3287–3294. [CrossRef]
9. Blank, U.; Ra, C.; Miller, L.; White, K.; Metzger, H.; Kinet, J.P. Complete structure and expression in transfected cells of high affinity IgE receptor. *Nature* **1989**, *337*, 187–189. [CrossRef]
10. Hallgren, J.; Gurish, M.F. Pathways of murine mast cell development and trafficking: Tracking the roots and routes of the mast cell. *Immunol. Rev.* **2007**, *217*, 8–18. [CrossRef]
11. Gurish, M.F.; Tao, H.; Abonia, J.P.; Arya, A.; Friend, D.S.; Parker, C.M.; Austen, K.F. Intestinal mast cell progenitors require CD49dβ7 (α4β7 integrin) for tissue-specific homing. *J. Exp. Med.* **2001**, *194*, 1243–1252. [CrossRef] [PubMed]
12. Abonia, J.P.; Austen, K.F.; Rollins, B.J.; Joshi, S.K.; Flavell, R.A.; Kuziel, W.A.; Koni, P.A.; Gurish, M.F. Constitutive homing of mast cell progenitors to the intestine depends on autologous expression of the chemokine receptor CXCR2. *Blood* **2005**, *105*, 4308–4313. [CrossRef] [PubMed]
13. Dahlin, J.S.; Ding, Z.; Hallgren, J. Distinguishing mast cell progenitors from mature mast cells in mice. *Stem Cells Dev.* **2015**, *24*, 1703–1711. [CrossRef] [PubMed]

14. Ochi, H.; Hirani, W.M.; Yuan, Q.; Friend, D.S.; Austen, K.F.; Boyce, J.A. T helper cell type 2 cytokine-mediated comitogenic responses and CCR3 expression during differentiation of human mast cells in vitro. *J. Exp. Med.* **1999**, *190*, 267–280. [CrossRef]
15. Gentek, R.; Ghigo, C.; Hoeffel, G.; Bulle, M.J.; Msallam, R.; Gautier, G.; Launay, P.; Chen, J.; Ginhoux, F.; Bajenoff, M. Hemogenic endothelial fate mapping reveals dual developmental origin of mast cells. *Immunity* **2018**, *48*, 1160–1171. [CrossRef]
16. Li, Z.; Liu, S.; Xu, J.; Zhang, X.; Han, D.; Liu, J.; Xia, M.; Yi, L.; Shen, Q.; Xu, S.; et al. Adult connective tissue-resident mast cells originate from late erythro-myeloid progenitors. *Immunity* **2018**, *49*, 640–653. [CrossRef]
17. Galli, S.J.; Maurer, M.; Lantz, C.S. Mast cells as sentinels of innate immunity. *Cur. Opin. Immunol.* **1999**, *11*, 53–59. [CrossRef]
18. Galli, S.J.; Nakae, S.; Tsai, M. Mast cells in the development of adaptive immune responses. *Nat. Immunol.* **2005**, *6*, 135–142. [CrossRef]
19. Metz, M.; Piliponsky, A.M.; Chen, C.C.; Lammel, V.; Abrink, M.; Pejler, G.; Tsai, M.; Galli, S.J. Mast cells can enhance resistance to snake and honeybee venoms. *Science* **2006**, *313*, 526–530. [CrossRef]
20. Maurer, M.; Wedemeyer, J.; Metz, M.; Piliponsky, A.M.; Weller, K.; Chatterjea, D.; Clouthier, D.E.; Yanagisawa, M.M.; Tsai, M.; Galli, S.J. Mast cells promote homeostasis by limiting endothelin-1-induced toxicity. *Nature* **2004**, *432*, 512–516. [CrossRef]
21. Schneider, L.A.; Schlenner, S.M.; Feyerabend, T.B.; Wunderlin, M.; Rodewald, H.R. Molecular mechanism of mast cell mediated innate defense against endothelin and snake venom sarafotoxin. *J. Exp. Med.* **2007**, *204*, 2629–2639. [CrossRef] [PubMed]
22. Ramirez-GarciaLuna, J.L.; Chan, D.; Samberg, R.; Abou-Rjeili, M.; Wong, T.H.; Li, A.; Feyerabend, T.B.; Rodewald, H.R.; Henderson, J.E.; Martineau, P.A. Defective bone repair in mast cell-deficient Cpa3Cre/+ mice. *PLoS ONE* **2017**, *12*, e0174396. [CrossRef] [PubMed]
23. Ngkelo, A.; Richart, A.; Kirk, J.A.; Bonnin, P.; Vilar, J.; Lemitre, M.; Marck, P.; Branchereau, M.; Le Gall, S.; Renault, N.; et al. Mast cells regulate myofilament calcium sensitization and heart function after myocardial infarction. *J. Exp. Med.* **2016**, *213*, 1353–1374. [CrossRef] [PubMed]
24. Reitz, M.; Brunn, M.L.; Rodewald, H.R.; Feyerabend, T.B.; Roers, A.; Dudeck, A.; Voehringer, D.; Jonsson, F.; Kuhl, A.A.; Breloer, M. Mucosal mast cells are indispensable for the timely termination of Strongyloides ratti infection. *Mucosal Immunol.* **2017**, *10*, 481–492. [CrossRef] [PubMed]
25. Galli, S.J.; Tsai, M. IgE and mast cells in allergic disease. *Nat. Med.* **2012**, *18*, 693–704. [CrossRef]
26. Schubert, N.; Dudeck, J.; Liu, P.; Karutz, A.; Speier, S.; Maurer, M.; Tuckermann, J.; Dudeck, A. Mast cell promotion of T cell-driven antigen-induced arthritis despite being dispensable for antibody-induced arthritis in which T cells are bypassed. *Arthritis Rheumatol.* **2015**, *67*, 903–913. [CrossRef]
27. Coussens, L.M.; Raymond, W.W.; Bergers, G.; Laig-Webster, M.; Behrendtsen, O.; Werb, Z.; Caughey, G.H.; Hanahan, D. Inflammatory mast cells up-regulate angiogenesis during squamous epithelial carcinogenesis. *Genes Dev.* **1999**, *13*, 1382–1397. [CrossRef]
28. Bradding, P.; Pejler, G. The controversial role of mast cells in fibrosis. *Immunol. Rev.* **2018**, *282*, 198–231. [CrossRef]
29. Dahdah, A.; Gautier, G.; Attout, T.; Fiore, F.; Lebourdais, E.; Msallam, R.; Daeron, M.; Monteiro, R.C.; Benhamou, M.; Charles, N.; et al. Mast cells aggravate sepsis by inhibiting peritoneal macrophage phagocytosis. *J. Clin. Investig.* **2014**, *124*, 4577–4589. [CrossRef]
30. Valent, P.; Akin, C.; Metcalfe, D.D. Mastocytosis: 2016 updated WHO classification and novel emerging treatment concepts. *Blood* **2017**, *129*, 1420–1427. [CrossRef]
31. Valent, P.; Akin, C.; Hartmann, K.; Nilsson, G.; Reiter, A.; Hermine, O.; Sotlar, K.; Sperr, W.R.; Escribano, L.; George, T.I.; et al. Advances in the classification and treatment of mastocytosis: Current status and outlook toward the future. *Cancer Res.* **2017**, *77*, 1261–1270. [CrossRef] [PubMed]
32. Valent, P. Mast cell activation syndromes: Definition and classification. *Allergy* **2013**, *68*, 417–424. [CrossRef] [PubMed]
33. Valent, P.; Akin, C.; Bonadonna, P.; Hartmann, K.; Brockow, K.; Niedoszytko, M.; Nedoszytko, B.; Siebenhaar, F.; Sperr, W.R.; Oude Elberink, J.N.G.; et al. Proposed diagnostic algorithm for patients with suspected mast cell activation syndrome. *J. Allergy Clin. Immunol. Pract.* **2019**, *7*, 1125–1133. [CrossRef] [PubMed]

34. Garcia-Faroldi, G.; Melo, F.R.; Ronnberg, E.; Grujic, M.; Pejler, G. Active caspase-3 is stored within secretory compartments of viable mast cells. *J. Immunol.* **2013**, *191*, 1445–1452. [CrossRef] [PubMed]
35. Pardo, J.; Wallich, R.; Ebnet, K.; Iden, S.; Zentgraf, H.; Martin, P.; Ekiciler, A.; Prins, A.; Mullbacher, A.; Huber, M.; et al. Granzyme B is expressed in mouse mast cells in vivo and in vitro and causes delayed cell death independent of perforin. *Cell Death Differ.* **2007**, *14*, 1768–1779. [CrossRef] [PubMed]
36. Wernersson, S.; Pejler, G. Mast cell secretory granules: Armed for battle. *Nat. Rev. Immunol.* **2014**, *14*, 478–494. [CrossRef]
37. Zorn, C.N.; Pardo, J.; Martin, P.; Kuhny, M.; Simon, M.M.; Huber, M. Secretory lysosomes of mouse mast cells store and exocytose active caspase-3 in a strictly granzyme B dependent manner. *Eur. J. Immunol.* **2013**, *43*, 3209–3218. [CrossRef]
38. Subramanian, H.; Gupta, K.; Ali, H. Roles of Mas-related G protein-coupled receptor X2 on mast cell-mediated host defense, pseudoallergic drug reactions, and chronic inflammatory diseases. *J. Allergy Clin. Immunol.* **2016**, *138*, 700–710. [CrossRef]
39. McNeil, B.D.; Pundir, P.; Meeker, S.; Han, L.; Undem, B.J.; Kulka, M.; Dong, X. Identification of a mast-cell-specific receptor crucial for pseudo-allergic drug reactions. *Nature* **2015**, *519*, 237–241. [CrossRef]
40. Boyce, J.A. Mast cells and eicosanoid mediators: A system of reciprocal paracrine and autocrine regulation. *Immunol. Rev.* **2007**, *217*, 168–185. [CrossRef]
41. Bischoff, S.C. Role of mast cells in allergic and non-allergic immune responses: Comparison of human and murine data. *Nat. Rev. Immunol.* **2007**, *7*, 93–104. [CrossRef] [PubMed]
42. Huber, M.; Kalis, C.; Keck, S.; Jiang, Z.; Georgel, P.; Du, X.; Shamel, L.; Sovath, S.; Mudd, S.; Beutler, B.; et al. R-form LPS, the master key to the activation of TLR4/MD2 positive cells. *Eur. J. Immunol.* **2006**, *36*, 701–711. [CrossRef] [PubMed]
43. Dietrich, N.; Rohde, M.; Geffers, R.; Kroger, A.; Hauser, H.; Weiss, S.; Gekara, N.O. Mast cells elicit proinflammatory but not type I interferon responses upon activation of TLRs by bacteria. *Proc. Natl. Acad. Sci. USA* **2010**, *107*, 8748–8753. [CrossRef] [PubMed]
44. Keck, S.; Muller, I.; Fejer, G.; Savic, I.; Tchaptchet, S.; Nielsen, P.J.; Galanos, C.; Huber, M.; Freudenberg, M.A. Absence of TRIF signaling in lipopolysaccharide-stimulated murine mast cells. *J. Immunol.* **2011**, *186*, 5478–5488. [CrossRef]
45. Duttlinger, R.; Manova, K.; Berrozpe, G.; Chu, T.Y.; DeLeon, V.; Timokhina, I.; Chaganti, R.S.; Zelenetz, A.D.; Bachvarova, R.F.; Besmer, P. The Wsh and Ph mutations affect the c-kit expression profile: C-kit misexpression in embryogenesis impairs melanogenesis in Wsh and Ph mutant mice. *Proc. Natl. Acad. Sci. USA* **1995**, *92*, 3754–3758. [CrossRef]
46. Grimbaldeston, M.A.; Chen, C.C.; Piliponsky, A.M.; Tsai, M.; Tam, S.Y.; Galli, S.J. Mast cell-deficient W-sash c-kit mutant Kit W-sh/W-sh mice as a model for investigating mast cell biology in vivo. *Am. J. Pathol.* **2005**, *167*, 835–848. [CrossRef]
47. Feyerabend, T.B.; Weiser, A.; Tietz, A.; Stassen, M.; Harris, N.; Kopf, M.; Radermacher, P.; Moller, P.; Benoist, C.; Mathis, D.; et al. Cre-mediated cell ablation contests mast cell contribution in models of antibody- and T cell-mediated autoimmunity. *Immunity* **2011**, *35*, 832–844. [CrossRef]
48. Scholten, J.; Hartmann, K.; Gerbaulet, A.; Krieg, T.; Muller, W.; Testa, G.; Roers, A. Mast cell-specific Cre/loxP-mediated recombination in vivo. *Transgenic Res.* **2008**, *17*, 307–315. [CrossRef]
49. Voehringer, D.; Liang, H.E.; Locksley, R.M. Homeostasis and effector function of lymphopenia-induced "memory-like" T cells in constitutively T cell-depleted mice. *J. Immunol.* **2008**, *180*, 4742–4753. [CrossRef]
50. Dudeck, A.; Dudeck, J.; Scholten, J.; Petzold, A.; Surianarayanan, S.; Kohler, A.; Peschke, K.; Vohringer, D.; Waskow, C.; Krieg, T.; et al. Mast cells are key promoters of contact allergy that mediate the adjuvant effects of haptens. *Immunity* **2011**, *34*, 973–984. [CrossRef]
51. Steimer, D.A.; Boyd, K.; Takeuchi, O.; Fisher, J.K.; Zambetti, G.P.; Opferman, J.T. Selective roles for antiapoptotic MCL-1 during granulocyte development and macrophage effector function. *Blood* **2009**, *113*, 2805–2815. [CrossRef] [PubMed]
52. Lilla, J.N.; Chen, C.C.; Mukai, K.; BenBarak, M.J.; Franco, C.B.; Kalesnikoff, J.; Yu, M.; Tsai, M.; Piliponsky, A.M.; Galli, S.J. Reduced mast cell and basophil numbers and function in Cpa3-Cre; Mcl-1fl/fl mice. *Blood* **2011**, *118*, 6930–6938. [CrossRef] [PubMed]
53. Reber, L.L.; Marichal, T.; Galli, S.J. New models for analyzing mast cell functions in vivo. *Am. J. Pathol.* **2012**, *33*, 613–625. [CrossRef] [PubMed]

54. Eming, S.A.; Wynn, T.A.; Martin, P. Inflammation and metabolism in tissue repair and regeneration. *Science* **2017**, *356*, 1026–1030. [CrossRef]
55. Weiskirchen, R.; Weiskirchen, S.; Tacke, F. Organ and tissue fibrosis: Molecular signals, cellular mechanisms and translational implications. *Mol. Asp. Med.* **2019**, *65*, 2–15. [CrossRef]
56. Potey, P.M.; Rossi, A.G.; Lucas, C.D.; Dorward, D.A. Neutrophils in the initiation and resolution of acute pulmonary inflammation: Understanding biological function and therapeutic potential. *J. Pathol.* **2019**, *247*, 672–685. [CrossRef]
57. Amarante-Mendes, G.P.; Adjemian, S.; Branco, L.M.; Zanetti, L.C.; Weinlich, R.; Bortoluci, K.R. Pattern recognition receptors and the host cell death molecular machinery. *Front Immunol.* **2018**, *9*, 2379. [CrossRef]
58. Gressner, A.M.; Weiskirchen, R. Modern pathogenetic concepts of liver fibrosis suggest stellate cells and TGF-β as major players and therapeutic targets. *J. Cell Mol. Med.* **2006**, *10*, 76–99. [CrossRef]
59. Abreu, J.G.; Ketpura, N.I.; Reversade, B.; De Robertis, E.M. Connective-tissue growth factor (CTGF) modulates cell signalling by BMP and TGF-β. *Nat. Cell Biol.* **2002**, *4*, 599–604. [CrossRef]
60. Mittal, M.; Siddiqui, M.R.; Tran, K.; Reddy, S.P.; Malik, A.B. Reactive oxygen species in inflammation and tissue injury. *Antioxid. Redox Signal.* **2014**, *20*, 1126–1167. [CrossRef]
61. Zlotnik, A.; Yoshie, O. Chemokines: A new classification system and their role in immunity. *Immunity* **2000**, *12*, 121–127. [CrossRef]
62. Weiskirchen, R. Hepatoprotective and anti-fibrotic agents: It's time to take the next step. *Front. Pharmacol.* **2016**, *6*, 303. [CrossRef] [PubMed]
63. Aggarwal, B.B.; Gupta, S.C.; Kim, J.H. Historical perspectives on tumor necrosis factor and its superfamily: 25 years later, a golden journey. *Blood* **2012**, *119*, 651–665. [CrossRef]
64. Doss, G.P.; Agoramoorthy, G.; Chakraborty, C. TNF/TNFR: Drug target for autoimmune diseases and immune-mediated inflammatory diseases. *Front. Biosci. (Landmark Ed)* **2014**, *19*, 1028–1040. [CrossRef]
65. De Bleser, P.J.; Xu, G.; Rombouts, K.; Rogiers, V.; Geerts, A. Glutathione levels discriminate between oxidative stress and transforming growth factor-β signaling in activated rat hepatic stellate cells. *J. Biol. Chem.* **1999**, *274*, 33881–33887. [CrossRef]
66. Manea, S.A.; Constantin, A.; Manda, G.; Sasson, S.; Manea, A. Regulation of Nox enzymes expression in vascular pathophysiology: Focusing on transcription factors and epigenetic mechanisms. *Redox Biol.* **2015**, *5*, 358–366. [CrossRef]
67. Romero, F.; Shah, D.; Duong, M.; Penn, R.B.; Fessler, M.B.; Madenspacher, J.; Stafstrom, W.; Kavuru, M.; Lu, B.; Kallen, C.B.; et al. A pneumocyte-macrophage paracrine lipid axis drives the lung toward fibrosis. *Am. J. Respir. Cell Mol. Biol.* **2015**, *53*, 74–86. [CrossRef]
68. Svegliati-Baroni, G.; Inagaki, Y.; Rincon-Sanchez, A.R.; Else, C.; Saccomanno, S.; Benedetti, A.; Ramirez, F.; Rojkind, M. Early response of α2(I) collagen to acetaldehyde in human hepatic stellate cells is TGF-β independent. *Hepatology* **2005**, *42*, 343–352. [CrossRef]
69. Kubo, H. Extracellular Vesicles in lung disease. *Chest* **2018**, *153*, 210–216. [CrossRef]
70. Momen-Heravi, F.; Bala, S.; Kodys, K.; Szabo, G. Exosomes derived from alcohol-treated hepatocytes horizontally transfer liver specific miRNA-122 and sensitize monocytes to LPS. *Sci. Rep.* **2015**, *5*, 9991. [CrossRef]
71. Heinrich, L.F.; Andersen, D.K.; Cleasby, M.E.; Lawson, C. Long-term high fat feeding of rats results in increased numbers of circulating microvesicles with pro-inflammatory effects on endothelial cells. *Br. J. Nutr.* **2015**, *113*, 1704–1711. [CrossRef] [PubMed]
72. Kim, D.K.; Cho, Y.E.; Komarow, H.D.; Bandara, G.; Song, B.J.; Olivera, A.; Metcalfe, D.D. Mastocytosis-derived extracellular vesicles exhibit a mast cell signature, transfer KIT to stellate cells, and promote their activation. *Proc. Natl. Acad. Sci. USA.* **2018**, *115*, E10692–E10701. [CrossRef] [PubMed]
73. Weiskirchen, R.; Weiskirchen, S.; Tacke, F. Recent advances in understanding liver fibrosis: Bridging basic science and individualized treatment concepts. *F1000Research* **2018**, *7*, 921. [CrossRef] [PubMed]
74. Campana, L.; Iredale, J.P. Regression of Liver Fibrosis. *Semin. Liver Dis.* **2017**, *37*, 1–10. [CrossRef]
75. Scholten, D.; Trebicka, J.; Liedtke, C.; Weiskirchen, R. The carbon tetrachloride model in mice. *Lab Anim.* **2015**, *49*, 4–11. [CrossRef]
76. Heymann, F.; Hamesch, K.; Weiskirchen, R.; Tacke, F. The concanavalin A model of acute hepatitis in mice. *Lab Anim.* **2015**, *49*, 12–20. [CrossRef]

77. Wallace, M.C.; Hamesch, K.; Lunova, M.; Kim, Y.; Weiskirchen, R.; Strnad, P.; Friedman, S.L. Standard operating procedures in experimental liver research: Thioacetamide model in mice and rats. *Lab Anim.* **2015**, *49*, 21–29. [CrossRef]
78. Mossanen, J.C.; Tacke, F. Acetaminophen-induced acute liver injury in mice. *Lab Anim.* **2015**, *49*, 30–36. [CrossRef]
79. Hamesch, K.; Borkham-Kamphorst, E.; Strnad, P.; Weiskirchen, R. Lipopolysaccharide-induced inflammatory liver injury in mice. *Lab Anim.* **2015**, *49*, 37–46. [CrossRef]
80. Ramadori, P.; Weiskirchen, R.; Trebicka, J.; Streetz, K. Mouse models of metabolic liver injury. *Lab Anim.* **2015**, *49*, 47–58. [CrossRef]
81. Tolba, R.; Kraus, T.; Liedtke, C.; Schwarz, M.; Weiskirchen, R. Diethylnitrosamine (DEN)-induced carcinogenic liver injury in mice. *Lab Anim.* **2015**, *49*, 59–69. [CrossRef]
82. Tag, C.G.; Weiskirchen, S.; Hittatiya, K.; Tacke, F.; Tolba, R.H.; Weiskirchen, R. Induction of experimental obstructive cholestasis in mice. *Lab Anim.* **2015**, *49*, 70–80. [CrossRef]
83. Tag, C.G.; Sauer-Lehnen, S.; Weiskirchen, S.; Borkham-Kamphorst, E.; Tolba, R.H.; Tacke, F.; Weiskirchen, R. Bile duct ligation in mice: Induction of inflammatory liver injury and fibrosis by obstructive cholestasis. *J. Vis. Exp.* **2015**. [CrossRef]
84. Nevzorova, Y.A.; Tolba, R.; Trautwein, C.; Liedtke, C. Partial hepatectomy in mice. *Lab Anim.* **2015**, *49*, 81–88. [CrossRef]
85. Smit, J.J.; Schinkel, A.H.; Oude Elferink, R.P.; Groen, A.K.; Wagenaar, E.; van Deemter, L.; Mol, C.A.; Ottenhoff, R.; Van Der Lugt, N.M.; van Roon, M.A.; et al. Homozygous disruption of the murine mdr2 P-glycoprotein gene leads to a complete absence of phospholipid from bile and to liver disease. *Cell* **1993**, *75*, 451–462. [CrossRef]
86. Kisseleva, T. The origin of fibrogenic myofibroblasts in fibrotic liver. *Hepatology* **2017**, *65*, 1039–1043. [CrossRef]
87. Gu, X.; Huang, D.; Ci, L.; Shi, J.; Zhang, M.; Yang, H.; Wang, Z.; Sheng, Z.; Sun, R.; Fei, J. Fate tracing of hepatocytes in mouse liver. *Sci. Rep.* **2017**, *7*, 16108. [CrossRef]
88. Seok, J.; Warren, H.S.; Cuenca, A.G.; Mindrinos, M.N.; Baker, H.V.; Xu, W.; Richards, D.R.; McDonald-Smith, G.P.; Gao, H.; Hennessy, L.; et al. Inflammation and Host Response to Injury, Large Scale Collaborative Research Program. Genomic responses in mouse models poorly mimic human inflammatory diseases. *Proc. Natl. Acad. Sci. USA* **2013**, *110*, 3507–3512. [CrossRef]
89. Metcalfe, D.D. The liver, spleen, and lymph nodes in mastocytosis. *J. Investig. Dermatol.* **1991**, *96*, 45S–46S. [CrossRef]
90. Mican, J.M.; Di Bisceglie, A.M.; Fong, T.L.; Travis, W.D.; Kleiner, D.E.; Baker, B.; Metcalfe, D.D. Hepatic involvement in mastocytosis: Clinicopathologic correlations in 41 cases. *Hepatology* **1995**, *22*, 1163–1170. [CrossRef]
91. Umezu, K.; Yuasa, S.; Sudoh, A. Change of hepatic histamine content during hepatic fibrosis. *Biochem. Pharmacol.* **1985**, *34*, 2007–2011. [CrossRef] [PubMed]
92. Gittlen, S.D.; Schulman, E.C.; Maddrey, W.C. Raised histamine concentrations in chronic cholestatic liver disease. *Gut* **1990**, *31*, 96–99. [CrossRef] [PubMed]
93. Peng, R.Y.; Wang, D.W.; Xu, Z.H.; Gao, Y.B.; Yang, R.B.; Liu, P.; Wang, Z.P.; Li, Y.P.J. The changes and significance of mast cells in irradiated rat liver. *Environ. Pathol. Toxicol. Oncol.* **1994**, *13*, 111–116.
94. Nakamura, A.; Yamazaki, K.; Suzuki, K.; Sato, S. Increased portal tract infiltration of mast cells and eosinophils in primary biliary cirrhosis. *Am. J. Gastroenterol.* **1997**, *92*, 2245–2249.
95. Rioux, K.P.; Sharkey, K.A.; Wallace, J.L.; Swain, M.G. Hepatic mucosal mast cell hyperplasia in rats with secondary biliary cirrhosis. *Hepatology* **1996**, *23*, 888–895. [CrossRef]
96. Armbrust, T.l.; Batusic, D.; Ringe, B.; Ramadori, G.J. Mast cells distribution in human liver disease and experimental rat liver fibrosis. Indications for mast cell participation in development of liver fibrosis. *Hepatology* **1997**, *26*, 1042–1054. [CrossRef]
97. Ozaki, S.; Sato, Y.; Yasoshima, M.; Harada, K.; Nakanuma, Y. Diffuse expression of heparan sulfate proteoglycan and connective tissue growth factor in fibrous septa with many mast cells relate to unresolving hepatic fibrosis of congenital hepatic fibrosis. *Liver Int.* **2005**, *25*, 817–828. [CrossRef]
98. Jarido, V.; Kennedy, L.; Hargrove, L.; Demieville, J.; Thomson, J.; Stephenson, K.; Francis, H. The emerging role of mast cells in liver disease. *Am. J. Physiol. Gastrointest. Liver Physiol.* **2017**, *313*, G89–G101. [CrossRef]

99. Thomson, J.; Hargrove, L.; Kennedy, L.; Demieville, J.; Francis, H. Cellular crosstalk during cholestatic liver injury. *Liver Res.* **2017**, *1*, 26–33. [CrossRef]
100. Nakano, T.; Lai, C.Y.; Goto, S.; Hsu, L.W.; Kawamoto, S.; Ono, K.; Chen, K.D.; Lin, C.C.; Chiu, K.W.; Wang, C.C.; et al. Immunological and regenerative aspects of hepatic mast cells in liver allograft rejection and tolerance. *PLoS ONE* **2012**, *7*, e37202. [CrossRef]
101. Shen, D.Z. A target role for mast cell in the prevention and therapy of hepatic fibrosis. *Med. Hypotheses* **2008**, *70*, 760–764. [CrossRef]
102. Hargrove, L.; Graf-Eaton, A.; Kennedy, L.; Demieville, J.; Owens, J.; Hodges, K.; Ladd, B.; Francis, H. Isolation and characterization of hepatic mast cells from cholestatic rats. *Lab. Investig.* **2016**, *96*, 1198–1210. [CrossRef] [PubMed]
103. Krystel-Whittemore, M.; Dileepan, K.N.; Wood, J.G. Mast cell: A multi-functional master cell. *Front. Immunol.* **2016**, *6*, 620. [CrossRef]
104. Matsunaga, Y.; Terada, T. Mast cell subpopulations in chronic inflammatory hepatobiliary diseases. *Liver* **2000**, *20*, 152–156. [CrossRef] [PubMed]
105. Halova, I.; Draberova, L.; Draber, P. Mast cell chemotaxis—Chemoattractants and signaling pathways. *Front. Immunol.* **2012**, *3*, 119. [CrossRef] [PubMed]
106. Gruber, B.L.; Marchese, M.J.; Kew, R.R. Transforming growth factor-β 1 mediates mast cell chemotaxis. *J. Immunol.* **1994**, *152*, 5860–5867. [PubMed]
107. Olsson, N.; Piek, E.; ten Dijke, P.; Nilsson, G. Human mast cell migration in response to members of the transforming growth factor-β family. *J. Leukoc. Biol.* **2000**, *67*, 350–356. [CrossRef]
108. Meininger, C.J.; Yano, H.; Rottapel, R.; Bernstein, A.; Zsebo, K.M.; Zetter, B.R. The c-kit receptor ligand functions as a mast cell chemoattractant. *Blood* **1992**, *79*, 958–963. [CrossRef]
109. Nilsson, G.; Butterfield, J.H.; Nilsson, K.; Siegbahn, A. Stem cell factor is a chemotactic factor for human mast cells. *J. Immunol.* **1994**, *153*, 3717–3723.
110. Gaça, M.D.; Pickering, J.A.; Arthur, M.J.; Benyon, R.C. Human and rat hepatic stellate cells produce stem cell factor: A possible mechanism for mast cell recruitment in liver fibrosis. *J. Hepatol.* **1999**, *30*, 850–858. [CrossRef]
111. Flanagan, J.G.; Chan, D.C.; Leder, P. Transmembrane form of the kit ligand growth factor is determined by alternative splicing and is missing in the Sld mutant. *Cell* **1991**, *64*, 1025–1035. [CrossRef]
112. Boyce, J.A.; Mellor, E.A.; Perkins, B.; Lim, Y.C.; Luscinskas, F.W. Human mast cell progenitors use α-integrin, VCAM-1, and PSGL-1 E-selectin for adhesive interactions with human vascular endothelium under flow conditions. *Blood* **2002**, *99*, 2890–2896. [CrossRef] [PubMed]
113. Brito, J.M.; Borojevic, R. Liver granulomas in schistosomiasis: Mast cell-dependent induction of SCF expression in hepatic stellate cells is mediated by TNF-α. *J. Leukoc. Biol.* **1997**, *62*, 389–396. [CrossRef] [PubMed]
114. Meadows, V.; Kennedy, L.; Hargrove, L.; Demieville, J.; Meng, F.; Virani, S.; Reinhart, E.; Kyritsi, K.; Invernizzi, P.; Yang, Z.; et al. Downregulation of hepatic stem cell factor by Vivo-Morpholino treatment inhibits mast cell migration and decreases biliary damage/senescence and liver fibrosis in *Mdr2*$^{-/-}$ mice. *Biochim. Biophys. Acta Mol. Basis Dis.* **2019**, *1865*, 165557. [CrossRef] [PubMed]
115. Faber, T.W.; Pullen, N.A.; Fernando, J.F.; Kolawole, E.M.; McLeod, J.J.; Taruselli, M.; Williams, K.L.; Rivera, K.O.; Barnstein, B.O.; Conrad, D.H.; et al. ADAM10 is required for SCF-induced mast cell migration. *Cell. Immunol.* **2014**, *290*, 80–88. [CrossRef]
116. Irani, A.A.; Craig, S.S.; Nilsson, G.; Ishizaka, T.; Schwartz, L.B. Characterization of human mast cells developed in vitro from fetal liver cells cocultured with murine 3T3 fibroblasts. *Immunology* **1992**, *77*, 136–143.
117. Irani, A.M.; Nilsson, G.; Miettinen, U.; Craig, S.S.; Ashman, L.K.; Ishizaka, T.; Zsebo, K.M.; Schwartz, L.B. Recombinant human stem cell factor stimulates differentiation of mast cells from dispersed human fetal liver cells. *Blood* **1992**, *80*, 3009–3021. [CrossRef]
118. Du, Z.; Li, Y.; Xia, H.; Irani, A.M.; Schwartz, L.B. Recombinant human granulocyte-macrophage colony-stimulating factor (CSF), but not recombinant human granulocyte CSF, down-regulates the recombinant human stem cell factor-dependent differentiation of human fetal liver-derived mast cells. *J. Immunol.* **1997**, *159*, 838–845.

119. Brito, J.M.; Mermelstein, C.S.; Tempone, A.J.; Borojevic, R. Mast cells can revert dexamethasone-mediated down-regulation of stem cell factor. *Eur. J. Pharmacol.* **2001**, *414*, 105–112. [CrossRef]
120. Wang, Y.Y.; Dahle, M.K.; Agren, J.; Myhre, A.E.; Reinholt, F.P.; Foster, S.J.; Collins, J.L.; Thiemermann, C.; Aasen, A.O.; Wang, J.E. Activation of the liver X receptor protects against hepatic injury in endotoxemia by suppressing Kupffer cell activation. *Shock* **2006**, *25*, 141–146. [CrossRef]
121. Nunomura, S.; Okayama, Y.; Matsumoto, K.; Hashimoto, N.; Endo-Umeda, K.; Terui, T.; Makishima, M.; Ra, C. Activation of LXRs using the synthetic agonist GW3965 represses the production of pro-inflammatory cytokines by murine mast cells. *Allergol. Int.* **2015**, *64*, S11–S17. [CrossRef] [PubMed]
122. Collins, A.M.; Leach, S.; Payne, J.; Mitchell, A.; Dai, Y.; Jackson, G.D. A role for the hepatobiliary system in IgE-mediated intestinal inflammation in the rat. *Clin. Exp. Allergy* **1999**, *29*, 262–270. [CrossRef] [PubMed]
123. Greenberg, G.; Burnstock, G. A novel cell-to-cell interaction between mast cells and other cell types. *Exp. Cell Res.* **1983**, *147*, 1–13. [CrossRef]
124. Grizzi, F.; Franceschini, B.; Gagliano, N.; Moscheni, C.; Annoni, G.; Vergani, C.; Hermonat, P.L.; Chiriva-Internati, M.; Dioguardi, N. Mast cell density, hepatic stellate cell activation and TGF-β transcripts in the aging Sprague-Dawley rat during early acute liver injury. *Toxicol. Pathol.* **2003**, *31*, 173–178. [CrossRef] [PubMed]
125. Takeshita, A. 1.; Shibayama, Y. Role of mast cells in hepatic remodeling during cholestasis and its resolution: Relevance to regulation of apoptosis. *Exp. Toxicol. Pathol.* **2005**, *56*, 273–280. [CrossRef] [PubMed]
126. Takahara, Y.; Takahashi, M.; Wagatsuma, H.; Yokoya, F.; Zhang, Q.W.; Yamaguchi, M.; Aburatani, H.; Kawada, N. Gene expression profiles of hepatic cell-type specific marker genes in progression of liver fibrosis. *World J. Gastroenterol.* **2006**, *12*, 6473–6499. [CrossRef]
127. Jeong, W.I.; Lee, C.S.; Park, S.J.; Chung, J.Y.; Jeong, K.S. Kinetics of macrophages, myofibroblasts and mast cells in carbon tetrachloride-induced rat liver cirrhosis. *Anticancer Res.* **2002**, *22*, 869–877.
128. Sugihara, A.; Tsujimura, T.; Fujita, Y.; Nakata, Y.; Terada, N. Evaluation of role of mast cells in the development of liver fibrosis using mast cell-deficient rats and mice. *J. Hepatol.* **1999**, *30*, 859–867. [CrossRef]
129. Amiot, L.; Vu, N.; Drenou, B.; Scrofani, M.; Chalin, A.; Devisme, C.; Samson, M. The anti-fibrotic role of mast cells in the liver is mediated by HLA-G and interaction with hepatic stellate cells. *Cytokine* **2019**, *117*, 50–58. [CrossRef]
130. Amiot, L.; Vu, N.; Rauch, M.; L'Helgoualc'h, A.; Chalmel, F.; Gascan, H.; Turlin, B.; Guyader, D.; Samson, M. Expression of HLA-G by mast cells is associated with hepatitis C virus-induced liver fibrosis. *J. Hepatol.* **2014**, *60*, 245–252. [CrossRef]
131. Miyazawa, S.; Hotta, O.; Doi, N.; Natori, Y.; Nishikawa, K.; Natori, Y. Role of mast cells in the development of renal fibrosis: Use of mast cell-deficient rats. *Kidney Int.* **2004**, *65*, 2228–2237. [CrossRef] [PubMed]
132. Hara, M.; Ono, K.; Hwang, M.W.; Iwasaki, A.; Okada, M.; Nakatani, K.; Sasayama, S.; Matsumori, A. Evidence for a role of mast cells in the evolution to congestive heart failure. *J. Exp. Med.* **2002**, *195*, 375–381. [CrossRef] [PubMed]
133. Veerappan, A.; O'Connor, N.J.; Brazin, J.; Reid, A.C.; Jung, A.; McGee, D.; Summers, B.; Branch-Elliman, D.; Stiles, B.; Worgall, S.; et al. Mast cells: A pivotal role in pulmonary fibrosis. *DNA Cell Biol.* **2013**, *32*, 206–218. [CrossRef] [PubMed]
134. Kong, P.; Christia, P.; Frangogiannis, N.G. The pathogenesis of cardiac fibrosis. *Cell Mol. Life Sci.* **2014**, *71*, 549–574. [CrossRef]
135. Shao, Z.; Nazari, M.; Guo, L.; Li, S.H.; Sun, J.; Liu, S.M.; Yuan, H.P.; Weisel, R.D.; Li, R.K. The cardiac repair benefits of inflammation do not persist: Evidence from mast cell implantation. *J. Cell Mol. Med.* **2015**, *19*, 2751–2762. [CrossRef]
136. Huang, Z.G.; Zhai, W.R.; Zhang, Y.E.; Zhang, X.R. Study of heteroserum-induced rat liver fibrosis model and its mechanism. *World J. Gastroenterol.* **1998**, *4*, 206–209. [CrossRef]
137. Akiyoshi, H.; Terada, T. Mast cell, myofibroblast and nerve terminal complexes in carbon tetrachloride-induced cirrhotic rat livers. *J. Hepatol.* **1998**, *29*, 112–119. [CrossRef]
138. Hargrove, L.; Kennedy, L.; Demieville, J.; Jones, H.; Meng, F.; DeMorrow, S.; Karstens, W.; Madeka, T.; Greene JJr Francis, H. Bile duct ligation-induced biliary hyperplasia, hepatic injury, and fibrosis are reduced in mast cell-deficient Kit(W-sh) mice. *Hepatology* **2017**, *65*, 1991–2004. [CrossRef]

139. Gordon, J.R.; Galli, S.J. Promotion of mouse fibroblast collagen gene expression by mast cells stimulated via the FcεRI. Role for mast cell-derived transforming growth factor β and tumor necrosis factor α. *J. Exp. Med.* **1994**, *180*, 2027–2037. [CrossRef]
140. Kendall, J.C.; Li, X.H.; Galli, S.J.; Gordon, J.R. Promotion of mouse fibroblast proliferation by IgE-dependent activation of mouse mast cells: Role for mast cell tumor necrosis factor-α and transforming growth factor-β1. *J. Allergy Clin. Immunol.* **1997**, *99*, 113–123. [CrossRef]
141. Gordon, J.R. TGFβ1 and TNFα secreted by mast cells stimulated via the FcεRI activate fibroblasts for high-level production of monocyte chemoattractant protein-1 (MCP-1). *Cell. Immunol.* **2000**, *201*, 42–49. [CrossRef] [PubMed]
142. Saito, H.; Matsumoto, K.; Okumura, S.; Kashiwakura, J.; Oboki, K.; Yokoi, H.; Kambe, N.; Ohta, K.; Okayama, Y. Gene expression profiling of human mast cell subtypes: An in silico study. *Allergol. Int.* **2006**, *55*, 173–179. [CrossRef] [PubMed]
143. Reynolds, D.S.; Stevens, R.L.; Lane, W.S.; Carr, M.H.; Austen, K.F.; Serafin, W.E. Different mouse mast cell populations express various combinations of at least six distinct mast cell serine proteases. *Proc. Natl. Acad. Sci. USA* **1990**, *87*, 3230–3234. [CrossRef]
144. Knight, V.; Tchongue, J.; Lourensz, D.; Tipping, P.; Sievert, W. Protease-activated receptor 2 promotes experimental liver fibrosis in mice and activates human hepatic stellate cells. *Hepatology* **2012**, *55*, 879–887. [CrossRef]
145. Gaça, M.D.; Zhou, X.; Benyon, R.C. Regulation of hepatic stellate cell proliferation and collagen synthesis by proteinase-activated receptors. *J. Hepatol.* **2002**, *36*, 362–369. [CrossRef]
146. Lu, J.; Chen, B.; Li, S.; Sun, Q. Tryptase inhibitor APC 366 prevents hepatic fibrosis by inhibiting collagen synthesis induced by tryptase/protease-activated receptor 2 interactions in hepatic stellate cells. *Int. Immunopharmacol.* **2014**, *20*, 352–357. [CrossRef]
147. Komeda, K.; Jin, D.; Takai, S.; Hayashi, M.; Takeshita, A.; Shibayama, Y.; Tanigawa, N.; Miyazaki, M. Significance of chymase-dependent angiotensin II formation in the progression of human liver fibrosis. *Hepatol. Res.* **2008**, *38*, 501–510. [CrossRef]
148. Urata, H.; Kinoshita, A.; Misono, K.S.; Bumpus, F.M.; Husain, A. Identification of a highly specific chymase as the major angiotensin II-forming enzyme in the human heart. *J. Biol. Chem.* **1990**, *265*, 22348–22357.
149. Yoshiji, H.; Kuriyama, S.; Yoshii, J.; Ikenaka, Y.; Noguchi, R.; Nakatani, T.; Tsujinoue, H.; Fukui, H. Angiotensin-II type 1 receptor interaction is a major regulator for liver fibrosis development in rats. *Hepatology* **2001**, *34*, 745–750. [CrossRef]
150. Ikura, Y.; Ohsawa, M.; Shirai, N.; Sugama, Y.; Fukushima, H.; Suekane, T.; Hirayama, M.; Ehara, S.; Naruko, T.; Ueda, M. Expression of angiotensin II type 1 receptor in human cirrhotic livers: Its relation to fibrosis and portal hypertension. *Hepatol. Res.* **2005**, *32*, 107–116. [CrossRef]
151. Yin, M.; Wu, L. Effect of mast cell chymase on activation, proliferation and transdifferentiation of hepatic stellate cells. *Hepatogastroenterology* **2015**, *62*, 1007–1010. [PubMed]
152. Kofford, M.W.; Schwartz, L.B.; Schechter, N.M.; Yager, D.R.; Diegelmann, R.F.; Graham, M.F. Cleavage of type I procollagen by human mast cell chymase initiates collagen fibril formation and generates a unique carboxyl-terminal propeptide. *J. Biol. Chem.* **1997**, *272*, 7127–7131. [CrossRef] [PubMed]
153. Takai, S.; Miyazaki, M. A novel therapeutic strategy against vascular disorders with chymase inhibitor. *Curr. Vasc. Pharmacol.* **2003**, *1*, 217–224. [CrossRef] [PubMed]
154. Furubayashi, K.; Takai, S.; Jin, D.; Miyazaki, M.; Katsumata, T.; Inagaki, S.; Kimura, M.; Tanaka, K.; Nishimoto, M.; Fukumoto, H. Chymase activates promatrix metalloproteinase-9 in human abdominal aortic aneurysm. *Clin. Chim. Acta* **2008**, *388*, 214–216. [CrossRef] [PubMed]
155. Longley, B.J.; Tyrrell, L.; Ma, Y.; Williams, D.A.; Halaban, R.; Langley, K.; Lu, H.S.; Schechter, N.M. Chymase cleavage of stem cell factor yields a bioactive, soluble product. *Proc. Natl. Acad. Sci. USA* **1997**, *94*, 9017–9021. [CrossRef] [PubMed]
156. Takai, S.; Jin, D. Chymase Inhibitor as a novel therapeutic agent for Non-alcoholic steatohepatitis. *Front. Pharmacol.* **2018**, *9*, 144. [CrossRef]
157. Johnson, C.; Huynh, V.; Hargrove, L.; Kennedy, L.; Graf-Eaton, A.; Owens, J.; Trzeciakowski, J.P.; Hodges, K.; DeMorrow, S.; Han, Y.; et al. Inhibition of mast cell-derived histamine decreases human cholangiocarcinoma growth and differentiation via c-Kit/Stem cell factor-dependent signaling. *Am. J. Pathol.* **2016**, *186*, 123–133. [CrossRef]

158. Jones, H.; Hargrove, L.; Kennedy, L.; Meng, F.; Graf-Eaton, A.; Owens, J.; Alpini, G.; Johnson, C.; Bernuzzi, F.; Demieville, J.; et al. Inhibition of mast cell-secreted histamine decreases biliary proliferation and fibrosis in primary sclerosing cholangitis Mdr2$^{-/-}$ mice. *Hepatology* **2016**, *64*, 1202–1216. [CrossRef]
159. Choi, J.S.; Kim, J.K.; Yang, Y.J.; Kim, Y.; Kim, P.; Park, S.G.; Cho, E.Y.; Lee, D.H.; Choi, J.W. Identification of cromolyn sodium as an anti-fibrotic agent targeting both hepatocytes and hepatic stellate cells. *Pharmacol. Res.* **2015**, *102*, 176–183. [CrossRef]
160. Kennedy, L.; Hargrove, L.; Demieville, J.; Karstens, W.; Jones, H.; DeMorrow, S.; Meng, F.; Invernizzi, P.; Bernuzzi, F.; Alpini, G.; et al. Blocking H1/H2 histamine receptors inhibits damage/fibrosis in *Mdr2*$^{-/-}$ mice and human cholangiocarcinoma tumorigenesis. *Hepatology* **2018**, *68*, 1042–1056. [CrossRef] [PubMed]
161. Boucek, R.J.; Noble, N.L. Histamine, norepinephrine, and bradykinin stimulation of fibroblast growth and modification of serotonin response. *Proc. Soc. Exp. Biol. Med.* **1973**, *144*, 929–933. [CrossRef]
162. Dayton, E.T.; Caulfield, J.P.; Hein, A.; Austen, K.F.; Stevens, R.L. Regulation of the growth rate of mouse fibroblasts by IL-3-activated mouse bone marrow-derived mast cells. *J. Immunol.* **1989**, *142*, 4307–4313.
163. Hatamochi, A.; Fujiwara, K.; Ueki, H. Effects of histamine on collagen synthesis by cultured fibroblasts derived from guinea pig skin. *Arch. Dermatol. Res.* **1985**, *277*, 60–64. [CrossRef]
164. Levi-Schaffer, F.; Rubinchik, E. Activated mast cells are fibrogenic for 3T3 fibroblasts. *J. Investig. Dermatol.* **1995**, *104*, 999–1003. [CrossRef]
165. Thompson, H.L.; Burbelo, P.D.; Gabriel, G.; Yamada, Y.; Metcalfe, D.D. Murine mast cells synthesize basement membrane components. A potential role in early fibrosis. *J. Clin. Investig.* **1991**, *87*, 619–623. [CrossRef]
166. Schon, H.T.; Weiskirchen, R. Immunomodulatory effects of transforming growth factor-β in the liver. *Hepatobiliary Surg. Nutr.* **2014**, *3*, 386–406. [CrossRef]
167. Miller, H.R.; Wright, S.H.; Knight, P.A.; Thornton, E.M. A novel function for transforming growth factor-β1, upregulation of the expression and the IgE-independent extracellular release of a mucosal mast cell granule-specific β-chymase, mouse mast cell protease-1. *Blood* **1999**, *93*, 3473–3486. [CrossRef]
168. Yamazaki, S.; Nakano, N.; Honjo, A.; Hara, M.; Maeda, K.; Nishiyama, C.; Kitaura, J.; Ohtsuka, Y.; Okumura, K.; Ogawa, H.; et al. The transcription factor Ehf is involved in TGF-β-induced suppression of FcεRI and c-Kit expression and FcεRI-mediated activation in mast cells. *J. Immunol.* **2015**, *195*, 3427–3435. [CrossRef]
169. Ndaw, V.S.; Abebayehu, D.; Spence, A.J.; Paez, P.A.; Kolawole, E.M.; Taruselli, M.T.; Caslin, H.L.; Chumanevich, A.P.; Paranjape, A.; Baker, B.; et al. TGF-β1 suppresses IL-33-induced mast cell function. *J. Immunol.* **2017**, *199*, 866–873. [CrossRef]
170. Norozian, F.; Kashyap, M.; Ramirez, C.D.; Patel, N.; Kepley, C.L.; Barnstein, B.O.; Ryan, J.J. TGFβ1 induces mast cell apoptosis. *Exp. Hematol.* **2006**, *34*, 579–587. [CrossRef]
171. Olsson, N.; Piek, E.; Sundström, M.; ten Dijke, P.; Nilsson, G. Transforming growth factor-β-mediated mast cell migration depends on mitogen-activated protein kinase activity. *Cell Signal.* **2001**, *13*, 483–490. [CrossRef]
172. Ramírez-Valadez, K.A.; Vázquez-Victorio, G.; Macías-Silva, M.; González-Espinosa, C. Fyn kinase mediates cortical actin ring depolymerization required for mast cell migration in response to TGF-β in mice. *Eur. J. Immunol.* **2017**, *47*, 1305–1316. [CrossRef]
173. Gebhardt, T.; Lorentz, A.; Detmer, F.; Trautwein, C.; Bektas, H.; Manns, M.P.; Bischoff, S.C. Growth, phenotype, and function of human intestinal mast cells are tightly regulated by transforming growth factor β1. *Gut* **2005**, *54*, 928–934. [CrossRef]
174. Kashyap, M.; Bailey, D.P.; Gomez, G.; Rivera, J.; Huff, T.F.; Ryan, J.J. TGF-β1 inhibits late-stage mast cell maturation. *Exp. Hematol.* **2005**, *33*, 1281–1291. [CrossRef]
175. Gomez, G.; Ramirez, C.D.; Rivera, J.; Patel, M.; Norozian, F.; Wright, H.V.; Kashyap, M.V.; Barnstein, B.O.; Fischer-Stenger, K.; Schwartz, L.B.; et al. TGF-β1 inhibits mast cell FcεRI expression. *J. Immunol.* **2005**, *174*, 5987–5993. [CrossRef]
176. Grizzi, F.; Di Caro, G.; Laghi, L.; Hermonat, P.; Mazzola, P.; Nguyen, D.D.; Radhi, S.; Figueroa, J.A.; Cobos, E.; Annoni, G.; et al. Mast cells and the liver aging process. *Immun. Ageing* **2013**, *10*, 9. [CrossRef]
177. Tolefree, J.A.; Garcia, A.J.; Farrell, J.; Meadows, V.; Kennedy, L.; Hargrove, L.; Demieville, J.; Francis, N. Mirabel, Francis. Alcoholic liver disease and mast cells: What's your gut got to do with it? *Liver Res.* **2019**, *3*, 46–54. [CrossRef]
178. Finn, D.F.; Walsh, J.J. Twenty-first century mast cell stabilizers. *Br. J. Pharmacol.* **2013**, *170*, 23–37. [CrossRef]

179. Bernstein, I.L.; Siegel, S.C.; Brandon, M.L.; Brown, E.B.; Evans, R.R.; Feinberg, A.R.; Friedlaender, S.; Krumholz, R.A.; Hadley, R.A.; Handelman, N.I.; et al. A controlled study of cromolyn sodium sponsored by the Drug Committee of the American Academy of Allergy. *J. Allergy Clin. Immunol.* **1972**, *50*, 235–245. [CrossRef]
180. Kusner, E.J.; Dubnick, B.; Herzig, D.J. The inhibition by disodium cromoglycate in vitro of anaphylactically induced histamine release from rat peritoneal mast cells. *J. Pharmacol. Exp. Ther.* **1973**, *184*, 41–46.
181. Oka, T.; Kalesnikoff, J.; Starkl, P.; Tsai, M.; Galli, S.J. Evidence questioning cromolyn's effectiveness and selectivity as a 'mast cell stabilizer' in mice. *Lab. Investig.* **2012**, *92*, 1472–1482. [CrossRef]
182. Mori, H.; Kawada, K.; Zhang, P.; Uesugi, Y.; Sakamoto, O.; Koda, A. Bleomycin-induced pulmonary fibrosis in genetically mast cell-deficient WBB6F1-W/Wv mice and mechanism of the suppressive effect of tranilast, an antiallergic drug inhibiting mediator release from mast cells, on fibrosis. *Int. Arch. Allergy Appl. Immunol.* **1991**, *95*, 195–201. [CrossRef]
183. Yan, Y.; Jun, C.; Lu, Y.; Jiangmei, S. Combination of metformin and luteolin synergistically protects carbon tetrachloride-induced hepatotoxicity: Mechanism involves antioxidant, anti-inflammatory, antiapoptotic, and Nrf2/HO-1 signaling pathway. *Biofactors* **2019**, *45*, 598–606. [CrossRef]
184. Abu-Elsaad, N.; El-Karef, A. Protection against nonalcoholic steatohepatitis through targeting IL-18 and IL-1alpha by luteolin. *Pharm. Rep.* **2019**, *71*, 688–694. [CrossRef]
185. He, Y.; Xia, Z.; Yu, D.; Wang, J.; Jin, L.; Huang, D.; Ye, X.; Li, X.; Zhang, B. Hepatoprotective effects and structure-activity relationship of five flavonoids against lipopolysaccharide/d-galactosamine induced acute liver failure in mice. *Int. Immunopharmacol.* **2019**, *68*, 171–178. [CrossRef]
186. Adewale, O.O.; Samuel, E.S.; Manubolu, M.; Pathakoti, K. Curcumin protects sodium nitrite-induced hepatotoxicity in Wistar rats. *Toxicol. Rep.* **2019**, *6*, 1006–1011. [CrossRef]
187. Al-Dossari, M.H.; Fadda, L.M.; Attia, H.A.; Hasan, I.H.; Mahmoud, A.M. Curcumin and selenium prevent lipopolysaccharide/diclofenac-induced liver injury by suppressing inflammation and oxidative stress. *Biol. Trace Elem. Res.* **2019**. [CrossRef]
188. Pereira, P.J.; Bergner, A.; Macedo-Ribeiro, S.; Huber, R.; Matschiner, G.; Fritz, H.; Sommerhoff, C.P.; Bode, W. Human β-tryptase is a ring-like tetramer with active sites facing a central pore. *Nature* **1998**, *392*, 306–311. [CrossRef]
189. Sommerhoff, C.P.; Bode, W.; Pereira, P.J.; Stubbs, M.T.; Sturzebecher, J.; Piechottka, G.P.; Matschiner, G.; Bergner, A. The structure of the human βII-tryptase tetramer: Fo(u)r better or worse. *Proc. Natl. Acad. Sci. USA* **1999**, *96*, 10984–10991. [CrossRef]
190. Sommerhoff, C.P.; Schaschke, N. Mast cell tryptase β as a target in allergic inflammation: An evolving story. *Curr. Pharm. Des.* **2007**, *13*, 313–332. [CrossRef]
191. Le, Q.T.; Lyons, J.J.; Naranjo, A.N.; Olivera, A.; Lazarus, R.A.; Metcalfe, D.D.; Milner, J.D.; Schwartz, L.B. Impact of naturally forming human α/β-tryptase heterotetramers in the pathogenesis of hereditary α-tryptasemia. *J. Exp. Med.* **2019**, *216*, 2348–2361. [CrossRef]
192. Steinhoff, M.; Buddenkotte, J.; Shpacovitch, V.; Rattenholl, A.; Moormann, C.; Vergnolle, N.; Luger, T.A.; Hollenberg, M.D. Proteinase-activated receptors: Transducers of proteinase-mediated signaling in inflammation and immune response. *Endocr. Rev.* **2005**, *26*, 1–43. [CrossRef]
193. Covic, L.; Gresser, A.L.; Talavera, J.; Swift, S.; Kuliopulos, A. Activation and inhibition of G protein-coupled receptors by cell-penetrating membrane-tethered peptides. *Proc. Natl. Acad. Sci. USA* **2002**, *99*, 643–648. [CrossRef]
194. Shearer, A.M.; Rana, R.; Austin, K.; Baleja, J.D.; Nguyen, N.; Bohm, A.; Covic, L.; Kuliopulos, A. Targeting liver fibrosis with a cell-penetrating protease-activated receptor-2 (PAR2) pepducin. *J. Biol. Chem.* **2016**, *291*, 23188–23198. [CrossRef]
195. Humphries, D.E.; Wong, G.W.; Friend, D.S.; Gurish, M.F.; Qiu, W.T.; Huang, C.; Sharpe, A.H.; Stevens, R.L. Heparin is essential for the storage of specific granule proteases in mast cells. *Nature* **1999**, *400*, 769–772. [CrossRef]
196. Fang, K.C.; Raymond, W.W.; Lazarus, S.C.; Caughey, G.H. Dog mastocytoma cells secrete a 92-kD gelatinase activated extracellularly by mast cell chymase. *J. Clin. Investig.* **1996**, *97*, 1589–1596. [CrossRef]
197. Lindstedt, K.A.; Wang, Y.; Shiota, N.; Saarinen, J.; Hyytiainen, M.; Kokkonen, J.O.; Keski-Oja, J.; Kovanen, P.T. Activation of paracrine TGF-β1 signaling upon stimulation and degranulation of rat serosal mast cells: A novel function for chymase. *FASEB J.* **2001**, *15*, 1377–1388. [CrossRef]

198. Masubuchi, S.; Takai, S.; Jin, D.; Tashiro, K.; Komeda, K.; Li, Z.L.; Otsuki, Y.; Okamura, H.; Hayashi, M.; Uchiyama, K. Chymase inhibitor ameliorates hepatic steatosis and fibrosis on established non-alcoholic steatohepatitis in hamsters fed a methionine- and choline-deficient diet. *Hepatol. Res.* **2013**, *43*, 970–978. [CrossRef]
199. Tashiro, K.; Takai, S.; Jin, D.; Yamamoto, H.; Komeda, K.; Hayashi, M.; Tanaka, K.; Tanigawa, N.; Miyazaki, M. Chymase inhibitor prevents the nonalcoholic steatohepatitis in hamsters fed a methionine- and choline-deficient diet. *Hepatol. Res.* **2010**, *40*, 514–523. [CrossRef]
200. Miyaoka, Y.; Jin, D.; Tashiro, K.; Komeda, K.; Masubuchi, S.; Hirokawa, F.; Hayashi, M.; Takai, S.; Uchiyama, K. Chymase inhibitor prevents the development and progression of non-alcoholic steatohepatitis in rats fed a high-fat and high-cholesterol diet. *J. Pharmacol. Sci.* **2017**, *134*, 139–146. [CrossRef]
201. Komeda, K.; Takai, S.; Jin, D.; Tashiro, K.; Hayashi, M.; Tanigawa, N.; Miyazaki, M. Chymase inhibition attenuates tetrachloride-induced liver fibrosis in hamsters. *Hepatol. Res.* **2010**, *40*, 832–840. [CrossRef]
202. Shimizu, S.; Satomura, K.; Aramaki, T.; Katsuta, Y.; Takano, T.; Omoto, Y. Hepatic chymase level in chronic hepatitis: Co-localization of chymase with fibrosis. *Hepatol. Res.* **2003**, *27*, 62–66. [CrossRef]
203. Alegre, F.; Pelegrin, P.; Feldstein, A.E. Inflammasomes in Liver Fibrosis. *Semin. Liver Dis.* **2017**, *37*, 119–127. [CrossRef]
204. Lopez-Castejon, G.; Brough, D. Understanding the mechanism of IL-1β secretion. *Cytokine Growth Factor Rev.* **2011**, *22*, 189–195. [CrossRef]
205. Mizutani, H.; Schechter, N.; Lazarus, G.; Black, R.A.; Kupper, T.S. Rapid and specific conversion of precursor interleukin 1β (IL-1β) to an active IL-1 species by human mast cell chymase. *J. Exp. Med.* **1991**, *174*, 821–825. [CrossRef]
206. Roy, A.; Ganesh, G.; Sippola, H.; Bolin, S.; Sawesi, O.; Dagalv, A.; Schlenner, S.M.; Feyerabend, T.; Rodewald, H.R.; Kjellén, L.; et al. Mast cell chymase degrades the alarmins heat shock protein 70, biglycan, HMGB1, and interleukin-33 (IL-33) and limits danger-induced inflammation. *J. Biol. Chem.* **2014**, *289*, 237–250. [CrossRef]
207. Marvie, P.; Lisbonne, M.; L'Helgoualc'h, A.; Rauch, M.; Turlin, B.; Preisser, L.; Bourd-Boittin, K.; Theret, N.; Gascan, H.; Piquet-Pellorce, C.; et al. Interleukin-33 overexpression is associated with liver fibrosis in mice and humans. *J. Cell Mol. Med.* **2010**, *14*, 1726–1739. [CrossRef]
208. Gao, Y.; Liu, Y.; Yang, M.; Guo, X.; Zhang, M.; Li, H.; Li, J.; Zhao, J. IL-33 treatment attenuated diet-induced hepatic steatosis but aggravated hepatic fibrosis. *Oncotarget* **2016**, *7*, 33649–33661. [CrossRef]
209. McHedlidze, T.; Waldner, M.; Zopf, S.; Walker, J.; Rankin, A.L.; Schuchmann, M.; Voehringer, D.; McKenzie, A.N.; Neurath, M.F.; Pflanz, S.; et al. Interleukin-33-dependent innate lymphoid cells mediate hepatic fibrosis. *Immunity* **2013**, *39*, 357–371. [CrossRef]
210. Tan, Z.; Liu, Q.; Jiang, R.; Lv, L.; Shoto, S.S.; Maillet, I.; Quesniaux, V.; Tang, J.; Zhang, W.; Sun, B.; et al. Interleukin-33 drives hepatic fibrosis through activation of hepatic stellate cells. *Cell. Mol. Immunol.* **2018**, *15*, 388–398. [CrossRef]
211. Arriazu, E.; Ge, X.; Leung, T.M.; Magdaleno, F.; Lopategi, A.; Lu, Y.; Kitamura, N.; Urtasun, R.; Theise, N.; Antoine, D.J.; et al. Signalling via the osteopontin and high mobility group box-1 axis drives the fibrogenic response to liver injury. *Gut* **2017**, *66*, 1123–1137. [CrossRef]
212. Ge, X.; Arriazu, E.; Magdaleno, F.; Antoine, D.J.; Dela Cruz, R.; Theise, N.; Nieto, N. High mobility group box-1 drives fibrosis progression signaling via the receptor for advanced glycation end products in mice. *Hepatology* **2018**, *68*, 2380–2404. [CrossRef]
213. Zhou, K.; Xie, G.; Wen, J.; Wang, J.; Pan, W.; Zhou, Y.; Xiao, Y.; Wang, Y.; Jia, W.; Cai, W. Histamine is correlated with liver fibrosis in biliary atresia. *Dig. Liver Dis.* **2016**, *48*, 921–926. [CrossRef]
214. Branco, A.C.C.C.; Yoshikawa, F.S.Y.; Pietrobon, A.J.; Sato, M.N. Role of histamine in modulating the immune response and inflammation. *Mediat. Inflamm.* **2018**, *2018*, 9524075. [CrossRef]
215. Popov, Y.; Patsenker, E.; Fickert, P.; Trauner, M.; Schuppan, D. *Mdr2* (*Abcb4*)$^{-/-}$ mice spontaneously develop severe biliary fibrosis via massive dysregulation of pro- and antifibrogenic genes. *J. Hepatol.* **2005**, *43*, 1045–1054. [CrossRef]
216. Jordana, M.; Befus, A.D.; Newhouse, M.T.; Bienenstock, J.; Gauldie, J. Effect of histamine on proliferation of normal human adult lung fibroblasts. *Thorax* **1988**, *43*, 552–558. [CrossRef]
217. Gailit, J.; Marchese, M.J.; Kew, R.R.; Gruber, B.L. The differentiation and function of myofibroblasts is regulated by mast cell mediators. *J. Investig. Dermatol.* **2001**, *117*, 1113–1119. [CrossRef]

218. Garbuzenko, E.; Nagler, A.; Pickholtz, D.; Gillery, P.; Reich, R.; Maquart, F.X.; Levi-Schaffer, F. Human mast cells stimulate fibroblast proliferation, collagen synthesis and lattice contraction: A direct role for mast cells in skin fibrosis. *Clin. Exp. Allergy* **2002**, *32*, 237–246. [CrossRef]
219. Lin, L.; Yamagata, K.; Nakayamada, S.; Sawamukai, N.; Yamaoka, K.; Sakata, K.; Nakano, K.; Tanaka, Y. Histamine inhibits differentiation of skin fibroblasts into myofibroblasts. *Biochem. Biophys. Res. Commun.* **2015**, *463*, 434–439. [CrossRef]

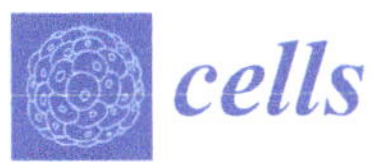

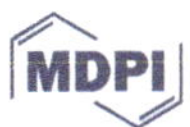

Review

The Role of Gut-Derived Microbial Antigens on Liver Fibrosis Initiation and Progression

Dishen Chen [1,†], Thanh H. Le [1,2,†], Haleh Shahidipour [1,3], Scott A. Read [1,3,*,†] and Golo Ahlenstiel [1,3,4,*,†]

1 Storr Liver Centre, The Westmead Institute for Medical Research, University of Sydney, Westmead 2145, NSW, Australia; dche9355@uni.sydney.edu.au (D.C.); 19664268@student.westernsydney.edu.au (T.H.L.); haleh.shahidipour@health.nsw.gov.au (H.S.)
2 School of Medicine, Western Sydney University, Campbelltown 2560, NSW, Australia
3 Blacktown Medical School, Western Sydney University, Blacktown 2148, NSW, Australia
4 Blacktown Hospital, Blacktown 2148, NSW, Australia
* Correspondence: s.read@westernsydney.edu.au (S.A.R.); g.ahlenstiel@westernsydney.edu.au (G.A.); Tel.: +61-2-8627-3000 (S.A.R.); +61-2-9851-6073 (G.A.)
† These authors contributed equally to this work.

Received: 30 September 2019; Accepted: 23 October 2019; Published: 27 October 2019

Abstract: Intestinal dysbiosis has recently become known as an important driver of gastrointestinal and liver disease. It remains poorly understood, however, how gastrointestinal microbes bypass the intestinal mucosa and enter systemic circulation to enact an inflammatory immune response. In the context of chronic liver disease (CLD), insults that drive hepatic inflammation and fibrogenesis (alcohol, fat) can drastically increase intestinal permeability, hence flooding the liver with gut-derived microbiota. Consequently, this may result in exacerbated liver inflammation and fibrosis through activation of liver-resident Kupffer and stellate cells by bacterial, viral, and fungal antigens transported to the liver via the portal vein. This review summarizes the current understanding of microbial translocation in CLD, the cell-specific hepatic response to intestinal antigens, and how this drives the development and progression of hepatic inflammation and fibrosis. Further, we reviewed current and future therapies targeting intestinal permeability and the associated, potentially harmful anti-microbial immune response with respect to their potential in terms of limiting the development and progression of liver fibrosis and end-stage cirrhosis.

Keywords: fibrosis; cirrhosis; alcoholic liver disease; NAFLD; NASH; intestinal permeability; bacterial translocation; innate immunity

1. Introduction

The progressive accumulation of extracellular matrix (ECM) in the liver, termed fibrosis, is the result of chronic liver damage due to a variety of insults: viral hepatitis (hepatitis B virus (HBV) and hepatitis C virus (HCV)), alcohol or fatty liver disease, drug-induced liver damage, or autoimmunity. While the prevalence of HCV- and HBV-mediated fibrosis has been on the decline since the advent of direct acting antivirals (DAAs) for HCV and improved vaccination/education strategies for HBV, other etiologies are on the rise [1]. The prevalence of non-alcoholic fatty liver disease (NAFLD) and its inflammatory form, non-alcoholic steatohepatitis (NASH), have increased in step with the obesity epidemic and are significant contributors to fibrosis, particularly in Western countries [1]. Indeed, while the prevalence of viral hepatitis dropped between 2000 and 2017, alcoholic cirrhosis increased by 16% and NASH cirrhosis by 33% [1].

The term gut–liver axis defines a bidirectional interaction between the gastrointestinal tract and the liver [2]. While the liver contributes bile acids, IgA, and antimicrobial peptides to the gut via the biliary tract, the portal vein transports gastrointestinal metabolites from the gut into the liver [2]. In the absence of disease, the mucosal barriers within the intestinal tract remain intact, preventing the transport of luminal microbes into the liver. In chronic liver disease (CLD) however, the intestinal barrier is impaired as a result of lifestyle choices (e.g., alcohol or obesity) or portal hypertension secondary to advanced fibrosis/cirrhosis, resulting in the translocation of microbes and their products into the blood.

Translocation of gut-derived antigens into the portal circulation enacts a potent inflammatory response in the liver, which has been well described in alcoholic and fatty liver disease, as well as liver cirrhosis [2]. These antigens not only drive hepatic inflammation and progressive fibrosis, but also contribute to mortality in end-stage liver disease due to their role in secondary infections such as spontaneous bacterial peritonitis (SBP) and hepatic encephalopathy [3]. While intestinal permeability is not the primary driver of liver inflammation and fibrosis, it has become evident that the inflammatory response to microbial antigens as a result of increased intestinal permeability strongly influences the progression of disease.

This review will focus on the multi-systemic nature of the gut–liver axis in health and disease. We have described (1) the intestinal barriers and mechanisms by which they become impaired in chronic liver disease, (2) the contribution of microbial antigens to liver inflammation and fibrosis, and (3), current therapies used to prevent either intestinal permeability or the hepatic inflammatory and fibrotic response.

2. Gut Microbiota and Bacterial Translocation in Chronic Liver Diseases

2.1. Gut Microbiota in Chronic Liver Diseases

The human gastrointestinal (GI) tract is estimated to contain more than 10^{14} microorganisms which collectively form the gut microbiota [4]. High motility and acidity within the esophagus and stomach limit colonization, however microbial numbers steadily increase throughout the small bowel, reaching the highest density in the colon where 10^{12} bacteria can be found in every gram of dry feces [5].

The intestinal microbiota is composed primarily of bacteria (60% of dry fecal mass), but is also abundant in archaea, eukarya, and viral species [6]. Sequencing of 16S ribosomal DNA from mucosal and stool samples has shown that Firmicutes and Bacteroidetes are the two most abundant phyla in human feces, followed by Proteobacteria, Actinobacteria, Fusobacteria, and Verrucomicrobia species [7]. Mucosal and fecal microbiota harbor distinct microbial profiles, characterized by an abundance of Bacteroidetes in stool, while human colonic crypts are colonized mainly with Firmicutes and Proteobacteria [8].

The non-bacterial intestinal microbiota contributes significantly to health and disease, but has been largely unappreciated to date. Eukaryotes account for less than 0.03% of fecal microbes and are primarily composed of 200–300 fungal species [9]. The study of intestinal viromes has been limited due to challenges in isolation and culture; however, recent metagenomic analyses have revealed that bacteriophages comprise ~90% of the gut virome and contribute significantly to bacterial dynamics [10].

The gut microbiota is essential for proper digestion and, furthermore, plays an important role in facilitating gut immune responses against potential pathogens. Indeed, commensal *Bacteroides* and *Lactobacillus* spp. can stimulate the release and activation of antimicrobial peptides such as C-type lectins and pro-defensins from intestinal Paneth cells [11,12], activate intestinal B cells to express secretory IgA [13,14], and stimulate the production of protective mucus from colonic goblet cells [15]—all mechanisms that prevent bacterial translocation across the mucosa [16]. Bacteriophage adherence to mucus layers has also been hypothesized to protect against bacterial colonization and infiltration [17].

Disturbances within the gut microbiota, termed "dysbiosis", are linked to numerous diseases, many of which are hepatic in nature [18]. This is likely due to the bidirectional nature of the gut–liver axis: nutrient rich portal vein blood entering the liver originates from the gut, while hepatic bile from gallbladder travels into the intestines to facilitate digestion [19]. Consequently, the insults that drive CLD, including caloric excess (NAFLD/NASH), alcoholism (ALD), and biliary damage (primary sclerosing cholangitis, primary biliary cirrhosis), can have significant effects on the gut microbiota, leading to intestinal permeability and exacerbation of inflammation and fibrosis.

Many studies have suggested an association between gut microbiome alteration and chronic liver diseases. Both Mouzaki et al. and Silva et al. demonstrated a reduction in *Bacteroidetes* and *Firmicutes* spp. in both NAFLD and NASH patients compared to adult healthy controls [20,21]. In pediatric studies, Zhu et al. measured a decrease in Firmicutes and increased Bacteroidetes in children with obesity or NASH [22]. A more recent, larger cohort study challenged these findings, finding a decrease of total Bacteroidetes in both NASH and NALFD pediatric patients, in agreement with adult studies [23].

In ALD, a reduction of *Lactobacillus* spp. has been recorded in both alcohol-consuming patients and mouse models [24,25]. Lactobacilli are beneficial bacteria commonly used in probiotics that have been shown to inhibit pathogen colonization [26]. Patients with ALD have also been found to have lower abundance of Bifidobacterium and Enterobacterium, and increased Proteobacteria, Fusobacteria, and Actinobacteria [27,28].

Changes in patient gut microbiota have also been measured in the context of worsening disease state. Indeed, significant differences in gut microbiota have been observed in NALFD subjects who had progressed to steatohepatitis or moderate fibrosis ($F \geq 2$) when compared to patients with earlier stages of the disease. Boursier et al. found that NASH patients possessed a significantly larger abundance of *Bacteroides* and a reduction in *Prevotella* compared to NAFLD patients [29]. Recently, Bastian et al. also confirmed a significantly higher proportion of *Bacteroides* in fibrotic (F2–F4) patients compared to patients with minimal fibrosis (F0–F1). Two large studies by Loomba et al. and Caussy et al. also found a reduction in *Firmicutes* spp. and an enrichment of *Proteobacteria* spp. in patients with cirrhosis compared to those with minimal fibrosis [30]. In addition, Bajaj et al. recently demonstrated that periodontal therapy improves gut dysbiosis and systemic inflammation in cirrhotic patients [31]. Cirrhotic patients treated with scaling and root planning followed by oral hygiene showed a reduction in Enterobacteriaceae and Streptococcaceae, and a decrease of inflammatory markers interleukin (IL)-1β and IL-6 [31]. Together, these findings suggest that certain bacteria, likely Bacteriodes and *Proteobacteria* spp., and other factors such as oral health may play important roles in liver fibrosis progression.

2.2. Physical and Chemical Barriers of the Intestinal Mucosa

To maintain a healthy coexistence with commensal microbes and prevent bacterial dissemination, the gastrointestinal tract is lined by a cellular epithelium. This physical barrier is composed primarily of epithelial cells, with the addition of specialized cell types that differ between the small and large intestine. While all epithelial cells arise from intestinal epithelial stem cells (IESC) at the base of crypts, they differentiate into a variety of cells, including enterocytes (colonocytes in the large intestine), goblet cells, Paneth cells, tuft cells, and Microfold cells (M cells) [32]. Apart from hormone-secreting enteroendocrine cells and nutrient-absorbing enterocytes, the remaining epithelial cells are largely responsible for defending against microbial invasion (Figure 1).

Goblet cells secret mucin proteins to form a highly glycosylated mucus layer over the vast epithelial surface, and this layer is significantly thinner in the small intestine compared to the colon due to a lower goblet cell density and bacterial colonization [33]. IgA secreted across the intestinal epithelium also comprises a significant component of the chemical defense. IgA is secreted by plasma cells in lymphoid follicles of the lamina propria, and transported via polymeric immunoglobulin receptors (pIgR) on the basolateral surface of epithelial cells into the lumen [34].

Epithelial integrity is maintained by junctions between intestinal epithelial cells (IECs) that provide selective nutrient permeability while preventing microbial translocation. There are three major types of cell junction that typically form near the apical end of the cells' side walls: tight junctions (TJs), gap junctions, and adherens junctions [35]. Among them, TJs form the most rigid and impenetrable seal, hence their name. This junction is a complex of more than 50 proteins, most of which are transmembrane proteins such as occludin, claudin, and the junctional adhesion molecule (JAM) family proteins such as zonula occludens (ZO)-1, which connect with the cytoskeleton and form fibrils with adjacent cells [36,37].

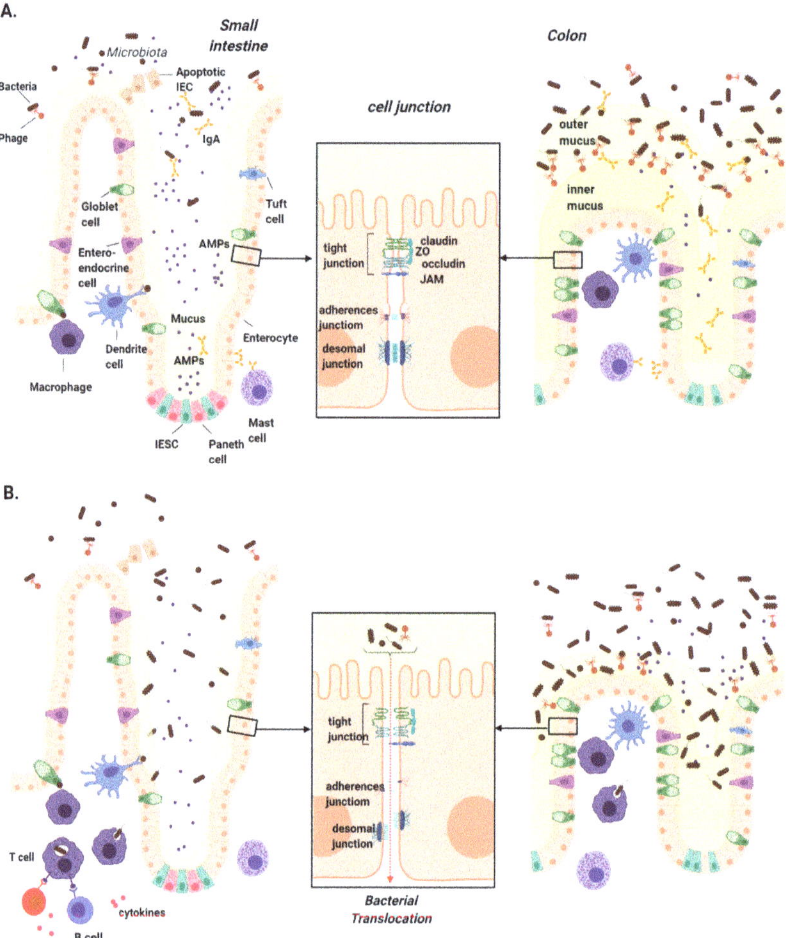

Figure 1. Intestinal mucosal barriers in health and chronic liver disease. (**A**) Several physical and chemical defenses make up the intestinal mucosa, which serves to protect us from luminal microbes. Intestinal epithelial stem cells (IESCs) located at the base of crypts give rise to all epithelial cells. Goblet cells secrete mucins to form a thin mucus layer in the small intestine and two thick layers in colon, the innermost of which is devoid of bacteria. Enterocytes/colonocytes and Paneth cells secrete antimicrobial peptides (AMPs) primarily in the small intestine, while mast cells secrete IgA, which travels through the epithelium and is concentrated in the colon. Underlying the epithelium, dendritic cells and macrophages continuously surveil luminal contents using trans-epithelial dendrites. (**B**) Disruption of these physical barriers can lead to intestinal permeability and increased microbial translocation in chronic liver disease. These include the reduction of secreted mucus, AMPs, and IgA, permitting microbial access to the epithelial layer. Downregulation, altered localization, or rearrangement of tight junction components can also significantly impact intestinal permeability, allowing microbial translocation into the portal circulation where they are transported into the liver.

2.3. Bacterial Translocation in Chronic Liver Disease

The intestinal mucosa represents the barrier protecting against luminal microbes while allowing the selective passage of digested nutrients into the circulation. This property, termed intestinal permeability, allows the intestinal tract to fulfill its absorptive function via two pathways [38]. The transcellular pathway enables macromolecules such as glucose, amino acids, or bacterial antigens to move through cells via enterocyte, M cell, and goblet cell transporter-mediated transcytosis or endocytosis. The paracellular pathway allows water and minerals to diffuse through the interspace between adjacent epithelial cells [39]. Passive transport in intestinal epithelium is, however, tightly controlled by the proteins making up the cell TJs [40]. Currently, intestinal permeability can be measured using in vivo or in vitro functional assays [39]. In vivo assays evaluate urinary or blood non-metabolized sugar such as lactulose/mannitol, polyethylene glycols (PEGs), Cr-labeled ethylenediaminetetraacetic acid (^{51}Cr-EDTA), ovalbumin (OVA), or Fluorescein isothiocyanate dextran (FITC-dextran) following ingestion. In vitro assays indirectly measure intestinal permeability by detecting biomarkers such as bacteria, lipopolysaccharides (LPS), endotoxin antibodies, or bacterial fermentation products in lymph/blood or by histologically examining TJ protein localization and expression.

Even in the absence of disease, bacteria can be transported across the intestinal epithelium into the lamina propria where they can interact with mesenteric lymph nodes (MLN) and extra-intestinal organs via the blood [41]. This process was termed bacterial translocation by Berg and Garlington in 1979, and has since been expanded to include other luminal microbes such as viruses and fungi [42]. In fact, sequencing and culture methods have detected low levels of viable and non-viable microbes, microbial DNA, and antigens in the MLN as well as in other "sterile" organs, including the liver [43,44]. Bacteriophages have also been detected in various sites within the human body including the blood, kidney, and liver [45], however their immunogenicity remains uncertain.

Increased bacterial translocation (BT) is associated with gastrointestinal diseases and the extra-intestinal conditions of the liver, kidney, and brain, among others [46–48]. As early as 1995, Berg et al. identified three factors that contribute to BT: bacterial growth or dysbiosis, intestinal permeability, and immune deficiency [41]. These factors have been identified in various forms of chronic liver disease, and are outlined below and in Table 1.

2.3.1. Alcoholic Liver Disease

In alcoholic fatty liver disease, viable bacteria, endotoxin, and LPS have been observed in the blood of both animal models and ALD patients, for which there are many potential mechanisms [49,50]. Small intestinal bacterial overgrowth (SIBO) in chronic alcoholics is more prevalent than healthy controls [51], perhaps due to extended orocaecal transit time in alcoholics compared to social drinkers [52]. SIBO has been suggested to mediate translocation due to differences in mucosal defense in the small intestine, primarily a reduction in mucus secretion. Increased intestinal permeability has also been reported in alcoholic cirrhosis, ALD, and even in non-cirrhotic alcoholics using in vivo assays [53–55].

In human studies, a reduction in the number of small intestinal villi, goblet cells, and TJ protein ZO-1 expression in the colon were observed in chronic alcoholics [56–58]. Furthermore, cell culture and animal studies suggest that ethanol and its metabolite, acetaldehyde, can alter intestinal barrier function by (1) inducing epithelial cell apoptosis, (2) disrupting TJs by downregulating ZO-1, occludin, and claudin and redistributing ZO-1 into cytoplasm, and (3) displacing the cytoplasmic skeleton [59–62].

Lastly, the production of intestinal IgA and the quantity of immune cells have been shown to be significantly altered in cases of chronic alcohol consumption and in ALD patients. While systematic IgA is increased in alcoholic liver diseases due to intestinal permeability, fecal IgA and IgA-producing B cells within the lamina propria are reduced in animal models of ALD [63,64]. Recently, a significant decrease in the number and activation state of mucosa-associated invariant T (MAIT) cells, a key component in antibacterial immune defense, was shown in ALD patients [65].

2.3.2. Non-Alcoholic Fatty Liver Disease

Multiple-pathogen-associated molecular patterns (PAMPs) such as peptidoglycan, LPS, and bacterial DNA have been detected in NALFD/NASH patient blood, and are linked to metabolic syndromes and obesity [66–68]. Two key drivers of bacterial translocation in NAFLD are SIBO and intestinal permeability, having been documented in numerous studies [69]. Increased intestinal permeability has been documented in both adult [70] and pediatric [71] NAFLD studies, as measured by 51Cr-EDTA and lactulose–mannitol assays, respectively. Moreover, intestinal permeability was associated with the severity of inflammation and fibrosis in children [71]. Clinical studies by Miele et al. and later by Xin et al. revealed that deregulation of TJ proteins may be responsible for intestinal permeability, demonstrating a reduction of ZO-1 and occludin expression in parallel with increased intestinal permeability in NAFLD patients [70,72]. Both in vitro and animal model studies of obesity further suggest that bile acids and leptin can stimulate intestinal permeability [73,74].

There is also an indication that liver damage as a result of NASH can directly contribute to loss of barrier integrity [67]. A meta-analysis performed by Luther et al. found a higher rate of intestinal permeability in NASH patients compared to NAFLD alone. A further study using a mouse model of NASH indicated that intestinal permeability occurs only after initial liver injury and the induction of pro-inflammatory cytokines [67].

Gut immune alteration is also a factor that can contribute to enhanced bacterial translocation in NAFLD. Luminal IgA and IgA-positive cells within ileal and colonic tissue are decreased in mouse models of NASH fed the methionine/choline-deficient diet [75]. Collective studies of innate and adaptive immunity on animals and patients with obesity have reported an increase in inflammatory cytokine expression and pro-inflammatory cluster differentiation (CD)4$^+$ and CD8$^+$ T cell, but an opposite trend in regulatory T cells [76]. These pro-inflammatory cytokines, such as interferon (IFN)-γ, IFN-α, and IL-6, have been shown to disturb intestinal TJs, allowing the translocation of luminal antigens across the intestinal barrier [77].

2.3.3. Liver Cirrhosis

Due to clinical associations with bacterial infection, microbial translocation is often examined in the context of liver cirrhosis. BT in cirrhosis has been identified using such methods as lymph node homogenate bacterial culture and bacterial DNA sequencing in cirrhotic patient blood [78,79]. Importantly, translocated bacteria, dominated by the Proteobacteria phylum, are abundant in the portal vein, as well as the hepatic and peripheral blood of decompensated cirrhotic patients [80]. When compared to healthy controls, SIBO is also significantly more common in patients with cirrhosis, particularly following decompensation [81,82]. Portal hypertension and abnormal small bowel motility are likely related to prevalent SIBO in decompensated cirrhosis [83].

Intestinal permeability as assessed by dual-sugar ingestion assays has been found to increase in both the small and large intestine of patients with decompensated/advanced cirrhosis [84–86]. Reduction in the expression of TJ proteins occludin and claudin-1 in cirrhotic patients may provide a mechanism for this increased permeability [87]. Nonetheless, electron microscopy experiments performed by Such et al. ten years prior demonstrated intact TJs in the duodenal epithelium of cirrhotic patients, but enlarged interspace between enterocytes [88]. More recently, an examination of cirrhotic mice treated with carbon tetrachloride (CCL_4) showed a reduction of mucin (MUC)2 expression, mucus thickness, and goblet cell number, as well as an increase in intestinal permeability associated with bacterial overgrowth and translocation. The authors also suggested a modulatory role of the bile acid receptor Farnesoid X receptor (FXR), due to the restoration of TJ protein expression, goblet cell number, and bacterial translocation following FXR agonist treatment [89].

Although clinical associations have yet to be found, alterations in intestinal humoral and cellular immunity within gut-associated lymphoid tissues (GALT) have also been observed in cirrhotic models. An increase in bacterial translocation in cirrhotic rat models can activate monocytes and dendritic cells in GALT, releasing pro-inflammatory cytokines such as tumour necrosis factor (TNF)-α and

IL-12 [90,91] that have been shown to increase intestinal permeability by deregulating ZO-1 and claudin 1 within the TJs [92,93]. While dendritic cells have been shown to open TJs to allow microbial sampling of the lumen, an increased incidence of DC sampling has been measured in cirrhotic rats, and is associated with increased translocation of bacterial DNA [91].

Table 1. Intestinal barrier deficiencies in chronic liver disease.

Intestinal Barriers	ALD	NAFLD/NASH	Cirrhosis
Mucus	Reduced mucus production [52], fewer goblet cells [56,57]	N/A	N/A
IgA	Increased systemic IgA, reduced luminal IgA [63,64]	Reduced luminal IgA [75]	N/A
Tight junctions	Downregulated ZO-1, occludin, claudin [58,60], redistributed ZO-1 into cytoplasm [94]	Downregulated ZO-1 and occludin claudin switching [70–72]	Reduced occludin and claudin-1 [87]
IECs	Apoptosis [61]	N/A	N/A
Gut immunity	Mucosal-associated invariant T-cell depletion and impaired activation thereof [65]	Fewer IgA-positive cells [75], increased production of inflammatory cytokines (IFN-γ, IFN-α, IL-6) [76], increase in $CD4^+$ and $CD8^+$ T cells [76]	Release of inflammatory cytokines (TNF-α, IL-12) [90], increased DC sampling [91]

ALD: alcohol liver disease; NAFLD: non-alcoholic fatty liver disease; NASH: non-alcoholic steatohepatitis; TJ: tight junction; ZO: zonula occludens; IFN: interferon; IL: interleukin; CD: cluster of differentiation; TNF: tumor necrosis factor; DC: dendritic cell.

Studies in recent years have provided sufficient evidence to suggest that microbial translocation can drive the development and exacerbation of chronic liver diseases. However, the detailed cellular and mechanisms implied by this association will need more efforts to elucidate.

3. Hepatic Recognition of Microbial Ligands: The Role of Pattern Recognition Receptors

Pattern recognition receptors (PRRs) are a group of host sensors that recognize antigens derived from both foreign and endogenous sources. PRRs are essential initiators of the inflammatory and immune responses that defend against foreign microbial invaders as well as endogenous cellular debris known as damage-associated molecular patterns (DAMPs). While these sensors are an essential component of hepatic immunity, they can contribute to chronic inflammation and fibrosis progression in response to prolonged activation. As outlined in the previous section, the intestinal barrier can become impaired in CLD, allowing continuous translocation of microbial antigens into the portal circulation. This section aimed to characterize the hepatic response to these antigens as it relates to inflammation and fibrosis.

The cellular drivers of liver fibrogenesis are the myofibroblast-like hepatic stellate cells (HSCs). They are largely responsible for wound healing in their steady state, but drive fibrogenesis through ECM deposition upon chronic activation [95]. HSC fibrogenesis can be triggered either directly, via induction of PRRs on HSCs, or indirectly via inflammatory signals produced by neighboring cells such as hepatocytes and Kupffer cells (KCs) [95]. This section covers PRRs that contribute to fibrosis development, with in vivo evidence of inflammatory and fibrogenic activity in CLDs, including toll-like receptor (TLR) 2, TLR3, TLR4, TLR5, TLR7 TLR9, nucleotide-binding and oligomerization domain (NOD)-like receptors (NLRs), c-type lectin receptors (CLRs), and stimulator of interferon genes (STING). General information regarding PRRs in CLD is summarized in Table 2.

Table 2. Pattern recognition receptors (PRRs) that contribute to hepatic inflammation and fibrogenesis.

PRRs	Hepatic Cell Expression	Ligands	Human Disease Involvement	Mouse Model	Role in Hepatic Inflammation and Fibrogenesis
TLR2	Hepatocyte, KC, HSC [96,97]	β-glycan, zymosan, LPS, HMGB1	↑ in NASH/NAFLD [98–100], ↓ in ALD [101].	**ALD**: Binge ethanol feeding	IL-1β, IL-6, and TNF-α ↑, hepatic neutrophil ↑ [102,103].
				NASH: MCD diet	Protective effect against NASH and inflammation [104].
				NASH: CDAA diet	KC activation and proinflammatory cytokine ↑ Activation of HSCs to directly promote fibrosis [96].
				Fibrosis: BDL	No effect [105]
				Fibrosis: CCl_4	CXCL2 ↑, neutrophil ↑ [106]. HSC ↑, α-SMA ↑ via MAPK and NF-κB pathways [107].
TLR3	Hepatocyte, KC, HSC, and LSEC [108–112]	dsRNA	N/A	**ALD**: HFD and binge drinking	IL-10 ↑ from KC and HSC, TNF-α, IL-2, CCL2 ↓ (anti-inflammatory) [113].
				Fibrosis: DDC/CCl_4	HSC killing via NK cell activation (anti-fibrotic) [114].
				Fibrosis: CCl_4	HSC activation, upregulated α-SMA, TGFβ, COL1A1 ↑ [115].
TLR4	Hepatocyte, KC, HSC, and LSEC [97,112]	LPS, HMGB1, and more	↑ in NASH ↑ circulating LPS [100,116]. PBMCs from ALD are sensitized to LPS [117]. NAFLD-associated [118].	**ALD**: Lieber–deCarli diet	ROS ↑ inflammation ↑, pro-inflammatory cytokine ↑ [119,120].
				NASH: HFHC-diet-fed ApoE KO	ROS ↑, inflammatory cytokine ↑ from KCs and hepatic macrophages [121,122].
				Fibrosis: Bile duct ligation	TLR4–MyD88–NF-κB pathway triggered HSC activation, pro-inflammatory cytokine, pro-fibrotic gene ↑ [105,123].
				Fibrosis: TAK1 KO	Directly activated HSC, pro-inflammatory cytokine, pro-fibrotic gene ↑ [124].
TLR5	Hepatocyte, LSEC, HSC [97,112,125]	Flagellin, HMGB1	N/A	**Inflammation**: Flagellin injection	Inflammatory cytokine ↑, macrophage and neutrophil recruitment [126].
				NASH: MCD diet	Hepatic inflammation ↓ inflammatory cytokines ↓, deactivating HSC [125].
				Fibrosis: CCl_4	Activated HSC via NF-κB and MAPK pathways to stimulate hepatic inflammation and collagen deposition [127].
TLR7	Hepatocyte, KC, and LSEC [112,128,129]	ssRNA	↑ in ALD [130,131]	**ALD**: 25% (w/v) ethanol diet	Inflammatory cytokine, TLR7 agonist let-7b ↑ [131].
				NASH: MCD diet	TNF-α and IFN-α ↑ in KC and DC respectively to stimulate hepatic inflammation [132].
				Fibrosis: CCl_4	Pro-inflammatory cytokine and pro-fibrotic gene ↑ [129].
TLR9	LSEC and KC [97]	Unmethylated CpG	↑ in NASH [100,133]. ↑ circulating bacterial DNA in ALD, liver fibrosis and cirrhosis [134–136].	**NASH**: CDAA diet	↑ IL-1β from KCs to ↑ hepatic inflammation. No direct fibrogenic effect [137,138].
				ALD: Chronic-binge ethanol feeding	IL-1β, CXCL1/2/5 ↑ from hepatocytes and HSC to recruit neutrophils [102,139].
				Fibrosis: BDL	Directly activated HSC [140].
				Fibrosis: Tak1ΔHep mice	Directly activated HSC [124].
NOD1	Hepatocyte, HSC, and KC [141,142].	LPS, flagellin, bacterial RNA, HMGB1, ATP	N/A	Mouse model of BDL/CCl_4-induced fibrosis	Recruited neutrophils to drive acute hepatic inflammation (CCl_4 model) [143]. CXCL1, CCL5, inflammation, fibrosis ↑ (BDL/ CCl_4 models).
NOD2				N/A	N/A
NLRP3				**NASH**: HFD	↑ NLRP3 caused ↑ inflammatory cytokine [144,145].

Table 2. *Cont.*

PRRs	Hepatic Cell Expression	Ligands	Human Disease Involvement	Mouse Model	Role in Hepatic Inflammation and Fibrogenesis
Dectin-1	Hepatocyte and LSEC [146].	β-glucans	N/A	**ALD**: Lieber-DeCarli diet (4.5% ethanol v/v) **Fibrosis**: TAA/CCl_4	Plasma β-glucan ↑ drove ↑ KC inflammatory cytokine [147]. Dectin-1 suppressed expression of TLR4 and CD14, inflammatory cytokine ↓ and activation of HSCs [146].
cGAS-cGAMP-STING	Hepatocyte, KC, HSC, and LSEC [112]	Cytosolic DNA and CDNs	STING ↑ in NAFLD [148]	**ALD**: Lieber–DeCarli diet (4.5% ethanol v/v) **NASH**: HFD and MCD diet **Fibrosis**: CCl_4	STING–IRF3 pathway triggered hepatic pro-inflammatory cytokine production [149]. mtDNA activated STING in KC [150]. STING–IRF3 pathway activated hepatocyte apoptosis, HSC, and fibrogenesis [151].

PRR: pattern recognition receptor; TLR: Toll-like receptor; KC: Kupffer cell; HSC: hepatic stellate cell; LPS: lipopolysaccharide; HMGB1: high mobility group box 1 protein; NASH: non-alcoholic steatohepatitis; NAFLD: non-alcoholic fatty liver disease; ALD: alcoholic liver disease; TNF-α: tumor necrosis factor; MCD diet: methionine/choline-deficient diet; LSEC: liver sinusoidal endothelial cell; CDAA: choline-deficient L-amino-defined; CCl_4: carbon tetrachloride; α-SMA: α-smooth muscle actin; MAPK: mitogen-activated protein kinase; NF-Kb: nuclear factor kappa-light-chain-enhancer of activated B cells; dsRNA: double-stranded RNA; HFD: highffat diet; DDC: 3,5-diethoxycarbonyl-1,4-dihydrocollidine; NK cell: natural killer cell; COL1A1: collagen type 1 A1; PBMC: peripheral blood mononuclear cell; ROS: reactive oxygen species; HFHC: high-fat, high-cholesterol; KO: knockout; TAK1: transforming growth factor beta-activated kinase 1; ssRNA: single-stranded RNA; IFN: interferon; DC: dendritic cell; NLR: NOD-like receptor; NOD: nucleotide-binding and oligomerization domain; NLRP: nucleotide-binding oligomerization domain, leucine-rich repeat- and pyrin-domain-containing; ATP: adenosine triphosphate; CLR: C-type lectin receptors; STING: Stimulator of Interferon Genes; cGAS: cyclic GMP-AMP Synthase; cGAMP: cyclic GMP-AMP; CDNs: cyclic dinucleotides; IRF3: interferon regulatory transcription factor 3; mtDNA: mitochondrial DNA. ↑: upregulation of expression; ↓: downregulation of expression.

3.1. Toll-Like Receptors

3.1.1. TLR2

Hepatic upregulation of TLR2 has been observed in patients with NAFLD/NASH [98,100] and fibrosis due to chronic viral infection [152]. In contrast, ALD patients show significantly lower expression of hepatic TLR2 compared to healthy controls [101].

In murine models of CLD, TLR2 significantly contributes to hepatic inflammation and fibrosis. In chronic ethanol-binge-fed mice, TLR2 is crucial for hepatic IL-1β, IL-6, and TNF-α-related liver injury and inflammation, as well as neutrophil-mediated hepatic injury [102,103]. In addition, using the choline-deficient L-amino-defined (CDAA)-diet-induced NASH model, TLR2 deficiency improved hepatic inflammation and injury by reducing Kupffer cell inflammasome activation and pro-inflammatory cytokine production, suggesting a KC-dependent inflammatory pathway mediated by TLR2 [96]. In contrast, TLR2 was protective in the NASH methionine/choline-deficient (MCD) diet model, as demonstrated by an increase in ALT and TNF-α in TLR2 KO mice [104].

In mouse models of fibrosis, TLR2 was reported to have limited contribution to fibrogenesis in bile duct ligation (BDL) mice [105]. In contrast, $TLR2^{-/-}$ mice treated with CCL_4, possessed significantly impaired HSC activation with reduced collagen deposition, pro-inflammatory cytokine and α-smooth muscle actin (SMA) expression [107]. In addition, they demonstrated attenuated mitogen-activated protein kinase (MAPK) and nuclear factor kappa-light-chain-enhancer of activated B cells (NF-κB) activation compared to wild type (WT) fibrotic mice. A neutrophil-driven mechanism of fibrogenesis in CCL_4-induced fibrosis has also been attributed to TLR2-mediated hepatic chemokine C–C motif ligand (CXCL)2 production [106]. Lastly, TLR2 knockout (KO) in CDAA-diet-induced NASH mice significantly dampened HSC activation, collagen deposition, α-SMA expression, and transforming growth factor (TGF)-β expression, thus, ameliorating NASH-associated fibrogenesis [96].

3.1.2. TLR3

The protective and anti-inflammatory role of TLR3 has been reported in mice fed with high-fat diet (HFD) followed by binge drinking to induce liver injury. Stimulating TLR3 using poly I:C resulted in elevated HSC and KC IL-10 expression, as well as reduced hepatic expression of TNF-α, IL-6, CXCL2 and impaired liver injury [113].

TLR3 signaling is well characterized in murine natural killer (NK) cells, where activation of TLR3 results in a potent anti-fibrotic effect in both 3,5-diethoxycarbonyl-1,4-dihydrocollidine (DDC)-diet- and CCl_4-induced murine fibrosis models [153,154]. TLR3 has been shown to work synergistically with IL-18 to activate the p38/PI3K/Akt pathway, thus stimulating NK cells to kill HSCs via TNF-related apoptosis-inducing ligand (TRAIL)-mediated degranulation [114]. In contrast, TLR3 is pro-fibrotic in the CCL_4 fibrosis model, where TLR3 KO results in downregulation of IL-6, TNF-α, and pro-fibrotic markers [115]. Interestingly, the authors concluded that CCL_4-treated hepatocyte exosomes stimulated HSC TLR3 signaling to drive $\gamma\delta$ T cell IL-17 production and fibrosis progression [115].

3.1.3. TLR4

TLR4 is the most thoroughly studied PRR in the setting of CLD. Hepatic and serum TLR4 is significantly upregulated in NASH patients, with elevated levels of circulating LPS in peripheral [100,116] and portal vein blood [155]. High serum levels of TLR4 have also been proposed as a predictive non-invasive marker for liver fibrosis development in NASH patients [156]. Although hepatic expression of TLR4 has not been studied in patients with ALD, peripheral blood mononuclear cells (PBMCs) from patients with ALD showed sensitized responses towards LPS treatment [117].

The role of TLR4 in murine models of liver inflammation has been well studied. TLR4-dependent ROS production and TLR4-dependent interferon regulatory factor (IRF)3 activation in the liver are required to drive hepatic inflammation in mice with alcoholic hepatitis [120]. A similar study showed that hepatic inflammatory cytokines were significantly downregulated in hepatocyte-selective-TLR4-deficient mice fed with a liquid diet containing 5% ethanol [119]. The importance of TLR4 in NASH development was further emphasized in a murine NASH model using high-fat, high-cholesterol (HFHC)-diet fed ApoE KO mice, showing a TLR4-mediated ROS production and triggering pro-inflammatory cytokine expression in KC [122]. Linking TLR4 to NAFLD pathogenesis, fatty acids such as palmitate can also trigger ROS production in a TLR4-dependent manner, inducing IL-1β and TNF-α production from liver macrophages [121].

TLR4-mediated fibrosis has been interrogated in a variety of mouse models. In BDL mice, the TLR4–MyD88–NF-κB pathway in HSCs has been shown to upregulate pro-inflammatory cytokine production, α-SMA, TIMP1, and TGF-β expression, and ECM deposition [105,123]. In addition, TLR4-mediated downregulation of Bambi (a TGFβ pseudoreceptor) was shown to sensitize quiescent HSCs for subsequent activation [105,123]. Using the transforming growth factor beta-activated kinase 1 (TAK1) KO murine model of fibrosis [124], TLR4 and MyD88 double KO mice also demonstrated reduced α-SMA, TIMP1, and TGFβ expression and collagen deposition, supporting the involvement of TLR4–MyD88–NF-κB signaling in hepatic fibrogenesis [124].

3.1.4. TLR5

Peritoneal injection with the TLR5 ligand flagellin has been shown to induce significant TLR5-mediated liver injury in mice, resulting in IL-6, IL-8, and IL-1β production, coupled with neutrophil and macrophage infiltration into the liver [126]. In the context of NASH, however, hepatocyte TLR5 may possess a protective effect. In mice fed with MCD diet to induce NASH, selective hepatocyte deficiency of TLR5 was shown to exacerbate liver inflammation and fibrosis via elevated expression of TNF-α, monocyte chemoattractant protein (MCP)1, and IL-1β, as well as Timp1, Mmp9, Col1, and collagen deposition [125]. These conflicting results may, however, be the result of hepatocyte versus whole-body knockout of TLR5 and require further study.

Unlike hepatocyte-specific TLR5 KO, whole-body KO ameliorates inflammation and fibrogenesis in the CCL_4 fibrosis model. TLR5 KO mice demonstrated a significant reduction of inflammatory mediators TNF-α, IL-6, and IL-1β and fibrogenesis, as indicated by downregulation in α-SMA, TGF-β, TIMP1, and collagen deposition compared to WT mice [127]. A significant reduction in NF-κB and MAPK signaling activity was measured in activated HSCs, suggesting a mechanism of hepatic fibrogenesis mediated by the TLR5-activated NF-κB/MAPK signaling pathway in HSCs [127].

3.1.5. TLR7

The role of TLR7 in NASH/NAFLD, liver fibrosis, or liver cirrhosis has been widely overlooked in the clinical setting; however, recent studies suggest that ALD-mediated inflammation and fibrosis is linked to hepatic TLR7 overexpression [130,131]. Moreover, TLR7-mediated IFN production is stimulated by alcohol in primary human hepatocytes and is correlated with patients with more advanced fibrosis as well as higher expression of fibrotic markers α-SMA, collagen I, and Timp1 [130].

The role of TLR7 in ALD, NASH/NAFLD, and fibrosis development has been established primarily in mouse models. A recent study using ethanol (25% w/v) feeding to stimulate alcoholic hepatitis showed that activation of TLR7 significantly upregulated expression of pro-inflammatory cytokines and the endogenous TLR-7 agonist let-7b from hepatocytes, hence exacerbating hepatic inflammation [131]. Roh et al. recently showed that TLR7 deficiency significantly reduced the degree of hepatic steatosis and inflammation in a MCD-diet-induced NASH mouse model, examined by H&E staining, as well as TNF-α and IFN-α production from KC and hepatic dendritic cells, respectively [132]. In contrast, TLR7 has been identified as a protective factor in hepatic fibrosis development in both CCL_4 and BDL murine fibrosis models. TLR7 KO mice expressed higher levels of hepatic pro-inflammatory cytokine and fibrosis marker expression as well as exacerbated collagen deposition [129]. Moreover, dendritic cell expressed type I IFNs upon TLR7 stimulation, triggered KC IL-1 receptor antagonist expression and ultimately suppressing IL-1-dependent liver injury and inflammation [129].

3.1.6. TLR9

In humans, hepatic TLR9 expression is upregulated in NASH patients [100,133], while high serum levels of bacterial DNA (TLR9 ligand) have also been linked with liver cirrhosis and liver fibrosis [134,135]. Indeed, an increase in circulating bacterial DNA has been measured in patients with alcoholic and fatty liver disease prior to fibrotic development [136]. In addition, acute binge drinking has been shown to significantly increase serum bacterial DNA and pro-inflammatory cytokines such as IL-6, TNF-α, and IL-1β to indirectly contribute to liver fibrosis [135,139,157].

The role of TLR9 in chronic liver inflammation has been well established in animal models. In mouse models of CDAA-induced NASH, activation of TLR9 can stimulate IL-1β expression in KCs, mediating steatohepatitis and hepatocyte apoptosis driven by lipid accumulation [137,138]. In addition, the pro-inflammatory role of TLR9 in NASH has been further confirmed in atherogenic diet-fed NASH and *foz* mouse models, demonstrating reduced pro-inflammatory cytokine production and attenuated hepatic neutrophil infiltration in $TLR9^{-/-}$ mice [133]. Similarly, evidence for TLR9-mediated liver injury and inflammation in chronic-binge-ethanol-fed mice was shown to be driven by IL-1β expression as well as TLR9/TLR2-dependent hepatic neutrophil infiltration mediated by CXCL1/2/5 expressed from hepatocytes and HSC [102,139].

Despite the inflammatory role of TLR9 in human NASH, TLR9 KO failed to improve hepatic fibrosis in murine NASH models [133]. TLR9 does, however, seem to influence fibrosis development in other models of fibrosis including murine BDL, where $TLR9^{-/-}$ mice demonstrated significantly alleviated fibrogenesis and HSC activation compared to WT mice [140]. Similar results were found using the spontaneous fibrosis Tak1ΔHep mouse model, also demonstrating a reduction in liver inflammation and fibrosis in TLR9 KO mice [124]. Moreover, stimulation of TLR9 using CpG DNA directly activated the fibrogenic phenotype in primary mouse HSCs and the immortalized human HSC LX-2 cell line [158].

3.2. NOD-Like Receptors

The influence of NLRs on liver inflammation and fibrosis was thoroughly reviewed recently by Xu et al. [145]. NOD1, NOD2, and nucleotide-binding oligomerization domain, leucine-rich repeat- and pyrin-domain-containing (NLRP)3 are the main NLRs driving hepatic inflammation, liver injury, and liver fibrogenesis. NOD1-mediated neutrophil recruitment has been described following acute liver injury and inflammation in a CCL_4-treated murine model [159]. In addition, activation of NOD-2 by muramyl dipeptide, a bacterial peptidoglycan motif, can induce NF-kB-dependent hepatic expression of pro-inflammatory cytokines to indirectly orchestrate liver inflammation and fibrosis [145,160]. Furthermore, it has been demonstrated that NLRP3–inflammasome pathway is activated in murine NASH to induce hepatic TNF-a, IL-6, and IL-8 production [144,145].

Hepatocyte stimulation of NOD1 via its ligands can activate the NF-kB and MAPK pathway to induce CXCL1 and CCL5 production, promoting wound healing and fibrogenesis [161]. NLRP3–inflammasome has been demonstrated to be a direct contributor in hepatic fibrogenesis. Activation of NLRP3 undoubtedly triggers direct activation of HSC to enhance matrix deposition, TGF-β expression, and fibrosis progression [142].

3.3. Anti-Fungal PRRs and Liver Fibrosis

The role of the CLR dectin-1 in liver inflammation and fibrosis development has been thoroughly studied. Ethanol-containing-diet-fed mice were found to have elevated serum β-glucan level and hepatic injury, which was significantly reduced upon treatment with anti-fungal agent [147]. More importantly, plasma β-glucans enhanced IL-1β expression in KC to drive hepatic inflammation that was absent in dectin-1 deficient mice [147]. A further study showed that hepatic expression of dectin-1 was upregulated in a thioacetamide (TAA)/CCL_4 fibrosis mouse model, and that dectin-1 negatively regulated the expression of TLR4 and its co-receptor CD14 to mitigate fibrosis development and hepatic inflammation [146]. Knocking out dectin-1 exacerbated liver fibrosis and inflammation, as demonstrated by increased expression of TNF-α, IL-6, and MCP-1, neutrophil and macrophage influx, and fibrosis progression [146].

3.4. STING

In view of its recent discovery, there have been a limited number of human studies exploring the role of STING in CLD. Luo et al. reported an overexpression of STING in the non-parenchymal cells within the liver tissue of NAFLD patients, albeit with no examination of their relationship to disease activity [148]. By utilizing the alcohol-fed mouse ALD model, Petrasek et al. demonstrated that activation of the STING–IRF3 pathway stimulates pro-inflammatory cytokine production in the liver [149]. In the same study, alcohol-induced liver injury was also shown to trigger the STING–IRF3 pathway by endoplasmic reticulum (ER) stress, promoting the mitochondrial apoptotic pathway in hepatocytes [149]. Knocking out STING in HFD-induced NAFLD and MCD-induced NASH murine models attenuated hepatic activation of IRF3 and NF-κB pathways, and significantly downregulated expression of pro-inflammatory cytokines to alleviate NAFLD/NASH severity [148]. Similar findings were reported by Yu et al. using HFD- and MCD-diet-induced NASH mice; hepatocytes releasing mitochondrial DNA during NASH development led to the activation of STING–IRF3 pathway on KC to trigger pro-inflammatory cytokine production and hepatic inflammation in NASH [150].

Taken together, the above studies suggest that STING plays an important role in both hepatic inflammation and hepatic fibrosis in NASH [148,150]. Similar findings were elucidated in a CCL_4-induced liver fibrosis murine model by Iracheta-Vellve et al. Hepatocytes were shown to undergo significant ER stress resulting in STING–IRF3 activation and induction of the mitochondria-dependent apoptosis pathway. Hepatocyte cell death was shown to activate HSC expression of α-SMA and COL1A2, collagen deposition, and fibrosis progression [151].

4. Therapies to Prevent Microbe-Driven Liver Inflammation and Fibrosis

The primary interventions for alcoholic and fatty liver disease have focused on lifestyle modifications: abstaining from alcohol and improving patient diet and exercise regimens. In more severe cases of obesity, surgical interventions (e.g., bariatric surgery) are required in combination with significant lifestyle adjustments. Unfortunately, even in the case of surgical interventions, patient compliance towards dietary and alcohol restrictions is often lacking, rendering the development of novel therapeutics a top priority.

In cirrhotic patients, dietary interventions and abstinence from alcohol drastically improve survival [162]. These patients also generally require treatment of portal hypertension, which is the contributing factor to intestinal permeability. Unfortunately, however, in decompensated cirrhosis, treatment of portal hypertension using beta-blockers and anti-hypertensives can dangerously reduce mean arterial pressure [163]. In addition, there is an increased risk of susceptibility to infections due to poor phagocytic capacity in the liver and increased likelihood of ascites: the accumulation of fluid in the peritoneal cavity [3]. These aspects further underline the vital need for novel therapies to prevent the progression of fibrosis, particularly in end-stage liver disease where there is currently a lack of effective treatment. Limiting the exacerbation of inflammation and fibrosis by microbial translocation into the liver is therefore an avenue that must be explored. We aimed to summarize current and potential therapies directed at (1) reducing microbial translocation, and (2) limiting the harmful response to microbial antigens in the liver.

4.1. Therapies to Reduce Intestinal Permeability

Studies examining intestinal permeability in ALD [24,53,54], NAFLD/NASH [67,70,164], and fibrotic liver disease/cirrhosis [86,87,165] have focused primarily on the reduction in TJ proteins such as ZO-1 and Claudin-1 [70,87,94], though the mechanisms by which this loss occurs remains largely unknown. Loss of intestinal mucus or mucosal IgA production [166] can also significantly increase intestinal permeability; however, these mechanisms have been largely overlooked in CLD.

Expansion of pathogenic bacterial species both within the colon and into the SIBO have been documented in CLD [70,167], motivating the examination of antibiotics and prebiotics as potential therapies. Antibiotic studies commonly use a broad spectrum and poorly absorbed antibiotics such as neomycin or rifaximin to achieve a gut-targeted intestinal decontamination. In rodent models of obesity [168], long-term ethanol exposure [169], NASH [170], and fibrosis [105], antibiotic treatment has been shown to reduce intestinal permeability and subsequent liver injury. In humans, a number of clinical trials are underway to assess the efficacy of antibiotics for the treatment of AH, NASH, and cirrhosis (reviewed in [171]). Early data suggests that short-term rifaximin treatment can reduce serum endotoxin and liver inflammation in NAFLD/NASH patients [172], whereas rifamixin prophylaxis over 24 weeks can significantly reduce hospitalization and mortality among cirrhotic patients [173]. These data support previous findings that rifaximin can reduce the risk of complications associated with cirrhosis, including hepatic encephalopathy, variceal bleeding, and SBP [174]. Importantly, antibiotics such as levofloxacin and metronidazole, but not rifaximin, can significantly increase gut proteases, thus contributing to intestinal permeability in both humans [175] and rats [176]. An antibiotic-mediated reduction in anti-proteolytic bacterial richness and abundance in the colon is thought to contribute to gut permeability.

Significant microbial perturbations caused by broad spectrum antibiotics have stimulated interest in probiotics (beneficial microbes) and prebiotics (beneficial microbial substrates) for the improvement of intestinal health. In mouse models of ethanol-induced liver injury, probiotic *Lactobacillus rhamnosus* strains have been shown to reduce serum endotoxin, hepatic oxidative stress, and inflammatory TNFα production [177,178]. While intestinal permeability was not assessed in these studies, Wang et al. demonstrated that *Lactobacillus* probiotics could prevent the alcohol-induced loss of intestinal ZO-1, Caludin-1, and Occludin-1, keeping the intestinal epithelium intact [179]. In rats, a similar reduction in ZO-1, intestinal permeability, steatosis, and fibrosis was observed in the choline-deficient/L-amino-acid-defined NASH diet, and was significantly attenuated by probiotic treatment with *Clostridium butyricum* MIYAIRI 588 strain. Interestingly, in mouse models of CCL_4-induced fibrosis, different probiotics achieve improved intestinal permeability via unique mechanisms: *Bifidobacterium* probiotics have been shown to increase intestinal TJ expression [180] whereas *Lactobacillus-paracasei*-fermented milk reduces intestinal permeability by increasing antimicrobial β-defensin expression [181].

The study of prebiotics allows researchers to understand the relationship between a substrate, microbial metabolism, gut health, and permeability. The majority of prebiotics used today are indigestible carbohydrate polymers (fibers) that become fermented by gut bacteria to produce, among other things, short chain fatty acids (SCFAs) consisting of acetate, propionate, and butyrate [182]. SCFAs are significant homeostatic and anti-inflammatory signaling molecules in the gut (reviewed in Reference [183]), but can also significantly alter intestinal permeability. In vitro, butyrate has been shown to increase ZO-1 expression in Caco-2 cells [184], and stimulate mucous secretion in E12 human colon cells [185]. In vivo, rats supplemented with oats rich in fermentable β-glucans were significantly more resistant to alcohol-induced oxidative stress and intestinal permeability [186]. In humans, increased fiber intake has also been associated with improved permeability (reduced circulating ZO-1) and reduced ALT/AST in NALFD patients [187]. These data are supported by two recent meta-analyses finding that both prebiotics and probiotics reduce liver enzymes ALT, AST, and GGT in NAFLD patients [188], with probiotics also reducing serum ammonia and hepatic encephalopathy in cirrhotic patients [189].

4.2. Therapies to Dampen the Hepatic Immune Response

Direct inhibition of PRRs for the treatment of chronic liver disease has not been a research priority due to their peripheral contribution to disease pathogenesis. It is, however, now becoming evident that PRR activation from both microbial and self-ligands can significantly contribute to liver inflammation and fibrogenesis. TLR-agonistic therapies are currently being actively pursued for cancer therapies/adjuvants (reviewed in Reference [190]). TLR inhibitors, on the other hand, have been studied to a lesser degree in a handful of studies assessing their efficacy in inflammatory and autoimmune disease. Even fewer therapies are being assessed in the context of chronic liver disease, with TLR2/4/9, NLRP3, and STING pathway inhibition garnering some interest from pharmaceutical companies [190].

The humanized TLR2 mAb OPN-305 can achieve significant blockade of TLR2 inflammatory signaling in response to bacterial stimuli in healthy subjects [191], and improved overall response rate in patients with myelodysplastic syndromes that had previously failed hypomethylating agent therapy [192]. While TLR2 blockade has not been assessed in human CLD, the pleiotropic nature of TLR2 suggests that it may benefit inflammatory and fibrotic progression.

Small molecule inhibitors of TLR4, i.e., NI-0101 [193] and Ibudilast [194], are being assessed in extrahepatic disease, and JKB-121, a weak TLR4 antagonist, is currently being assessed in NASH [195]: preliminary results do not support a significant therapeutic benefit of JKB-121, though the study was confounded by a notable improvement in liver inflammation within the placebo group.

TLR9 blockade represents perhaps the most exciting TLR-targeting therapy. The TLR9 inhibitor hydroxychloroquine is currently used as treatment for autoimmune diseases such as rheumatoid arthritis and lupus, allowing potential repurposing for CLD. Furthermore, the novel TLR9 antagonist COV08-0064 has shown promise in animal models of sterile liver inflammation, particularly in the context of fatty liver where it limits inflammasome activation [196,197]. While TLR9 inhibition has yet to be assessed in human CLD, its diversity of microbial ligands, including bacterial, fungal, and phage DNA, will surely make it a candidate for future trials.

Research targeting the NLRP3–inflammasome pathway is undergoing rapid expansion alongside the number of inflammasome-associated diseases. While the NLRP3 inhibitor CP-456,773 was removed from phase II trials for rheumatoid arthritis due to supposed liver toxicity, other inhibitors are in different stages of development for the treatment of gout and Parkinson's disease, among others [198].

In 2018, Genentec acquired San Diego-based Jecure Therapeutics and their portfolio of preclinical NLRP3 inhibitors as a treatment for NASH and hepatic fibrosis [199].

Lastly, the intracellular DNA sensor STING has become a popular target due to its association with autoimmune disease. STING inhibitors have been recently developed [200], and are being actively generated by a number of pharmaceutical companies with the aim of targeting STING-related genetic disease. This compound would have the potential to move towards therapies for CLDs such as NASH and fibrosis in the future [201].

5. Conclusions and Future Perspectives

In summary, this review has highlighted the strong connection between the liver and gut in the context of liver disease. Indeed, CLD does not occur in isolation, but is accompanied by disturbances of the complex balance of gastrointestinal microbiota, architecture, and immunity. Similarly, gut microbiota can play a significant role in liver health by altering host metabolism and immunity. While such associations are strong, it is much less certain whether the distinct disease states in CLD and fibrosis stimulate changes in microbiota, or if gut microbiota exacerbate inflammatory and fibrotic progression.

Host, microbiomic, and lifestyle factors that influence intestinal permeability are beginning to be understood, but there is still much to be learned. Specifically, there is poor understanding of the exact mechanisms by which intestinal permeability is altered and the physiological reasons for it. TJ expression and localization are often examined in isolation, while overlooking the numerous additional barriers that prevent microbial translocation in the gut. Antimicrobial peptides, IgA, and mucus abundance and localization are rarely examined in this context, and a better understanding of their regulation in health and disease is warranted.

Lastly, along with public health initiatives aimed at reducing the causative lifestyle factors of fibrosis, i.e., alcohol and obesity, we must focus research on the development of novel PRR-antagonizing therapies. Murine studies have highlighted the contribution of individual PRRs to the development and progression of liver inflammation and fibrosis (as summarized in Figure 2); however, it remains unclear how multiple sensors collectively drive disease and may potentiate each signal. Human trials are pending to examine microbial sensors such as TLR9 and STING as well as inflammasome components to determine their contribution, whether alone or in concert, to fibrosis progression.

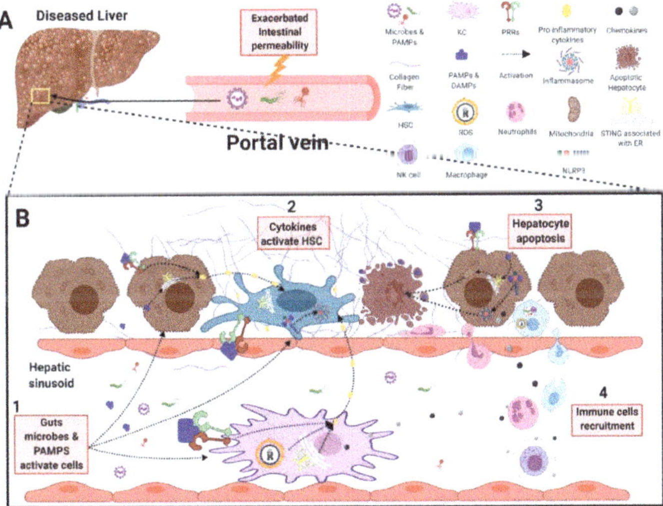

Figure 2. Gastrointestinal microbes and their contribution to liver inflammation and fibrosis. (**A**) In chronic liver disease, gut microbes and PAMPs can cross the intestinal barrier due to an increase in

intestinal permeability, resulting in their transport into the liver through the hepatic portal vein. (**B1**) Gut-derived antigens are recognized by, and activate HSCs, KCs, and hepatocytes, resulting in the secretion of pro-inflammatory cytokines and chemokines. (**B2**) Pro-inflammatory cytokines produced from KCs and hepatocytes further activate HSCs to further exacerbate fibrogenesis. (**B3**) In addition, activation of STING– and NLRP3–inflammasome pathways in hepatocytes can trigger apoptosis and release of DAMPs to further activate HSCs. (**B4**) Chemokines produced by activated KCs, HSCs, and hepatocytes recruit immune cells such as neutrophils, NK cells, and monocytes to further exacerbate liver inflammation and injury. PAMP: pathogen associated molecular pattern; KC: Kupffer cell; HSC: hepatic stellate cell; NK cell: natural killer cell; PRR: pattern recognition receptor; TLR: Toll-like receptor; NOD: nucleotide-binding oligomerization domain-containing protein 1; NLRP3: nucleotide-binding oligomerization domain, leucine-rich repeat- and pyrin-domain-containing 3; STING: stimulator of interferon genes; DAMP: damage associate molecular pattern.

Author Contributions: Writing—original draft preparation (S.A.R., T.H.L., D.C.); writing—review and editing (S.A.R., H.S., G.A.); supervision (S.A.R., G.A.).

Funding: This research received no external funding.

Acknowledgments: Figures were created with Biorender.com (©BioRender-biorender.com).

Conflicts of Interest: The authors declare no conflict of interest.

References

1. Loomba, R.; Sanyal, A.J. The global NAFLD epidemic. *Nat. Rev. Gastroenterol. Hepatol.* **2013**, *10*, 686–690. [CrossRef] [PubMed]
2. Tripathi, A.; Debelius, J.; Brenner, D.A.; Karin, M.; Loomba, R.; Schnabl, B.; Knight, R. The gut-liver axis and the intersection with the microbiome. *Nat. Rev. Gastroenterol. Hepatol.* **2018**, *15*, 397–411. [CrossRef] [PubMed]
3. Iebba, V.; Guerrieri, F.; Di Gregorio, V.; Levrero, M.; Gagliardi, A.; Santangelo, F.; Sobolev, A.P.; Circi, S.; Giannelli, V.; Mannina, L.; et al. Combining amplicon sequencing and metabolomics in cirrhotic patients highlights distinctive microbiota features involved in bacterial translocation, systemic inflammation and hepatic encephalopathy. *Sci. Rep.* **2018**, *8*. [CrossRef] [PubMed]
4. Doré, J.; Simrén, M.; Buttle, L.; Guarner, F. Hot topics in gut microbiota. *United Eur. Gastroenterol. J.* **2013**, *1*, 311–318. [CrossRef] [PubMed]
5. Sekirov, I.; Russell, S.L.; Antunes, L.C.M.; Finlay, B.B. Gut Microbiota in Health and Disease. *Physiol. Rev.* **2010**, *90*, 859–904. [CrossRef]
6. Cani, P.D. Human gut microbiome: Hopes, threats and promises. *Gut* **2018**, *67*, 1716. [CrossRef]
7. Eckburg, P.B.; Bik, E.M.; Bernstein, C.N.; Purdom, E.; Dethlefsen, L.; Sargent, M.; Gill, S.R.; Nelson, K.E.; Relman, D.A. Diversity of the human intestinal microbial flora. *Science (New York, NY)* **2005**, *308*, 1635–1638. [CrossRef]
8. Saffarian, A.; Mulet, C.; Regnault, B.; Amiot, A.; Tran-Van-Nhieu, J.; Ravel, J.; Sobhani, I.; Sansonetti, P.J.; Pédron, T. Crypt- and Mucosa-Associated Core Microbiotas in Humans and Their Alteration in Colon Cancer Patients. *MBio* **2019**, *10*, e01315-19. [CrossRef]
9. Hillman, E.T.; Lu, H.; Yao, T.; Nakatsu, C.H. Microbial Ecology along the Gastrointestinal Tract. *Microbes Envrion.* **2017**, *32*, 300–313. [CrossRef]
10. Reyes, A.; Semenkovich, N.P.; Whiteson, K.; Rohwer, F.; Gordon, J.I. Going viral: Next-generation sequencing applied to phage populations in the human gut. *Nat. Rev. Microbiol.* **2012**, *10*, 607–617. [CrossRef]
11. Cash, H.L.; Whitham, C.V.; Behrendt, C.L.; Hooper, L.V. Symbiotic bacteria direct expression of an intestinal bactericidal lectin. *Science (New York, NY)* **2006**, *313*, 1126–1130. [CrossRef] [PubMed]
12. Aguilera, M.; Cerda-Cuellar, M.; Martinez, V. Antibiotic-induced dysbiosis alters host-bacterial interactions and leads to colonic sensory and motor changes in mice. *Gut Microbes* **2015**, *6*, 10–23. [CrossRef] [PubMed]
13. Yanagibashi, T.; Hosono, A.; Oyama, A.; Tsuda, M.; Hachimura, S.; Takahashi, Y.; Itoh, K.; Hirayama, K.; Takahashi, K.; Kaminogawa, S. Bacteroides induce higher IgA production than Lactobacillus by increasing activation-induced cytidine deaminase expression in B cells in murine Peyer's patches. *Biosci. Biotechnol. Biochem.* **2009**, *73*, 372–377. [CrossRef] [PubMed]

14. Macpherson, A.J.; Gatto, D.; Sainsbury, E.; Harriman, G.R.; Hengartner, H.; Zinkernagel, R.M. A primitive T cell-independent mechanism of intestinal mucosal IgA responses to commensal bacteria. *Science* **2000**, *288*, 2222–2226. [CrossRef]
15. Mack, D.R.; Michail, S.; Wei, S.; McDougall, L.; Hollingsworth, M.A. Probiotics inhibit enteropathogenic *E. coli* adherence in vitro by inducing intestinal mucin gene expression. *Am. J. Physiol.* **1999**, *276*, G941–G950. [CrossRef]
16. Jandhyala, S.M.; Talukdar, R.; Subramanyam, C.; Vuyyuru, H.; Sasikala, M.; Nageshwar Reddy, D. Role of the normal gut microbiota. *World J. Gastroentero* **2015**, *21*, 8787–8803. [CrossRef]
17. Barr, J.J.; Auro, R.; Sam-Soon, N.; Kassegne, S.; Peters, G.; Bonilla, N.; Hatay, M.; Mourtada, S.; Bailey, B.; Youle, M.; et al. Subdiffusive motion of bacteriophage in mucosal surfaces increases the frequency of bacterial encounters. *Proc. Natl. Acad. Sci. USA* **2015**, *112*, 13675. [CrossRef]
18. Henao-Mejia, J.; Elinav, E.; Thaiss, C.A.; Flavell, R.A. Chapter Three—The Intestinal Microbiota in Chronic Liver Disease. In *Advances in Immunology*; Alt, F.W., Ed.; Academic Press: Cambridge, MA, USA, 2013; Volume 117, pp. 73–97.
19. Adawi, D.; Molin, G.; Jeppsson, B. Gut–liver axis. *HPB* **1999**, *1*, 173–186. [CrossRef]
20. Mouzaki, M.; Comelli, E.M.; Arendt, B.M.; Bonengel, J.; Fung, S.K.; Fischer, S.E.; McGilvray, I.D.; Allard, J.P. Intestinal microbiota in patients with nonalcoholic fatty liver disease. *Hepatology* **2013**, *58*, 120–127. [CrossRef]
21. Da Silva, H.E.; Teterina, A.; Comelli, E.M.; Taibi, A.; Arendt, B.M.; Fischer, S.E.; Lou, W.; Allard, J.P. Nonalcoholic fatty liver disease is associated with dysbiosis independent of body mass index and insulin resistance. *Sci Rep.* **2018**, *8*, 1466. [CrossRef]
22. Zhu, L.; Baker, S.S.; Gill, C.; Liu, W.; Alkhouri, R.; Baker, R.D.; Gill, S.R. Characterization of gut microbiomes in nonalcoholic steatohepatitis (NASH) patients: A connection between endogenous alcohol and NASH. *Hepatology* **2013**, *57*, 601–609. [CrossRef] [PubMed]
23. Del Chierico, F.; Nobili, V.; Vernocchi, P.; Russo, A.; De Stefanis, C.; Gnani, D.; Furlanello, C.; Zandonà, A.; Paci, P.; Capuani, G.; et al. Gut microbiota profiling of pediatric nonalcoholic fatty liver disease and obese patients unveiled by an integrated meta-omics-based approach. *Hepatology* **2017**, *65*, 451–464. [CrossRef] [PubMed]
24. Leclercq, S.; Matamoros, S.; Cani, P.D.; Neyrinck, A.M.; Jamar, F.; Stärkel, P.; Windey, K.; Tremaroli, V.; Bäckhed, F.; Verbeke, K.; et al. Intestinal permeability, gut-bacterial dysbiosis, and behavioral markers of alcohol-dependence severity. *Proc. Natl. Acad. Sci. USA* **2014**, *111*, E4485–E4493. [CrossRef] [PubMed]
25. Yan, A.W.; Fouts, D.E.; Brandl, J.; Stärkel, P.; Torralba, M.; Schott, E.; Tsukamoto, H.; Nelson, K.E.; Brenner, D.A.; Schnabl, B. Enteric dysbiosis associated with a mouse model of alcoholic liver disease. *Hepatology* **2011**, *53*, 96–105. [CrossRef] [PubMed]
26. Gaspar, C.; Donders, G.G.; Palmeira-de-Oliveira, R.; Queiroz, J.A.; Tomaz, C.; Martinez-de-Oliveira, J.; Palmeira-de-Oliveira, A. Bacteriocin production of the probiotic Lactobacillus acidophilus KS400. *Amb Express* **2018**, *8*, 153. [CrossRef] [PubMed]
27. Schwenger, K.J.P.; Clermont-Dejean, N.; Allard, J.P. The role of the gut microbiome in chronic liver disease: The clinical evidence revised. *Jhep Rep.* **2019**. [CrossRef]
28. Bull-Otterson, L.; Feng, W.; Kirpich, I.; Wang, Y.; Qin, X.; Liu, Y.; Gobejishvili, L.; Joshi-Barve, S.; Ayvaz, T.; Petrosino, J.; et al. Metagenomic Analyses of Alcohol Induced Pathogenic Alterations in the Intestinal Microbiome and the Effect of Lactobacillus rhamnosus GG Treatment. *PLoS ONE* **2013**, *8*, e53028. [CrossRef]
29. Boursier, J.; Mueller, O.; Barret, M.; Machado, M.; Fizanne, L.; Araujo-Perez, F.; Guy, C.D.; Seed, P.C.; Rawls, J.F.; David, L.A.; et al. The severity of nonalcoholic fatty liver disease is associated with gut dysbiosis and shift in the metabolic function of the gut microbiota. *Hepatology* **2016**, *63*, 764–775. [CrossRef]
30. Bastian, W.P.; Hasan, I.; Lesmana, C.R.A.; Rinaldi, I.; Gani, R.A. Gut Microbiota Profiles in Nonalcoholic Fatty Liver Disease and Its Possible Impact on Disease Progression Evaluated with Transient Elastography: Lesson Learnt from 60 Cases. *Case Rep. Gastroenterol.* **2019**, *13*, 125–133. [CrossRef]
31. Bajaj, J.S.; Matin, P.; White, M.B.; Fagan, A.; Deeb, J.G.; Acharya, C.; Dalmet, S.S.; Sikaroodi, M.; Gillevet, P.M.; Sahingur, S.E. Periodontal therapy favorably modulates the oral-gut-hepatic axis in cirrhosis. *Am. J. Physiol. Gastrointest. Liver Physiol.* **2018**, *315*, G824–G837. [CrossRef]
32. Umar, S. Intestinal stem cells. *Curr. Gastroenterol. Rep.* **2010**, *12*, 340–348. [CrossRef] [PubMed]

33. Johansson, M.E.V.; Phillipson, M.; Petersson, J.; Velcich, A.; Holm, L.; Hansson, G.C. The inner of the two Muc2 mucin-dependent mucus layers in colon is devoid of bacteria. *Proc. Natl. Acad. Sci. USA* **2008**, *105*, 15064–15069. [CrossRef] [PubMed]
34. Cerutti, A.; Rescigno, M. The biology of intestinal immunoglobulin A responses. *Immunity* **2008**, *28*, 740–750. [CrossRef] [PubMed]
35. Farquhar, M.G.; Palade, G.E. JUNCTIONAL COMPLEXES IN VARIOUS EPITHELIA. *J. Cell Biol.* **1963**, *17*, 375–412. [CrossRef] [PubMed]
36. Ulluwishewa, D.; Anderson, R.C.; McNabb, W.C.; Moughan, P.J.; Wells, J.M.; Roy, N.C. Regulation of Tight Junction Permeability by Intestinal Bacteria and Dietary Components. *J. Nutr.* **2011**, *141*, 769–776. [CrossRef] [PubMed]
37. Fanning, A.S.; Jameson, B.J.; Jesaitis, L.A.; Anderson, J.M. The Tight Junction Protein ZO-1 Establishes a Link between the Transmembrane Protein Occludin and the Actin Cytoskeleton. *J. Biol. Chem.* **1998**, *273*, 29745–29753. [CrossRef] [PubMed]
38. Chelakkot, C.; Ghim, J.; Ryu, S.H. Mechanisms regulating intestinal barrier integrity and its pathological implications. *Exp. Mol. Med.* **2018**, *50*, 103. [CrossRef]
39. Galipeau, H.J.; Verdu, E.F. The complex task of measuring intestinal permeability in basic and clinical science. *Neurogastroenterol. Motil.* **2016**, *28*, 957–965. [CrossRef]
40. Groschwitz, K.R.; Hogan, S.P. Intestinal barrier function: Molecular regulation and disease pathogenesis. *J. Allergy Clin. Immunol.* **2009**, *124*, 3–22. [CrossRef]
41. Berg, R.D. Bacterial translocation from the gastrointestinal tract. *Trends Microbiol.* **1995**, *3*, 149–154. [CrossRef]
42. Berg, R.D.; Garlington, A.W. Translocation of certain indigenous bacteria from the gastrointestinal tract to the mesenteric lymph nodes and other organs in a gnotobiotic mouse model. *Infect. Immun.* **1979**, *23*, 403–411. [PubMed]
43. Garcia-Tsao, G.; Lee, F.-Y.; Barden, G.E.; Cartun, R.; Brian West, A. Bacterial translocation to mesenteric lymph nodes is increased in cirrhotic rats with ascites. *Gastroenterology* **1995**, *108*, 1835–1841. [CrossRef]
44. MacFie, J.; O'Boyle, C.; Mitchell, C.J.; Buckley, P.M.; Johnstone, D.; Sudworth, P. Gut origin of sepsis: A prospective study investigating associations between bacterial translocation, gastric microflora, and septic morbidity. *Gut* **1999**, *45*, 223–228. [CrossRef] [PubMed]
45. Barr, J.J. A bacteriophages journey through the human body. *Immunol. Rev.* **2017**, *279*, 106–122. [CrossRef] [PubMed]
46. Wiest, R.; Rath, H.C. Bacterial translocation in the gut. *Best Pract. Res. Clin. Gastroenterol.* **2003**, *17*, 397–425. [CrossRef]
47. Lehto, M.; Groop, P.H. The Gut-Kidney Axis: Putative Interconnections Between Gastrointestinal and Renal Disorders. *Front. Endocrinol. (Lausanne)* **2018**, *9*, 553. [CrossRef]
48. Kohler, C.A.; Maes, M.; Slyepchenko, A.; Berk, M.; Solmi, M.; Lanctot, K.L.; Carvalho, A.F. The Gut-Brain Axis, Including the Microbiome, Leaky Gut and Bacterial Translocation: Mechanisms and Pathophysiological Role in Alzheimer's Disease. *Curr. Pharm. Des.* **2016**, *22*, 6152–6166. [CrossRef]
49. Yan, A.W.; Schnabl, B. Bacterial translocation and changes in the intestinal microbiome associated with alcoholic liver disease. *World J. Hepatol.* **2012**, *4*, 110–118. [CrossRef]
50. Zhou, Z.; Zhong, W. Targeting the gut barrier for the treatment of alcoholic liver disease. *Liver Res.* **2017**, *1*, 197–207. [CrossRef]
51. Bode, J.C.; Bode, C.; Heidelbach, R.; Durr, H.K.; Martini, G.A. Jejunal microflora in patients with chronic alcohol abuse. *Hepatogastroenterology* **1984**, *31*, 30–34.
52. Hartmann, P.; Seebauer, C.T.; Schnabl, B. Alcoholic liver disease: The gut microbiome and liver cross talk. *Alcohol. Clin. Exp. Res.* **2015**, *39*, 763–775. [CrossRef] [PubMed]
53. Leclercq, S.; Cani, P.D.; Neyrinck, A.M.; Starkel, P.; Jamar, F.; Mikolajczak, M.; Delzenne, N.M.; de Timary, P. Role of intestinal permeability and inflammation in the biological and behavioral control of alcohol-dependent subjects. *Brain Behav. Immun.* **2012**, *26*, 911–918. [CrossRef] [PubMed]
54. Llopis, M.; Cassard, A.M.; Wrzosek, L.; Boschat, L.; Bruneau, A.; Ferrere, G.; Puchois, V.; Martin, J.C.; Lepage, P.; Le Roy, T.; et al. Intestinal microbiota contributes to individual susceptibility to alcoholic liver disease. *Gut* **2016**, *65*, 830–839. [CrossRef] [PubMed]
55. Keshavarzian, A.; Holmes, E.W.; Patel, M.; Iber, F.; Fields, J.Z.; Pethkar, S. Leaky gut in alcoholic cirrhosis: A possible mechanism for alcohol-induced liver damage. *Am. J. Gastroenterol.* **1999**, *94*, 200–207. [CrossRef]

56. Bode, J.C.; Knuppel, H.; Schwerk, W.; Lorenz-Meyer, H.; Durr, H.K. Quantitative histomorphometric study of the jejunal mucosa in chronic alcoholics. *Digestion* **1982**, *23*, 265–270. [CrossRef] [PubMed]
57. Brozinsky, S.; Fani, K.; Grosberg, S.J.; Wapnick, S. Alcohol ingestion-induced changes in the human rectal mucosa: Light and electron microscopic studies. *Dis. Colon Rectum* **1978**, *21*, 329–335. [CrossRef]
58. Tang, Y.; Banan, A.; Forsyth, C.B.; Fields, J.Z.; Lau, C.K.; Zhang, L.J.; Keshavarzian, A. Effect of Alcohol on miR-212 Expression in Intestinal Epithelial Cells and Its Potential Role in Alcoholic Liver Disease. *Alcohol. Clin. Exp. Res.* **2008**, *32*, 355–364. [CrossRef]
59. Zhong, W.; McClain, C.J.; Cave, M.; Kang, Y.J.; Zhou, Z. The role of zinc deficiency in alcohol-induced intestinal barrier dysfunction. *Am. J. Physiol. Gastrointest. Liver Physiol.* **2010**, *298*, G625–G633. [CrossRef]
60. Ma, T.Y.; Nguyen, D.; Bui, V.; Nguyen, H.; Hoa, N. Ethanol modulation of intestinal epithelial tight junction barrier. *Am. J. Physiol.* **1999**, *276*, G965–G974. [CrossRef]
61. Asai, K.; Buurman, W.A.; Reutelingsperger, C.P.; Schutte, B.; Kaminishi, M. Low concentrations of ethanol induce apoptosis in human intestinal cells. *Scand. J. Gastroenterol.* **2003**, *38*, 1154–1161. [CrossRef]
62. Elamin, E.E.; Masclee, A.A.; Dekker, J.; Jonkers, D.M. Ethanol metabolism and its effects on the intestinal epithelial barrier. *Nutr. Rev.* **2013**, *71*, 483–499. [CrossRef] [PubMed]
63. Moro-Sibilot, L.; Blanc, P.; Taillardet, M.; Bardel, E.; Couillault, C.; Boschetti, G.; Traverse-Glehen, A.; Defrance, T.; Kaiserlian, D.; Dubois, B. Mouse and Human Liver Contain Immunoglobulin A-Secreting Cells Originating From Peyer's Patches and Directed Against Intestinal Antigens. *Gastroenterology* **2016**, *151*, 311–323. [CrossRef] [PubMed]
64. Inamine, T.; Yang, A.M.; Wang, L.; Lee, K.C.; Llorente, C.; Schnabl, B. Genetic Loss of Immunoglobulin A Does Not Influence Development of Alcoholic Steatohepatitis in Mice. *Alcohol. Clin. Exp. Res.* **2016**, *40*, 2604–2613. [CrossRef] [PubMed]
65. Riva, A.; Patel, V.; Kurioka, A.; Jeffery, H.C.; Wright, G.; Tarff, S.; Shawcross, D.; Ryan, J.M.; Evans, A.; Azarian, S.; et al. Mucosa-associated invariant T cells link intestinal immunity with antibacterial immune defects in alcoholic liver disease. *Gut* **2018**, *67*, 918–930. [CrossRef] [PubMed]
66. Volynets, V.; Kuper, M.A.; Strahl, S.; Maier, I.B.; Spruss, A.; Wagnerberger, S.; Konigsrainer, A.; Bischoff, S.C.; Bergheim, I. Nutrition, intestinal permeability, and blood ethanol levels are altered in patients with nonalcoholic fatty liver disease (NAFLD). *Dig. Dis. Sci.* **2012**, *57*, 1932–1941. [CrossRef]
67. Luther, J.; Garber, J.J.; Khalili, H.; Dave, M.; Bale, S.S.; Jindal, R.; Motola, D.L.; Luther, S.; Bohr, S.; Jeoung, S.W.; et al. Hepatic Injury in Nonalcoholic Steatohepatitis Contributes to Altered Intestinal Permeability. *Cell Mol. Gastroenterol. Hepatol.* **2015**, *1*, 222–232. [CrossRef]
68. Hawkesworth, S.; Moore, S.E.; Fulford, A.J.C.; Barclay, G.R.; Darboe, A.A.; Mark, H.; Nyan, O.A.; Prentice, A.M. Evidence for metabolic endotoxemia in obese and diabetic Gambian women. *Nutr. Diabetes* **2013**, *3*, e83. [CrossRef]
69. Nazim, M.; Stamp, G.; Hodgson, H.J. Non-alcoholic steatohepatitis associated with small intestinal diverticulosis and bacterial overgrowth. *Hepatogastroenterology* **1989**, *36*, 349–351.
70. Miele, L.; Valenza, V.; La Torre, G.; Montalto, M.; Cammarota, G.; Ricci, R.; Masciana, R.; Forgione, A.; Gabrieli, M.L.; Perotti, G.; et al. Increased Intestinal Permeability and Tight Junction Alterations in Nonalcoholic Fatty Liver Disease. *Hepatology* **2009**, *49*, 1877–1887. [CrossRef]
71. Giorgio, V.; Miele, L.; Principessa, L.; Ferretti, F.; Villa, M.P.; Negro, V.; Grieco, A.; Alisi, A.; Nobili, V. Intestinal permeability is increased in children with non-alcoholic fatty liver disease, and correlates with liver disease severity. *Dig. Liver Dis.* **2014**, *46*, 556–560. [CrossRef]
72. Xin, D.; Zong-Shun, L.; Bang-Mao, W.; Lu, Z. Expression of intestinal tight junction proteins in patients with non-alcoholic fatty liver disease. *Hepatogastroenterology* **2014**, *61*, 136–140. [PubMed]
73. Suzuki, T.; Hara, H. Dietary fat and bile juice, but not obesity, are responsible for the increase in small intestinal permeability induced through the suppression of tight junction protein expression in LETO and OLETF rats. *Nutr. Metab. (Lond.)* **2010**, *7*, 19. [CrossRef] [PubMed]
74. Ahmad, R.; Rah, B.; Bastola, D.; Dhawan, P.; Singh, A.B. Obesity-induces Organ and Tissue Specific Tight Junction Restructuring and Barrier Deregulation by Claudin Switching. *Sci. Rep.* **2017**, *7*, 5125. [CrossRef] [PubMed]
75. Matsumoto, K.; Ichimura, M.; Tsuneyama, K.; Moritoki, Y.; Tsunashima, H.; Omagari, K.; Hara, M.; Yasuda, I.; Miyakawa, H.; Kikuchi, K. Fructo-oligosaccharides and intestinal barrier function in a methionine-choline-deficient mouse model of nonalcoholic steatohepatitis. *PLoS ONE* **2017**, *12*, e0175406. [CrossRef]

76. Winer, D.A.; Luck, H.; Tsai, S.; Winer, S. The Intestinal Immune System in Obesity and Insulin Resistance. *Cell Metab.* **2016**, *23*, 413–426. [CrossRef]
77. Al-Sadi, R.; Boivin, M.; Ma, T. Mechanism of cytokine modulation of epithelial tight junction barrier. *Front. Biosci. (Landmark Ed.)* **2009**, *14*, 2765–2778. [CrossRef]
78. Teltschik, Z.; Wiest, R.; Beisner, J.; Nuding, S.; Hofmann, C.; Schoelmerich, J.; Bevins, C.L.; Stange, E.F.; Wehkamp, J. Intestinal bacterial translocation in rats with cirrhosis is related to compromised Paneth cell antimicrobial host defense. *Hepatology* **2012**, *55*, 1154–1163. [CrossRef]
79. Alvarez-Silva, C.; Schierwagen, R.; Pohlmann, A.; Magdaleno, F.; Uschner, F.E.; Ryan, P.; Vehreschild, M.J.G.T.; Claria, J.; Latz, E.; Lelouvier, B.; et al. Compartmentalization of Immune Response and Microbial Translocation in Decompensated Cirrhosis. *Front. Immunol.* **2019**, *10*. [CrossRef]
80. Schierwagen, R.; Alvarez-Silva, C.; Madsen, M.S.A.; Kolbe, C.C.; Meyer, C.; Thomas, D.; Uschner, F.E.; Magdaleno, F.; Jansen, C.; Pohlmann, A.; et al. Circulating microbiome in blood of different circulatory compartments. *Gut* **2019**, *68*, 578–580. [CrossRef]
81. Casafont Morencos, F.; de las Heras Castano, G.; Martin Ramos, L.; Lopez Arias, M.J.; Ledesma, F.; Pons Romero, F. Small bowel bacterial overgrowth in patients with alcoholic cirrhosis. *Dig. Dis. Sci.* **1996**, *41*, 552–556. [CrossRef]
82. Maslennikov, R.; Pavlov, C.; Ivashkin, V. Small intestinal bacterial overgrowth in cirrhosis: Systematic review and meta-analysis. *Hepatol. Int.* **2018**, *12*, 567–576. [CrossRef] [PubMed]
83. Gunnarsdottir, S.A.; Sadik, R.; Shev, S.; Simren, M.; Sjovall, H.; Stotzer, P.O.; Abrahamsson, H.; Olsson, R.; Bjornsson, E.S. Small intestinal motility disturbances and bacterial overgrowth in patients with liver cirrhosis and portal hypertension. *Am. J. Gastroenterol.* **2003**, *98*, 1362–1370. [CrossRef] [PubMed]
84. Campillo, B.; Pernet, P.; Bories, P.N.; Richardet, J.P.; Devanlay, M.; Aussel, C. Intestinal permeability in liver cirrhosis: Relationship with severe septic complications. *Eur. J. Gastroenterol. Hepatol.* **1999**, *11*, 755–759. [CrossRef] [PubMed]
85. Pascual, S.; Such, J.; Esteban, A.; Zapater, P.; Casellas, J.A.; Aparicio, J.R.; Girona, E.; Gutierrez, A.; Carnices, F.; Palazon, J.M.; et al. Intestinal permeability is increased in patients with advanced cirrhosis. *Hepatogastroenterology* **2003**, *50*, 1482–1486. [PubMed]
86. Pijls, K.E.; Koek, G.H.; Elamin, E.E.; de Vries, H.; Masclee, A.A.; Jonkers, D.M. Large intestine permeability is increased in patients with compensated liver cirrhosis. *Am. J. Physiol. Gastrointest. Liver Physiol.* **2014**, *306*, G147–G153. [CrossRef]
87. Assimakopoulos, S.F.; Tsamandas, A.C.; Tsiaoussis, G.I.; Karatza, E.; Triantos, C.; Vagianos, C.E.; Spiliopoulou, I.; Kaltezioti, V.; Charonis, A.; Nikolopoulou, V.N.; et al. Altered intestinal tight junctions' expression in patients with liver cirrhosis: A pathogenetic mechanism of intestinal hyperpermeability. *Eur. J. Clin. Investig.* **2012**, *42*, 439–446. [CrossRef]
88. Such, J.; Guardiola, J.V.; de Juan, J.; Casellas, J.A.; Pascual, S.; Aparicio, J.R.; Sola-Vera, J.; Perez-Mateo, M. Ultrastructural characteristics of distal duodenum mucosa in patients with cirrhosis. *Eur. J. Gastroenterol. Hepatol.* **2002**, *14*, 371–376. [CrossRef]
89. Sorribas, M.; Jakob, M.O.; Yilmaz, B.; Li, H.; Stutz, D.; Noser, Y.; De Gottardi, A.; Moghadamrad, S.; Hassan, M.; Albillos, A.; et al. FXR-modulates the gut-vascular barrier by regulating the entry sites for bacterial translocation in experimental cirrhosis. *J. Hepatol.* **2019**. [CrossRef]
90. Muñoz, L.; Albillos, A.; Nieto, M.; Reyes, E.; Lledó, L.; Monserrat, J.; Sanz, E.; de la Hera, A.; Alvarez-Mon, M. Mesenteric Th1 polarization and monocyte TNF-α production: First steps to systemic inflammation in rats with cirrhosis. *Hepatology* **2005**, *42*, 411–419. [CrossRef]
91. Munoz, L.; Jose Borrero, M.; Ubeda, M.; Lario, M.; Diaz, D.; Frances, R.; Monserrat, J.; Pastor, O.; Aguado-Fraile, E.; Such, J.; et al. Interaction between intestinal dendritic cells and bacteria translocated from the gut in rats with cirrhosis. *Hepatology* **2012**, *56*, 1861–1869. [CrossRef]
92. Ma, T.Y.; Iwamoto, G.K.; Hoa, N.T.; Akotia, V.; Pedram, A.; Boivin, M.A.; Said, H.M. TNF-alpha-induced increase in intestinal epithelial tight junction permeability requires NF-kappa B activation. *Am. J. Physiol. Gastrointest. Liver Physiol.* **2004**, *286*, G367–G376. [CrossRef] [PubMed]
93. Al-Sadi, R.; Ye, D.; Boivin, M.; Guo, S.; Hashimi, M.; Ereifej, L.; Ma, T.Y. Interleukin-6 modulation of intestinal epithelial tight junction permeability is mediated by JNK pathway activation of claudin-2 gene. *PLoS ONE* **2014**, *9*, e85345. [CrossRef] [PubMed]

94. Elamin, E.; Masclee, A.; Troost, F.; Pieters, H.J.; Keszthelyi, D.; Aleksa, K.; Dekker, J.; Jonkers, D. Ethanol impairs intestinal barrier function in humans through mitogen activated protein kinase signaling: A combined in vivo and in vitro approach. *PLoS ONE* **2014**, *9*, e107421. [CrossRef] [PubMed]
95. Elpek, G.O. Cellular and molecular mechanisms in the pathogenesis of liver fibrosis: An update. *World J. Gastroenterol.* **2014**, *20*, 7260–7276. [CrossRef] [PubMed]
96. Miura, K.; Yang, L.; Van Rooijen, N.; Brenner, D.A.; Ohnishi, H.; Seki, E. Toll-like receptor 2 and palmitic acid cooperatively contribute to the development of nonalcoholic steatohepatitis through inflammasome activation in mice. *Hepatology* **2013**, *57*, 577–589. [CrossRef] [PubMed]
97. Kiziltas, S. Toll-like receptors in pathophysiology of liver diseases. *World J. Hepatol.* **2016**, *8*, 1354–1369. [CrossRef]
98. Thuy, S.; Ladurner, R.; Volynets, V.; Wagner, S.; Strahl, S.; KöNigsrainer, A.; Maier, K.-P.; Bischoff, S.C.; Bergheim, I. Nonalcoholic Fatty Liver Disease in Humans Is Associated with Increased Plasma Endotoxin and Plasminogen Activator Inhibitor 1 Concentrations and with Fructose Intake. *J. Nutr.* **2008**, *138*, 1452–1455. [CrossRef]
99. Singh, R.; Bullard, J.; Kalra, M.; Assefa, S.; Kaul, A.K.; Vonfeldt, K.; Strom, S.C.; Conrad, R.S.; Sharp, H.L.; Kaul, R. Status of bacterial colonization, Toll-like receptor expression and nuclear factor-kappa B activation in normal and diseased human livers. *Clin. Immunol.* **2011**, *138*, 41–49. [CrossRef]
100. Aragonès, G.; Colom-Pellicer, M.; Aguilar, C.; Guiu-Jurado, E.; Martínez, S.; Sabench, F.; Antonio Porras, J.; Riesco, D.; Del Castillo, D.; Richart, C.; et al. Circulating microbiota-derived metabolites: A "liquid biopsy? *Int. J. Obes.* **2019**. [CrossRef]
101. Stärkel, P.; De Saeger, C.; Strain, A.J.; Leclercq, I.; Horsmans, Y. NFκB, cytokines, TLR 3 and 7 expression in human end-stage HCV and alcoholic liver disease. *Eur. J. Clin. Investig.* **2010**, *40*, 575–584. [CrossRef]
102. Roh, Y.S.; Zhang, B.; Loomba, R.; Seki, E. TLR2 and TLR9 contribute to alcohol-mediated liver injury through induction of CXCL1 and neutrophil infiltration. *Am. J. Physiol. Gastrointest. Liver Physiol.* **2015**, *309*, G30–G41. [CrossRef] [PubMed]
103. Goodridge, H.S.; Underhill, D.M. Fungal Recognition by TLR2 and Dectin-1. In *Toll-like Receptors (TLRs) and Innate Immunity*; Stefan Bauer, G.H., Ed.; Springer: Berlin/Heidelberg, Germany, 2008; pp. 87–109. [CrossRef]
104. Szabo, G.; Velayudham, A.; Romics, L.; Mandrekar, P. Modulation of non-alcoholic steatohepatitis by pattern recognition receptors in mice: The role of toll-like receptors 2 and 4. *Alcohol. Clin. Exp. Res.* **2005**, *29*, 140S–145S. [CrossRef] [PubMed]
105. Seki, E.; De Minicis, S.; Österreicher, C.H.; Kluwe, J.; Osawa, Y.; Brenner, D.A.; Schwabe, R.F. TLR4 enhances TGF-β signaling and hepatic fibrosis. *Nat. Med.* **2007**, *13*, 1324–1332. [CrossRef] [PubMed]
106. Moles, A.; Murphy, L.; Wilson, C.L.; Chakraborty, J.B.; Fox, C.; Park, E.J.; Mann, J.; Oakley, F.; Howarth, R.; Brain, J.; et al. A TLR2/S100A9/CXCL-2 signaling network is necessary for neutrophil recruitment in acute and chronic liver injury in the mouse. *J. Hepatol.* **2014**, *60*, 782–791. [CrossRef]
107. Ji, L.; Xue, R.; Tang, W.; Wu, W.; Hu, T.; Liu, X.; Peng, X.; Gu, J.; Chen, S.; Zhang, S. Toll like receptor 2 knock-out attenuates carbon tetrachloride (CCl4)-induced liver fibrosis by downregulating MAPK and NF-κB signaling pathways. *Febs Lett.* **2014**, *588*, 2095–2100. [CrossRef] [PubMed]
108. Yano, T.; Ohira, M.; Nakano, R.; Tanaka, Y.; Ohdan, H. Hepatectomy leads to loss of TRAIL-expressing liver NK cells via downregulation of the CXCL9-CXCR3 axis in mice. *PLoS ONE* **2017**, *12*, e0186997. [CrossRef] [PubMed]
109. Li, K.; Chen, Z.; Kato, N.; Gale, M.; Lemon, S.M. Distinct Poly(I-C) and Virus-activated Signaling Pathways Leading to Interferon- Production in Hepatocytes. *J. Biol. Chem.* **2005**, *280*, 16739–16747. [CrossRef]
110. Wang, B.; Trippler, M.; Pei, R.; Lu, M.; Broering, R.; Gerken, G.; Schlaak, J.F. Toll-like receptor activated human and murine hepatic stellate cells are potent regulators of hepatitis C virus replication. *J. Hepatol.* **2009**, *51*, 1037–1045. [CrossRef]
111. Tu, Z.; Bozorgzadeh, A.; Pierce, R.H.; Kurtis, J.; Crispe, I.N.; Orloff, M.S. TLR-dependent cross talk between human Kupffer cells and NK cells. *JEM* **2008**, *205*, 233–244. [CrossRef]
112. Faure-Dupuy, S.; Vegna, S.; Aillot, L.; Dimier, L.; Esser, K.; Broxtermann, M.; Bonnin, M.; Bendriss-Vermare, N.; Rivoire, M.; Passot, G.; et al. Characterization of Pattern Recognition Receptor Expression and Functionality in Liver Primary Cells and Derived Cell Lines. *J. Innate Immun.* **2018**, *10*, 339–348. [CrossRef]

113. Byun, J.-S.; Suh, Y.-G.; Yi, H.-S.; Lee, Y.-S.; Jeong, W.-I. Activation of toll-like receptor 3 attenuates alcoholic liver injury by stimulating Kupffer cells and stellate cells to produce interleukin-10 in mice. *J. Hepatol.* **2012**. [CrossRef] [PubMed]
114. Li, T.; Yang, Y.; Song, H.; Li, H.; Cui, A.; Liu, Y.; Su, L.; Crispe, I.N.; Tu, Z. Activated NK cells kill hepatic stellate cells via p38/PI3K signaling in a TRAIL-involved degranulation manner. *J. Leukoc. Biol.* **2019**. [CrossRef] [PubMed]
115. Seo, W.; Eun, H.S.; Kim, S.Y.; Yi, H.-S.; Lee, Y.-S.; Park, S.-H.; Jang, M.-J.; Jo, E.; Kim, S.C.; Han, Y.-M.; et al. Exosome-mediated activation of toll-like receptor 3 in stellate cells stimulates interleukin-17 production by $\gamma\delta$ T cells in liver fibrosis. *Hepatology* **2016**, *64*, 616–631. [CrossRef] [PubMed]
116. Sharifnia, T.; Antoun, J.; Verriere, T.G.C.; Suarez, G.; Wattacheril, J.; Wilson, K.T.; Peek, R.M.; Abumrad, N.N.; Flynn, C.R. Hepatic TLR4 signaling in obese NAFLD. *Am. J. Physiol. Gastrointest. Liver Physiol.* **2015**, *309*, G270–G278. [CrossRef]
117. Saikia, P.; Roychowdhury, S.; Bellos, D.; Pollard, K.A.; McMullen, M.R.; McCullough, R.L.; McCullough, A.J.; Gholam, P.; De La Motte, C.; Nagy, L.E. Hyaluronic acid 35 normalizes TLR4 signaling in Kupffer cells from ethanol-fed rats via regulation of microRNA291b and its target Tollip. *Sci. Rep.* **2017**, *7*, 15671. [CrossRef]
118. Yi, M.; Zhou, J.; Sun, H.; Shi, L.; Wu, Y.; Zhang, J.; Chen, Q. Correlation between TLR4 expression and gene polymorphism in peripheral blood mononuclear cells and condition of nonalcoholic fatty acid disease in Han people of Shaanxi. *Int. J. Clin. Exp. Pathol.* **2017**, *10*, 3496–3502.
119. Jia, L.; Chang, X.; Qian, S.; Liu, C.; Lord, C.C.; Ahmed, N.; Lee, C.E.; Lee, S.; Gautron, L.; Mitchell, M.C.; et al. Hepatocyte toll-like receptor 4 deficiency protects against alcohol-induced fatty liver disease. *Mol. Metab.* **2018**, *14*, 121–129. [CrossRef]
120. Hritz, I.; Mandrekar, P.; Velayudham, A.; Catalano, D.; Dolganiuc, A.; Kodys, K.; Kurt-Jones, E.; Szabo, G. The critical role of toll-like receptor (TLR) 4 in alcoholic liver disease is independent of the common TLR adapter MyD88. *Hepatology* **2008**, *48*, 1224–1231. [CrossRef]
121. Kim, S.Y.; Jeong, J.-M.; Kim, S.J.; Seo, W.; Kim, M.-H.; Choi, W.-M.; Yoo, W.; Lee, J.-H.; Shim, Y.-R.; Yi, H.-S.; et al. Pro-inflammatory hepatic macrophages generate ROS through NADPH oxidase 2 via endocytosis of monomeric TLR4–MD2 complex. *Nat. Commun.* **2017**, *8*. [CrossRef]
122. Ye, D.; Li, F.Y.L.; Lam, K.S.L.; Li, H.; Jia, W.; Wang, Y.; Man, K.; Lo, C.M.; Li, X.; Xu, A. Toll-like receptor-4 mediates obesity-induced non-alcoholic steatohepatitis through activation of X-box binding protein-1 in mice. *Gut* **2012**, *61*, 1058–1067. [CrossRef]
123. Dattaroy, D.; Seth, R.K.; Sarkar, S.; Kimono, D.; Albadrani, M.; Chandrashekaran, V.; Hasson, F.A.; Singh, U.P.; Seth, R.K.; Scappinie, E.; et al. Sparstolonin B (SSnB) attenuates liver fibrosisvia a parallel conjugate pathway involving P53-P21 axis, TGF-beta signaling and focal adhesion that is TLR4 dependent. *Eur. J. Pharmacol.* **2018**. [CrossRef] [PubMed]
124. Song, I.J.; Yang, Y.M.; Inokuchi-Shimizu, S.; Roh, Y.S.; Yang, L.; Seki, E. The contribution of toll-like receptor signaling to the development of liver fibrosis and cancer in hepatocyte-specific TAK1-deleted mice. *Int. J. Cancer* **2018**, *142*, 81–91. [CrossRef] [PubMed]
125. Etienne-Mesmin, L.; Vijay-Kumar, M.; Gewirtz, A.T.; Chassaing, B. Hepatocyte Toll-Like Receptor 5 Promotes Bacterial Clearance and Protects Mice Against High-Fat Diet–Induced Liver Disease. *Cell. Mol. Gastroenterol. Hepatol.* **2016**, *2*, 584–604. [CrossRef] [PubMed]
126. Xiao, Y.; Liu, F.; Yang, J.; Zhong, M.; Zhang, E.; Li, Y.; Zhou, D.; Cao, Y.; Li, W.; Yu, J.; et al. Over-activation of TLR5 signaling by high-dose flagellin induces liver injury in mice. *Cell. Mol. Immunol.* **2015**, *12*, 729–742. [CrossRef] [PubMed]
127. Shu, M.; Huang, D.-D.; Hung, Z.-a.; Hu, X.-R.; Zhang, S. Inhibition of MAPK and NF-κB signaling pathways alleviate carbon tetrachloride (CCl4)-induced liver fibrosis in Toll-like receptor 5 (TLR5) deficiency mice. *Biochem. Biophys. Res. Commun.* **2016**, *471*, 233–239. [CrossRef]
128. Kim, S.; Park, S.; Kim, B.; Kwon, J. Toll-like receptor 7 affects the pathogenesis of non-alcoholic fatty liver disease. *Sci. Rep.* **2016**, *6*, 27849. [CrossRef]
129. Roh, Y.S.; Park, S.; Kim, J.W.; Lim, C.W.; Seki, E.; Kim, B. Toll-like receptor 7-mediated type I interferon signaling prevents cholestasis- and hepatotoxin-induced liver fibrosis. *Hepatology* **2014**, *60*, 237–249. [CrossRef]

130. Stärkel, P.; Schnabl, B.; Leclercq, S.; Komuta, M.; Bataller, R.; Argemi, J.; Palma, E.; Chokshi, S.; Hellerbrand, C.; Maccioni, L.; et al. Deficient IL-6/Stat3 Signaling, High TLR7, and Type I Interferons in Early Human Alcoholic Liver Disease: A Triad for Liver Damage and Fibrosis. *Hepatol. Commun.* **2019**, *3*, 867–882. [CrossRef]
131. Massey, V.L.; Qin, L.; Cabezas, J.; Caballeria, J.; Sancho-Bru, P.; Bataller, R.; Crews, F.T. TLR7-let-7 Signaling Contributes to Ethanol-Induced Hepatic Inflammatory Response in Mice and in Alcoholic Hepatitis. *Alcohol. Clin. Exp. Res.* **2018**. [CrossRef]
132. Roh, Y.S.; Kim, J.W.; Park, S.; Shon, C.; Kim, S.; Eo, S.K.; Kwon, J.K.; Lim, C.W.; Kim, B. Toll-Like Receptor-7 Signaling Promotes Nonalcoholic Steatohepatitis by Inhibiting Regulatory T Cells in Mice. *Am. J. Pathol.* **2018**, *188*, 2574–2588. [CrossRef]
133. Mridha, A.R.; Haczeyni, F.; Yeh, M.M.; Haigh, W.G.; Ioannou, G.N.; Barn, V.; Ajamieh, H.; Adams, L.; Hamdorf, J.M.; Teoh, N.C.; et al. TLR9 is up-regulated in human and murine NASH: Pivotal role in inflammatory recruitment and cell survival. *Clin. Sci. (London, England: 1979)* **2017**, *131*, 2145. [CrossRef] [PubMed]
134. Wiest, R.; Lawson, M.; Geuking, M. Pathological bacterial translocation in liver cirrhosis. *J. Hepatol.* **2014**, *60*, 197–209. [CrossRef] [PubMed]
135. Koutsounas, I.; Kaltsa, G.; Siakavellas, S.I.; Bamias, G. Markers of bacterial translocation in end-stage liver disease. *World J. Hepatol.* **2015**, *7*, 2264–2273. [CrossRef] [PubMed]
136. Vergis, N.; Atkinson, S.R.; Knapp, S.; Maurice, J.; Allison, M.; Austin, A.; Forrest, E.H.; Masson, S.; McCune, A.; Patch, D.; et al. In Patients With Severe Alcoholic Hepatitis, Prednisolone Increases Susceptibility to Infection and Infection-Related Mortality, and Is Associated With High Circulating Levels of Bacterial DNA. *Gastroenterology* **2017**, *152*, 1068–1077.e4. [CrossRef] [PubMed]
137. Miura, K.; Kodama, Y.; Inokuchi, S.; Schnabl, B.; Aoyama, T.; Ohnishi, H.; Olefsky, J.M.; Brenner, D.A.; Seki, E. Toll-Like Receptor 9 Promotes Steatohepatitis by Induction of Interleukin-1β in Mice. *Gastroenterology* **2010**, *139*, 323–334.e7. [CrossRef]
138. Gieling, R.; Wallace, K.; Han, Y.-P. Interleukin-1 participates in the progression from liver injury to fibrosis. *Am. J. Physiol.* **2009**, *296*, G1324. [CrossRef]
139. Bala, S.; Marcos, M.; Gattu, A.; Catalano, D.; Szabo, G. Acute Binge Drinking Increases Serum Endotoxin and Bacterial DNA Levels in Healthy Individuals. *PLoS ONE* **2014**, *9*, e96864. [CrossRef]
140. Gabele, E.; Muhlbauer, M.; Dorn, C.; Weiss, T.S.; Froh, M.; Schnabl, B.; Wiest, R.; Scholmerich, J.; Obermeier, F.; Hellerbrand, C. Role of TLR9 in hepatic stellate cells and experimental liver fibrosis. *Biochem. Biophys. Res. Commun.* **2008**, *376*, 271–276. [CrossRef]
141. Boaru, S.G.; Borkham-Kamphorst, E.; Tihaa, L.; Haas, U.; Weiskirchen, R. Expression analysis of inflammasomes in experimental models of inflammatory and fibrotic liver disease. *J. Inflamm.* **2012**, *9*, 49. [CrossRef]
142. Watanabe, A.; Sohail, M.A.; Gomes, D.A.; Hashmi, A.; Nagata, J.; Sutterwala, F.S.; Mahmood, S.; Jhandier, M.N.; Shi, Y.; Flavell, R.A.; et al. Inflammasome-mediated regulation of hepatic stellate cells. *Am. J. Physiol. Gastrointest. Liver Physiol.* **2009**, *296*, G1248–G1257. [CrossRef]
143. Nicoletti, F.; Zaccone, P.; Xiang, M.; Magro, G.; Di Mauro, M.; Di Marco, R.; Garotta, G.; Meroni, P. ESSENTIAL PATHOGENETIC ROLE FOR INTERFERON (IFN-)γ IN CONCANAVALIN A-INDUCED T CELL-DEPENDENT HEPATITIS: EXACERBATION BY EXOGENOUS IFN-γ AND PREVENTION BY IFN-γ RECEPTOR-IMMUNOGLOBULIN FUSION PROTEIN. *Cytokine* **2000**, *12*, 315–323. [CrossRef] [PubMed]
144. Wang, Y.-G.; Fang, W.-L.; Wei, J.; Wang, T.; Wang, N.; Ma, J.-L.; Shi, M. The involvement of NLRX1 and NLRP3 in the development of nonalcoholic steatohepatitis in mice. *J. Chin. Med. Assoc.* **2013**, *76*, 686–692. [CrossRef]
145. Xu, T.; Du, Y.; Fang, X.-B.; Chen, H.; Zhou, D.-D.; Wang, Y.; Zhang, L. New insights into Nod-like receptors (NLRs) in liver diseases. *Int. J. Physiol. Pathophysiol. Pharmacol.* **2018**, *10*, 1–16. [PubMed]
146. Seifert, L.; Deutsch, M.; Alothman, S.; Alqunaibit, D.; Werba, G.; Pansari, M.; Pergamo, M.; Ochi, A.; Torres-Hernandez, A.; Levie, E.; et al. Dectin-1 Regulates Hepatic Fibrosis and Hepatocarcinogenesis by Suppressing TLR4 Signaling Pathways. *Cell Rep.* **2015**, *13*, 1909–1921. [CrossRef] [PubMed]
147. Yang, A.M.; Inamine, T.; Hochrath, K.; Chen, P.; Wang, L.; Llorente, C.; Bluemel, S.; Hartmann, P.; Xu, J.; Koyama, Y.; et al. Intestinal fungi contribute to development of alcoholic liver disease. *J. Clin. Investig.* **2017**, *127*, 2829–2841. [CrossRef] [PubMed]

148. Luo, X.; Li, H.; Ma, L.; Zhou, J.; Guo, X.; Woo, S.-L.; Pei, Y.; Knight, L.R.; Deveau, M.; Chen, Y.; et al. Expression of STING Is Increased in Liver Tissues From Patients With NAFLD and Promotes Macrophage-Mediated Hepatic Inflammation and Fibrosis in Mice. *Gastroenterology* **2018**, *155*, 1971–1984.e4. [CrossRef]
149. Petrasek, J.; Iracheta-Vellve, A.; Csak, T.; Satishchandran, A.; Kodys, K.; Kurt-Jones, E.; Fitzgerald, K.; Szabo, G. STING-IRF3 pathway links endoplasmic reticulum stress with hepatocyte apoptosis in early alcoholic liver disease. *Proc. Natl. Acad. Sci. USA* **2013**, *110*, 16544–16549. [CrossRef]
150. Yu, Y.; Liu, Y.; An, W.; Song, J.; Zhang, Y.; Zhao, X. STING-mediated inflammation in Kupffer cells contributes to progression of nonalcoholic steatohepatitis.(RESEARCH ARTICLE). *J. Clin. Investig.* **2019**, *129*, 546. [CrossRef]
151. Iracheta-Vellve, A.; Petrasek, J.; Gyongyosi, B.; Satishchandran, A.; Lowe, P.; Kodys, K.; Catalano, D.; Calenda, C.D.; Kurt-Jones, E.A.; Fitzgerald, K.A.; et al. Endoplasmic Reticulum Stress-induced Hepatocellular Death Pathways Mediate Liver Injury and Fibrosis via Stimulator of Interferon Genes. *J. Biol. Chem.* **2016**, *291*, 26794–26805. [CrossRef]
152. Soares, J.-B.; Pimentel-Nunes, P.; Afonso, L.; Rolanda, C.; Lopes, P.; Roncon-Albuquerque, R.; Gonçalves, N.; Boal-Carvalho, I.; Pardal, F.; Lopes, S.; et al. Increased hepatic expression of TLR2 and TLR4 in the hepatic inflammation-fibrosis-carcinoma sequence. *Innate Immun.* **2012**, *18*, 700–708. [CrossRef]
153. Radaeva, S.; Sun, R.; Jaruga, B.; Nguyen, V.T.; Tian, Z.; Gao, B. Natural Killer Cells Ameliorate Liver Fibrosis by Killing Activated Stellate Cells in NKG2D-Dependent and Tumor Necrosis Factor–Related Apoptosis-Inducing Ligand–Dependent Manners. *Gastroenterology* **2006**, *130*, 435–452. [CrossRef] [PubMed]
154. Jeong, W.-I.; Park, O.; Radaeva, S.; Gao, B. STAT1 inhibits liver fibrosis in mice by inhibiting stellate cell proliferation and stimulating NK cell cytotoxicity. *Hepatology* **2006**, *44*, 1441–1451. [CrossRef]
155. Queck, A.; Carnevale, R.; Uschner, F.E.; Schierwagen, R.; Klein, S.; Jansen, C.; Meyer, C.; Praktiknjo, M.; Thomas, D.; Strassburg, C.; et al. Role of portal venous platelet activation in patients with decompensated cirrhosis and TIPS. *Gut* **2019**. [CrossRef] [PubMed]
156. Cengiz, M.; Ozenirler, S.; Elbeg, S. Role of serum toll-like receptors 2 and 4 in non-alcoholic steatohepatitis and liver fibrosis. *J. Gastroenterol. Hepatol.* **2015**, *30*, 1190–1196. [CrossRef] [PubMed]
157. González-Navajas, J.M.; Bellot, P.; Francés, R.; Zapater, P.; Muñoz, C.; García-Pagán, J.C.; Pascual, S.; Pérez-Mateo, M.; Bosch, J.; Such, J. Presence of bacterial-DNA in cirrhosis identifies a subgroup of patients with marked inflammatory response not related to endotoxin. *J. Hepatol.* **2008**, *48*, 61–67. [CrossRef]
158. Watanabe, A.; Hashmi, A.; Gomes, D.A.; Town, T.; Badou, A.; Flavell, R.A.; Mehal, W.Z. Apoptotic hepatocyte DNA inhibits hepatic stellate cell chemotaxis via toll-like receptor 9. *Hepatology* **2007**, *46*, 1509–1518. [CrossRef]
159. Dharancy, S.; Body-Malapel, M.; Louvet, A.; Berrebi, D.; Gantier, E.; Gosset, P.; Viala, J.; Hollebecque, A.; Moreno, C.; Philpott, D.J.; et al. Neutrophil Migration During Liver Injury Is Under Nucleotide-Binding Oligomerization Domain 1 Control. *Gastroenterology* **2010**, *138*, 1546–1556.e5. [CrossRef]
160. Kobayashi, K.S.; Chamaillard, M.; Ogura, Y.; Henegariu, O.; Inohara, N.; Nuñez, G.; Flavell, R.A. Nod2-dependent regulation of innate and adaptive immunity in the intestinal tract. *Science (New York, NY)* **2005**, *307*, 731–734. [CrossRef]
161. Seki, E.; De Minicis, S.; Gwak, G.-Y.; Kluwe, J.; Inokuchi, S.; Bursill, C.A.; Llovet, J.M.; Brenner, D.A.; Schwabe, R.F. CCR1 and CCR5 promote hepatic fibrosis in mice.(Research article)(Chemokine (C-C motif) receptor)(Report). *J. Clin. Investig.* **2009**, *119*, 1858. [CrossRef]
162. Veldt, B.J.; Laine, F.; Guillygomarc'h, A.; Lauvin, L.; Boudjema, K.; Messner, M.; Brissot, P.; Deugnier, Y.; Moirand, R. Indication of liver transplantation in severe alcoholic liver cirrhosis: Quantitative evaluation and optimal timing. *J. Hepatol.* **2002**, *36*, 93–98. [CrossRef]
163. Ge, P.S.; Runyon, B.A. Treatment of Patients with Cirrhosis. *N. Engl. J. Med.* **2016**, *375*, 2104–2105. [CrossRef] [PubMed]
164. Nier, A.; Engstler, A.J.; Maier, I.B.; Bergheim, I. Markers of intestinal permeability are already altered in early stages of non-alcoholic fatty liver disease: Studies in children. *PLoS ONE* **2017**, *12*, e0183282. [CrossRef] [PubMed]
165. Tuomisto, S.; Pessi, T.; Collin, P.; Vuento, R.; Aittoniemi, J.; Karhunen, P.J. Changes in gut bacterial populations and their translocation into liver and ascites in alcoholic liver cirrhotics. *BMC Gastroenterol.* **2014**, 14. [CrossRef] [PubMed]

166. Floreani, A.; Baragiotta, A.; Pizzuti, D.; Martines, D.; Cecchetto, A.; Chiarelli, S. Mucosal IgA defect in primary biliary cirrhosis. *Am. J. Gastroenterol.* **2002**, *97*, 508–510. [CrossRef]
167. Schwimmer, J.B.; Johnson, J.S.; Angeles, J.E.; Behling, C.; Belt, P.H.; Borecki, I.; Bross, C.; Durelle, J.; Goyal, N.P.; Hamilton, G.; et al. Microbiome Signatures Associated with Steatohepatitis and Moderate to Severe Fibrosis in Children With Nonalcoholic Fatty Liver Disease. *Gastroenterology* **2019**. [CrossRef]
168. Cani, P.D.; Bibiloni, R.; Knauf, C.; Waget, A.; Neyrinck, A.M.; Delzenne, N.M.; Burcelin, R. Changes in gut microbiota control metabolic endotoxemia-induced inflammation in high-fat diet-induced obesity and diabetes in mice. *Diabetes* **2008**, *57*, 1470–1481. [CrossRef]
169. Adachi, Y.; Moore, L.E.; Bradford, B.U.; Gao, W.; Thurman, R.G. Antibiotics prevent liver injury in rats following long-term exposure to ethanol. *Gastroenterology* **1995**, *108*, 218–224. [CrossRef]
170. Douhara, A.; Moriya, K.; Yoshiji, H.; Noguchi, R.; Namisaki, T.; Kitade, M.; Kaji, K.; Aihara, Y.; Nishimura, N.; Takeda, K.; et al. Reduction of endotoxin attenuates liver fibrosis through suppression of hepatic stellate cell activation and remission of intestinal permeability in a rat non-alcoholic steatohepatitis model. *Mol. Med. Rep.* **2015**, *11*, 1693–1700. [CrossRef]
171. Wiest, R.; Albillos, A.; Trauner, M.; Bajaj, J.S.; Jalan, R. Targeting the gut-liver axis in liver disease. *J. Hepatol.* **2017**, *67*, 1084–1103. [CrossRef]
172. Gangarapu, V.; Ince, A.T.; Baysal, B.; Kayar, Y.; Kilic, U.; Gok, O.; Uysal, O.; Senturk, H. Efficacy of rifaximin on circulating endotoxins and cytokines in patients with nonalcoholic fatty liver disease. *Eur. J. Gastroenterol. Hepatol.* **2015**, *27*, 840–845. [CrossRef]
173. Bajaj, J.S.; Heimanson, Z.; Israel, R.; Sanyal, A. Efficacy of rifaximin soluble solid dispersion in patients with early decompensated cirrhosis and a Conn score of 0: A post hoc analysis of a randomized, double-blind, placebo-controlled trial. *J. Hepatol.* **2019**, *70*, E631. [CrossRef]
174. Kang, S.H.; Lee, Y.B.; Lee, J.H.; Nam, J.Y.; Chang, Y.; Cho, H.; Yoo, J.J.; Cho, Y.Y.; Cho, E.J.; Yu, S.J.; et al. Rifaximin treatment is associated with reduced risk of cirrhotic complications and prolonged overall survival in patients experiencing hepatic encephalopathy. *Aliment. Pharmacol. Ther.* **2017**, *46*, 845–855. [CrossRef] [PubMed]
175. Yoon, H.; Schaubeck, M.; Lagkouvardos, I.; Blesl, A.; Heinzlmeir, S.; Hahne, H.; Clavel, T.; Panda, S.; Ludwig, C.; Kuster, B.; et al. Increased Pancreatic Protease Activity in Response to Antibiotics Impairs Gut Barrier and Triggers Colitis. *Cell. Mol. Gastroenterol. Hepatol.* **2018**, *6*, 370. [CrossRef] [PubMed]
176. Tulstrup, M.V.L.; Christensen, E.G.; Carvalho, V.; Linninge, C.; Ahrne, S.; Hojberg, O.; Licht, T.R.; Bahl, M.I. Antibiotic Treatment Affects Intestinal Permeability and Gut Microbial Composition in Wistar Rats Dependent on Antibiotic Class. *PLoS ONE* **2015**, *10*. [CrossRef] [PubMed]
177. Wang, Y.H.; Liu, Y.L.; Kirpich, I.; Ma, Z.H.; Wang, C.L.; Zhang, M.; Suttles, J.; McClain, C.; Feng, W.K. Lactobacillus rhamnosus GG reduces hepatic TNF alpha production and inflammation in chronic alcohol-induced liver injury. *J. Nutr. Biochem.* **2013**, *24*, 1609–1615. [CrossRef]
178. Tian, F.W.; Chi, F.F.; Wang, G.; Liu, X.M.; Zhang, Q.X.; Chen, Y.Q.; Zhang, H.; Chen, W. Lactobacillus rhamnosus CCFM1107 treatment ameliorates alcohol -induced liver injury in a mouse model of chronic alcohol feeding. *J. Microbiol.* **2015**, *53*, 856–863. [CrossRef]
179. Wang, Y.H.; Liu, Y.L.; Kirpich, I.; McClain, C.; Feng, W.K. Lactobacillus rhamnosus GG treatment potentiates intestinal hypoxia-inducible factor, promotes intestinal integrity, prevents inflammation, and ameliorates alcohol-induced liver injury. *Faseb J.* **2012**, *26*.
180. Moratalla, A.; Gomez-Hurtado, I.; Santacruz, A.; Moya, A.; Peiro, G.; Zapater, P.; Gonzalez-Navajas, J.M.; Gimenez, P.; Such, J.; Sanz, Y.; et al. Protective effect of Bifidobacterium pseudocatenulatum CECT7765 against induced bacterial antigen translocation in experimental cirrhosis. *Liver Int.* **2014**, *34*, 850–858. [CrossRef]
181. Sanchez, E.; Nieto, J.C.; Vidal, S.; Santiago, A.; Martinez, X.; Sancho, F.J.; Sancho-Bru, P.; Mirelis, B.; Corominola, H.; Juarez, C.; et al. Fermented milk containing Lactobacillus paracasei subsp paracasei CNCM I-1518 reduces bacterial translocation in rats treated with carbon tetrachloride. *Sci. Rep.* **2017**, *7*. [CrossRef]
182. Holscher, H.D. Dietary fiber and prebiotics and the gastrointestinal microbiota. *Gut Microbes* **2017**, *8*, 172–184. [CrossRef]
183. Koh, A.; De Vadder, F.; Kovatcheva-Datchary, P.; Backhed, F. From Dietary Fiber to Host Physiology: Short-Chain Fatty Acids as Key Bacterial Metabolites. *Cell* **2016**, *165*, 1332–1345. [CrossRef] [PubMed]

184. Peng, L.Y.; Li, Z.R.; Green, R.S.; Holzman, I.R.; Lin, J. Butyrate Enhances the Intestinal Barrier by Facilitating Tight Junction Assembly via Activation of AMP-Activated Protein Kinase in Caco-2 Cell Monolayers. *J. Nutr.* **2009**, *139*, 1619–1625. [CrossRef] [PubMed]
185. Nielsen, D.S.G.; Jensen, B.B.; Theil, P.K.; Nielsen, T.S.; Knudsen, K.E.B.; Purup, S. Effect of butyrate and fermentation products on epithelial integrity in a mucus-secreting human colon cell line. *J. Funct. Foods* **2018**, *40*, 9–17. [CrossRef]
186. Tang, Y.M.; Forsyth, C.B.; Banan, A.; Fields, J.Z.; Keshavarzian, A. Oats Supplementation Prevents Alcohol-Induced Gut Leakiness in Rats by Preventing Alcohol-Induced Oxidative Tissue Damage. *J. Pharm. Exp.* **2009**, *329*, 952–958. [CrossRef]
187. Krawczyk, M.; Maciejewska, D.; Ryterska, K.; Czerwinka-Rogowska, M.; Jamiol-Milc, D.; Skonieczna-Zydecka, K.; Milkiewicz, P.; Raszeja-Wyszomirska, J.; Stachowska, E. Gut Permeability Might be Improved by Dietary Fiber in Individuals with Nonalcoholic Fatty Liver Disease (NAFLD) Undergoing Weight Reduction. *Nutrients* **2018**, *10*. [CrossRef]
188. Loman, B.R.; Hernandez-Saavedra, D.; An, R.P.; Rector, R.S. Prebiotic and probiotic treatment of nonalcoholic fatty liver disease: A systematic review and meta-analysis. *Nutr. Rev.* **2018**, *76*, 822–839. [CrossRef]
189. Cao, Q.; Yu, C.B.; Yang, S.G.; Cao, H.C.; Chen, P.; Deng, M.; Li, L.J. Effect of probiotic treatment on cirrhotic patients with minimal hepatic encephalopathy: A meta-analysis. *Hepatob. Pancreat Dis.* **2018**, *17*, 9–16. [CrossRef]
190. Anwar, M.A.; Shah, M.; Kim, J.; Choi, S. Recent clinical trends in Toll-like receptor targeting therapeutics. *Med. Res. Rev.* **2019**, *39*, 1053–1090. [CrossRef]
191. Reilly, M.; Miller, R.M.; Thomson, M.H.; Patris, V.; Ryle, P.; McLoughlin, L.; Mutch, P.; Gilboy, P.; Miller, C.; Broekema, M.; et al. Randomized, Double-Blind, Placebo-Controlled, Dose-Escalating Phase I, Healthy Subjects Study of Intravenous OPN-305, a Humanized Anti-TLR2 Antibody. *Clin. Pharm.* **2013**, *94*, 593–600. [CrossRef]
192. Garcia-Manero, G.; Jabbour, E.J.; Konopleva, M.Y.; Daver, N.G.; Borthakur, G.; DiNardo, C.D.; Bose, P.; Patel, P.; Komrokji, R.S.; Shastri, A.; et al. A Clinical Study of Tomaralimab (OPN-305), a Toll-like Receptor 2 (TLR-2) Antibody, in Heavily Pre-Treated Transfusion Dependent Patients with Lower Risk Myelodysplastic Syndromes (MDS) That Have Received and Failed on Prior Hypomethylating Agent (HMA) Therapy. *Blood* **2018**, *132*. [CrossRef]
193. Monnet, E.; Lapeyre, G.; van Poelgeest, E.; Jacqmin, P.; de Graaf, K.; Reijers, J.; Moerland, M.; Burggraaf, J.; de Min, C. Evidence of NI-0101 Pharmacological Activity, an Anti-TLR4 Antibody, in a Randomized Phase I Dose Escalation Study in Healthy Volunteers Receiving LPS. *Clin. Pharm.* **2017**, *101*, 200–208. [CrossRef] [PubMed]
194. Fox, R.J.; Coffey, C.S.; Conwit, R.; Cudkowicz, M.E.; Gleason, T.; Goodman, A.; Klawiter, E.C.; Matsuda, K.; McGovern, M.; Naismith, R.T.; et al. Phase 2 Trial of Ibudilast in Progressive Multiple Sclerosis. *N. Engl. J. Med.* **2018**, *379*, 846–855. [CrossRef] [PubMed]
195. Diehl, A.M.; Harrison, S.; Caldwell, S.; Rinella, M.; Paredes, A.; Moylan, C.; Guy, C.; Bashir, M.; Wang, Y.; Miller, L.; et al. JKB-121 in patients with nonalcoholic steatohepatitis: A phase 2 double blind randomized placebo control study. *J. Hepatol.* **2018**, *68*, S103. [CrossRef]
196. Hoque, R.; Farooq, A.; Malik, A.; Trawick, B.N.; Berberich, D.W.; McClurg, J.P.; Galen, K.P.; Mehal, W. A Novel Small-Molecule Enantiomeric Analogue of Traditional (-)-Morphinans Has Specific TLR9 Antagonist Properties and Reduces Sterile Inflammation-Induced Organ Damage. *J. Immunol.* **2013**, *190*, 4297–4304. [CrossRef] [PubMed]
197. Shaker, M.E.; Trawick, B.N.; Mehal, W.Z. The novel TLR9 antagonist COV08-0064 protects from ischemia/reperfusion injury in non-steatotic and steatotic mice livers. *Biochem Pharm.* **2016**, *112*, 90–101. [CrossRef] [PubMed]
198. Jansen, T.L.; Kluck, V.; Janssen, M.; Comarniceanu, A.; Efde, M.; Scribner, C.L.; Barrow, R.B.; Skouras, D.B.; Dinarello, C.A.; Joosten, L.A. The First Phase 2a Proof-of-Concept Study of a Selective Nlrp3 Inflammasome Inhibitor, Dapansutrile (Tm) (Olt1177 (Tm)), in Acute Gout. *Ann. Rheum. Dis.* **2019**, *78*, A70–A71. [CrossRef]
199. Mullard, A. NLRP3 inhibitors stoke anti-inflammatory ambitions. *Nat. Rev. Drug Discov.* **2019**, *18*, 405–410. [CrossRef]

200. Haag, S.M.; Gulen, M.F.; Reymond, L.; Gibelin, A.; Abrami, L.; Decout, A.; Heymann, M.; van der Goot, F.G.; Turcatti, G.; Behrendt, R.; et al. Targeting STING with covalent small-molecule inhibitors. *Nature* **2018**, *559*, 269–273. [CrossRef]
201. Sheridan, C. Drug developers switch gears to inhibit STING. *Nat. Biotechnol.* **2019**, *37*, 199–201. [CrossRef]

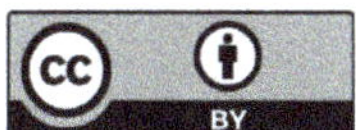

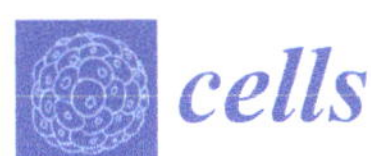
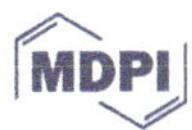

Review

Roles of the Hepatic Endocannabinoid and Apelin Systems in the Pathogenesis of Liver Fibrosis

Pedro Melgar-Lesmes [1,2,3], Meritxell Perramon [1] and Wladimiro Jiménez [1,2,*]

1 Biochemistry and Molecular Genetics Service, Hospital Clínic Universitari, IDIBAPS, CIBERehd, Villarroel 170, 08036 Barcelona, Spain; pmelgar@clinic.cat (P.M.-L.); mperramon@clinic.cat (M.P.)
2 Department of Biomedicine, University of Barcelona, 08036 Barcelona, Spain
3 Institute for Medical Engineering and Science, Massachusetts Institute of Technology, Cambridge, MA 02139, USA
* Correspondence: wjimenez@clinic.cat; Tel.: +34-93-227-5400 (ext. 3091); Fax: +34-93-227-5697

Received: 25 September 2019; Accepted: 23 October 2019; Published: 24 October 2019

Abstract: Hepatic fibrosis is the consequence of an unresolved wound healing process in response to chronic liver injury and involves multiple cell types and molecular mechanisms. The hepatic endocannabinoid and apelin systems are two signalling pathways with a substantial role in the liver fibrosis pathophysiology—both are upregulated in patients with advanced liver disease. Endogenous cannabinoids are lipid-signalling molecules derived from arachidonic acid involved in the pathogenesis of cardiovascular dysfunction, portal hypertension, liver fibrosis, and other processes associated with hepatic disease through their interactions with the CB_1 and CB_2 receptors. Apelin is a peptide that participates in cardiovascular and renal functions, inflammation, angiogenesis, and hepatic fibrosis through its interaction with the APJ receptor. The endocannabinoid and apelin systems are two of the multiple cell-signalling pathways involved in the transformation of quiescent hepatic stellate cells into myofibroblast like cells, the main matrix-producing cells in liver fibrosis. The mechanisms underlying the control of hepatic stellate cell activity are coincident despite the marked dissimilarities between the endocannabinoid and apelin signalling pathways. This review discusses the current understanding of the molecular and cellular mechanisms by which the hepatic endocannabinoid and apelin systems play a significant role in the pathophysiology of liver fibrosis.

Keywords: endocannabinoids; apelin; liver fibrosis; CB_1; CB_2; APJ

---

1. Introduction

Hepatic fibrosis is the excessive accumulation of connective tissue proteins, particularly collagens, in the liver extracellular matrix [1]. This process is the result of chronic liver injury that may be of different aetiologies: viruses, ethanol, toxins, drugs, or cholestasis [1]. Non-alcoholic fatty liver disease (NAFLD) is the most common cause of chronic liver disease worldwide with a prevalence of 20 to 40% in the general population and up to 95% in subjects with obesity and diabetes [2]. NAFLD is characterized by an abnormal accumulation of fatty acids into hepatocytes and includes a wide spectrum of liver diseases, ranging from mild to severe steatosis and non-alcoholic steatohepatitis (NASH) [3]. Both NAFLD and NASH have the potential to evolve into liver fibrosis and cirrhosis. Liver fibrosis involves multiple cell types and molecular mechanisms and processes. Hepatocellular injury unleashes a complex inflammatory response and the release of a plethora of cytokines and growth factors that, on one hand, trigger transformation of quiescent hepatic stellate cells (HSC) into myofibroblast-like cells and, on the other hand, stimulate inflammation and angiogenesis [4]. Chronic inflammation and the long-term injury and regeneration processes perpetuate liver fibrosis and eventually results in distortion of lobular architecture, nodular formation, and cirrhosis [5]. Documented reversibility of advanced liver fibrosis in patients [6–8] has encouraged research on anti-fibrotic drugs and novel therapeutic strategies [9–15], which are effective in experimental models of liver fibrosis, but their utility in humans is still unknown. Most strategies aimed at interfering with liver fibrosis focus on the inhibition of HSC activation, the modulation of inflammatory response, or the reduction of hepatocyte damage by targeting and modulating multiple cell signalling pathways [4]. Two of these signalling pathways, which have significant impact on the pathophysiology of liver fibrosis, are the endocannabinoid and apelin systems. Patients with advanced liver disease show high circulating levels of both endocannabinoids and apelin, and their respective signalling pathways appear to be upregulated in advanced liver disease [16–18].

This review focuses on recent advances in elucidating the roles of the endocannabinoid and apelin systems in liver fibrosis and their potential clinical relevance. We emphasize recent findings regarding the cellular and molecular mechanisms by which these endogenous systems are involved in liver fibrosis.

2. Overview of the Endogenous Cannabinoid System

Since its discovery in the 80s, the cannabinoid system has been extensively studied and described as being a relevant modulator of numerous physiological and pathological functions. This system comprises endogenous cannabinoids (endocannabinoids, EC), their receptors (CB), and the enzymes responsible for their synthesis and degradation. EC have a multifaceted role: in physiological conditions as psychoactive, analgesic, antiemetic, anti-inflammatory, vasorelaxant, orexigenic [19–22] and in a myriad of pathological states such as neurodegenerative disorders [23–25], myocardial infarction [25], liver fibrosis [26], and cancer [27,28]. Therefore, pharmacologic intervention of the EC system is a promising strategy for the management of many diseases. In fact, a substantial number of pharmacological agents that interfere with this system has been developed to date. Herein, we describe the most recent findings on the EC system, focusing on the pathogenesis of liver disease.

2.1. Endocannabinoids

EC are a class of arachidonic acid (AA) derivatives that interact with CB and were originally described as targets of Δ9-Tetrahydrocannabinol (THC), the main psychoactive constituent of *Cannabis sativa* [29]. EC share a common backbone structure resulting from their synthesis from membrane phospholipid precursors that contain AA and are conjugated either with ethanolamine or glycerol [22,26,30]. They are synthetized on demand, often in response to increased intracellular calcium concentrations [31]. EC amount is tightly regulated by changes in its catabolism rather by their synthesis. Figure 1 depicts the chemical structure of the main EC. Other less-characterized CB-interacting peptides and a series of AA derivatives that generate endocannabinoid-like effects such as N-palmitoylethanolamine (PEA) and Oleoylethanolamine (OEA) have also been described [32]. Most investigations focus on the first discovered and best studied EC: N-arachidonoylethanolamine (anandamide, AEA) and 2-arachidonoylglycerol (2-AG) [33,34].

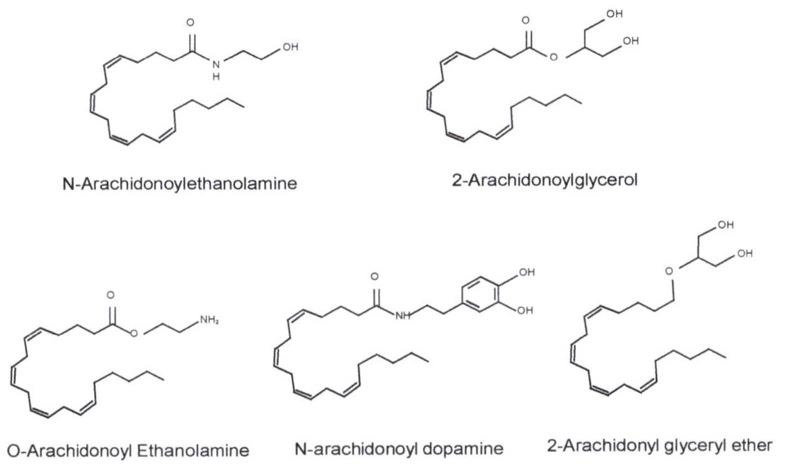

N-Arachidonoylethanolamine 2-Arachidonoylglycerol

O-Arachidonoyl Ethanolamine N-arachidonoyl dopamine 2-Arachidonyl glyceryl ether

Figure 1. Chemical structures of endogenous cannabinoids: *N*-arachidonoylethanolamine (AEA, anandamide), 2-arachidonoylglycerol (2-AG), *O*-arachidonoyl-ethanolamine (*O*-AEA, virodhamine), *N*-arachidonoyl dopamine (NADA), and 2-arachidonyl-glyceryl ether (2-AGE, noladin ether).

AEA is a *N*-(polyunsaturated fatty acyl) generated from *N*-arachidonoyl phosphatidylethanolamine (NAPE) through multiple different pathways: cleavage by phospholipase D (PLD), sequential deacylation of NAPE by α,β-hydrolase followed by the cleavage of glycerophosphate, and phospholipase C-mediated hydrolysis of NAPE, which is then dephosphorylated by phosphatases [35]. It is a partial agonist of CB_1 and CB_2, presenting a lower intrinsic activity for the latter [29]. Fatty acid amino hydrolase (FAAH) is the main enzyme responsible for AEA degradation. However, it can also be catabolized via oxidation by cyclooxygenase-2 (COX-2) and by N-acylethanolamine-hydrolysing acid amidase (NAAA) [31]. 2-AG is an ester formed from AA-containing phospholipids and glycerol [31] via three major pathways: sequential activation of a phospholipase Cβ and a diacylglycerol lipase, sequential action of phospholipase A1 and a lyso phospholipase C, and by dephosphorylation of arachidonoyl- lysophosphatidic acid [36–38]. 2-AG is a full agonist of both CB receptors with moderate-to-low affinity [32]. Monoacylglycerol lipase (MAGL) is its principal degradation enzyme. 2-AG is also degraded by alpha/beta domain hydrolases 6 and 12 (ABHD6 and 12), oxidized by COX-2 and hydrolysed under some conditions by FAAH [31]. Although AEA and 2-AG are involved in similar processes such as the control of redox homeostasis and display anti-inflammatory effects, both agents are implicated in a myriad of different activities. For instance, AEA participates in cell cycle regulation and apoptosis, whereas 2-AG is important in synaptic signalling.

2.2. EC Canonical Receptors

EC mediate their cellular effects through two canonical CB: CB_1 and CB_2, numbered in the order of their discovery [20]. Both CB are seven transmembrane class A metabotropic G-protein-coupled receptors (GPCRs) but differ in amino acid sequence (48% homology in humans), tissue distribution, and signalling mechanisms [39]. Some EC actions may be mediated by other non-CB receptors including: G protein-coupled receptors (GPR3, GPR6, GPR12, GPR18, GPR55, and GPR119), transient receptor potential channels (TRPV1, TRPV2, TRPA1, TRPM8), ligand-gated ion channels, and nuclear receptors (for example, the peroxisome proliferator-activated receptor) [24,26,30,32,35,39–41]. Indeed, non-receptor targets such as cholesterol and cyclooxygenase-2 (COX-2) have been identified as interacting with them as well [40–43].

The CNR1 gene encodes a 472 amino-acid protein corresponding to CB_1 in humans [32]. One canonical and two additional isoforms result from alternative splicing [44,45]. CB_1 is the most abundant EC receptor and is exclusively responsible of the psychoactive effects of cannabinoids [22]. Its highest expression is found in the nervous system [31,39]. CB_1 is also found to a lesser extent in vessels and peripheral tissues: skeletal muscle, spleen, tonsils, adrenal gland, bone marrow, liver, heart, lung, prostate, kidney, pancreatic islet, testis, and female reproductive tissues [32,39]. Mice deficient in CB_1 have reduced progeny [46–48], show hypoactivity, hypoalgesia, enhanced spatial working memory, impaired contextual fear memory [48,49], and decreased insulin and leptin plasma levels [50].

CB_2, encoded by the CNR2 gene, is composed of 360 amino acids in humans [32]. Two isoforms have been identified. CB_2 is primarily expressed in the immune system: B cells, natural killer cells, spleen, bone marrow, tonsils, and pancreatic mast cells [51,52]. Functionally relevant expression has also been found in brain, myocardium, gut, endothelium, vascular smooth muscle and Kupffer cells, pancreas, bone, and reproductive organs [53]. CB_2 knock-out mice display increased neuropathic pain, impaired formation of numerous immune cell populations such as splenic memory $CD4^+$, and exacerbated inflammation as a result of enhanced monocyte and neutrophil recruitment [54–56].

CB can exist in dimers and complexes of higher magnitude [57], but the physiological relevance of dimerization has not yet been fully established. However, the expression of some heterodimers has been associated with different pathologies, for instance, cancer [58]. This suggests that EC can interact with multiple endogenous systems adding a higher level of complexity to the understanding of EC molecular mechanisms. Nevertheless, more data are needed to identify their specific biological functions.

2.3. *Cell Signalling Pathways Activated by CB_1 and CB_2*

Both CB are GPCRs that couple similar transduction systems of heterotrimeric G proteins [59]. Intracellular signalling is complex because it includes both G protein dependent and independent pathways, as well as ceramide signalling [53]. Figure 2 illustrates the main molecular pathways. Activation of CB decreases the intracellular accumulation of cyclic adenosine monophosphate (cAMP). This results in the inhibition of the adenylyl cyclase activity and a reduction in intracellular Ca^{2+}, which eventually leads to the inhibition of protein kinase A and the dephosphorylation of K^+ channel type A [60,61], a critical process that modulates the responses to ionotropic neurotransmitters in neurons. Moreover, CB_1 negatively binds certain Ca^{2+} voltage dependent channels, induces G-protein-coupled modulating K^+ channels (GIRK), and subsequently inhibits neurotransmitter release independently of cAMP [55]. CB also activate mitogen-activated protein kinase (MAPK) pathways, including extracellular signal-regulated kinase 1 or 2 (ERK1/2), p38, and c-Jun N-terminal kinase (JNK), which are important for orchestrating cellular functions such as cell growth, cellular transformation, and apoptosis [56]. It has been proposed that two signal transduction pathways activate MAPK in response to CB activation: one involves the activation of phosphatidylinositide-3-kinase (PI3K), and the second, sphingomyelin, hydrolysis and release of ceramide [57]. PI3K has also been reported to induce AKT-mediated cell survival by inhibiting apoptosis [56]. De novo ceramide synthesis promoted by CB is known to directly trigger apoptosis in a G protein-independent manner [62]. CB is also associated with β-arrestin, a key mediator of GPCR desensitization [32]. β-arrestin binds to the phosphorylated receptor and initiates its internalization process, during which it can mediate different signalling pathways [32].

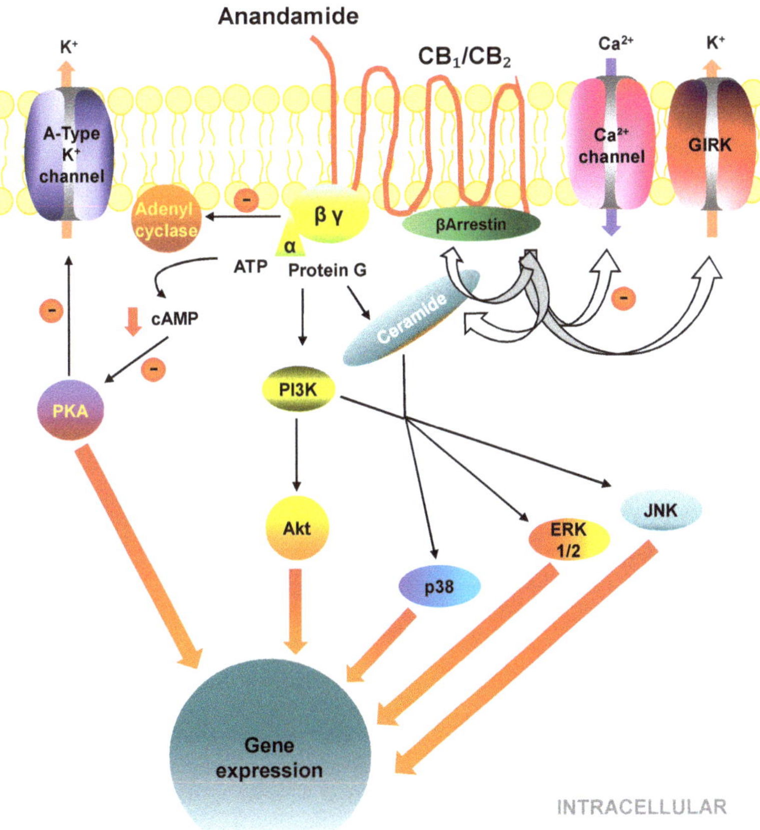

Figure 2. Molecular and cell signalling pathways of cannabinoid receptors.

3. The Endocannabinoid System (ECS) in Health and Disease

The ECS is widely distributed in the body and is involved in a wide array of physiological functions including pain, sleep, arousal, body temperature, feeding, and emotional regulation [63]. Disequilibrium of the ECS results in a myriad of pathological states. In the nervous system, CB_1 activation is anti-emetic, enhances eating, causes changes in short-term and working memory, inhibits the release of neurotransmitters involved in anxiety and depression, attenuates nociception, and is protective against excitotoxicity [64–66]. In neurodegenerative diseases and psychiatric disorders, such as Alzheimer's disease and schizophrenia, CB_1 expression is reduced, whereas CB_2 is induced in an attempt to halt inflammatory response [67,68]. Indeed, upon injury or inflammation, CB_2 is highly induced to dampen inflammatory response [51]. CB_2 activation decreases the production of reactive oxygen species (ROS) and the release of inflammatory mediators such as tumour necrosis factor α (TNF-α), and nitric oxide (NO) [68]. It activates immune cell apoptosis and suppresses immune cell activation, proliferation, and migration [69]. In the central nervous system, treatment with CB_1 inverse agonists reduces the behavioural effects associated with drugs of abuse [63] and produces appetite suppression decreasing food intake, partially due to drug-induced food aversions such as nausea or vomiting [70]. In contrast, CB_2 agonists block defecation, increase urination frequency, and produce analgesia [71]. Inhibition of EC catabolic enzymes such as FAAH seems also a good strategy to increase EC concentration and treat diseases such as anxiety, sleep disorders, and neuropathic pain [72].

In physiological conditions, the modulation of the ECS has a minor impact on the regulation of the cardiovascular system even though the ECS is widely distributed in the heart and blood vessels [17]. In contrast, ECS dysregulation results in disorders such as hypertension, myocardial infarction (MI), and chronic heart failure [62]. The activation of CB_2 is cardioprotective, reducing cardiac fibrosis and infarcted areas during ischemia-reperfusion (I/R) and, at the same time, increasing the activation of cardiac progenitor cells and cardiomyocyte proliferation [73,74].

The ECS also plays a crucial role in lipid and glucose metabolism [63], displays orexigenic effects, and modulates peripheral energy metabolism [20]. In obese mice, stearoyl-CoA desaturase-1 generates monounsaturated fatty acids, which inhibit FAAH, resulting in increased AEA hepatic levels promoting excessive energy storage and insulin resistance [26]. In liver, CB_1 stimulation increases de novo lipogenesis [20]. It has been suggested that CB_1 has a key role in the development of diet-induced obesity and fatty liver disease [20]. Treatment with a CB_1 inverse agonist SR141716 (rimonabant) improves glycaemic control, insulin resistance, and dyslipidemia [75]. However, it has no clinical use due to the significant psychiatric side effects: anxiety, depression, and suicidal ideation [63]. CB_2 inverse agonists have also been proposed to modulate the metabolic syndrome, in particular triglycerides, insulin, adipose tissue, and arterial pressure [76].

The ECS also plays important roles in the gastrointestinal tract [77] and in oncology, not only as palliative but also as anti-emetic and anti-tumoural agents (due to their effect in controlling cellular proliferation, angiogenesis, and metastasis in experimental models of cancer [21,41,78]). However, there is controversy regarding their role as oncogenes or tumour suppressors [79,80].

4. Involvement of the ECS in the Pathogenesis of Liver Fibrosis

The role of ECS in fibrosis is complex and not yet completely understood since EC may mediate their effects in a CB receptor-dependent and independent manner. In early stages of liver disease, AEA and 2-AG levels are increased in rodents [81]. Furthermore, their serum and hepatic levels together with PEA and OEA are augmented in cirrhotic (CH) patients [82,83]. EC display a wide array of activities including anti-inflammatory, pro-apoptotic, and anti-proliferative [84]. Healthy hepatocytes have the highest level of expression and activity of FAAH in the body to tightly regulate AEA, PEA, and OEA levels in order to shield against cell death independently of CB receptors [85]. FAAH is decreased in murine models of BDL and CCl_4, which promotes EC accumulation and, consequently, increased ROS and hepatocellular injury [86]. Activated HSC do not produce FAAH, and therefore, they are sensitive to EC-mediated apoptosis, a phenomenon which could be used as a promising therapeutic approach to attenuate the fibrogenic response [87]. Among all EC, 2-AG is known to be mainly metabolized by COX-2 to pro-apoptotic prostaglandin glycerol esters, which selectively induce HSC apoptosis [85,88]. OEA also ameliorates hepatic fibrosis by directly inhibiting tumour growth factor beta 1 (TGFβ1), signalling through the suppression of SMAD2/3 phosphorylation, a phenomenon inhibited in peroxisome proliferator-activated receptor alpha (PPAR-α) knock-out mice [89].

During acute and chronic liver injury, the expression of CB_1 and CB_2 is also augmented [90,91]. CB_1 is strongly induced in hepatocytes, HSC, endothelial, inflammatory, and ductular proliferating cells, whereas CB_2 is mainly induced in inflammatory cells and HSC [92]. A large number of studies have addressed the role of CB in liver pathogenesis elucidating that both exhibit opposite effects. CB_1 activation promotes hepatic steatosis, inflammation, and fibrosis in non- and alcoholic fatty liver diseases [93,94]. CB_1 stimulation also contributes to the progression of cirrhosis by triggering fibrogenesis. In contrast, genetic and pharmacological inactivation of CB_1 with rimonabant enhances HSC apoptosis and decreases the proliferative response to platelet-derived growth factor (PDGF), reducing TGFβ1 levels and liver fibrosis [92]. Systemic administration of rimonabant also results in increased arterial pressure and peripheral resistance and a reduced mesenteric blood flow and portal pressure in CCl_4-exposed rats, an effect not seen in healthy animals [95,96]. In line with these results, rimonabant reduces the incidence and accumulation of ascites and also improves sodium balance, delaying decompensation in CH rats [97]. Rimonabant has also been shown to reduce the matrix methaloproteinase (MMP) abundance and activity, the expression of the pro-fibrogenic factors endothelin 1 (ET-1) and TGF-β, and the synthesis of the pro-inflammatory factors TNF-α and monocyte chemoattractant protein-1 (MCP-1) in CCl_4-treated cirrhotic rats [98]. In addition, CB_1 antagonism with rimonabant protects against lipopolysaccharide (LPS)-enhanced liver injury by interfering with inflammatory response [99]. Circulating LPS, which is common in CH patients, has been reported to increase de novo AEA and 2-AG production in monocytes and platelets and activates CB_1, suggesting a key role of LPS in triggering the EC synthesis in the fibrotic liver [100]. These EC are also highly synthesized in adventitial cells and detected at a lower concentration in endothelial cells from CH mesenteric vessels, although they can also be found at lesser amounts in healthy vessels [101]. Monocytes isolated from CH patients and then injected to control rats promote CB_1-mediated hypotension [90]. CB_1 is also involved in other complications associated with liver cirrhosis, including cardiomyopathy and encephalopathy [102], and at the same time, in the process of liver regeneration [103].

CB_2 exerts anti-fibrogenic and anti-inflammatory effects [104] and protects against liver I/R injury [105]. CB_2 knock-out mice exhibit enhanced fibrosis, inflammation, and steatosis compared to wild type animals [19]. These mice are more susceptible to hepatic insult, enhancing MMP-2 activity as a consequence of IL-6 down-regulation [92]. Activation of CB_2 by the selective agonist JWH-133 reduces inflammation and fibrosis and increases arterial pressure and non-parenchymal cell apoptosis in CH rats [106]. JWH-133 administration in CCl_4-treated mice reduces liver injury and accelerates the regenerative response [92]. JWH-133 also reduces liver fibrosis and inflammation by decreasing IL-17 production via STAT5-dependent signalling in BDL rats [107]. In agreement with these findings, long-term administration of the CB_2 agonist AM-1241 significantly inhibits PDGF signalling, reduces HSC activation and hepatic fibrosis, and improves hemodynamic function in fibrotic rats [104].

Increased levels of endogenous AEA have also been found in the heart of cirrhotic rats, where it contributes to the reduced cardiac contractile function that leads to cirrhotic cardiomyopathy [90]. In the brain of mice, 2-AG has also been found to be elevated with thioacetamide-induced hepatic encephalopathy. Indeed, the administration of a CB_2 selective agonist improves the cognitive function in these mice [108]. These findings point to ECS as a potential target for the treatment of hepatic encephalopathy secondary to decompensated cirrhosis.

All the investigations and evidence so far suggest that the ECS may be a crucial regulator in different liver diseases. Both CB_1 blockade and CB_2 receptor stimulation have been successful in preventing fibrosis progression in experimental animal models. Figure 3 illustrates the potential roles of CB_1 antagonists and CB_2 agonists in the intervention algorithm for the treatment of liver steatosis, fibrosis, cirrhosis, and its complications. CB_1 antagonists additionally ameliorate systemic haemodynamics. However, since CB_1 is highly expressed in the central nervous system, treatment with antagonists is often associated with undesirable central effects. Therefore, to date, treatment with CB_2 agonists seems to be a more feasible approach to treat liver fibrosis and cirrhosis and its complications.

Further studies are required to elucidate the precise mechanism by which EC participate in the pathophysiology of liver disease and more long-term studies are needed to confirm the absence of central effects of selective CB_1 antagonists. In addition, further efforts should be made in the generation of specific compounds able to modulate EC anabolism, transport, or catabolism since this could be a promising strategy to modulate the ECS activation tone. The future of EC therapeutics in fibrosis might be addressed to combine a CB_2 agonist with another efficient anti-fibrotic agent to synergize activities. In line with this, one study has shown that the CB_2 agonist AM-1241 and the apelin receptor antagonist F13A display similar mechanisms of control of HSC cell activity despite the clear differences between the CB_2 and APJ signalling pathways [104]. The combination of different drugs with anti-fibrotic activity could be an interesting approach to improve pharmacological therapies in liver fibrosis.

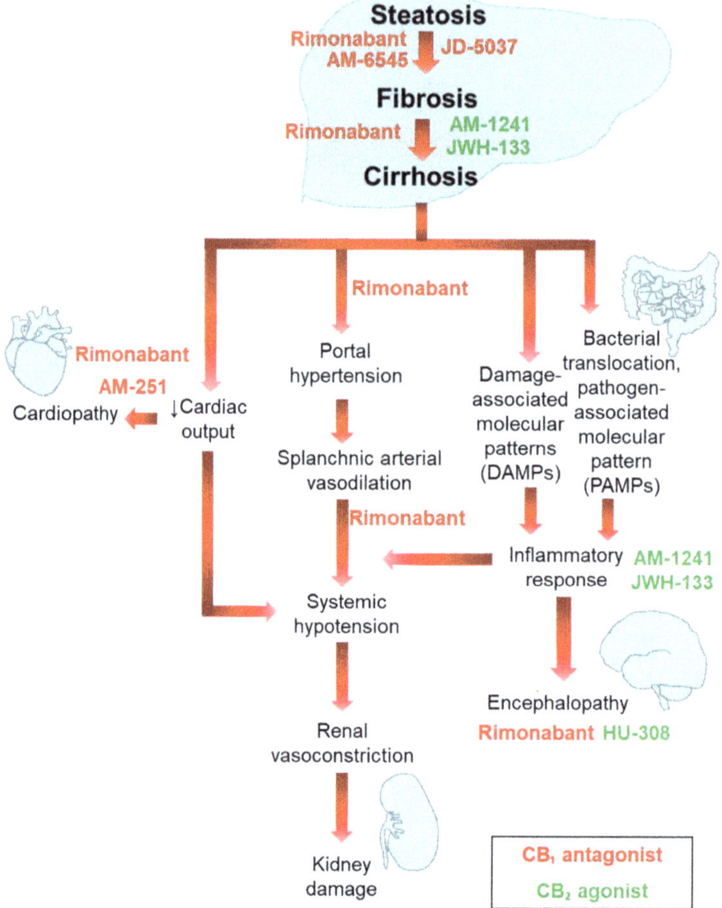

Figure 3. CB_1 antagonists and CB_2 agonists as potential drugs for the treatment of liver cirrhosis.

5. Overview of the Apelin System

Apelin is a peptide that was first described in 1998 as the endogenous ligand for an orphan receptor called angiotensin-like-receptor 1 (AGTRL1, also known as APJ), a G-protein-coupled receptor [109]. During the last two decades, this receptor has been involved in an array of physiologic events, such as water homeostasis [110], regulation of cardiovascular tone [111], and cardiac contractility [112] as well as in chronic liver disease [18]. Apelin and its receptor are expressed in the central nervous system and in peripheral tissues, especially in endothelial cells as well as in HSC, leukocytes, enterocytes, adipocytes, and cardiomyocytes [113–118]. Since the discovery of the apelin/APJ interaction, numerous investigations have emerged highlighting new roles for the apelin system in the regulation of different homeostatic processes or involving apelin/APJ in disease. Here, we briefly review the components of the apelin/APJ system as well as the molecular mechanisms involved in the diverse cellular effects observed so far before focusing on the relationship between the apelin system and the pathogenesis of liver fibrosis.

5.1. Apelin: Peptide Isoforms

The human apelin gene (APLN) encodes a 77 amino acid prepropeptide that can be cleaved into different fragments [119]. Endopeptidases cleave the apelin prepropeptide into a 55 amino acid molecule, which in turn is fragmented by the angiotensin-converting enzyme 2 (ACE2) generating the following bioactive isoforms: apelin 36, apelin 17, apelin 13, and apelin 12 (Figure 4). This family of apelin peptides displays a wide array of biological functions in mammals including the neuroendocrine, cardiovascular, and immune systems [120] that can be explained by their asymmetric tissue distribution, activity and receptor binding affinity. Indeed, the shortest apelin isoforms (apelin 12 and 13) demonstrate the highest agonist activity on APJ [117,121]. Apelin 13 can act via autocrine, paracrine, endocrine, and exocrine signalling and is the main agent responsible for the APJ stimulation and downstream biological activities of mature apelin [122]. Several investigations have reported that the transcriptional regulation of apelin expression is modulated by some conditions, hormones, and inflammatory factors. Induction of apelin expression has been associated with hypoxia [123–125], activity of hormones [118,126–132], and inflammatory factors [115,133,134] in different cell types and tissues. Apelin knock-out mice show reduced retinal vascularization and ocular development, denoting its major role in angiogenesis [135], which is independent of VEGF and FGF receptors [136]. Moreover, a lack of apelin in knock-out mice increases angiotensin II-induced dysfunction and pathological remodelling [137].

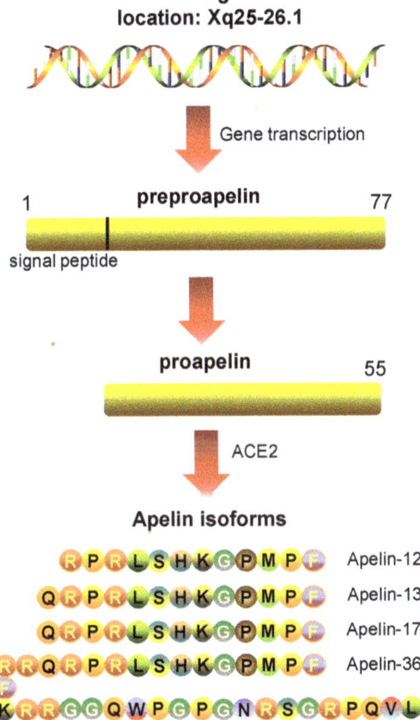

Figure 4. Apelin peptide isoforms.

5.2. APJ, the Apelin Receptor

APJ is a G-protein-coupled receptor composed of seven transmembrane domains with a 31% of homology with the receptor 1 of angiotensin [138]. For this reason, it was initially called angiotensin-like-receptor 1. However, it has been demonstrated that angiotensin II (AII) has no affinity for APJ. In fact, the activation of vascular APJ displays a counterregulatory effect against the activation of the AII receptor [139]. In normal conditions, lung, spleen, and mammary glands show the highest APJ expression [117,121]. APJ is coupled to an activator G protein (Gq) and to an inhibitor G protein (Gi), the activation of which results in an array of physiological effects such as the regulation of hydrosaline equilibrium, vascular tone, cardiac formation and contractility, angiogenesis, and HSC activation [111,124,132,140,141]. The APJ gene sequence has no introns. APJ gene expression is modulated by hypoxia [124,142], insulin [143], stress, and glucocorticoids [144]. However, the molecular mechanisms of APJ transcriptional regulation have not been extensively characterised to date. Mice deficient in APJ do not show any relevant phenotype apart from a higher vasoconstrictor response to AII [110]. During the last few years, another peptide called Apela/ELABELA has been described as an APJ activator, displaying similar effects to apelin on the cardiovascular system [145–147]. The possible interactions of this new APJ agonist and the clinical implications of Apela in the apelin system are still under investigation.

5.3. Cell Signalling Pathways Activated by the APJ Receptor

On one hand, APJ activation leads to the activation of phospholipase Cβ, the phosphatidylinositol-3-kinase (PI3K)/Akt pathways and the Na/H exchanger type 1 and, on the other hand, inhibits adenylyl cyclase and subsequent cyclic adenosine monophosphate production [111,148–151]. Phospholipase Cβ triggers protein kinase C (PKC) and downstream Ras/Raf/MEK/Erk, which together with Akt via mTOR are involved in the activation of P70S6K [152] and the endothelial NO synthase, promoting the release of NO, vascular dilatation, and cell proliferation [149]. The activation of the Na/H exchanger type 1 via PKC in cardiomyocytes is responsible for the dose-dependent increase in in vivo and in vitro myocardial contractility [153]. Moreover, some studies associate APJ activation with inflammation [113,115,134]. Actually, APJ induces the expression of vascular cell adhesion molecule-1 (VCAM-1), MCP-1 and intercellular adhesion molecule-1 (ICAM-1) via the NF-κB and the Jnk signalling pathway [154] (Figure 5).

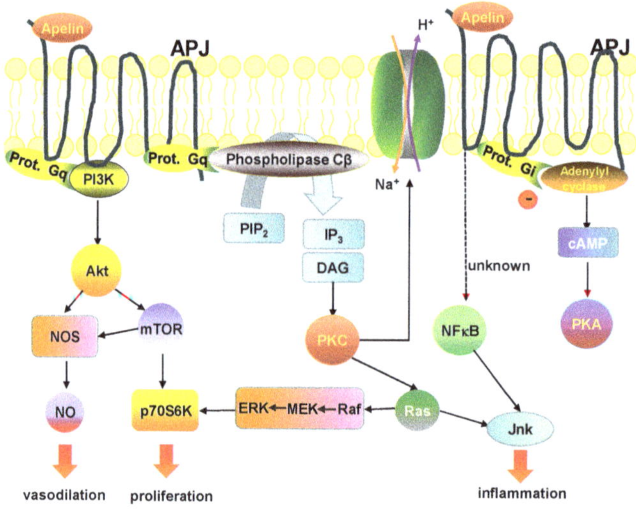

Figure 5. Molecular and cell signalling pathways of APJ.

6. The Apelin System in Health and Disease

The apelin system displays major physiological roles in vascular and lymphatic development [155,156], in neurology [157], and in the digestive system [158]. The activation of the apelin system has demonstrated many beneficial effects in cardiovascular, kidney, skin, and metabolic diseases [128,142,150,159–164]. Apelin has aroused a special interest in the field of cardiology since it is one of the most powerful dose-dependent positive inotropic agents known to date, as demonstrated in perfused hearts [153]. Moreover, apelin is a very-well known vasodilator involved in the stimulation of NO vascular release [165]. Indeed, APJ agonism shows sustained and preserved local vascular and systemic hemodynamic responses in patients with stable symptomatic chronic heart failure and standard medical therapy [166]. However, there are some controversial data on the precise role of the apelin system in the pathogenesis of human heart failure. Some reports suggest that the apelin/APJ system is down-regulated in heart failure and upregulated in left ventricular remodelling [167,168]. This might point to a systemic compensatory effect to recover cardiac contractility. Indeed, acute administration of apelin restores cardiovascular functions in chronic heart failure [169]. However, the potential utility of apelin in cardiovascular disease needs further investigation.

The use of apelin as a biomarker in human heart failure has been challenging. Some reports point out that apelin does not reliably predict acute heart failure in patients presenting dyspnoea, and it is not a prognostic marker in those with confirmed heart failure or with chronic heart failure secondary to idiopathic dilated cardiomyopathy [170,171]. In contrast, plasma apelin concentrations add prognostic value in conjunction with brain natriuretic peptide (BNP) to the risk of mortality at 6 months in patients with ST-segment elevation myocardial infarction [172].

7. Involvement of the Apelin System in the Pathogenesis of Liver Fibrosis

The apelin system has certain therapeutic abilities, but it may also play a role in disease depending on the cellular and molecular milieu. A clear example of this is the role of apelin in tissue fibrosis. Apelin displays anti-fibrotic actions counteracting AII in models of cardiac fibrosis [173,174] and renal fibrosis [175,176]. In contrast, the scenario and role of the apelin system are completely different in liver disease. Apelin is a hepatic pro-fibrotic agent, in part by mediating some of the fibrogenic effects triggered by AII and ET-1 in the activation of HSC occurring in liver fibrosis [118]. These outcomes highlight the intriguing difference between myofibroblastic-cell types in liver compared to myofibroblasts in heart, kidney, or skin in which apelin acts by decreasing myofibroblast accumulation and activity [137,176–178]. In vitro, apelin has also demonstrated a significant potential to promote liver fibrosis. It acts directly on LX-2 cells (a cell line used as a reliable in vitro model of HSC) through Erk signalling [179], stimulating cell survival and the synthesis of PDGF-β receptor and collagen-I in these cells [118]. In turn, PDGF-β and LPS can stimulate the expression of APJ, expanding and perpetuating HSC activation [180]. Therefore, apelin may, in theory, induce HSC to a pro-fibrogenic profile and prolong its stimulation autocrinally during all stages of liver fibrosis in chronic liver disease (Figure 6). In fact, some data have revealed that the inhibition of APJ using F13A (an APJ antagonist) prevents fibrosis progression in rats under a non discontinued fibrosis induction program using CCl_4 [101].

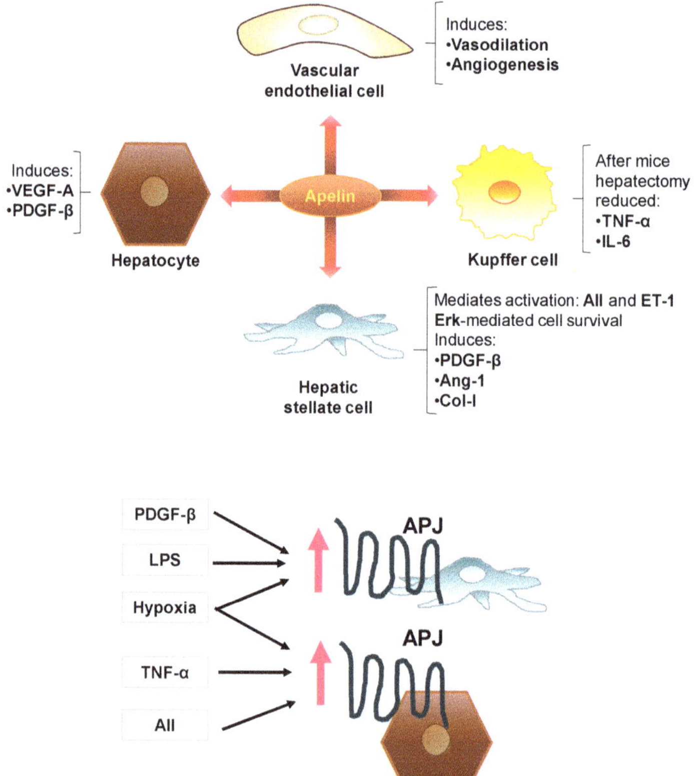

Figure 6. Overview of the roles of the apelin system in liver fibrosis.

Several investigations have uncovered the close and integrated relationship between pathological angiogenesis and fibrosis [12,181–186]. As mentioned above, apelin is a powerful angiogenic agent through the activation of endothelial APJ and different downstream signalling pathways. Two reports have associated the inhibition of APJ with a reduction in angiogenesis and with a concomitant drop in fibrosis in CH and fibrotic rats [18,104]. Although a direct relationship was not established between the two phenomena, there are evidence pointing out that APJ activation by apelin stimulates the expression of a well-known pro-angiogenic factor, angiopoietin-1 (from the angiopoietin family involved in pathological angiogenesis in chronic liver disease) [185,187] in LX-2 cells [118]. This suggests that fibrogenic cells such as HSC may participate in hepatic angiogenesis by secreting angiogenic factors such as angiopoietin 1. Indeed, the inhibition of HSC-secreted angiopietin-1 has shown to drastically reduce pathological angiogenesis and liver fibrosis induced in mice by either CCl_4 or BDL [187].

Aside from HSC, hepatocytes have also been related to contribute to both phenomena, pathological angiogenesis and liver fibrosis, by releasing pro-angiogenic and pro-fibrogenic factors [186]. There is a growing belief that local hypoxia is the link interconnecting both pathological angiogenesis and liver fibrogenesis, orchestrating the harmonic and coordinated activation of HSC, hepatocytes and other hepatic cells [188]. Detection of hypoxic areas is a common trait at any stage of chronic liver disease, expanding progressively from early injury to the development of cirrhosis [189]., Through the action of hypoxia-inducible factors (HIF), hepatic hypoxia up-regulates the expression of a wide array of growth factors and mediators of liver repair and angiogenesis [189]. However, pathological angiogenesis can be inefficient due to the immaturity and permeability of vascular endothelial growth factor (VEGF)-induced new vessels [190] and, consequently, the liver may be unable to reduce hypoxia.

Hypoxia up-regulates in vitro the expression of APJ in LX-2 (HSC) and in HepG2 (hepatocytes) [124]. Interestingly, the pro-inflammatory and pro-fibrogenic agents TNF-α and AII also induce the expression of APJ in HepG2 cells [124]. APJ activation in HepG2 cells triggers the expression of VEGF-A and PDGF-β, factors that in turn may promote angiogenesis and activation of HSC and, consequently, liver fibrosis [15,191]. According to these data, hypoxia, inflammation and pro-fibrogenic factors up-regulate APJ in HSC and hepatocytes, which can release different pro-angiogenic and pro-fibrogenic factors such as apelin (from activated HSC) together to perpetuate fibrosis while injury and these stimuli remain. In vivo, APJ is upregulated preferentially in hepatocytes and HSC, while apelin levels are increased and localized in HSC in cirrhotic rats and in patients with liver cirrhosis caused by hepatitis C virus or ethanol [18,124]. High apelin levels and liver damage have also been observed in human non-alcoholic fatty liver disease [192]. A contemporary clinical investigation revealed that circulating apelin levels are associated with histological and hemodynamic features of chronic liver disease [193], but more clinical studies are needed to confirm the major relevance of apelin system in human liver fibrosis.

One study suggested that apelin may play a different role in liver fibrosis by being an initiator of hepatic injury instead of merely a HSC activator following exogenous injury [194]. In this study, the authors described that the apelin system may stimulate Fas-induced liver injury via the phosphorylation of Jnk in mice intraperitoneally injected with an agonistic anti-Fas antibody. Similar results have been obtained when acute liver injury was promoted by hepatectomy. Blockade of the apelin system resulted in mouse liver regeneration via activation of Kupffer cells and by increasing TNF-α and IL-6 levels in hepatectomized mice [195]. These results suggest that the apelin system may interfere with hepatocyte proliferation after partial hepatectomy in mice. However, a recent study has shown that the administration of a long-acting apelin fusion protein resulted in attenuated hepatocyte damage, diminished apoptosis and ROS production in a mouse model of LPS-induced liver injury [196]. Altogether, these findings suggest that the apelin system may be involved in the processes of hepatic injury and regeneration, but these specific aspects need further investigation.

8. Conclusions

The EC and apelin systems are two of the multiple cell-signalling pathways involved in the pathogenesis of liver fibrosis. Both systems play a major role in the pathophysiological mechanisms underlying the control of HSC activity, involving different receptors and molecules, but with a common significant impact in the development of liver fibrosis.

The ECS is upregulated in liver disease and has been associated with hepatic steatosis, regeneration, fibrosis, and cirrhosis. In liver fibrosis, the cannabinoid receptors CB_1 and CB_2 exhibit opposite roles: CB_1 activation accentuates hepatic fibrosis progression whereas CB_2 displays anti-fibrogenic and anti-inflammatory activities. CB_1 also contributes significantly to cirrhosis complications including portal hypertension, splanchnic vasodilation, cardiomyopathy, and encephalopathy. More specific CB_1 antagonists and CB_2 agonists need to be developed as current CB_1 antagonists are able to cross the blood–brain barrier causing psychotic side effects. Compounds targeting EC synthesis, degradation, and cellular transport pathways could also be a valuable approach to modulate the ECS. Several efforts have been devoted to understanding the specific pathways regulated by this system but there is still a long way to go in the development of drugs targeting the ECS.

Recent studies have reported multiple roles for the apelin/APJ system in liver disease, including acute liver injury, regeneration, fibrosis progression, and cirrhosis. Apelin/APJ has unique functions as a regulator of cell proliferation, apoptosis, pro-inflammatory activity, and revascularization. Apelin/APJ gene expression is temporally increased during liver cirrhotic development and is decreased in stabilized liver fibrosis. The validation of using apelin/APJ as a biomarker in different liver diseases would also be a crucial step toward its clinical use. Further experimental or clinical findings will help to determine the potential of therapeutic strategies targeting the apelin/APJ system for the treatment of liver disease.

Future investigations to further define the mechanisms by which the EC and apelin systems contribute to modulate liver fibrosis will enhance our understanding of their cellular and molecular mechanisms and possible therapeutic targets. This understanding will eventually help in the development of novel therapeutic strategies and drug candidates for treating liver fibrosis in patients with chronic liver disease.

Author Contributions: Writing—review and editing, P.M.-L., M.P., and W.J.; P.M.-L. and M.P. composed the figures.

Funding: This work was supported by grants to W.J. and P.M.-L. from the Ministerio de Ciencia, Innovación y Universidades (grant RTI2018-094734-B-C21), and the AGAUR Beatriu de Pinos Program 2016 (BP-00236) and then from the Ramón y Cajal Program 2018 (Ministerio de Ciencia, Innovación y Universidades, Reference: RYC2018-023971-I) to P.M-L. The Centro de Investigación Biomédica en Red de Enfermedades Hepáticas y Digestivas (CIBERehd) is funded by the Instituto de Salud Carlos III.

Conflicts of Interest: The authors declare no conflict of interest.

References

1. Lee, Y.A.; Wallace, M.C.; Friedman, S.L. Pathobiology of liver fibrosis: A translational success story. *Gut* **2015**, *64*, 830–841. [CrossRef] [PubMed]
2. Levene, A.P.; Goldin, R.D. The epidemiology, pathogenesis and histopathology of fatty liver disease. *Histopathology* **2012**, *61*, 141–152. [CrossRef] [PubMed]
3. Vernon, G.; Baranova, A.; Younossi, Z.M. Systematic review: The epidemiology and natural history of non-alcoholic fatty liver disease and non-alcoholic steatohepatitis in adults. *Aliment. Pharmacol. Ther.* **2011**, *34*, 274–285. [CrossRef] [PubMed]
4. Tsuchida, T.; Friedman, S.L. Mechanisms of hepatic stellate cell activation. *Nat. Rev. Gastroenterol. Hepatol.* **2017**, *14*, 397–411. [CrossRef]
5. Cordero-Espinoza, L.; Huch, M. The balancing act of the liver: Tissue regeneration versus fibrosis. *J. Clin. Investig.* **2018**, *128*, 85–96. [CrossRef]
6. Rout, G.; Nayak, B.; Patel, A.H.; Gunjan, D.; Singh, V.; Kedia, S.; Shalimar. Therapy with oral directly acting agents in hepatitis C infection is associated with reduction in fibrosis and increase in hepatic steatosis on transient elastography. *J. Clin. Exp. Hepatol.* **2019**, *9*, 207–214. [CrossRef]
7. Grgurevic, I.; Bozin, T.; Madir, A. Hepatitis C is now curable, but what happens with cirrhosis and portal hypertension afterwards? *Clin. Exp. Hepatol.* **2017**, *3*, 181–186. [CrossRef]
8. Arthur, M.J. Reversibility of liver fibrosis and cirrhosis following treatment for hepatitis C. *Gastroenterology* **2002**, *122*, 1525–1528. [CrossRef]
9. Melgar-Lesmes, P.; Luquero, A.; Parra-Robert, M.; Mora, A.; Ribera, J.; Edelman, E.R.; Jimenez, W. Graphene-dendrimer nanostars for targeted macrophage overexpression of metalloproteinase 9 and hepatic fibrosis precision therapy. *Nano Lett.* **2018**, *18*, 5839–5845. [CrossRef]
10. Oro, D.; Yudina, T.; Fernandez-Varo, G.; Casals, E.; Reichenbach, V.; Casals, G.; Gonzalez de la Presa, B.; Sandalinas, S.; Carvajal, S.; Puntes, V.; et al. Cerium oxide nanoparticles reduce steatosis, portal hypertension and display anti-inflammatory properties in rats with liver fibrosis. *J. Hepatol.* **2016**, *64*, 691–698. [CrossRef]
11. Schuppan, D.; Ashfaq-Khan, M.; Yang, A.T.; Kim, Y.O. Liver fibrosis: Direct antifibrotic agents and targeted therapies. *Matrix Biol.* **2018**, *68*, 435–451. [CrossRef] [PubMed]
12. Tugues, S.; Fernandez-Varo, G.; Munoz-Luque, J.; Ros, J.; Arroyo, V.; Rodes, J.; Friedman, S.L.; Carmeliet, P.; Jimenez, W.; Morales-Ruiz, M. Antiangiogenic treatment with sunitinib ameliorates inflammatory infiltrate, fibrosis, and portal pressure in cirrhotic rats. *Hepatology* **2007**, *46*, 1919–1926. [CrossRef] [PubMed]
13. Sancho-Bru, P.; Bataller, R.; Fernandez-Varo, G.; Moreno, M.; Ramalho, L.N.; Colmenero, J.; Mari, M.; Claria, J.; Jimenez, W.; Arroyo, V.; et al. Bradykinin attenuates hepatocellular damage and fibrosis in rats with chronic liver injury. *Gastroenterology* **2007**, *133*, 2019–2028. [CrossRef] [PubMed]
14. Titos, E.; Claria, J.; Planaguma, A.; Lopez-Parra, M.; Villamor, N.; Parrizas, M.; Carrio, A.; Miquel, R.; Jimenez, W.; Arroyo, V.; et al. Inhibition of 5-lipoxygenase induces cell growth arrest and apoptosis in rat Kupffer cells: Implications for liver fibrosis. *FASEB J.* **2003**, *17*, 1745–1747. [CrossRef] [PubMed]

15. Reichenbach, V.; Fernandez-Varo, G.; Casals, G.; Oro, D.; Ros, J.; Melgar-Lesmes, P.; Weiskirchen, R.; Morales-Ruiz, M.; Jimenez, W. Adenoviral dominant-negative soluble PDGFRbeta improves hepatic collagen, systemic hemodynamics, and portal pressure in fibrotic rats. *J. Hepatol.* **2012**, *57*, 967–973. [CrossRef] [PubMed]
16. Biswas, K.K.; Sarker, K.P.; Abeyama, K.; Kawahara, K.; Iino, S.; Otsubo, Y.; Saigo, K.; Izumi, H.; Hashiguchi, T.; Yamakuchi, M.; et al. Membrane cholesterol but not putative receptors mediates anandamide-induced hepatocyte apoptosis. *Hepatology* **2003**, *38*, 1167–1177. [CrossRef] [PubMed]
17. Fernandez-Rodriguez, C.M.; Romero, J.; Petros, T.J.; Bradshaw, H.; Gasalla, J.M.; Gutierrez, M.L.; Lledo, J.L.; Santander, C.; Fernandez, T.P.; Tomas, E.; et al. Circulating endogenous cannabinoid anandamide and portal, systemic and renal hemodynamics in cirrhosis. *Liver Int.* **2004**, *24*, 477–483. [CrossRef]
18. Principe, A.; Melgar-Lesmes, P.; Fernandez-Varo, G.; del Arbol, L.R.; Ros, J.; Morales-Ruiz, M.; Bernardi, M.; Arroyo, V.; Jimenez, W. The hepatic apelin system: A new therapeutic target for liver disease. *Hepatology* **2008**, *48*, 1193–1201. [CrossRef]
19. Julien, B.; Grenard, P.; Teixeira-Clerc, F.; Van Nhieu, J.T.; Li, L.; Karsak, M.; Zimmer, A.; Mallat, A.; Lotersztajn, S. Antifibrogenic role of the cannabinoid receptor CB2 in the liver. *Gastroenterology* **2005**, *128*, 742–755. [CrossRef]
20. Osei-Hyiaman, D.; DePetrillo, M.; Pacher, P.; Liu, J.; Radaeva, S.; Batkai, S.; Harvey-White, J.; Mackie, K.; Offertaler, L.; Wang, L.; et al. Endocannabinoid activation at hepatic CB1 receptors stimulates fatty acid synthesis and contributes to diet-induced obesity. *J. Clin. Investig.* **2005**, *115*, 1298–1305. [CrossRef]
21. Velasco, G.; Sanchez, C.; Guzman, M. Anticancer mechanisms of cannabinoids. *Curr. Oncol.* **2016**, *23*, S23–S32. [CrossRef] [PubMed]
22. Pacher, P.; Batkai, S.; Kunos, G. The endocannabinoid system as an emerging target of pharmacotherapy. *Pharmacol. Rev.* **2006**, *58*, 389–462. [CrossRef] [PubMed]
23. Poleszak, E.; Wosko, S.; Slawinska, K.; Szopa, A.; Wrobel, A.; Serefko, A. Cannabinoids in depressive disorders. *Life Sci.* **2018**, *213*, 18–24. [CrossRef] [PubMed]
24. Schmole, A.C.; Lundt, R.; Toporowski, G.; Hansen, J.N.; Beins, E.; Halle, A.; Zimmer, A. Cannabinoid receptor 2-deficiency ameliorates disease symptoms in a mouse model with Alzheimer's Disease-like pathology. *J. Alzheimers Dis.* **2018**, *64*, 379–392. [CrossRef]
25. Lamontagne, D.; Lepicier, P.; Lagneux, C.; Bouchard, J.F. The endogenous cardiac cannabinoid system: A new protective mechanism against myocardial ischemia. *Arch. Mal. Coeur. Vaiss.* **2006**, *99*, 242–246.
26. Bazwinsky-Wutschke, I.; Zipprich, A.; Dehghani, F. Endocannabinoid system in hepatic glucose metabolism, fatty liver disease, and cirrhosis. *Int. J. Mol. Sci.* **2019**, *20*. [CrossRef]
27. Perez-Gomez, E.; Andradas, C.; Blasco-Benito, S.; Caffarel, M.M.; Garcia-Taboada, E.; Villa-Morales, M.; Moreno, E.; Hamann, S.; Martin-Villar, E.; Flores, J.M.; et al. Role of cannabinoid receptor CB2 in HER2 pro-oncogenic signaling in breast cancer. *J. Natl. Cancer. Inst.* **2015**, *107*, djv077. [CrossRef]
28. Ramer, R.; Schwarz, R.; Hinz, B. Modulation of the endocannabinoid system as a potential anticancer strategy. *Front. Pharmacol.* **2019**, *10*, 430. [CrossRef]
29. Mechoulam, R.; Hanus, L.O.; Pertwee, R.; Howlett, A.C. Early phytocannabinoid chemistry to endocannabinoids and beyond. *Nat. Rev. Neurosci.* **2014**, *15*, 757–761. [CrossRef]
30. Piomelli, D. The molecular logic of endocannabinoid signalling. *Nat. Rev. Neurosci.* **2003**, *4*, 873–884. [CrossRef]
31. Lu, H.C.; Mackie, K. An introduction to the endogenous cannabinoid system. *Biol. Psychiatry* **2016**, *79*, 516–525. [CrossRef] [PubMed]
32. Zou, S.; Kumar, U. Cannabinoid receptors and the endocannabinoid system: Signaling and function in the central nervous system. *Int. J. Mol. Sci.* **2018**, *19*. [CrossRef]
33. Hillard, C.J. Circulating endocannabinoids: From whence do they come and where are they going? *Neuropsychopharmacology* **2018**, *43*, 155–172. [CrossRef] [PubMed]
34. Di Marzo, V.; Fontana, A.; Cadas, H.; Schinelli, S.; Cimino, G.; Schwartz, J.C.; Piomelli, D. Formation and inactivation of endogenous cannabinoid anandamide in central neurons. *Nature* **1994**, *372*, 686–691. [CrossRef]
35. Liu, J.; Wang, L.; Harvey-White, J.; Huang, B.X.; Kim, H.Y.; Luquet, S.; Palmiter, R.D.; Krystal, G.; Rai, R.; Mahadevan, A.; et al. Multiple pathways involved in the biosynthesis of anandamide. *Neuropharmacology* **2008**, *54*, 1–7. [CrossRef]

36. Stella, N.; Schweitzer, P.; Piomelli, D. A second endogenous cannabinoid that modulates long-term potentiation. *Nature* **1997**, *388*, 773–778. [CrossRef]
37. Nakane, S.; Oka, S.; Arai, S.; Waku, K.; Ishima, Y.; Tokumura, A.; Sugiura, T. 2-Arachidonoyl-sn-glycero-3-phosphate, an arachidonic acid-containing lysophosphatidic acid: Occurrence and rapid enzymatic conversion to 2-arachidonoyl-sn-glycerol, a cannabinoid receptor ligand, in rat brain. *Arch. Biochem. Biophys.* **2002**, *402*, 51–58. [CrossRef]
38. Bisogno, T.; Howell, F.; Williams, G.; Minassi, A.; Cascio, M.G.; Ligresti, A.; Matias, I.; Schiano-Moriello, A.; Paul, P.; Williams, E.J.; et al. Cloning of the first sn1-DAG lipases points to the spatial and temporal regulation of endocannabinoid signaling in the brain. *J. Cell Biol.* **2003**, *163*, 463–468. [CrossRef]
39. Howlett, A.C.; Barth, F.; Bonner, T.I.; Cabral, G.; Casellas, P.; Devane, W.A.; Felder, C.C.; Herkenham, M.; Mackie, K.; Martin, B.R.; et al. International union of pharmacology. XXVII. Classification of cannabinoid receptors. *Pharmacol. Rev.* **2002**, *54*, 161–202. [CrossRef]
40. De Petrocellis, L.; Ligresti, A.; Moriello, A.S.; Allara, M.; Bisogno, T.; Petrosino, S.; Stott, C.G.; Di Marzo, V. Effects of cannabinoids and cannabinoid-enriched Cannabis extracts on TRP channels and endocannabinoid metabolic enzymes. *Br. J. Pharmacol.* **2011**, *163*, 1479–1494. [CrossRef]
41. Baram, L.; Peled, E.; Berman, P.; Yellin, B.; Besser, E.; Benami, M.; Louria-Hayon, I.; Lewitus, G.M.; Meiri, D. The heterogeneity and complexity of Cannabis extracts as antitumor agents. *Oncotarget* **2019**, *10*, 4091–4106. [CrossRef] [PubMed]
42. Kozak, K.R.; Rowlinson, S.W.; Marnett, L.J. Oxygenation of the endocannabinoid, 2-arachidonylglycerol, to glyceryl prostaglandins by cyclooxygenase-2. *J. Biol. Chem.* **2000**, *275*, 33744–33749. [CrossRef] [PubMed]
43. Di Pasquale, E.; Chahinian, H.; Sanchez, P.; Fantini, J. The insertion and transport of anandamide in synthetic lipid membranes are both cholesterol-dependent. *PLoS ONE* **2009**, *4*, e4989. [CrossRef] [PubMed]
44. Ryberg, E.; Vu, H.K.; Larsson, N.; Groblewski, T.; Hjorth, S.; Elebring, T.; Sjogren, S.; Greasley, P.J. Identification and characterisation of a novel splice variant of the human CB1 receptor. *FEBS Lett.* **2005**, *579*, 259–264. [CrossRef]
45. Shire, D.; Carillon, C.; Kaghad, M.; Calandra, B.; Rinaldi-Carmona, M.; Le Fur, G.; Caput, D.; Ferrara, P. An amino-terminal variant of the central cannabinoid receptor resulting from alternative splicing. *J. Biol. Chem.* **1995**, *270*, 3726–3731. [CrossRef] [PubMed]
46. Correa, F.; Wolfson, M.L.; Valchi, P.; Aisemberg, J.; Franchi, A.M. Endocannabinoid system and pregnancy. *Reproduction* **2016**, *152*, R191–R200. [CrossRef]
47. Sun, X.; Dey, S.K. Aspects of endocannabinoid signaling in periimplantation biology. *Mol. Cell Endocrinol.* **2008**, *286*, S3–S11. [CrossRef]
48. Zimmer, A.; Zimmer, A.M.; Hohmann, A.G.; Herkenham, M.; Bonner, T.I. Increased mortality, hypoactivity, and hypoalgesia in cannabinoid CB1 receptor knockout mice. *Proc. Natl. Acad. Sci. USA* **1999**, *96*, 5780–5785. [CrossRef]
49. Li, Y.; Kim, J. CB2 Cannabinoid receptor knockout in mice impairs contextual long-term memory and enhances spatial working memory. *Neural Plast* **2016**, *2016*, 9817089. [CrossRef]
50. Ravinet Trillou, C.; Delgorge, C.; Menet, C.; Arnone, M.; Soubrie, P. CB1 cannabinoid receptor knockout in mice leads to leanness, resistance to diet-induced obesity and enhanced leptin sensitivity. *Int. J. Obes. Relat. Metab. Disord.* **2004**, *28*, 640–648. [CrossRef]
51. Mallat, A.; Lotersztajn, S. Endocannabinoids and liver disease. I. Endocannabinoids and their receptors in the liver. *Am. J. Physiol. Gastrointest Liver Physiol.* **2008**, *294*, G9–G12. [CrossRef] [PubMed]
52. Piomelli, D.; Giuffrida, A.; Calignano, A.; Rodriguez de Fonseca, F. The endocannabinoid system as a target for therapeutic drugs. *Trends Pharmacol. Sci.* **2000**, *21*, 218–224. [CrossRef]
53. Pacher, P.; Kunos, G. Modulating the endocannabinoid system in human health and disease–successes and failures. *FEBS J.* **2013**, *280*, 1918–1943. [CrossRef] [PubMed]
54. Ibsen, M.S.; Connor, M.; Glass, M. Cannabinoid CB1 and CB2 receptor signaling and bias. *Cannabis Cannabinoid Res.* **2017**, *2*, 48–60. [CrossRef]
55. Demuth, D.G.; Molleman, A. Cannabinoid signalling. *Life Sci.* **2006**, *78*, 549–563. [CrossRef]
56. Ozaita, A.; Puighermanal, E.; Maldonado, R. Regulation of PI3K/Akt/GSK-3 pathway by cannabinoids in the brain. *J. Neurochem.* **2007**, *102*, 1105–1114. [CrossRef]
57. Morales, P.; Reggio, P.H. An update on non-CB1, non-CB2 cannabinoid related G-protein-coupled receptors. *Cannabis Cannabinoid Res.* **2017**, *2*, 265–273. [CrossRef]

58. Moreno, E.; Cavic, M.; Krivokuca, A.; Casado, V.; Canela, E. The endocannabinoid system as a target in cancer diseases: Are we there yet? *Front. Pharmacol.* **2019**, *10*, 339. [CrossRef]
59. Li, X.; Hua, T.; Vemuri, K.; Ho, J.H.; Wu, Y.; Wu, L.; Popov, P.; Benchama, O.; Zvonok, N.; Locke, K.; et al. Crystal structure of the human cannabinoid receptor CB2. *Cell* **2019**, *176*, 459–467. [CrossRef]
60. Howlett, A.C.; Fleming, R.M. Cannabinoid inhibition of adenylate cyclase. Pharmacology of the response in neuroblastoma cell membranes. *Mol. Pharmacol.* **1984**, *26*, 532–538.
61. Mlost, J.; Wasik, A.; Starowicz, K. Role of endocannabinoid system in dopamine signalling within the reward circuits affected by chronic pain. *Pharmacol. Res.* **2019**, *143*, 40–47. [CrossRef] [PubMed]
62. Yang, J.; Tian, Y.; Zheng, R.; Li, L.; Qiu, F. Endocannabinoid system and the expression of endogenous ceramides in human hepatocellular carcinoma. *Oncol. Lett.* **2019**, *18*, 1530–1538. [CrossRef] [PubMed]
63. Kirilly, E.; Gonda, X.; Bagdy, G. CB1 receptor antagonists: New discoveries leading to new perspectives. *Acta Physiol.* **2012**, *205*, 41–60. [CrossRef]
64. Ranganathan, M.; D'Souza, D.C. The acute effects of cannabinoids on memory in humans: A review. *Psychopharmacology* **2006**, *188*, 425–444. [CrossRef] [PubMed]
65. Sanchez-Blazquez, P.; Rodriguez-Munoz, M.; Vicente-Sanchez, A.; Garzon, J. Cannabinoid receptors couple to NMDA receptors to reduce the production of NO and the mobilization of zinc induced by glutamate. *Antioxid Redox Signal.* **2013**, *19*, 1766–1782. [CrossRef] [PubMed]
66. Khaspekov, L.G.; Brenz Verca, M.S.; Frumkina, L.E.; Hermann, H.; Marsicano, G.; Lutz, B. Involvement of brain-derived neurotrophic factor in cannabinoid receptor-dependent protection against excitotoxicity. *Eur. J. Neurosci.* **2004**, *19*, 1691–1698. [CrossRef]
67. Parolaro, D.; Realini, N.; Vigano, D.; Guidali, C.; Rubino, T. The endocannabinoid system and psychiatric disorders. *Exp. Neurol.* **2010**, *224*, 3–14. [CrossRef]
68. Scotter, E.L.; Abood, M.E.; Glass, M. The endocannabinoid system as a target for the treatment of neurodegenerative disease. *Br. J. Pharmacol.* **2010**, *160*, 480–498. [CrossRef]
69. Donvito, G.; Nass, S.R.; Wilkerson, J.L.; Curry, Z.A.; Schurman, L.D.; Kinsey, S.G.; Lichtman, A.H. The endogenous cannabinoid system: A budding source of targets for treating inflammatory and neuropathic pain. *Neuropsychopharmacology* **2018**, *43*, 52–79. [CrossRef]
70. Salamone, J.D.; McLaughlin, P.J.; Sink, K.; Makriyannis, A.; Parker, L.A. Cannabinoid CB1 receptor inverse agonists and neutral antagonists: Effects on food intake, food-reinforced behavior and food aversions. *Physiol. Behav.* **2007**, *91*, 383–388. [CrossRef]
71. Smoum, R.; Baraghithy, S.; Chourasia, M.; Breuer, A.; Mussai, N.; Attar-Namdar, M.; Kogan, N.M.; Raphael, B.; Bolognini, D.; Cascio, M.G.; et al. CB2 cannabinoid receptor agonist enantiomers HU-433 and HU-308: An inverse relationship between binding affinity and biological potency. *Proc. Natl. Acad. Sci. USA* **2015**, *112*, 8774–8779. [CrossRef] [PubMed]
72. Mallet, C.; Dubray, C.; Dualé, C. FAAH inhibitors in the limelight, but regrettably. *Int. J. Clin. Pharmacol. Ther.* **2016**, *54*, 498–501. [CrossRef] [PubMed]
73. Wang, Y.; Ma, S.; Wang, Q.; Hu, W.; Wang, D.; Li, X.; Su, T.; Qin, X.; Zhang, X.; Ma, K.; et al. Effects of cannabinoid receptor type 2 on endogenous myocardial regeneration by activating cardiac progenitor cells in mouse infarcted heart. *Sci. China Life Sci.* **2014**, *57*, 201–208. [CrossRef]
74. Ward, S.J.; Castelli, F.; Reichenbach, Z.W.; Tuma, R.F. Surprising outcomes in cannabinoid CB1/CB2 receptor double knockout mice in two models of ischemia. *Life Sci.* **2018**, *195*, 1–5. [CrossRef]
75. Kunos, G.; Tam, J. The case for peripheral CB(1) receptor blockade in the treatment of visceral obesity and its cardiometabolic complications. *Br. J. Pharmacol.* **2011**, *163*, 1423–1431. [CrossRef]
76. Morales, P.; Hernandez-Folgado, L.; Goya, P.; Jagerovic, N. Cannabinoid receptor 2 (CB2) agonists and antagonists: A patent update. *Expert Opin. Ther. Pat.* **2016**, *26*, 843–856. [CrossRef]
77. Izzo, A.A.; Sharkey, K.A. Cannabinoids and the gut: New developments and emerging concepts. *Pharmacol. Ther.* **2010**, *126*, 21–38. [CrossRef]
78. Velasco, G.; Sanchez, C.; Guzman, M. Towards the use of cannabinoids as antitumour agents. *Nat. Rev. Cancer* **2012**, *12*, 436–444. [CrossRef]
79. Wang, D.; Wang, H.; Ning, W.; Backlund, M.G.; Dey, S.K.; DuBois, R.N. Loss of cannabinoid receptor 1 accelerates intestinal tumor growth. *Cancer Res.* **2008**, *68*, 6468–6476. [CrossRef]

80. Orellana-Serradell, O.; Poblete, C.E.; Sanchez, C.; Castellon, E.A.; Gallegos, I.; Huidobro, C.; Llanos, M.N.; Contreras, H.R. Proapoptotic effect of endocannabinoids in prostate cancer cells. *Oncol. Rep.* **2015**, *33*, 1599–1608. [CrossRef]
81. Siegmund, S.V.; Schwabe, R.F. Endocannabinoids and liver disease. II. Endocannabinoids in the pathogenesis and treatment of liver fibrosis. *Am. J. Physiol. Gastrointest. Liver Physiol.* **2008**, *294*, G357–G362. [CrossRef] [PubMed]
82. Patsenker, E.; Stoll, M.; Millonig, G.; Agaimy, A.; Wissniowski, T.; Schneider, V.; Mueller, S.; Brenneisen, R.; Seitz, H.K.; Ocker, M.; et al. Cannabinoid receptor type I modulates alcohol-induced liver fibrosis. *Mol. Med.* **2011**, *17*, 1285–1294. [CrossRef] [PubMed]
83. Caraceni, P.; Viola, A.; Piscitelli, F.; Giannone, F.; Berzigotti, A.; Cescon, M.; Domenicali, M.; Petrosino, S.; Giampalma, E.; Riili, A.; et al. Circulating and hepatic endocannabinoids and endocannabinoid-related molecules in patients with cirrhosis. *Liver Int.* **2010**, *30*, 816–825. [CrossRef] [PubMed]
84. Patsenker, E.; Sachse, P.; Chicca, A.; Gachet, M.S.; Schneider, V.; Mattsson, J.; Lanz, C.; Worni, M.; de Gottardi, A.; Semmo, M.; et al. Elevated levels of endocannabinoids in chronic hepatitis C may modulate cellular immune response and hepatic stellate cell activation. *Int. J. Mol. Sci.* **2015**, *16*, 7057–7076. [CrossRef]
85. Siegmund, S.V.; Wojtalla, A.; Schlosser, M.; Zimmer, A.; Singer, M.V. Fatty acid amide hydrolase but not monoacyl glycerol lipase controls cell death induced by the endocannabinoid 2-arachidonoyl glycerol in hepatic cell populations. *Biochem. Biophys. Res. Commun.* **2013**, *437*, 48–54. [CrossRef]
86. Siegmund, S.V.; Seki, E.; Osawa, Y.; Uchinami, H.; Cravatt, B.F.; Schwabe, R.F. Fatty acid amide hydrolase determines anandamide-induced cell death in the liver. *J. Biol. Chem.* **2006**, *281*, 10431–10438. [CrossRef]
87. Siegmund, S.V.; Uchinami, H.; Osawa, Y.; Brenner, D.A.; Schwabe, R.F. Anandamide induces necrosis in primary hepatic stellate cells. *Hepatology* **2005**, *41*, 1085–1095. [CrossRef]
88. Siegmund, S.V.; Wojtalla, A.; Schlosser, M.; Schildberg, F.A.; Knolle, P.A.; Nusing, R.M.; Zimmer, A.; Strassburg, C.P.; Singer, M.V. Cyclooxygenase-2 contributes to the selective induction of cell death by the endocannabinoid 2-arachidonoyl glycerol in hepatic stellate cells. *Biochem. Biophys. Res. Commun.* **2016**, *470*, 678–684. [CrossRef]
89. Chen, L.; Li, L.; Chen, J.; Li, L.; Zheng, Z.; Ren, J.; Qiu, Y. Oleoylethanolamide, an endogenous PPAR-alpha ligand, attenuates liver fibrosis targeting hepatic stellate cells. *Oncotarget* **2015**, *6*, 42530–42540. [CrossRef]
90. Batkai, S.; Mukhopadhyay, P.; Harvey-White, J.; Kechrid, R.; Pacher, P.; Kunos, G. Endocannabinoids acting at CB1 receptors mediate the cardiac contractile dysfunction in vivo in cirrhotic rats. *Am. J. Physiol. Heart Circ. Physiol.* **2007**, *293*, H1689–H1695. [CrossRef]
91. Dai, E.; Zhang, L.; Ye, L.; Wan, S.; Feng, L.; Qi, Q.; Yao, F.; Li, Z. Hepatic expression of cannabinoid receptors CB1 and CB2 correlate with fibrogenesis in patients with chronic hepatitis B. *Int. J. Infect. Dis* **2017**, *59*, 124–130. [CrossRef] [PubMed]
92. Teixeira-Clerc, F.; Belot, M.P.; Manin, S.; Deveaux, V.; Cadoudal, T.; Chobert, M.N.; Louvet, A.; Zimmer, A.; Tordjmann, T.; Mallat, A.; et al. Beneficial paracrine effects of cannabinoid receptor 2 on liver injury and regeneration. *Hepatology* **2010**, *52*, 1046–1059. [CrossRef] [PubMed]
93. Hezode, C.; Zafrani, E.S.; Roudot-Thoraval, F.; Costentin, C.; Hessami, A.; Bouvier-Alias, M.; Medkour, F.; Pawlostky, J.M.; Lotersztajn, S.; Mallat, A. Daily cannabis use: A novel risk factor of steatosis severity in patients with chronic hepatitis C. *Gastroenterology* **2008**, *134*, 432–439. [CrossRef]
94. Dibba, P.; Li, A.A.; Cholankeril, G.; Iqbal, U.; Gadiparthi, C.; Khan, M.A.; Kim, D.; Ahmed, A. The role of cannabinoids in the setting of cirrhosis. *Medicines* **2018**, *5*. [CrossRef]
95. Batkai, S.; Jarai, Z.; Wagner, J.A.; Goparaju, S.K.; Varga, K.; Liu, J.; Wang, L.; Mirshahi, F.; Khanolkar, A.D.; Makriyannis, A.; et al. Endocannabinoids acting at vascular CB1 receptors mediate the vasodilated state in advanced liver cirrhosis. *Nat. Med.* **2001**, *7*, 827–832. [CrossRef]
96. Ros, J.; Claria, J.; To-Figueras, J.; Planaguma, A.; Cejudo-Martin, P.; Fernandez-Varo, G.; Martin-Ruiz, R.; Arroyo, V.; Rivera, F.; Rodes, J.; et al. Endogenous cannabinoids: A new system involved in the homeostasis of arterial pressure in experimental cirrhosis in the rat. *Gastroenterology* **2002**, *122*, 85–93. [CrossRef]
97. Domenicali, M.; Caraceni, P.; Giannone, F.; Pertosa, A.M.; Principe, A.; Zambruni, A.; Trevisani, F.; Croci, T.; Bernardi, M. Cannabinoid type 1 receptor antagonism delays ascites formation in rats with cirrhosis. *Gastroenterology* **2009**, *137*, 341–349. [CrossRef]

98. Giannone, F.A.; Baldassarre, M.; Domenicali, M.; Zaccherini, G.; Trevisani, F.; Bernardi, M.; Caraceni, P. Reversal of liver fibrosis by the antagonism of endocannabinoid CB1 receptor in a rat model of CCl(4)-induced advanced cirrhosis. *Lab. Invest.* **2012**, *92*, 384–395. [CrossRef]
99. Caraceni, P.; Pertosa, A.M.; Giannone, F.; Domenicali, M.; Grattagliano, I.; Principe, A.; Mastroleo, C.; Perrelli, M.G.; Cutrin, J.; Trevisani, F.; et al. Antagonism of the cannabinoid CB-1 receptor protects rat liver against ischaemia-reperfusion injury complicated by endotoxaemia. *Gut* **2009**, *58*, 1135–1143. [CrossRef]
100. Liu, J.; Batkai, S.; Pacher, P.; Harvey-White, J.; Wagner, J.A.; Cravatt, B.F.; Gao, B.; Kunos, G. Lipopolysaccharide induces anandamide synthesis in macrophages via CD14/MAPK/phosphoinositide 3-kinase/NF-kappaB independently of platelet-activating factor. *J. Biol. Chem.* **2003**, *278*, 45034–45039. [CrossRef]
101. Domenicali, M.; Ros, J.; Fernandez-Varo, G.; Cejudo-Martin, P.; Crespo, M.; Morales-Ruiz, M.; Briones, A.M.; Campistol, J.M.; Arroyo, V.; Vila, E.; et al. Increased anandamide induced relaxation in mesenteric arteries of cirrhotic rats: Role of cannabinoid and vanilloid receptors. *Gut* **2005**, *54*, 522–527. [CrossRef] [PubMed]
102. Izzo, A.A.; Deutsch, D.G. Unique pathway for anandamide synthesis and liver regeneration. *Proc. Natl. Acad. Sci. USA* **2011**, *108*, 6339–6340. [CrossRef] [PubMed]
103. Pisanti, S.; Picardi, P.; Pallottini, V.; Martini, C.; Petrosino, S.; Proto, M.C.; Vitale, M.; Laezza, C.; Gazzerro, P.; Di Marzo, V.; et al. Anandamide drives cell cycle progression through CB1 receptors in a rat model of synchronized liver regeneration. *J. Cell Physiol.* **2015**, *230*, 2905–2914. [CrossRef] [PubMed]
104. Reichenbach, V.; Ros, J.; Fernandez-Varo, G.; Casals, G.; Melgar-Lesmes, P.; Campos, T.; Makriyannis, A.; Morales-Ruiz, M.; Jimenez, W. Prevention of fibrosis progression in CCl4-treated rats: Role of the hepatic endocannabinoid and apelin systems. *J. Pharmacol. Exp. Ther.* **2012**, *340*, 629–637. [CrossRef]
105. Horvath, B.; Magid, L.; Mukhopadhyay, P.; Batkai, S.; Rajesh, M.; Park, O.; Tanchian, G.; Gao, R.Y.; Goodfellow, C.E.; Glass, M.; et al. A new cannabinoid CB2 receptor agonist HU-910 attenuates oxidative stress, inflammation and cell death associated with hepatic ischaemia/reperfusion injury. *Br. J. Pharmacol.* **2012**, *165*, 2462–2478. [CrossRef]
106. Munoz-Luque, J.; Ros, J.; Fernandez-Varo, G.; Tugues, S.; Morales-Ruiz, M.; Alvarez, C.E.; Friedman, S.L.; Arroyo, V.; Jimenez, W. Regression of fibrosis after chronic stimulation of cannabinoid CB2 receptor in cirrhotic rats. *J. Pharmacol. Exp. Ther.* **2008**, *324*, 475–483. [CrossRef]
107. Guillot, A.; Hamdaoui, N.; Bizy, A.; Zoltani, K.; Souktani, R.; Zafrani, E.S.; Mallat, A.; Lotersztajn, S.; Lafdil, F. Cannabinoid receptor 2 counteracts interleukin-17-induced immune and fibrogenic responses in mouse liver. *Hepatology* **2014**, *59*, 296–306. [CrossRef]
108. Avraham, Y.; Israeli, E.; Gabbay, E.; Okun, A.; Zolotarev, O.; Silberman, I.; Ganzburg, V.; Dagon, Y.; Magen, I.; Vorobia, L.; et al. Endocannabinoids affect neurological and cognitive function in thioacetamide-induced hepatic encephalopathy in mice. *Neurobiol. Dis.* **2006**, *21*, 237–245. [CrossRef]
109. Tatemoto, K.; Hosoya, M.; Habata, Y.; Fujii, R.; Kakegawa, T.; Zou, M.X.; Kawamata, Y.; Fukusumi, S.; Hinuma, S.; Kitada, C.; et al. Isolation and characterization of a novel endogenous peptide ligand for the human APJ receptor. *Biochem. Biophys. Res. Commun.* **1998**, *251*, 471–476. [CrossRef]
110. De Mota, N.; Reaux-Le Goazigo, A.; El Messari, S.; Chartrel, N.; Roesch, D.; Dujardin, C.; Kordon, C.; Vaudry, H.; Moos, F.; Llorens-Cortes, C. Apelin, a potent diuretic neuropeptide counteracting vasopressin actions through inhibition of vasopressin neuron activity and vasopressin release. *Proc. Natl. Acad. Sci. USA* **2004**, *101*, 10464–10469. [CrossRef]
111. Szokodi, I.; Tavi, P.; Foldes, G.; Voutilainen-Myllyla, S.; Ilves, M.; Tokola, H.; Pikkarainen, S.; Piuhola, J.; Rysa, J.; Toth, M.; et al. Apelin, the novel endogenous ligand of the orphan receptor APJ, regulates cardiac contractility. *Circ. Res.* **2002**, *91*, 434–440. [CrossRef]
112. Ishida, J.; Hashimoto, T.; Hashimoto, Y.; Nishiwaki, S.; Iguchi, T.; Harada, S.; Sugaya, T.; Matsuzaki, H.; Yamamoto, R.; Shiota, N.; et al. Regulatory roles for APJ, a seven-transmembrane receptor related to angiotensin-type 1 receptor in blood pressure in vivo. *J. Biol. Chem.* **2004**, *279*, 26274–26279. [CrossRef] [PubMed]
113. Horiuchi, Y.; Fujii, T.; Kamimura, Y.; Kawashima, K. The endogenous, immunologically active peptide apelin inhibits lymphocytic cholinergic activity during immunological responses. *J. Neuroimmunol.* **2003**, *144*, 46–52. [CrossRef] [PubMed]
114. Dray, C.; Sakar, Y.; Vinel, C.; Daviaud, D.; Masri, B.; Garrigues, L.; Wanecq, E.; Galvani, S.; Negre-Salvayre, A.; Barak, L.S.; et al. The intestinal glucose-apelin cycle controls carbohydrate absorption in mice. *Gastroenterology* **2013**, *144*, 771–780. [CrossRef]

115. Daviaud, D.; Boucher, J.; Gesta, S.; Dray, C.; Guigne, C.; Quilliot, D.; Ayav, A.; Ziegler, O.; Carpene, C.; Saulnier-Blache, J.S.; et al. TNFalpha up-regulates apelin expression in human and mouse adipose tissue. *FASEB J.* **2006**, *20*, 1528–1530. [CrossRef]
116. Scott, I.C.; Masri, B.; D'Amico, L.A.; Jin, S.W.; Jungblut, B.; Wehman, A.M.; Baier, H.; Audigier, Y.; Stainier, D.Y. The G protein-coupled receptor agtrl1b regulates early development of myocardial progenitors. *Dev. Cell* **2007**, *12*, 403–413. [CrossRef]
117. Kawamata, Y.; Habata, Y.; Fukusumi, S.; Hosoya, M.; Fujii, R.; Hinuma, S.; Nishizawa, N.; Kitada, C.; Onda, H.; Nishimura, O.; et al. Molecular properties of apelin: Tissue distribution and receptor binding. *Biochim. Biophys Acta* **2001**, *1538*, 162–171. [CrossRef]
118. Melgar-Lesmes, P.; Casals, G.; Pauta, M.; Ros, J.; Reichenbach, V.; Bataller, R.; Morales-Ruiz, M.; Jimenez, W. Apelin mediates the induction of profibrogenic genes in human hepatic stellate cells. *Endocrinology* **2010**, *151*, 5306–5314. [CrossRef]
119. Tatemoto, K.; Takayama, K.; Zou, M.X.; Kumaki, I.; Zhang, W.; Kumano, K.; Fujimiya, M. The novel peptide apelin lowers blood pressure via a nitric oxide-dependent mechanism. *Regul. Pept.* **2001**, *99*, 87–92. [CrossRef]
120. Masri, B.; Knibiehler, B.; Audigier, Y. Apelin signalling: A promising pathway from cloning to pharmacology. *Cell Signal.* **2005**, *17*, 415–426. [CrossRef]
121. Hosoya, M.; Kawamata, Y.; Fukusumi, S.; Fujii, R.; Habata, Y.; Hinuma, S.; Kitada, C.; Honda, S.; Kurokawa, T.; Onda, H.; et al. Molecular and functional characteristics of APJ. Tissue distribution of mRNA and interaction with the endogenous ligand apelin. *J. Biol. Chem.* **2000**, *275*, 21061–21067. [CrossRef]
122. Akcilar, R.; Turgut, S.; Caner, V.; Akcilar, A.; Ayada, C.; Elmas, L.; Ozcan, T.O. The effects of apelin treatment on a rat model of type 2 diabetes. *Adv. Med. Sci.* **2015**, *60*, 94–100. [CrossRef]
123. Casals, G.; Fernandez-Varo, G.; Melgar-Lesmes, P.; Marfa, S.; Reichenbach, V.; Morales-Ruiz, M.; Jimenez, W. Factors involved in extracellular matrix turnover in human derived cardiomyocytes. *Cell Physiol. Biochem.* **2013**, *32*, 1125–1136. [CrossRef]
124. Melgar-Lesmes, P.; Pauta, M.; Reichenbach, V.; Casals, G.; Ros, J.; Bataller, R.; Morales-Ruiz, M.; Jimenez, W. Hypoxia and proinflammatory factors upregulate apelin receptor expression in human stellate cells and hepatocytes. *Gut* **2011**, *60*, 1404–1411. [CrossRef]
125. Eyries, M.; Siegfried, G.; Ciumas, M.; Montagne, K.; Agrapart, M.; Lebrin, F.; Soubrier, F. Hypoxia-induced apelin expression regulates endothelial cell proliferation and regenerative angiogenesis. *Circ. Res.* **2008**, *103*, 432–440. [CrossRef]
126. Glassford, A.J.; Yue, P.; Sheikh, A.Y.; Chun, H.J.; Zarafshar, S.; Chan, D.A.; Reaven, G.M.; Quertermous, T.; Tsao, P.S. HIF-1 regulates hypoxia- and insulin-induced expression of apelin in adipocytes. *Am. J. Physiol. Endocrinol. Metab.* **2007**, *293*, E1590–E1596. [CrossRef]
127. Mazzucotelli, A.; Ribet, C.; Castan-Laurell, I.; Daviaud, D.; Guigne, C.; Langin, D.; Valet, P. The transcriptional co-activator PGC-1alpha up regulates apelin in human and mouse adipocytes. *Regul. Pept.* **2008**, *150*, 33–37. [CrossRef]
128. Zhang, L.; Li, F.; Su, X.; Li, Y.; Wang, Y.; Fang, R.; Guo, Y.; Jin, T.; Shan, H.; Zhao, X.; et al. Melatonin prevents lung injury by regulating apelin 13 to improve mitochondrial dysfunction. *Exp. Mol. Med.* **2019**, *51*, 73. [CrossRef]
129. Wei, L.; Hou, X.; Tatemoto, K. Regulation of apelin mRNA expression by insulin and glucocorticoids in mouse 3T3-L1 adipocytes. *Regul. Pept.* **2005**, *132*, 27–32. [CrossRef]
130. Kralisch, S.; Lossner, U.; Bluher, M.; Paschke, R.; Stumvoll, M.; Fasshauer, M. Growth hormone induces apelin mRNA expression and secretion in mouse 3T3-L1 adipocytes. *Regul. Pept.* **2007**, *139*, 84–89. [CrossRef]
131. Jiang, H.; Ye, X.P.; Yang, Z.Y.; Zhan, M.; Wang, H.N.; Cao, H.M.; Xie, H.J.; Pan, C.M.; Song, H.D.; Zhao, S.X. Aldosterone directly affects apelin expression and secretion in adipocytes. *J. Mol. Endocrinol.* **2013**, *51*, 37–48. [CrossRef]
132. Llorens-Cortes, C.; Moos, F. Opposite potentiality of hypothalamic coexpressed neuropeptides, apelin and vasopressin in maintaining body-fluid homeostasis. *Prog. Brain Res.* **2008**, *170*, 559–570. [CrossRef]
133. Rastellini, C.; Han, S.; Bhatia, V.; Cao, Y.; Liu, K.; Gao, X.; Ko, T.C.; Greeley, G.H., Jr.; Falzon, M. Induction of chronic pancreatitis by pancreatic duct ligation activates BMP2, apelin, and PTHrP expression in mice. *Am. J. Physiol. Gastrointest Liver Physiol.* **2015**, *309*, G554–G565. [CrossRef]

134. Han, S.; Englander, E.W.; Gomez, G.A.; Aronson, J.F.; Rastellini, C.; Garofalo, R.P.; Kolli, D.; Quertermous, T.; Kundu, R.; Greeley, G.H., Jr. Pancreatitis activates pancreatic apelin-APJ axis in mice. *Am. J. Physiol. Gastrointest Liver Physiol.* **2013**, *305*, G139–G150. [CrossRef]
135. Kasai, A.; Shintani, N.; Kato, H.; Matsuda, S.; Gomi, F.; Haba, R.; Hashimoto, H.; Kakuda, M.; Tano, Y.; Baba, A. Retardation of retinal vascular development in apelin-deficient mice. *Arterioscler Thromb Vasc. Biol.* **2008**, *28*, 1717–1722. [CrossRef]
136. Cox, C.M.; D'Agostino, S.L.; Miller, M.K.; Heimark, R.L.; Krieg, P.A. Apelin, the ligand for the endothelial G-protein-coupled receptor, APJ, is a potent angiogenic factor required for normal vascular development of the frog embryo. *Dev. Biol.* **2006**, *296*, 177–189. [CrossRef]
137. Sato, T.; Kadowaki, A.; Suzuki, T.; Ito, H.; Watanabe, H.; Imai, Y.; Kuba, K. Loss of apelin augments angiotensin II-induced cardiac dysfunction and pathological remodeling. *Int. J. Mol. Sci.* **2019**, *20*. [CrossRef]
138. O'Dowd, B.F.; Heiber, M.; Chan, A.; Heng, H.H.; Tsui, L.C.; Kennedy, J.L.; Shi, X.; Petronis, A.; George, S.R.; Nguyen, T. A human gene that shows identity with the gene encoding the angiotensin receptor is located on chromosome 11. *Gene* **1993**, *136*, 355–360. [CrossRef]
139. Siddiquee, K.; Hampton, J.; McAnally, D.; May, L.; Smith, L. The apelin receptor inhibits the angiotensin II type 1 receptor via allosteric trans-inhibition. *Br. J. Pharmacol.* **2013**, *168*, 1104–1117. [CrossRef]
140. Zhang, Z.Z.; Wang, W.; Jin, H.Y.; Chen, X.; Cheng, Y.W.; Xu, Y.L.; Song, B.; Penninger, J.M.; Oudit, G.Y.; Zhong, J.C. Apelin is a negative regulator of angiotensin II-mediated adverse myocardial remodeling and dysfunction. *Hypertension* **2017**, *70*, 1165–1175. [CrossRef]
141. Falcao-Pires, I.; Goncalves, N.; Henriques-Coelho, T.; Moreira-Goncalves, D.; Roncon-Albuquerque, R., Jr.; Leite-Moreira, A.F. Apelin decreases myocardial injury and improves right ventricular function in monocrotaline-induced pulmonary hypertension. *Am. J. Physiol. Heart Circ. Physiol.* **2009**, *296*, H2007–H2014. [CrossRef]
142. Hou, J.; Wang, L.; Long, H.; Wu, H.; Wu, Q.; Zhong, T.; Chen, X.; Zhou, C.; Guo, T.; Wang, T. Hypoxia preconditioning promotes cardiac stem cell survival and cardiogenic differentiation in vitro involving activation of the HIF-1alpha/apelin/APJ axis. *Stem Cell Res. Ther.* **2017**, *8*, 215. [CrossRef]
143. Dray, C.; Debard, C.; Jager, J.; Disse, E.; Daviaud, D.; Martin, P.; Attane, C.; Wanecq, E.; Guigne, C.; Bost, F.; et al. Apelin and APJ regulation in adipose tissue and skeletal muscle of type 2 diabetic mice and humans. *Am. J. Physiol. Endocrinol. Metab.* **2010**, *298*, E1161–E1169. [CrossRef]
144. O'Carroll, A.M.; Don, A.L.; Lolait, S.J. APJ receptor mRNA expression in the rat hypothalamic paraventricular nucleus: Regulation by stress and glucocorticoids. *J. Neuroendocrinol.* **2003**, *15*, 1095–1101. [CrossRef]
145. Deng, C.; Chen, H.; Yang, N.; Feng, Y.; Hsueh, A.J. Apela regulates fluid homeostasis by binding to the APJ receptor to activate Gi signaling. *J. Biol. Chem.* **2015**, *290*, 18261–18268. [CrossRef]
146. Yang, P.; Read, C.; Kuc, R.E.; Buonincontri, G.; Southwood, M.; Torella, R.; Upton, P.D.; Crosby, A.; Sawiak, S.J.; Carpenter, T.A.; et al. Elabela/toddler is an endogenous agonist of the apelin APJ receptor in the adult cardiovascular system, and exogenous administration of the peptide compensates for the downregulation of its expression in pulmonary arterial hypertension. *Circulation* **2017**, *135*, 1160–1173. [CrossRef]
147. Ho, L.; Tan, S.Y.; Wee, S.; Wu, Y.; Tan, S.J.; Ramakrishna, N.B.; Chng, S.C.; Nama, S.; Szczerbinska, I.; Chan, Y.S.; et al. ELABELA is an endogenous growth factor that sustains hESC self-renewal via the PI3K/AKT pathway. *Cell Stem Cell* **2015**, *17*, 435–447. [CrossRef]
148. Langelaan, D.N.; Reddy, T.; Banks, A.W.; Dellaire, G.; Dupre, D.J.; Rainey, J.K. Structural features of the apelin receptor N-terminal tail and first transmembrane segment implicated in ligand binding and receptor trafficking. *Biochim. Biophys. Acta* **2013**, *1828*, 1471–1483. [CrossRef]
149. Liu, C.; Su, T.; Li, F.; Li, L.; Qin, X.; Pan, W.; Feng, F.; Chen, F.; Liao, D.; Chen, L. PI3K/Akt signaling transduction pathway is involved in rat vascular smooth muscle cell proliferation induced by apelin-13. *Acta Biochim. Biophys. Sin.* **2010**, *42*, 396–402. [CrossRef]
150. Chaves-Almagro, C.; Castan-Laurell, I.; Dray, C.; Knauf, C.; Valet, P.; Masri, B. Apelin receptors: From signaling to antidiabetic strategy. *Eur. J. Pharmacol.* **2015**, *763*, 149–159. [CrossRef]
151. Li, Y.; Chen, J.; Bai, B.; Du, H.; Liu, Y.; Liu, H. Heterodimerization of human apelin and kappa opioid receptors: Roles in signal transduction. *Cell Signal.* **2012**, *24*, 991–1001. [CrossRef]
152. Masri, B.; Morin, N.; Cornu, M.; Knibiehler, B.; Audigier, Y. Apelin (65-77) activates p70 S6 kinase and is mitogenic for umbilical endothelial cells. *FASEB J.* **2004**, *18*, 1909–1911. [CrossRef]

153. Berry, M.F.; Pirolli, T.J.; Jayasankar, V.; Burdick, J.; Morine, K.J.; Gardner, T.J.; Woo, Y.J. Apelin has in vivo inotropic effects on normal and failing hearts. *Circulation* **2004**, *110*, II187–II193. [CrossRef]
154. Lu, Y.; Zhu, X.; Liang, G.X.; Cui, R.R.; Liu, Y.; Wu, S.S.; Liang, Q.H.; Liu, G.Y.; Jiang, Y.; Liao, X.B.; et al. Apelin-APJ induces ICAM-1, VCAM-1 and MCP-1 expression via NF-kappaB/JNK signal pathway in human umbilical vein endothelial cells. *Amino Acids* **2012**, *43*, 2125–2136. [CrossRef]
155. Kim, J.D.; Kang, Y.; Kim, J.; Papangeli, I.; Kang, H.; Wu, J.; Park, H.; Nadelmann, E.; Rockson, S.G.; Chun, H.J.; et al. Essential role of Apelin signaling during lymphatic development in zebrafish. *Arterioscler Thromb Vasc. Biol.* **2014**, *34*, 338–345. [CrossRef]
156. Mughal, A.; O'Rourke, S.T. Vascular effects of apelin: Mechanisms and therapeutic potential. *Pharmacol. Ther.* **2018**, *190*, 139–147. [CrossRef]
157. Xiao, Z.Y.; Wang, B.; Fu, W.; Jin, X.; You, Y.; Tian, S.W.; Kuang, X. The hippocampus is a critical site mediating antidepressant-like activity of apelin-13 in rats. *Neuroscience* **2018**, *375*, 1–9. [CrossRef]
158. Huang, Z.; Luo, X.; Liu, M.; Chen, L. Function and regulation of apelin/APJ system in digestive physiology and pathology. *J. Cell Physiol.* **2019**, *234*, 7796–7810. [CrossRef]
159. Ureche, C.; Tapoi, L.; Volovat, S.; Voroneanu, L.; Kanbay, M.; Covic, A. Cardioprotective apelin effects and the cardiac-renal axis: Review of existing science and potential therapeutic applications of synthetic and native regulated apelin. *J. Hum. Hypertens* **2019**, *33*, 429–435. [CrossRef]
160. Yin, J.; Wang, Y.; Chang, J.; Li, B.; Zhang, J.; Liu, Y.; Lai, S.; Jiang, Y.; Li, H.; Zeng, X. Apelin inhibited epithelial-mesenchymal transition of podocytes in diabetic mice through downregulating immunoproteasome subunits beta5i. *Cell Death Dis.* **2018**, *9*, 1031. [CrossRef]
161. Wang, W.; Zhang, D.; Yang, R.; Xia, W.; Qian, K.; Shi, Z.; Brown, R.; Zhou, H.; Xi, Y.; Shi, L.; et al. Hepatic and cardiac beneficial effects of a long-acting Fc-apelin fusion protein in diet-induced obese mice. *Diabetes Metab. Res. Rev.* **2018**, *34*, e2997. [CrossRef] [PubMed]
162. Renaud-Gabardos, E.; Tatin, F.; Hantelys, F.; Lebas, B.; Calise, D.; Kunduzova, O.; Masri, B.; Pujol, F.; Sicard, P.; Valet, P.; et al. Therapeutic benefit and gene network regulation by combined gene transfer of apelin, FGF2, and SERCA2a into ischemic heart. *Mol. Ther.* **2018**, *26*, 902–916. [CrossRef] [PubMed]
163. Tatin, F.; Renaud-Gabardos, E.; Godet, A.C.; Hantelys, F.; Pujol, F.; Morfoisse, F.; Calise, D.; Viars, F.; Valet, P.; Masri, B.; et al. Apelin modulates pathological remodeling of lymphatic endothelium after myocardial infarction. *JCI Insight* **2017**, *2*. [CrossRef] [PubMed]
164. Pang, H.; Han, B.; Yu, T.; Zong, Z. Effect of apelin on the cardiac hemodynamics in hypertensive rats with heart failure. *Int. J. Mol. Med.* **2014**, *34*, 756–764. [CrossRef] [PubMed]
165. Zhong, J.C.; Yu, X.Y.; Huang, Y.; Yung, L.M.; Lau, C.W.; Lin, S.G. Apelin modulates aortic vascular tone via endothelial nitric oxide synthase phosphorylation pathway in diabetic mice. *Cardiovasc. Res.* **2007**, *74*, 388–395. [CrossRef] [PubMed]
166. Barnes, G.D.; Alam, S.; Carter, G.; Pedersen, C.M.; Lee, K.M.; Hubbard, T.J.; Veitch, S.; Jeong, H.; White, A.; Cruden, N.L.; et al. Sustained cardiovascular actions of APJ agonism during renin-angiotensin system activation and in patients with heart failure. *Circ. Heart Fail.* **2013**, *6*, 482–491. [CrossRef]
167. Foldes, G.; Horkay, F.; Szokodi, I.; Vuolteenaho, O.; Ilves, M.; Lindstedt, K.A.; Mayranpaa, M.; Sarman, B.; Seres, L.; Skoumal, R.; et al. Circulating and cardiac levels of apelin, the novel ligand of the orphan receptor APJ, in patients with heart failure. *Biochem. Biophys. Res. Commun.* **2003**, *308*, 480–485. [CrossRef]
168. Chong, K.S.; Gardner, R.S.; Morton, J.J.; Ashley, E.A.; McDonagh, T.A. Plasma concentrations of the novel peptide apelin are decreased in patients with chronic heart failure. *Eur. J. Heart Fail.* **2006**, *8*, 355–360. [CrossRef]
169. Japp, A.G.; Cruden, N.L.; Barnes, G.; van Gemeren, N.; Mathews, J.; Adamson, J.; Johnston, N.R.; Denvir, M.A.; Megson, I.L.; Flapan, A.D.; et al. Acute cardiovascular effects of apelin in humans: Potential role in patients with chronic heart failure. *Circulation* **2010**, *121*, 1818–1827. [CrossRef]
170. Perea, R.J.; Morales-Ruiz, M.; Ortiz-Perez, J.T.; Bosch, X.; Andreu, D.; Borras, R.; Acosta, J.; Penela, D.; Prat-Gonzalez, S.; de Caralt, T.M.; et al. Utility of galectin-3 in predicting post-infarct remodeling after acute myocardial infarction based on extracellular volume fraction mapping. *Int. J. Cardiol.* **2016**, *223*, 458–464. [CrossRef]
171. Miettinen, K.H.; Magga, J.; Vuolteenaho, O.; Vanninen, E.J.; Punnonen, K.R.; Ylitalo, K.; Tuomainen, P.; Peuhkurinen, K.J. Utility of plasma apelin and other indices of cardiac dysfunction in the clinical assessment of patients with dilated cardiomyopathy. *Regul. Pept.* **2007**, *140*, 178–184. [CrossRef] [PubMed]

172. Sans-Rosello, J.; Casals, G.; Rossello, X.; Gonzalez de la Presa, B.; Vila, M.; Duran-Cambra, A.; Morales-Ruiz, M.; Ferrero-Gregori, A.; Jimenez, W.; Sionis, A. Prognostic value of plasma apelin concentrations at admission in patients with ST-segment elevation acute myocardial infarction. *Clin. Biochem.* **2017**, *50*, 279–284. [CrossRef] [PubMed]
173. Siddiquee, K.; Hampton, J.; Khan, S.; Zadory, D.; Gleaves, L.; Vaughan, D.E.; Smith, L.H. Apelin protects against angiotensin II-induced cardiovascular fibrosis and decreases plasminogen activator inhibitor type-1 production. *J. Hypertens* **2011**, *29*, 724–731. [CrossRef] [PubMed]
174. Fukushima, H.; Kobayashi, N.; Takeshima, H.; Koguchi, W.; Ishimitsu, T. Effects of olmesartan on Apelin/APJ and Akt/endothelial nitric oxide synthase pathway in Dahl rats with end-stage heart failure. *J. Cardiovasc. Pharmacol.* **2010**, *55*, 83–88. [CrossRef] [PubMed]
175. Nishida, M.; Okumura, Y.; Oka, T.; Toiyama, K.; Ozawa, S.; Itoi, T.; Hamaoka, K. The role of apelin on the alleviative effect of Angiotensin receptor blocker in unilateral ureteral obstruction-induced renal fibrosis. *Nephron Extra* **2012**, *2*, 39–47. [CrossRef] [PubMed]
176. Wang, L.Y.; Diao, Z.L.; Zhang, D.L.; Zheng, J.F.; Zhang, Q.D.; Ding, J.X.; Liu, W.H. The regulatory peptide apelin: A novel inhibitor of renal interstitial fibrosis. *Amino Acids* **2014**, *46*, 2693–2704. [CrossRef]
177. Yokoyama, Y.; Sekiguchi, A.; Fujiwara, C.; Uchiyama, A.; Uehara, A.; Ogino, S.; Torii, R.; Ishikawa, O.; Motegi, S.I. Inhibitory regulation of skin fibrosis in systemic sclerosis by Apelin/APJ signaling. *Arthritis Rheumatol.* **2018**, *70*, 1661–1672. [CrossRef]
178. Wang, L.Y.; Diao, Z.L.; Zheng, J.F.; Wu, Y.R.; Zhang, Q.D.; Liu, W.H. Apelin attenuates TGF-beta1-induced epithelial to mesenchymal transition via activation of PKC-epsilon in human renal tubular epithelial cells. *Peptides* **2017**, *96*, 44–52. [CrossRef]
179. Wang, Y.; Song, J.; Bian, H.; Bo, J.; Lv, S.; Pan, W.; Lv, X. Apelin promotes hepatic fibrosis through ERK signaling in LX-2 cells. *Mol. Cell Biochem.* **2019**, *460*, 205–215. [CrossRef]
180. Yokomori, H.; Oda, M.; Yoshimura, K.; Machida, S.; Kaneko, F.; Hibi, T. Overexpression of apelin receptor (APJ/AGTRL1) on hepatic stellate cells and sinusoidal angiogenesis in human cirrhotic liver. *J. Gastroenterol.* **2011**, *46*, 222–231. [CrossRef]
181. Van Steenkiste, C.; Ribera, J.; Geerts, A.; Pauta, M.; Tugues, S.; Casteleyn, C.; Libbrecht, L.; Olievier, K.; Schroyen, B.; Reynaert, H.; et al. Inhibition of placental growth factor activity reduces the severity of fibrosis, inflammation, and portal hypertension in cirrhotic mice. *Hepatology* **2011**, *53*, 1629–1640. [CrossRef] [PubMed]
182. Liu, L.; You, Z.; Yu, H.; Zhou, L.; Zhao, H.; Yan, X.; Li, D.; Wang, B.; Zhu, L.; Xu, Y.; et al. Mechanotransduction-modulated fibrotic microniches reveal the contribution of angiogenesis in liver fibrosis. *Nat. Mater.* **2017**, *16*, 1252–1261. [CrossRef] [PubMed]
183. Wang, Z.; Li, J.; Xiao, W.; Long, J.; Zhang, H. The STAT3 inhibitor S3I-201 suppresses fibrogenesis and angiogenesis in liver fibrosis. *Lab. Investig.* **2018**, *98*, 1600–1613. [CrossRef] [PubMed]
184. Zhang, F.; Hao, M.; Jin, H.; Yao, Z.; Lian, N.; Wu, L.; Shao, J.; Chen, A.; Zheng, S. Canonical hedgehog signalling regulates hepatic stellate cell-mediated angiogenesis in liver fibrosis. *Br. J. Pharmacol.* **2017**, *174*, 409–423. [CrossRef]
185. Pauta, M.; Ribera, J.; Melgar-Lesmes, P.; Casals, G.; Rodriguez-Vita, J.; Reichenbach, V.; Fernandez Varo, G.; Morales-Romero, B.; Bataller, R.; Michelena, J.; et al. Overexpression of angiopoietin-2 in rats and patients with liver fibrosis. Therapeutic consequences of its inhibition. *Liver Int.* **2015**, *35*, 1383–1392. [CrossRef]
186. Bocca, C.; Novo, E.; Miglietta, A.; Parola, M. Angiogenesis and fibrogenesis in chronic liver diseases. *Cell Mol. Gastroenterol. Hepatol.* **2015**, *1*, 477–488. [CrossRef]
187. Taura, K.; De Minicis, S.; Seki, E.; Hatano, E.; Iwaisako, K.; Osterreicher, C.H.; Kodama, Y.; Miura, K.; Ikai, I.; Uemoto, S.; et al. Hepatic stellate cells secrete angiopoietin 1 that induces angiogenesis in liver fibrosis. *Gastroenterology* **2008**, *135*, 1729–1738. [CrossRef]
188. Rosmorduc, O.; Housset, C. Hypoxia: A link between fibrogenesis, angiogenesis, and carcinogenesis in liver disease. *Semin. Liver Dis.* **2010**, *30*, 258–270. [CrossRef]
189. Cannito, S.; Paternostro, C.; Busletta, C.; Bocca, C.; Colombatto, S.; Miglietta, A.; Novo, E.; Parola, M. Hypoxia, hypoxia-inducible factors and fibrogenesis in chronic liver diseases. *Histol. Histopathol.* **2014**, *29*, 33–44. [CrossRef]

190. Melgar-Lesmes, P.; Tugues, S.; Ros, J.; Fernandez-Varo, G.; Morales-Ruiz, M.; Rodes, J.; Jimenez, W. Vascular endothelial growth factor and angiopoietin-2 play a major role in the pathogenesis of vascular leakage in cirrhotic rats. *Gut* **2009**, *58*, 285–292. [CrossRef]
191. Ying, H.Z.; Chen, Q.; Zhang, W.Y.; Zhang, H.H.; Ma, Y.; Zhang, S.Z.; Fang, J.; Yu, C.H. PDGF signaling pathway in hepatic fibrosis pathogenesis and therapeutics (Review). *Mol. Med. Rep.* **2017**, *16*, 7879–7889. [CrossRef] [PubMed]
192. Ercin, C.N.; Dogru, T.; Tapan, S.; Kara, M.; Haymana, C.; Karadurmus, N.; Karslioglu, Y.; Acikel, C. Plasma apelin levels in subjects with nonalcoholic fatty liver disease. *Metabolism* **2010**, *59*, 977–981. [CrossRef] [PubMed]
193. Lim, Y.L.; Choi, E.; Jang, Y.O.; Cho, Y.Z.; Kang, Y.S.; Baik, S.K.; Kwon, S.O.; Kim, M.Y. Clinical implications of the serum apelin level on portal hypertension and prognosis of liver cirrhosis. *Gut Liver* **2016**, *10*, 109–116. [CrossRef]
194. Yasuzaki, H.; Yoshida, S.; Hashimoto, T.; Shibata, W.; Inamori, M.; Toya, Y.; Tamura, K.; Maeda, S.; Umemura, S. Involvement of the apelin receptor APJ in Fas-induced liver injury. *Liver Int.* **2013**, *33*, 118–126. [CrossRef]
195. Yoshiya, S.; Shirabe, K.; Imai, D.; Toshima, T.; Yamashita, Y.; Ikegami, T.; Okano, S.; Yoshizumi, T.; Kawanaka, H.; Maehara, Y. Blockade of the apelin-APJ system promotes mouse liver regeneration by activating Kupffer cells after partial hepatectomy. *J. Gastroenterol.* **2015**, *50*, 573–582. [CrossRef]
196. Zhou, H.; Yang, R.; Wang, W.; Xu, F.; Xi, Y.; Brown, R.A.; Zhang, H.; Shi, L.; Zhu, D.; Gong, D.W. Fc-apelin fusion protein attenuates lipopolysaccharide-induced liver injury in mice. *Sci. Rep.* **2018**, *8*, 11428. [CrossRef]

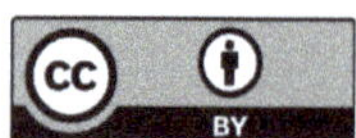

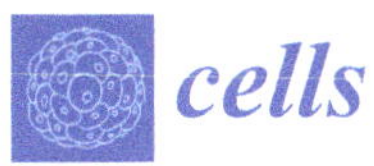
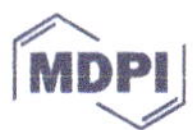

Review

Magnetic-Assisted Treatment of Liver Fibrosis

Kateryna Levada [1], Alexander Omelyanchik [1], Valeria Rodionova [1,2], Ralf Weiskirchen [3] and Matthias Bartneck [4,*]

1 Institute of Physics, Mathematics and Information Technology, Immanuel Kant Baltic Federal University, 236016 Kaliningrad, Russia; kateryna.levada@gmail.com (K.L.); asomelyanchik@kantiana.ru (A.O.); valeriarodionova@gmail.com (V.R.)
2 National University of Science and Technology "MISiS", 119049 Moscow, Russia
3 Institute of Molecular Pathobiochemistry, Experimental Gene Therapy and Clinical Chemistry, RWTH University Hospital Aachen, D-52074 Aachen, Germany; rweiskirchen@ukaachen.de
4 Department of Medicine III, Medical Faculty, RWTH Aachen, D-52074 Aachen, Germany
* Correspondence: mbartneck@ukaachen.de; Tel.: +49-241-80-80611

Received: 19 September 2019; Accepted: 15 October 2019; Published: 19 October 2019

Abstract: Chronic liver injury can be induced by viruses, toxins, cellular activation, and metabolic dysregulation and can lead to liver fibrosis. Hepatic fibrosis still remains a major burden on the global health systems. Nonalcoholic fatty liver disease (NAFLD) and nonalcoholic steatohepatitis (NASH) are considered the main cause of liver fibrosis. Hepatic stellate cells are key targets in antifibrotic treatment, but selective engagement of these cells is an unresolved issue. Current strategies for antifibrotic drugs, which are at the critical stage 3 clinical trials, target metabolic regulation, immune cell activation, and cell death. Here, we report on the critical factors for liver fibrosis, and on prospective novel drugs, which might soon enter the market. Apart from the current clinical trials, novel perspectives for anti-fibrotic treatment may arise from magnetic particles and controlled magnetic forces in various different fields. Magnetic-assisted techniques can, for instance, enable cell engineering and cell therapy to fight cancer, might enable to control the shape or orientation of single cells or tissues mechanically. Furthermore, magnetic forces may improve localized drug delivery mediated by magnetism-induced conformational changes, and they may also enhance non-invasive imaging applications.

Keywords: liver fibrosis; magnetic fields; nanomedicines; immune cells; macrophages; hepatic stellate cells; RNA-based medicines; drug delivery; magnetic nanoparticles

---

1. Introduction

The liver has a unique capability for regeneration, which has been known since Greek mythology. Strikingly, up to 70% of healthy liver tissue loss can be regenerated by its cells [1]. Regardless of the part, the liver of Prometheus regenerated overnight [1]. In evolutionary terms, the liver is the only organ in mammals that has preserved a high potential for regeneration to be replaceable after injury [2]. Despite this unique role, liver diseases are becoming an increasing burden of the health system. There are currently three stage 3 clinical trials with promising data. Future developments may include cell-selective targeting of key cell types of fibrogenesis, such as hepatic stellate cells (HSC). Here, we discuss magnetic-assisted applications including microfluidics technology, which have broadly enriched cancer therapy, including for instance in leukocyte engineering, i.e., in generating chimeric antigen receptor T (CAR T) cells. Microfluidic technologies have enabled the use of magnetic fields to control cell isolation, motility and directed migration, and modulating mechanical forces may also improve the methods to manipulate single cells. Medical applications of amplifying the precision of drug delivery towards tumor or dying cells at inflammatory sites are urgently needed. Directed use of magnetism may also further improve non-invasive imaging methodologies.

1.1. Liver Fibrosis

The capacity of the liver for regeneration is unique, but repeated and chronic liver injury frequently results in liver fibrosis. Fibrosis, which often precedes cancer, is characterized by the continuous accumulation of extracellular matrix (ECM), which is extremely rich in collagen I and III, leads to the deposition of scars and progressing on liver fibrosis [3]. This disease is characterized by an excessive accumulation of extracellular matrix (ECM) in the space of Disse. The accumulation of ECM has a negative effect on diverse functions of the organ such as detoxification and other liver functions, and it disturbs the hepatic blood flow. The recruitment of inflammatory immune cells, which can also amplify tumor development, represents another key event of fibrosis [4,5]. Untreated liver fibrosis can develop into cirrhosis and is accompanied by portal hypertension, hepatic encephalopathy, liver failure, and also is associated with an increased risk for the development of hepatocellular carcinoma (HCC) [6,7]. Liver injury usually is initiated by a noxa, virtually anything which can harm or kill the sensitive hepatocytes. Disease factors are viral hepatitis, chronic alcohol abuse, cholestatic disorders, genetic heritage, and autoimmune diseases. Apparently, nonalcoholic fatty liver disease (NAFLD) and nonalcoholic steatohepatitis (NASH) represent the major etiology of liver fibrosis. The demographic change caused by the ageing population and the growing epidemic of obesity lead to increased prevalence of liver fibrosis [8]. NAFLD is regarded as the main inducer of chronic liver disease in industrialized countries. It is assumed that NAFLD will be the leading indication for liver transplantation [9]. A significant number of as much as 20–30% of adults have NAFLD. Additional factors in disease, particularly immune cell infiltration, can lead to the progression of NAFLD to NASH and fibrosis. Fibrosis severity has been linked to mortality related to hepatic and other diseases, as evidenced in several longitudinal clinical studies and correspondingly, the effectiveness for the evaluation of drugs against NAFLD is their impact on liver fibrosis [9], which may also have a positive outcome on nonhepatic diseases [10]. It was estimated that liver-related mortality will increase dramatically in the next decade [9]. Fibrosis can be considered a dysregulated wound-healing response which leads to scarring of tissues. Different disease etiologies exhibit specific hallmarks, but advanced stages are commonly characterized by bridging fibers between portal fields [11].

1.2. Roles of Different Hepatic Cell Types in Liver Fibrosis

The process of fibrosis development, fibrogenesis, can be analyzed from a cellular perspective. The regeneration of hepatocytes works in a streaming fashion, as shown in a rat model by Zajicek and colleagues in 1985. Hepatocytes located at the portal space gradually stream towards the hepatic vein where they are eliminated by apoptosis. This cellular traveling was estimated to last 201 days in rats [2]. However, during liver fibrosis, the empty spaces left by the missing hepatocytes are frequently replenished with ECM by HSC, rather than with fresh hepatocytes. During the course of cell death, certain molecules are released by hepatocytes, which function as danger signals for other cell types, for instance for HSC [12]. These "alarm bells" also attract immune cells which themselves secrete pathogenic factors that can induce apoptosis of hepatocytes. These processes result in an amplification of the fibrogenic response. Innate immune cells are well known to initiate liver inflammation in NAFLD and they express pattern recognition receptors (PRR) which can sense danger-associated and pathogen-associated molecular pattern molecules (DAMP and PAMP), as well as inflammatory mediators [12].

In recent years, the roles of cholangiocytes, particularly in cholestatic liver injury, started to be explored. For instance, cholangiocyte proliferation is a substantial driver of liver fibrosis in biliary atresia. Researchers demonstrated that a long non-coding RNA has a major impact on the proliferation of cholangiocytes and thus represents a therapeutic target in this regard [13]. Damage of cholangiocytes in toxic liver injury leads to a hampered production of bile acids. Sato and colleagues further revealed that extracellular vesicles and microRNAs might be critical factors which regulate cyclic adenosine monophosphate (cAMP) metabolism in cholangiocytes [14].

Mast cells are another cell type reported to further amplify hepatic fibrosis and injury. Particularly, mast cell-deficient mice exhibited less pronounced fibrosis. It was reported that mast cells regulate the proliferation of cholangiocytes and contribute to the activation of HSC [15]. A means to specific deactivation of mast cells might therefore represent a novel therapeutic strategy. However, the involvement of mast cells in fibrosis remains controversial since they have been reported to be both harmful and protective [16].

The hepatic macrophages form a complex mixture of cells of various activation stages and cellular origin. They can be distinguished as resident macrophages, which were originally defined as Kupffer cells, as well as monocyte-derived macrophages (MoMF). These cells can be separated using cell sorting applications [17]. Kupffer cells were first discovered by Karl Wilhelm von Kupffer in 1876 [18], even before the relevance of phagocytic cells was first published by Metchnikoff in 1888 in Tuberculosis [19]. While cell sorting has unraveled hepatic macrophage subpopulations that were characterized in RNA bulk sequencing where thousands of cells are analyzed in a single RNA isolate [17], single cell RNA sequencing has begun to start unraveling the real complexity of hepatic macrophage subtypes [20]. Single cell RNA sequencing has also enabled identification of subpopulations of HSC [21]. The so-called resting or quiescent HSC (qHSC) form a homogenous population characterized by high platelet-derived growth factor receptor β (PDGFRβ) expression. However, the activated HSC, which are also called myofibroblasts, can further be sub-divided into populations expressing α-smooth muscle actin (α-SMA), collagens, or immunological markers. The S100 calcium binding protein A6 (S100A6) was identified as a universal marker of activated HSC, myofibroblasts (MFB), for both mRNA and protein expression [21]. The so-called transdifferentiation of the resting and vitamin A storing HSC into MFB, which are proliferative and which express huge amounts of collagen, is central for fibrogenesis [22]. The activation of HSC can be induced through a variety of extracellular signals from other liver cell types like hepatocytes and macrophages. Further, intracellular processes like oxidative stress, autophagy, endoplasmatic reticulum stress, or metabolic dysregulations, have been studied in great detail and are regarded as causative for HSC activation [23]. The fact that fibrosis is a bidirectional path is evidenced by reports on fibrosis regression [24]. HSC thus represent a valuable target for fibrosis therapy since they are the source of excessive matrix production. Inhibiting the construction of different collagens, which in part takes place in the extracellular space by specific inhibitors, for example, Lysyl oxidase-like 2 (LOXL2), has recently been proposed to be done by small molecules [25].

It was shown that, if a circumvention of the inflammatory insult is achieved, among other factors, the anti-inflammatory and restorative activities of macrophages persist and impact the hepatic microenvironment [26]. During fibrosis regression, MFB are eliminated through cell death induction, become senescent, or may even revert into cells which resemble quiescent HSC [27]. The excessively deposited ECM was shown to be degraded, i.e., by matrix metalloproteinases (MMP) that are released by certain subtypes of macrophages [24] (Figure 1).

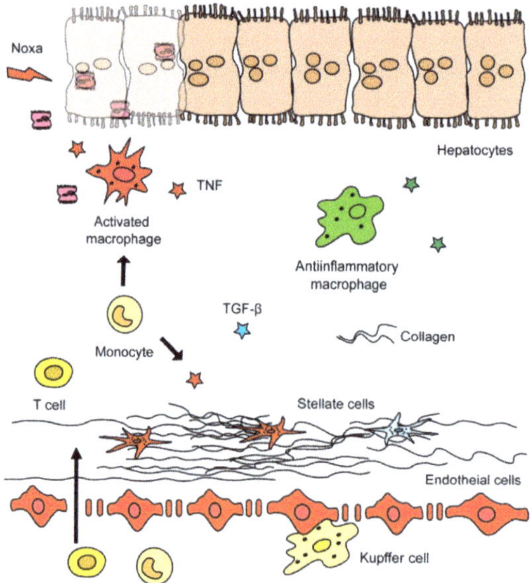

Figure 1. Cells, their roles, and potential targets in liver fibrosis. Liver disease is in most cases initiated by a noxa that leads to hepatocyte cell death. Cytokines secreted by immune and other cell types promote hepatocyte cell injury, i.e., the tumor necrosis factor (TNF) triggers apoptosis of hepatocytes. Hepatic collagen deposition by activated hepatic stellate cells is a hallmark of fibrosis and in part is facilitated by extracellular enzymes.

1.3. Current Clinical Trials on Liver Fibrosis

Nowadays, the treatment options for liver fibrosis remain scarce and the most efficient strategy remains to overcome the vicious circle of liver injury. This results in an eradication of viruses or weight reduction and dietary changes in NAFLD, in order to stop disease progression or in the ideal case, by inducing fibrosis regression [28–30]. Currently, three stage 3 clinical trials are ongoing, which will be ready in the next years. Importantly, none of these focus on the direct modification of the pathogenic mechanisms of fibrosis, but on other mechanistic links such as the cause for the underlying liver injury, signals from other organs, for instance, derived from the intestine (i.e., bile acids), or from immune cells, metabolic activation, or cell death. The cell death of hepatocytes represents a key mechanism for liver fibrosis [31]. The inhibition of cell death has emerged as a therapeutic strategy in the treatment of liver fibrosis [32]. The classical definition of cell death separates necrosis (uncontrolled death of cells, autolysis) from apoptosis (regulated cell death). However, it has become apparent that many types of necrosis in fact are specifically regulated, and the terms necroptosis, ferroptosis, or autophagy have been brought up [33]. However, a general inhibition of cell death might be problematic because apoptosis of HSC is also required in fibrosis regression [23,31]. Furthermore, cell death induction is also required to trigger the death of cancer cells. During oncogenesis, cancer cells can overcome apoptosis to escape from elimination by immune cells. Many candidate drugs have been developed to interfere with the development or progression of hepatic fibrogenesis (Table 1).

Table 1. Selected candidate drugs for treatment of hepatic injury and fibrosis.

Molecular Target	Compound	Effect
Apoptosis signal-regulating kinase 1 (ASK1)	Selonsertib (GS-4997)	oral bioavailable inhibitor of ASK1, thereby preventing the production of inflammatory and fibrotic acting cytokines
Hepatic metabolism	Obeticholic acid	synthetically modified bile acid and potent agonist of the farnesoid X nuclear receptor (FXR)
	Elafibranor	Orally administered drug acting on the 3 sub-types of PPAR (PPARα, PPARγ, PPARδ)
	Tropifexor	Investigational drug which acts as an agonist of the farnesoid X nuclear receptor (FXR)
	Cilofexor (GS-9674)	agonist of the farnesoid X nuclear receptor (FXR) which improves cholestasis and liver injury
	AKN-083	farnesoid X receptor (FXR) agonist
	INT-767	a dual agonist targeting the farnesoid X receptor (FXR) and the G protein-coupled bile acid receptor 1 (GPBAR1)
	Aramchol	An orally active fatty acid bile acid conjugate that inhibits stearoyl coenzyme A desaturase 1 (SCD1)
	Saroglitazar	Agonist of PPARα (and PPARγ)
	Lanifibranor	Orally administered drug acting on the 3 sub-types of PPAR (PPARα, PPARγ, PPARδ)
	Firsocostat (GS-0976)	Liver-targeted acetyl-CoA carboxylase (ACC) inhibitor
	PF-05221304	Liver-targeted acetyl-CoA carboxylase (ACC) inhibitor
Chemokine receptors	Cenicriviroc	blocks the chemokine receptors CC chemokine receptor 2 (CCR2) and CCR5
Caspases	Emricasan	Prevents cells death by inhibition of caspases
	VX-166	The drug has anti-apoptotic activity and prevents release of interleukins
	Nivocasan (GS-9450)	hepatoprotective activity preventing fibrosis and apoptosis
Fibroblast growth factor 21 (FGF21)	Pegbelfermin (BMS-986036)	PEGylated FGF21 analogue that improves metabolic parameters
Fibroblast growth factor 19 (FGF19)	Aldafermin (NGM282)	Synthetic FGF19 analogue preventing hepatic fat accumulation and liver damage
Glucagon-like peptide-1 receptor	Liraglutide	GLP-1 receptor agonist triggering insulin synthesis
	Semaglutide	GLP-1 receptor agonist triggering insulin synthesis

An ideal treatment strategy would be cell-type specific, and, in the case of targeting cell death, should be hepatocyte-specific. In line with these conclusions, the ASK1 inhibitor Selonsertib (GS-4997, Gilead), which has been studied in NASH patients in a stage 3 clinical trial (STELLAR 4) has not been successful. Selonsertib exerts its activity by inhibiting an important cell death switch of Apoptosis-signal-regulating kinase 1 (ASK1). ASK1 is induced by oxidative stress and enhances hepatocyte death, inflammation, and fibrosis [34]. However, there is still new hope from three other stage 3 clinical trials on liver fibrosis. Targeting another facet of the disease, two drugs target hepatic metabolism: the drug obeticholic acid (OCA) and Elafibranor (ELA). OCA is a synthetic lipophilic bile acid which is already approved for the treatment of primary biliary cholangitis (PBC). OCA acts via activating the nuclear bile acid receptor Farnesoid X receptor (FXR), and this in turn leads to a reduction of bile acids (which are produced in the liver and the small intestine. OCA is a semi-synthetic analogue of natural bile acids and exhibits a more than 100-fold increased stimulation of FXR compared to the natural bile acids. OCA leads to reduced bile acid production, and also to a reduction in the uptake of glucose and lipids from food [35]. This drug is currently tested in a huge phase III trial in NASH patients (REGENERATE). The drug ELA is an Insulin-sensitizer which aims to improve the action of natural insulin. ELA activates Peroxisome-proliferator-activated receptors (PPAR). The concept of ELA is to prevent fat deposition in hepatocytes and thereby steatosis, by removing glucose from circulation. It acts on (PPARα/δ R) via agonism. The phase III trial on NASH patients is performed by the company Genfit (RESOLVE-IT). There are also attempts to combine both OCA and ELA, which further improve liver histology in fibrosis models [36].

a high surface to volume ratio, meaning that the comparatively high surface can be functionalized with ligands. These ligands can change the pharmacokinetics of the particles, i.e., polyethylene glycol (PEG) can increase the circulation time of nanoparticles [58–60]. Specific ligands for cellular receptors can enable specific binding to specific cell types. Moreover, this valuable surface can be conjugated via drugs for their delivery and on-demand release [59,61], or with fluorescence marker and other molecules for multimodal imaging or therapy [62,63]. The prefix "magnetic" means that MNPs are sensitive to the magnetic field. This field brings numerous options that are attractive for biomedical applications since this field can easily penetrate the body and interact with MNPs, for example, for their detection, visualization, manipulation, or heating.

The magnetite Fe_3O_4 and magnetite γ-Fe_2O_3 are the most applicable magnetic materials in the biomedical field. Bulk magnetite has a cubic inverted spinel structure and exhibits a ferrimagnetic behavior at room temperature. The nano-sized magnetite oxidizes rapidly into maghemite, which also has similar ferrimagnetic properties and spinel structures with some valences. The iron oxide-based MNPs of a diameter (d) below 30 nm act in the SPM regime at room temperature and are abbreviated as SPIONs (superparamagnetic iron oxide nanoparticles) [53]. Particles sized less than 10 nm are usually attributed to ultra-small SPIONs (USPIONs [53]) and are characterized by reduced magnetization and increased anisotropy because of the influence of non-collinear spins at the surface [64,65]. The SPIONs and USPIONs are in the frame of interest for biomedical applications, especially for magnetic resonance imaging (MRI) where they are applied as contrast agents for both T1 and T2 relaxation times [66–68]. For specific applications, for instance, magnetic hyperthermia, the adjustable anisotropy of MNPs, is needed [69,70]. For this reason, magnetic anisotropy can be tuned, for instance, by variation of the chemical composition of ferrites ($Me^{2+}Fe_2O_4$) by doping the spinel structure of ferrite with the ions of transition metals (Me^{2+} = Co, Mn, Zn, and others [71].

2.1.1. Methods for Synthesis of Magnetic Nanomedicines

The various types of synthesis strategies for MNP can be separated into two approaches: top-down and bottom-up. The "bottom-up approach" starts from metal ions in solution via chemical methods and is probably the most commonly used strategy. The top-down approach starts with bulk material, which is further processed, i.e., by laser ablation [72–76] or lithography [77–79] including that of nanospheres [80]. The lithography techniques have broad control on the shape of nano or microstructures; however, the scaling of this method to large-scale production was reported to be challenging [81]. The laser ablation method offers the building of quite complicated structures such as core-shell MNPs and has a lot of degrees of freedom for adjustment by variation of the environment, material of target, laser regime, as well as external stimulus, for example, magnetic or electrical field to change the shape and structural properties of MNPs [72,75]. This method beats some drawbacks of more common chemical methods; for example, it does not require high temperature, pressure, or organometallic precursors to obtain MNPs with excellent magnetic properties [76,82]. Thus, the laser ablation method has great potential to set higher standards in nanoparticle production.

However, many methods are combinations of both types of methods. For example, the known ball milling method of the MNP preparation is popular for permanent magnet fabrication [83]. It allows one to scale up the synthesis to an industrial scale, although the control of particle shape and size is difficult. Potential agglomerations of nanoparticles can occur which makes the particles unsuitable for biomedical applications [83]. Nevertheless, in combination with chemistry, the ball milling equipment can be used in the so-called mechanochemical process. Here, for instance, a nanocomposite of MNPs in the benzene-1,3,5-tricarboxylic acid matrix was obtained via a mechanochemical process [84]. The obtained material was porous and defined as a metal-organic framework. This nanocomposite was tested for a drug delivery application to release doxorubicin as a model drug. The authors noted that the high surface area of such porous materials favors an increased loading rate, while the magnetic properties of this material offer novel perspectives for diagnostic systems [84].

Typical synthesis steps of chemical methods consist of different steps, particularly burst nucleation, and the following nanocrystal grow, which is called Ostwald ripening [85,86]. Control of reaction kinetics by varying temperature, solvent or other conditions, and operation with the Ostwald process by pH control and electrostatic repulsion of nuclei allow us to systematically vary the size of the particles [86]. It is of utmost importance to obtain nanoparticles with precise and predefined size, shape, and phase composition [87,88]. It was suggested to evaluate the most commonly used synthesis strategies by the four-word strengths, weaknesses, opportunities, and threats (SWOT) analysis for applications in molecular recognition [88]. The research group evaluated the co-precipitation, thermal decomposition (HTD), microemulsion, and microfluidic synthesis method and studied dual-particles consisting of several materials. The first one, co-precipitation, is an easy to use technique to obtain large amounts of MNPs by alkalization of metal salt solutions. First demonstrated in 1981 by Massart, this method is beneficial and allows us to produce well-crystallized iron oxide or ferrite MNPs in the size range of 10–30 nm [89–91]. The drawbacks of this method are the poor control of shape and size distribution; moreover, for smaller particles, less than 10 nm, the quality of crystals decreases and the number of disordered spins leads to a change in the magnetic properties [64,92]. Advanced co-precipitation methods are performed at high temperature and pressure, by hydrothermal surface treatment, or hydrothermal routes [93–95], as well as in non-aqueous medium by solvothermal methods [96–98]. The polyol process is another interesting method which is a cost-effective and easily scalable method to produce MNPs of high quality and variety morphology, from simple pseudo-spherical to multi-core nanoflowers of core-shell MNPs [99–101]. In the polyol process, solvents also play the role of a reducing agent and a surfactant.

Invented in 2004 for the synthesis of MNPs, the HTD method allows us to obtain MNPs with a narrow size distribution and high crystallinity [102–104]. MNPs produced with this method have a high value of magnetization, favoring their use in many biological applications, including sensors and detection [92,105]. According to the SWOT analysis above described [88], a drawback of this method is that it is time consuming and expensive. Precise shape control can be achieved by varying the experimental conditions. For instance, a variation of ligands and surfactants offers advantages for both magnetic properties and the related behavior in biological environments [87,106,107]. The group of Jinwoo Cheon [108] demonstrated higher magnetization values of cubic MNPs (165 emu/g_{Fe+Zn}) compared to spherical (145 emu/g_{Fe+Zn}) particles. The difference can be attributed to the lower amount of disordered spins on the surface. It was also reported that cubic shaped MNPs on the sensor's surface exhibit a higher binding ability because of the higher contact area of planar interface compared to the spherical one [106]. Furthermore, cubic MNPs exhibited stronger signals, as evaluated by giant magnetoresistive sensing (GMR) and force-induced remnant magnetization spectroscopy (FIRMS).

There are various methods for co-precipitation with different modifications, which, together with HTD, are the most frequently used methods for MNP synthesis [60,88]. Co-precipitation represents the most important production method. it is easy, cheap, and enables a rapid synthesis. The generated particles have hydrophilic surfaces, which can be functionalized in situ. The second most important method, HTD, allows one to produce MNPs with well-defined shape and narrow size distribution. However, the low amount of reaction products, high-cost reagents, and hydrophobic surfaces, which can be functionalized in the multi-step process, make this method currently mostly interesting only for research activity.

2.1.2. Clinical Use and Further Perspectives Iron Oxide

Currently, Feraheme® (ferumoxytol) which is approved by the U.S. Food and Drug Administration (FDA) as well as in Europe and Canada is the most successful iron oxide-based drug. It is prescribed to patients with iron deficiency anemia and chronic kidney disease. It can be considered as a great advantage that iron is a naturally occurring element of the body which also leaves the body via natural pathways of iron metabolism [109]. Feraheme is based on non-stoichiometric magnetite MNPs with diameter (d) ~ 7 nm and hydrodynamic diameter (d_H) = 28–33 nm coated with carboxy-dextran [66].

Feraheme is also an 'off label' magnetic resonance angiography (MRA) and magnetic resonance imaging (MRI) contrast agent [66,110]. In order to study MNP uptake by macrophages in vivo, high-resolution 3D-maps of pancreatic inflammation were generated using MRI and it showed that the MNP uptake by macrophages was higher in the inflamed pancreatic lesion in T1D-models [111]. Therefore, the special properties of the inflammatory setting on noninvasive imaging have to be considered. The capability of iron oxide to produce reactive oxygen species (ROS) was recently discovered to be usable in order to treat leukaemia [112]. In contrast to intravenously administrated drugs, the oral delivery (OD) is more popular with patients. Yet, the passage of the gastrointestinal (GI) tract, which has a very low pH level, [113] is a problem for iron oxides since they degrade at this pH. Thus, to overcome this limitation, a coating is required which is stable in the wide pH range of 2–8. Coatings such as gold or silica oxide are applicable for this purpose since these materials are stable in the GI tract.

Mesenchymal stem cells (MSC) have been demonstrated to be a promising tool for the treatment of many types of human diseases, including liver fibrosis and hepatocellular carcinoma (HCC) [114–118]. Labeling of MCS with MNPs can be used as a supplementary diagnostic approach. Recently, Faidah at al., proved that application of MNPs have not changed the viability and proliferative capabilities of MSCs in a rat cirrhosis model based on a carbon tetrachloride (CCl_4) model for toxic liver injury [119]. Additionally, similar results by Lai and co-authors have shown that MSCs that overexpress human hepatocyte growth factor (HGF) promote liver recovery in a rat liver fibrosis model [120]. Further, labeling of MSC with NP led to an accumulation of the cells in MRI-based imaging [119,120], which seems to confirm the idea that magnetic NPs in liver fibrosis can be used as a diagnostic agent for MRI.

The off-label use of feraheme is continuing to grow. The assessment of the stage of liver fibrosis remains a key issue in patient diagnostics. Currently, the gold standard is still given by a liver biopsy while imaging techniques as elastography and relaxometry have not been elaborated in this regard, particularly, for proving moderate fibrosis [121]. A recent study showed that patients with different stages of liver fibrosis exhibited MRI-assessible differences. One should, however, be aware that T2 parameters can be quantified via a dual echo turbo-spin echo technique. Besides, these applications can also help to understand different stages of fibrosis patients [121]. It is noticeable that T2 or negative contrast agents possess superparamagnetic properties and are represented by nanoparticles with iron oxide core or other magnetic materials [122]. For this purpose, researchers are using different types of synthesis, shapes and covering of nanoparticles with magnetic cores. One should, nevertheless, consider the associated problems from another perspective: Li and coworkers proposed to conjugate Fe_3O_4 NPs with immunofluorescence markers (indocyanine green (ICG). Further, a targeting ligand for integrin avb3, arginine–glycine–aspartic acid (RGD) expressed by HSCs to detect early stages of liver fibrosis, was used [123]. A similar approach was used by Zhang and coauthors, who investigated diagnostic of liver fibrosis stages in a rat model induced by CCl_4 injection. Although they were using molecular MRI with RGD peptide, modified ultrasmall superparamagnetic iron oxide nanoparticles (USPIO) were demonstrated to be a promising tool for noninvasive imaging of the progression of the liver fibrosis [124].

Furthermore, one should note that together with the advantageous properties of magnetic materials which makes them usable as MRI contrast agents, the iron overload in tissues can be really harmful. Thus, Wei and coauthors reported that a single dose of MNP application at a high concentration (5 mg Fe/kg) induced a septic shock response at 24 h and provoked high levels of serum markers (ALT, AST, cholesterol and other markers), which was noted within 14 days. Moreover, a high dose of MNPs activated significant expression changes of a distinct subset of genes in cirrhosis liver compared with a normal dose of MNP application (0.5 mg Fe/kg) [125]. Furthermore, Lunov et. al. analyzed the impact of MNPs on macrophages and demonstrated that overload of iron leads to apoptosis in these cells, which is mediated via activation of the c-Jun N-terminal kinase (JNK) pathway [126]. This investigation demonstrated that iron overload caused by MNP application may have dramatic effects, particularly on the liver, which contains a large numbers of macrophages.

2.1.3. Magnetic Hybrid Nanomaterials

Iron oxides exhibit moderate cytotoxicity; however, for their use in biomedicine, such aspects as biotransformation, biodistribution and in-blood circulating time should be controlled [60,127]. Because of this reason, the iron oxide MNPs can be hybridized, i.e., with certain polymers (dextran, chitosan, PEG) [128], noble metals (Au, Ag) [129,130], non-magnetic oxides (MgO, ZnO) [131,132], or silica dioxide (SiO_2) [133]. Apart from polysaccharides, PEG is more often used for organic coating of MNPs. By varying the molecular weight of the PEG from 6000 to 50,000, it is possible to prolong the circulation time (blood half-life) from 30 min to one day [134]. The coating leads to a change in the surface charge of MNPs and, therefore, also significantly affects the pharmacokinetic behavior [60]. Typically, the negatively charged MNPs exhibit a longer blood half-life [60]. The coating also makes it easier to modify the surface for modifications with biomolecules, genes, or drugs. Furthermore, hybrid materials possess additional functionalities, for instance, nano-dimensional gold exhibits the surface plasmon resonance phenomenon changing the optical properties of the material, which can be exploited for the detection in photothermal therapy [129,135,136]. Maria Efremova and her colleagues reported on nanohybrids of magnetite and gold in the form of Janus-like MNPs [129]. Two district surfaces established a platform for conjugation with two different molecules, for example, with fluorescent dyes or drugs. These nanohybrids exhibited enhanced contrast for MRI and allowed tracking delivery of the attached drug in a real-time fashion via intravital fluorescent microscopy.

Lipid-based nanomedicines represent the nanomedicines with the highest market value. Via a combination of SPIONs embedded into the lipid membrane of liposomes, the desired properties of both materials can be combined. One example of an application with magnetoliposomes is the application of a magnetic field to induce release of nucleic acids, such as DNA, which might be useful in drug release. Salvatore et al. demonstrated that SPIONs can trigger release of DNA from a multifunctional hybrid nanomaterial composed of liposome components, double-stranded DNA, and hydrophobic SPIONs [137].

There is a huge and virtually an endless number of options for hybrid nanomaterials and we only shed light on these. Their numbers are very likely to further increase in future nanomedicines.

2.2. *Magnetic Materials in Drug Delivery*

2.2.1. Magnetic-Assisted Medical Applications

The size of nanomaterials is a critical factor for their behavior and distribution in the body. Small particles in the blood tend to aggregate or to be decorated with a protein corona and, because of their charge, create an electrical double layer. In this sense, the total size of particles characterized by the hydrodynamic diameter (d_H) can be measured i.e., using dynamic light scattering (DLS) [138]. Both the hydrodynamic and physical size of MNPs determine their magnetic properties. In circulation, systemically injected MNPs circulate in the lumen of blood vessels, interacting with macrophages of the reticuloendothelial system (RES). Smaller USPIONs with $d_H > 10$ nm were characterized by longer blood half-life than SPIONs $d_H > 50$ nm [66,134]. Depending on the hydrodynamic size as well as the electrical charge and other properties, pharmacokinetics and biodistribution of MNPs are rendered [60,139]. MNPs with a d_H below than 15 nm are filtered by the kidney; MNPs with a d_H less than 100 nm accumulate in the liver in hepatocytes and Disse space; a d_H of 100–150 nm leads to the primary accumulation in liver that is based on the uptake by Kupffer cells and these larger hydrodynamic particles can also be trapped by splenic macrophages.

Since the liver and spleen are primary targets for MPN accumulation, they can also be targeted with these particles. The hydrodynamic size of 10–50 nm seems optimal for longer circulation time, but it should be stressed that not only size matters, but properties of the surface such as zeta-potential and hydrophilic/hydrophobic properties are critical factors for biodistribution [60,134]. Non-specific biodistribution of MNPs was used for MRI enhancement of liver disease [139,140]. Ferrucci and Starkre reported that 80% of intravenously injected non-specific SPIONs were internalized by Kupffer cells. Thereby, the MNPs create an MR-contrast that enables us to trace hepatic neoplasms [140].

We would like to highlight four non-exhaustive areas in which magnetic materials are important (Table 2). The first area includes the biggest success story for using magnetic fields for binding-mediated cell capturing. The chimeric antigen receptor (CAR) T cells have significantly advanced tumor therapies. This technology is based on the isolation of T cells from autologous donors and these cells are genetically engineered to target a specific antigen. The isolation of T cells is currently approved for treatment of B cell lymphoma, and it is expected that T cell engineering will enrich many other fields as well; clinical studies are ongoing in liver cancer. The group of Michael Sadelain pioneered T cell engineering and they have recently shown that macrophages play a key role in mediating the side effects of CAR T cell therapy [141]. Other groups also attempt to manipulate other immune cells, such as natural killer cells [142]. Microfluidics that facilitate binding-mediated cell capturing and release is a key technology for sorting cells in closed systems [143–145]. The microfluidic concept for manufacturing lab-on-a-chip devices use MNPs and these allow for a quick analysis and an automated composition of an individual treatment. Currently, the CAR T cell therapies are mainly focused on B cell malignancies, but other types of cancer are being explored in clinical trials.

Tissue engineering has been given further opportunities by magnetic fields, i.e., by facilitating the arrangement of different cellular layers [146–148]. Magnetic fields have been used to establish three-dimenstional cell culture arrays, to enable cell patterning for the evaluation of the effect of fibroblasts on their capability of infiltration [149–151]. Rieck et al. recently demonstrated that magnetic nanocarriers can be localized in specific areas of the body using magnetic fields. Their approach was done using complexes of lentivirus and MNPs in combination with magnetic fields. The group highlighted that using this method in the murine embryonic stem cell system offers the opportunity to site-specifically downregulate protein tyrosine phosphatase SHP2 by RNAi technology in selected areas with the pathogenic vessel formation [152]. Using this principle would allow us to selectively transmit a specific payload to immune cells based on phagocytic uptake to diseased sites in the liver. Muthana et al. demonstrated that even magnetic resonance imaging machines might be usable to control the spatial concentration of MNPs [153].

The second field of application that we would like to emphasize is mechanical cell control. Here, the aim is to get control over the mechanical properties of cells. In the near future, the technology may be used to measure the stiffness of biological molecules or cellular organelles in vivo. Magnetic tweezers are used as a simple tool to study mechanical forces of biological molecules and cells [154]. Low-frequency magnetic fields are applicable for directed cell destruction and induction of apoptosis [78,155,156]. The concept of mechanical cell control has already been used to function as a cellular remote control, to modulate the stem cells differentiation, or to modulate the behavior of single cells [157–159]. Magnetic micromanipulation based on the application of magnetic tweezers is a potent biophysical technique that is applicable for single-molecule unfolding, rheology measurements, and analyses of force-regulated processes in living cells [160,161].

The third type of application is drug delivery. MNPs are a powerful tool for therapy to target killing of injured or infected cells, which may be achieved by, for example, native toxicity of the MNPs, thermomagnetic effect in magnetic hyperthermia, or targeted drug delivery and release [135,162,163]. In particular, the field of drug delivery can potentially be highly enriched by magnetism-based applications. In addition to the above-mentioned application of MRI scanners to spatially concentrate magnetic particles, magnetic fluids, meaning magnetic particles in a dispersion, might be controlled magnetically. The release of drugs, for example, mediated by magnetism-enhanced thermosensitive polymers, might also be enriched by magnetic actions, for example, to trigger the release of different drugs from a single carrier from porous materials, remote-controlled drug release using azo-functionalized iron oxide nanoparticles, or in order to trigger heat and drug release from magnetically controlled nanocarriers [133,164,165]. In addition to particulate or crystal-based systems, surface immobilized iron might be controlled using noninvasive magnetic stimulation [166–169].

The fourth area in which magnetism has been used intensively is applications based on imaging. For instance, MRI-based imaging of liver fibrosis can be enabled by visualizing fibrosis based on non-invasive analysis of collagen or elastin. Fibrosis might even be visualized by labeling HSC, i.e., by monitoring a specific surface marker such as the folate-receptor, that has already been used for this purpose. Folate receptor-targeted particles have also led to improved specificity of tissue binding [66,124,170]. In order to enable an early therapy of fibrosis, it is critical that it is also diagnosed at early stages. However, there is currently no established early stage marker. In the future, improved early recognition techniques such as circulating collagen fragments, i.e., the N-terminal propeptide of collagen III (Pro-C3) will very likely enable to perform "liquid biopsies" for early detection of fibrosis. Screening of Pro-C3 in plasma of patients has already been done in hepatitis C patients and has been demonstrated to be able to predict fibrosis progression [171]. Other biomarkers might be circulating micro-RNA, and other types of RNA, such as long non-coding RNA (LncRNA), epigenetic analyses, and microbiome studies. Usually, biomarkers work best if they are combined to calculate a specific score such as the NAFLD fibrosis score, the fibrosis 4 (FIB-4) index, or the aspartate aminotransferase to platelet ratio index (APRI) score.

Non-invasive imaging techniques have high potential to confirm the findings from biomarker screening. Consequently, there is a high unmet need for the development of improved techniques for non-invasive diagnosis of liver fibrosis [116]. In ref. [116], the molecular MRI was used for distinguishing different fibrosis stages in a CCl_4-based rat model. Enhanced accuracy of detection was achieved by using a targeted USPIO-based contrast agent for MRI. The MRI contrast depends on the time of relaxation of protons that alters in the presence of a magnetic field generated by MNPs and it depends on the degree of interaction of the MNPs with protons. Furthermore, direct imaging of the distribution of MNPs is possible by magnetic particle imaging (MPI) introduced in 2005 and based on measurements of the nonlinear magnetic signal of MNPs [172,173]. Potentially, MPI can enable an improved spatial and temporal resolution than the resolution of the MRI and because of the native biodistribution of iron oxide-based MNPs, the use of this technique for liver seems promising. Improved detection methodologies may also further improve the usage of magnetic particles as biosensors [174]. Imaging probes such as those monitoring Elastin will very likely also improve imaging of liver fibrosis at later stages of the disease, as Elastin appears in late-stage fibrosis [175] (Table 2).

The tripeptide arginine-glycine-aspartic acid (RGD) binds to integrin $\alpha v\beta 3$ expressed on HSCs [124]. Conjugation with RGD significantly improved targeting of administrated USPIONs [124]. This allowed authors of ref. [124] to differentiate various liver fibrosis stages with MRI. The relaxivity of developed nanoparticles was higher than, for example, the earlier reported collagen-specific contrast agent based on Gd^{3+}. Further improvement was done by multimodal imaging with nanohybrids [123]. In this study, it was suggested that the conjugation of USPIONs-SiO_2 with indocyanine green (ICG) dye may further improve near-infrared fluorescence imaging and RGD for targeting. This combination of imaging modalities enables it to perform multimodal imaging (NIR and MRI). To establish theranostic platforms, an additional drug should be attached [176,177].

In order to further visualize some selected applications of magnetic fields, we have illustrated these with a sketch. In particular, cell sorting technology which is currently enabling breakthroughs in cancer therapy is largely based on magnetic forces to sort cells, i.e., the magnetic-assisted cell sorting technology (MACS). These technologies are based on magnetic fields and enable sorting and manipulate cells in closed systems. Mechanical cell control is still in its infancy, but may significantly enrich single cell analysis methods. The field of drug delivery may assumingly expect high potential for breakthroughs due to the potential localized targeting of tissues or cells in vivo, to reduce side effects on non-target cells with enhanced specificity. Imaging applications are already profiting from steadily improved probes, improved methods for signal detection, and better biological targets. In fibrosis imaging, non-invasive assessment of Collagen and Elastin might in future enable significantly improved and more specific assessment of liver fibrosis (Figure 2).

Table 2. Selected areas of applications for magnetic nanoparticles.

Role of MNP [1]	Area of Biomedical Application	Literature
Binding-mediated cell capturing	Cell isolation and separation	[141,143–145]
	Cell and tissue engineering	[146–148]
	Cell patterning and concentration	[149–153]
Mechanical cell control	Low-frequency magnetic field for cell destruction and induction of apoptosis	[78,155,156]
	Differentiation of stem cells, modulation of cell division and motility	[157–159]
	Fundamental study of macromolecules and cell's mechanical properties	[160,161]
Drug delivery	Magnetic fluid hyperthermia of cancer	[135,162,163]
	On-demand release of drugs via thermosensitive polymers or azo molecules from hybrid nanoplatforms	[133,164,165]
	Targeting or delivery of drug or genes immobilized on surfaces	[166–169]
Imaging applications	Reduction of T_1 and T_2 relaxation time of the water protons for the MRI-contrast	[66,124,170]
	Imaging and detection via a non-linear magnetic signal	[172,173]
	Improved detection of magnetic signals, imaging of liver fibrosis	[174,175]

[1] MNP: Magnetic nanoparticle(s).

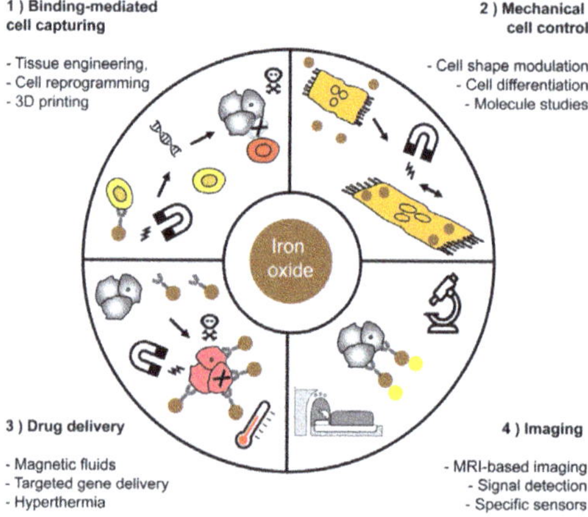

Figure 2. Applications of magnetic nanoparticles in medicine and biotechnology. We would like to highlight four main fields of application for magnetic materials and have chosen some representative schemes for each field of application.

2.2.2. Selective Targeting of Hepatic Stellate Cells—Mission Impossible?

Cell type-specific treatment of disease was first proposed by Paul Ehrlich, who suggested the development of magic bullets which aim at the pathogens only [178]. Ehrlich assumed that people would in the near future be able to specifically target cells or tissues to cure disease with unmet specificity. However, such directed therapies for cancer have been challenged in the past with unexpected problems. One example of a company focusing on cell targeting is BIND therapeutics which went bankrupt in 2016 [179]. Through re-investments, its drug, encapsulated Docetaxel targeting the prostate-specific membrane antigen (PSA), has entered clinical testing again and is currently evaluated in a phase 2 trials in patients with metastatic castration-resistant prostate cancer [180]. It can be assumed that targeting liver fibrosis might face similar difficulties like cancer. However, without any doubt, HSCs as the key cells for fibrosis, represent an ideal target in this regard since they are the main source of activated myofibroblasts and portal fibroblasts that control the fibrogenic process [181].

However, reaching HSCs with drugs is intrinsically difficult since they are located in the perisinusoidal space between hepatocytes and sinusoidal endothelial cells. Under normal physiological conditions, one major function of qHSCs is a depository for vitamin A [182]. In response to liver damage, inflammatory mediators promote HSC activation and their subsequent differentiation into myofibroblasts [183]. Activated HSCs (aHSC) are the main source of collagen in the liver and can abundantly secrete ECM proteins, tissue inhibitors of metalloproteinases and matrix metalloproteinases (MMPs), which cause remodeling of the liver architecture [184]. It is important to note that HSCs are responsible for 80% of the total fibrillar collagen I in the fibrous liver [185]. Thus, inactivation or modulation of HSC is a one of the key aspects in the development of innovative fibrosis therapy.

HSC and MFB express/upregulate diverse specific receptors, such as the mannose-6-phosphate/insulin-like growth factor II receptor (M6P/IGFII) [186,187], PPAR [188], integrins [189], platelet-derived growth factor receptor (PDGFR) [181], or a peptide receptor of the relaxin 1 family (RXFP1) [182]. Various receptors of HSC have been engaged with specific drugs directed to these. The mannose 6-phosphate/Insulin-like growth factor receptor (M6P/IGFR) is among the most popular targeting structures for HSC. The strategy of eliminating the HSC was investigated in a study 2006 by Greupink et al., in which a nanocarrier consisting of human serum albumin (HSA) was used as a carrier, and functionalized with mannose-6-phosphate (M6P) for this purpose. In order to eliminate these cells, the authors employed doxorubicin, which is used in cancer therapy to kill tumor cells [190]. However, side effects were noted from using the M6P-directed carriers, and in search for a better target, researchers have turned towards PDGFβR since it was also observed that it is specifically upregulated in liver fibrosis [191]. It is known that interferon γ (IFNγ) has exhibited side effects when administered systemically. The research group of Klaas Poelstra therefore created a fusion protein composed of IFNγ and PDGFβR bicyclic peptide. These fusion proteins were demonstrated to inhibit liver fibrogenesis in vivo, based on a significant increase in pSTAT1α activation, compared to the single unit of the fusion protein [192]. A drawback of these fusion proteins is their limited bioavailability, and therefore, a strategy to deposit them in the body is desirable. Van Dijk et al. thus developed biodegradable polymeric microspheres for the sustained release of such protein-based drugs [193].

Integrins have also been explored as potential targeting moieties in this regard. Integrins fulfil important roles by connecting the intracellular cytoskeleton of cells to the ECM. Many integrins were reported to activate the transforming growth factor β (TGF-β), which is another critical factor in fibrogenesis [194]. However, direct inhibition of TGF-β is critical since it is involved in many anti-inflammatory processes. Thus, integrin targeting is in fact a type of indirect targeting of TGF-β. This was pioneered by Henderson et al. in 2013, showing that the pharmacological inhibition of αv integrins by a small molecule (CWHM-12) attenuated both liver and lung fibrosis [195]. Bansal and colleagues, in 2017, further explored the role of integrins in liver fibrosis. They observed that integrin α 11 (IαV) is critically involved in the regulation of the myofibroblast phenotype and that is colocalizes with α-smooth muscle actin-positive myofibroblasts. They further assumed that IαV apparently is involved in fibrogenic signaling and might act downstream of the hedgehog signaling pathway [196]. However, a drawback of integrin targeting is that integrins are important for many vital functions in the body. A scheme for several different ligands to target HSC receptors has been generated (Figure 3).

The hormone relaxin represents a potential anti-fibrotic ligand which binds to its receptor on HSC [197]. One of the important effects of relaxin is the widespread remodeling of the extracellular matrix, which includes altered secretion and degradation of its components [188]. The role of relaxin as an anti-fibrotic agent has been demonstrated in experiments on genetically engineered mice that are deficient in the relaxin gene. These mice spontaneously developed age-related fibrosis of the lungs, heart, skin, and kidneys [198]. It turned out that relaxin also affects the processes of fibrogenesis in the liver. Treatment with relaxin in rats caused acute changes in the microcirculation of the liver [198], and morphological changes were found in non-parenchymal sinusoidal cells [199]. The effects of relaxin were mediated by activation of the receptor for the peptide 1 family of relaxins (RXFP1), which is expressed predominantly in HSC in the liver [197]. Finally, using an in vivo model of experimental liver fibrosis, it was shown that relaxin prevented the content of liver collagen and was effective in treating established liver fibrosis [200]. Thus, relaxin has established itself as an active therapeutic agent in the treatment of liver fibrosis. However, free relaxin has a very short half-life due to its small size (6 kDa) and rapid renal clearance [201]. Frequent administration of relaxin in chronic fibrosis increases systemic vasodilation, which adversely affects the general condition of the body [199].

When studying the effects of relaxin on fibrosis, it was shown that relaxin conjugated nanoparticles significantly inhibited differentiation, TGF-β-induced migration, and contractile ability of human HSC in contrast to the control, where free relaxin was used; in addition, they drastically reduced collagen gel contraction with maximum inhibitory effects [176].

The evolving and expanding field of RNA technologies has a huge potential to bring up novel drugs. Recently, the first siRNA-based drug, Patisiran, was approved [202]. In the area of liver fibrosis research, Bangen and colleagues demonstrated that inhibiting the cell cycle protein cyclin E1 during liver fibrosis progression in CCl_4-induced fibrosis significantly reduced disease severity [203]. RNA interference may also make use of nucleic acids to manipulate micro-RNA, which is known to also regulate the inflammatory processes in liver fibrosis [204]. Local release of therapeutic RNA might further improve efficiency of RNA interference technology.

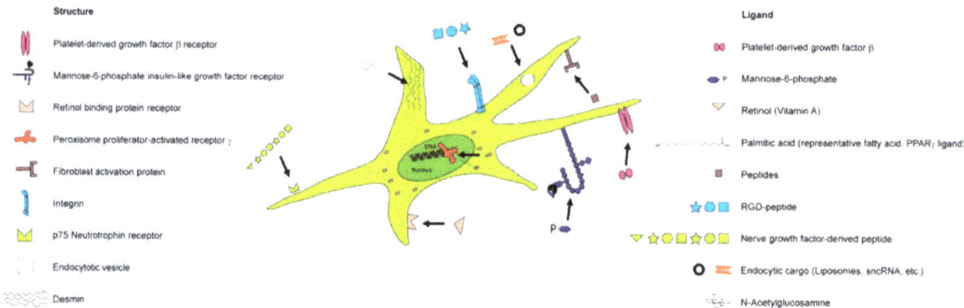

Figure 3. Ligand-based targeting of hepatic stellate cells. Hepatic stellate cells can be targeted based on their expression of receptors on their surface, in the cytoplasm, or inside the cell nucleus. The endocytic route allows the transport of HSC-directed sncRNA, small molecules, or liposomal carriers.

In conclusion, the path towards an efficient treatment of fibrosis remains a rocky road equipped with many pitfalls. However, the high number of drugs evaluated for novel therapies is encouraging. Targeted drugs that might be further improved by magnetism may represent anti-fibrotic drugs of the upcoming generations.

Author Contributions: Writing—original draft preparation, K.L., A.O. and M.B.; writing—review and editing, M.B., V.R., R.W.

Funding: Research in the group of M.B. was funded by the German Research Foundation (DFG), BA 6226/2-1 and the Wilhelm Sander Foundation (2018.129.1). R.W. is supported by the German Research Foundation (SFB/TRR57, projects P13 and Q3) and the Interdisciplinary Centre for Clinical Research (IZKF) within the Faculty of Medicine at the RWTH Aachen University (Project O3-1). K.L., A.O. and V.R., are supported by the Ministry of Education and Science of the Russian Federation in the framework of government assignment 3.4168.2017/4.6 and by the support of the 5 top 100 Russian Academic Excellence Project at the Immanuel Kant Baltic Federal University.

Conflicts of Interest: The authors declare no conflict of interest.

References

1. Hodgson, H.J. Basic and clinical aspects of liver growth: Prometheus revisited. Humphry Davy Rolleston Lecture 1992. *J. Roy. Coll. Phys. Lond.* **1993**, *27*, 278–283.
2. Zajicek, G.; Oren, R.; Weinreb, M., Jr. The streaming liver. *Liver* **1985**, *5*, 293–300. [CrossRef] [PubMed]
3. Van Dijk, F.; Teekamp, N.; Beljaars, L.; Post, E.; Schuppan, D.; Kim, Y.; Poelstra, K.; Frijlink, E.; Hinrichs, W.; Olinga, P. Towards clinical use of targeted therapies for liver fibrosis: Development of a sustained release formulation for therapeutic proteins. *J. Hepatol.* **2017**, *66*, S44. [CrossRef]
4. Lee, Y.A.; Wallace, M.C.; Friedman, S.L. Pathobiology of liver fibrosis: A translational success story. *Gut* **2015**, *64*, 830–841. [CrossRef] [PubMed]

5. Weiskirchen, R.; Tacke, F. Liver Fibrosis: From Pathogenesis to Novel Therapies. *Digest. Dis.* **2016**, *34*, 410–422. [CrossRef]
6. Pinzani, M. Pathophysiology of liver fibrosis. *Digest. Dis.* **2015**, *33*, 492–497. [CrossRef]
7. Schuppan, D. Liver fibrosis: Common mechanisms and antifibrotic therapies. *Clin. Res. Hepatol. Gastroenterol.* **2015**, *39*, S51–S59. [CrossRef]
8. Ng, M.; Fleming, T.; Robinson, M.; Thomson, B.; Graetz, N.; Margono, C.; Mullany, E.C.; Biryukov, S.; Abbafati, C.; Abera, S.F.; et al. Global, regional, and national prevalence of overweight and obesity in children and adults during 1980-2013: A systematic analysis for the Global Burden of Disease Study 2013. *Lancet* **2014**, *384*, 766–781. [CrossRef]
9. Dulai, P.S.; Singh, S.; Patel, J.; Soni, M.; Prokop, L.J.; Younossi, Z.; Sebastiani, G.; Ekstedt, M.; Hagstrom, H.; Nasr, P.; et al. Increased risk of mortality by fibrosis stage in nonalcoholic fatty liver disease: Systematic review and meta-analysis. *Hepatology* **2017**, *65*, 1557–1565. [CrossRef]
10. Siddiqui, M.S.; Harrison, S.A.; Abdelmalek, M.F.; Anstee, Q.M.; Bedossa, P.; Castera, L.; Dimick-Santos, L.; Friedman, S.L.; Greene, K.; Kleiner, D.E.; et al. Case definitions for inclusion and analysis of endpoints in clinical trials for nonalcoholic steatohepatitis through the lens of regulatory science. *Hepatology* **2018**, *67*, 2001–2012. [CrossRef]
11. Tapper, E.B.; Lok, A.S. Use of Liver Imaging and Biopsy in Clinical Practice. *N. Engl. J. Med.* **2017**, *377*, 756–768. [CrossRef] [PubMed]
12. Seki, E.; De Minicis, S.; Osterreicher, C.H.; Kluwe, J.; Osawa, Y.; Brenner, D.A.; Schwabe, R.F. TLR4 enhances TGF-beta signaling and hepatic fibrosis. *Nat. Med.* **2007**, *13*, 1324–1332. [CrossRef] [PubMed]
13. Xiao, Y.; Liu, R.; Li, X.; Gurley, E.C.; Hylemon, P.B.; Lu, Y.; Zhou, H.; Cai, W. Long Noncoding RNA H19 Contributes to Cholangiocyte Proliferation and Cholestatic Liver Fibrosis in Biliary Atresia. *Hepatology* **2019**. [CrossRef] [PubMed]
14. Sato, K.; Meng, F.; Giang, T.; Glaser, S.; Alpini, G. Mechanisms of cholangiocyte responses to injury. *Biochim. Biophys. Acta Mol. Basis Dis.* **2018**, *1864*, 1262–1269. [CrossRef]
15. Hargrove, L.; Kennedy, L.; Demieville, J.; Jones, H.; Meng, F.; DeMorrow, S.; Karstens, W.; Madeka, T.; Greene, J., Jr.; Francis, H. Bile duct ligation-induced biliary hyperplasia, hepatic injury, and fibrosis are reduced in mast cell-deficient Kit(W-sh) mice. *Hepatology* **2017**, *65*, 1991–2004. [CrossRef]
16. Bradding, P.; Pejler, G. The controversial role of mast cells in fibrosis. *Immunol. Rev.* **2018**, *282*, 198–231. [CrossRef]
17. Bartneck, M.; Ritz, T.; Keul, H.A.; Wambach, M.; Bornemann, J.; Gbureck, U.; Ehling, J.; Lammers, T.; Heymann, F.; Gassler, N.; et al. Peptide-functionalized gold nanorods increase liver injury in hepatitis. *ACS Nano* **2012**, *6*, 8767–8777. [CrossRef]
18. Kupffer, K.W.v. Über Sternzellen der Leber. Arch Mikroskop Anat., 1876; Volume 12, pp. 353–358. Available online: http://www.springerlink.com/index/F7X6532P76172836.pdf (accessed on 17 October 2019).
19. Metchnikof, E. Ueber die phagocytäre Rolle der Tuberkelriesenzellen. Archiv für pathologische Anatomie und Physiologie und für klinische Medecin, 1888; Volume 113, pp. 63–94. Available online: http://www.springerlink.com/index/70U3823357485325.pdf (accessed on 17 October 2019).
20. Krenkel, O.; Puengel, T.; Govaere, O.; Abdallah, A.T.; Mossanen, J.C.; Kohlhepp, M.; Liepelt, A.; Lefebvre, E.; Luedde, T.; Hellerbrand, C.; et al. Therapeutic inhibition of inflammatory monocyte recruitment reduces steatohepatitis and liver fibrosis. *Hepatology* **2018**, *67*, 1270–1283. [CrossRef]
21. Krenkel, O.; Hundertmark, J.; Ritz, T.P.; Weiskirchen, R.; Tacke, F. Single Cell RNA Sequencing Identifies Subsets of Hepatic Stellate Cells and Myofibroblasts in Liver Fibrosis. *Cells* **2019**, *8*, 503. [CrossRef]
22. Trautwein, C.; Friedman, S.L.; Schuppan, D.; Pinzani, M. Hepatic fibrosis: Concept to treatment. *J. Hepatol.* **2015**, *62*, S15–S24. [CrossRef]
23. Tsuchida, T.; Friedman, S.L. Mechanisms of hepatic stellate cell activation. *Nat. Rev. Gastroenterol. Hepatol.* **2017**, *14*, 397–411. [CrossRef] [PubMed]
24. Campana, L.; Iredale, J.P. Regression of Liver Fibrosis. *Semin. Liver Dis.* **2017**, *37*, 1–10. [PubMed]
25. Hutchinson, J.H.; Rowbottom, M.W.; Lonergan, D.; Darlington, J.; Prodanovich, P.; King, C.D.; Evans, J.F.; Bain, G. Small Molecule Lysyl Oxidase-like 2 (LOXL2) Inhibitors: The Identification of an Inhibitor Selective for LOXL2 over LOX. *ACS Med. Chem. Lett.* **2017**, *8*, 423–427. [CrossRef] [PubMed]

26. Bartneck, M.; Fech, V.; Ehling, J.; Govaere, O.; Warzecha, K.T.; Hittatiya, K.; Vucur, M.; Gautheron, J.; Luedde, T.; Trautwein, C.; et al. Histidine-rich glycoprotein promotes macrophage activation and inflammation in chronic liver disease. *Hepatology* **2016**, *63*, 1310–1324. [CrossRef] [PubMed]
27. Jun, J.I.; Lau, L.F. Resolution of organ fibrosis. *J. Clin. Invest.* **2018**, *128*, 97–107. [CrossRef] [PubMed]
28. Vilar-Gomez, E.; Martinez-Perez, Y.; Calzadilla-Bertot, L.; Torres-Gonzalez, A.; Gra-Oramas, B.; Gonzalez-Fabian, L.; Friedman, S.L.; Diago, M.; Romero-Gomez, M. Weight Loss Through Lifestyle Modification Significantly Reduces Features of Nonalcoholic Steatohepatitis. *Gastroenterology* **2015**, *149*, 367–378. [CrossRef] [PubMed]
29. Marcellin, P.; Gane, E.; Buti, M.; Afdhal, N.; Sievert, W.; Jacobson, I.M.; Washington, M.K.; Germanidis, G.; Flaherty, J.F.; Aguilar Schall, R.; et al. Regression of cirrhosis during treatment with tenofovir disoproxil fumarate for chronic hepatitis B: A 5-year open-label follow-up study. *Lancet* **2013**, *381*, 468–475. [CrossRef]
30. Ellis, E.L.; Mann, D.A. Clinical evidence for the regression of liver fibrosis. *J. Hepatol.* **2012**, *56*, 1171–1180. [CrossRef]
31. Luedde, T.; Kaplowitz, N.; Schwabe, R.F. Cell death and cell death responses in liver disease: Mechanisms and clinical relevance. *Gastroenterology* **2014**, *147*, 765–783. [CrossRef]
32. Wree, A.; Mehal, W.Z.; Feldstein, A.E. Targeting Cell Death and Sterile Inflammation Loop for the Treatment of Nonalcoholic Steatohepatitis. *Semin. Liver Dis.* **2016**, *36*, 27–36. [CrossRef]
33. Vanden Berghe, T.; Linkermann, A.; Jouan-Lanhouet, S.; Walczak, H.; Vandenabeele, P. Regulated necrosis: The expanding network of non-apoptotic cell death pathways. *Nat. Rev. Mol. Cell Biol.* **2014**, *15*, 135–147. [CrossRef] [PubMed]
34. Loomba, R.; Lawitz, E.; Mantry, P.S.; Jayakumar, S.; Caldwell, S.H.; Arnold, H.; Diehl, A.M.; Djedjos, C.S.; Han, L.; Myers, R.P.; et al. The ASK1 inhibitor selonsertib in patients with nonalcoholic steatohepatitis: A randomized, phase 2 trial. *Hepatology* **2018**, *67*, 549–559. [CrossRef] [PubMed]
35. Fickert, P.; Fuchsbichler, A.; Moustafa, T.; Wagner, M.; Zollner, G.; Halilbasic, E.; Stoger, U.; Arrese, M.; Pizarro, M.; Solis, N.; et al. Farnesoid X receptor critically determines the fibrotic response in mice but is expressed to a low extent in human hepatic stellate cells and periductal myofibroblasts. *Am. J. Pathol.* **2009**, *175*, 2392–2405. [CrossRef] [PubMed]
36. Roth, J.D.; Veidal, S.S.; Fensholdt, L.K.D.; Rigbolt, K.T.G.; Papazyan, R.; Nielsen, J.C.; Feigh, M.; Vrang, N.; Young, M.; Jelsing, J.; et al. Combined obeticholic acid and elafibranor treatment promotes additive liver histological improvements in a diet-induced ob/ob mouse model of biopsy-confirmed NASH. *Sci. Rep.* **2019**, *9*, 9046. [CrossRef]
37. Lefebvre, E.; Moyle, G.; Reshef, R.; Richman, L.P.; Thompson, M.; Hong, F.; Chou, H.L.; Hashiguchi, T.; Plato, C.; Poulin, D.; et al. Antifibrotic Effects of the Dual CCR2/CCR5 Antagonist Cenicriviroc in Animal Models of Liver and Kidney Fibrosis. *PLoS ONE* **2016**, *11*, e0158156. [CrossRef]
38. Friedman, S.; Sanyal, A.; Goodman, Z.; Lefebvre, E.; Gottwald, M.; Fischer, L.; Ratziu, V. Efficacy and safety study of cenicriviroc for the treatment of non-alcoholic steatohepatitis in adult subjects with liver fibrosis: CENTAUR Phase 2b study design. *Contemp. Clin. Trials* **2016**, *47*, 356–365. [CrossRef]
39. Fisher, F.M.; Chui, P.C.; Nasser, I.A.; Popov, Y.; Cunniff, J.C.; Lundasen, T.; Kharitonenkov, A.; Schuppan, D.; Flier, J.S.; Maratos-Flier, E. Fibroblast growth factor 21 limits lipotoxicity by promoting hepatic fatty acid activation in mice on methionine and choline-deficient diets. *Gastroenterology* **2014**, *147*, 1073–1083. [CrossRef]
40. Armstrong, M.J.; Gaunt, P.; Aithal, G.P.; Barton, D.; Hull, D.; Parker, R.; Hazlehurst, J.M.; Guo, K.; Abouda, G.; Aldersley, M.A.; et al. Liraglutide safety and efficacy in patients with non-alcoholic steatohepatitis (LEAN): A multicentre, double-blind, randomised, placebo-controlled phase 2 study. *Lancet* **2016**, *387*, 679–690. [CrossRef]
41. Stiede, K.; Miao, W.; Blanchette, H.S.; Beysen, C.; Harriman, G.; Harwood, H.J., Jr.; Kelley, H.; Kapeller, R.; Schmalbach, T.; Westlin, W.F. Acetyl-coenzyme A carboxylase inhibition reduces de novo lipogenesis in overweight male subjects: A randomized, double-blind, crossover study. *Hepatology* **2017**, *66*, 324–334. [CrossRef]
42. Harrison, S.A.; Rinella, M.E.; Abdelmalek, M.F.; Trotter, J.F.; Paredes, A.H.; Arnold, H.L.; Kugelmas, M.; Bashir, M.R.; Jaros, M.J.; Ling, L.; et al. NGM282 for treatment of non-alcoholic steatohepatitis: A multicentre, randomised, double-blind, placebo-controlled, phase 2 trial. *Lancet* **2018**, *391*, 1174–1185. [CrossRef]
43. Gubin, S.P.; Koksharov, Y.A.; Khomutov, G.; Yurkov, G.Y. Magnetic nanoparticles: Preparation, structure and properties. *Russ. Chem. Rev.* **2005**, *74*, 489. [CrossRef]
44. Krishnan, K.M. *Fundamentals and Applications of Magnetic Materials*; Oxford University Press: Oxford, UK, 2016.

45. Cullity, B.D.; Graham, C.D. *Introduction to Magnetic Materials*; John Wiley & Sons: Hoboken, NJ, USA, 2011.
46. Peddis, D.; Jönsson, P.E.; Laureti, S.; Varvaro, G. Magnetic interactions: A tool to modify the magnetic properties of materials based on nanoparticles. In *Frontiers of Nanoscience*; Elsevier: Amsterdam, The Netherlands, 2014; pp. 129–188.
47. Liu, J.P.; Fullerton, E.; Gutfleisch, O.; Sellmyer, D.J. *Nanoscale Magnetic Materials and Applications*; Springer: Berlin, Germany, 2009.
48. Pankhurst, Q.; Thanh, N.; Jones, S.; Dobson, J. Progress in applications of magnetic nanoparticles in biomedicine. *J. Phys. D Appl. Phys.* **2009**, *42*, 224001. [CrossRef]
49. Pankhurst, Q.A.; Connolly, J.; Jones, S.; Dobson, J. Applications of magnetic nanoparticles in biomedicine. *J. Phys. D Appl. Phys.* **2003**, *36*, R167. [CrossRef]
50. De Crozals, G.; Bonnet, R.; Farre, C.; Chaix, C. Nanoparticles with multiple properties for biomedical applications: A strategic guide. *Nano Today* **2016**, *11*, 435–463. [CrossRef]
51. Stoner, E.C.; Wohlfarth, E. A mechanism of magnetic hysteresis in heterogeneous alloys. *Philos. Trans. R. Soc. Lond. Ser. A Math. Phys. Sci.* **1948**, *240*, 599–642. [CrossRef]
52. Dormann, J.L.; Fiorani, D.; Tronc, E. Magnetic relaxation in fine-particle systems. *Adv. Chem. Phys.* **1997**, *283*. [CrossRef]
53. Angelakeris, M. Magnetic nanoparticles: A multifunctional vehicle for modern theranostics. *Biochim. Biophys. Acta* **2017**, *1861*, 1642–1651. [CrossRef]
54. Knobel, M.; Nunes, W.; Socolovsky, L.; De Biasi, E.; Vargas, J.; Denardin, J. Superparamagnetism and other magnetic features in granular materials: A review on ideal and real systems. *J. Nanosci. Nanotechnol.* **2008**, *8*, 2836–2857. [CrossRef]
55. Di Corato, R.; Espinosa, A.; Lartigue, L.; Tharaud, M.; Chat, S.; Pellegrino, T.; Ménager, C.; Gazeau, F.; Wilhelm, C. Magnetic hyperthermia efficiency in the cellular environment for different nanoparticle designs. *Biomaterials* **2014**, *35*, 6400–6411. [CrossRef]
56. Bartneck, M. Immunomodulatory Nanomedicine. *Macromol. Biosci.* **2017**. Published online on 6 April. [CrossRef]
57. Salas, G.; Veintemillas-Verdaguer, S.; Morales, M.d.P. Relationship between physico-chemical properties of magnetic fluids and their heating capacity. *Int. J. Hyperthermia* **2013**, *29*, 768–776. [CrossRef] [PubMed]
58. Weissleder, R.; Bogdanov, A.; Neuwelt, E.A.; Papisov, M. Long-circulating iron oxides for MR imaging. *Adv. Drug Deliv. Rev.* **1995**, *16*, 321–334. [CrossRef]
59. Peer, D.; Karp, J.M.; Hong, S.; Farokhzad, O.C.; Margalit, R.; Langer, R. Nanocarriers as an emerging platform for cancer therapy. *Nat. Nanotechnol.* **2007**, *2*, 751. [CrossRef] [PubMed]
60. Arami, H.; Khandhar, A.; Liggitt, D.; Krishnan, K.M. In vivo delivery, pharmacokinetics, biodistribution and toxicity of iron oxide nanoparticles. *Chem. Soc. Rev.* **2015**, *44*, 8576–8607. [CrossRef] [PubMed]
61. Thomas, C.R.; Ferris, D.P.; Lee, J.-H.; Choi, E.; Cho, M.H.; Kim, E.S.; Stoddart, J.F.; Shin, J.-S.; Cheon, J.; Zink, J.I. Noninvasive remote-controlled release of drug molecules in vitro using magnetic actuation of mechanized nanoparticles. *J. Am. Chem. Soc.* **2010**, *132*, 10623–10625. [CrossRef] [PubMed]
62. Cheon, J.; Lee, J.-H. Synergistically integrated nanoparticles as multimodal probes for nanobiotechnology. *Acc. Chem. Res.* **2008**, *41*, 1630–1640. [CrossRef] [PubMed]
63. McCarthy, J.R.; Weissleder, R. Multifunctional magnetic nanoparticles for targeted imaging and therapy. *Adv. Drug Deliv. Rev.* **2008**, *60*, 1241–1251. [CrossRef]
64. Batlle, X.; Pérez, N.; Guardia, P.; Iglesias, O.; Labarta, A.; Bartolomé, F.; García, L.; Bartolomé, J.; Roca, A.; Morales, M. Magnetic nanoparticles with bulklike properties. *J. Appl. Phys.* **2011**, *109*, 07B524. [CrossRef]
65. Lacroix, L.-M.; Lachaize, S.; Falqui, A.; Blon, T.; Carrey, J.; Respaud, M.; Dumestre, F.; Amiens, C.; Margeat, O.; Chaudret, B. Ultrasmall iron nanoparticles: Effect of size reduction on anisotropy and magnetization. *J. Appl. Phys.* **2008**, *103*, 07D521. [CrossRef]
66. Iv, M.; Telischak, N.; Feng, D.; Holdsworth, S.J.; Yeom, K.W.; Daldrup-Link, H.E. Clinical applications of iron oxide nanoparticles for magnetic resonance imaging of brain tumors. *Nanomedicine* **2015**, *10*, 993–1018. [CrossRef]
67. Weissleder, R.; Elizondo, G.; Wittenberg, J.; Rabito, C.; Bengele, H.; Josephson, L. Ultrasmall superparamagnetic iron oxide: Characterization of a new class of contrast agents for MR imaging. *Radiology* **1990**, *175*, 489–493. [CrossRef] [PubMed]

68. Laurent, S.; Vander Elst, L.; Muller, R.N. Superparamagnetic iron oxide nanoparticles for MRI. In *The Chemistry of Contrast Agents in Medical Magmetic Resonance Imaging*; John Wiley & Sons, Ltd.: Hoboken, NJ, USA, 2013; pp. 427–447.
69. Morales, I.; Costo, R.; Mille, N.; Silva, G.B.d.; Carrey, J.; Hernando, A.; Presa, P.d.l. High Frequency Hysteresis Losses on γ-Fe2O3 and Fe3O4: Susceptibility as a Magnetic Stamp for Chain Formation. *Nanomaterials* **2018**, *8*, 970. [CrossRef]
70. Carrey, J.; Mehdaoui, B.; Respaud, M. Simple models for dynamic hysteresis loop calculations of magnetic single-domain nanoparticles: Application to magnetic hyperthermia optimization. *J. Appl. Phys.* **2011**, *109*, 083921. [CrossRef]
71. da Silva, F.; Depeyrot, J.; Campos, A.; Aquino, R.; Fiorani, D.; Peddis, D. Structural and Magnetic Properties of Spinel Ferrite Nanoparticles. *J. Nanosci. Nanotechnol.* **2019**, *19*, 4888–4902. [CrossRef] [PubMed]
72. Wagener, P.; Jakobi, J.; Rehbock, C.; Chakravadhanula, V.S.K.; Thede, C.; Wiedwald, U.; Bartsch, M.; Kienle, L.; Barcikowski, S. Solvent-surface interactions control the phase structure in laser-generated iron-gold core-shell nanoparticles. *Sci. Rep.* **2016**, *6*, 23352. [CrossRef] [PubMed]
73. Maneeratanasarn, P.; Khai, T.V.; Kim, S.Y.; Choi, B.G.; Shim, K.B. Synthesis of phase-controlled iron oxide nanoparticles by pulsed laser ablation in different liquid media. *Phys. Status Solidi A* **2013**, *210*, 563–569. [CrossRef]
74. Fazio, E.; Santoro, M.; Lentini, G.; Franco, D.; Guglielmino, S.P.P.; Neri, F. Iron oxide nanoparticles prepared by laser ablation: Synthesis, structural properties and antimicrobial activity. *Colloids Surf. A* **2016**, *490*, 98–103. [CrossRef]
75. Xiao, J.; Liu, P.; Wang, C.; Yang, G. External field-assisted laser ablation in liquid: An efficient strategy for nanocrystal synthesis and nanostructure assembly. *Prog. Mater. Sci.* **2017**, *87*, 140–220. [CrossRef]
76. Amendola, V.; Meneghetti, M.; Granozzi, G.; Agnoli, S.; Polizzi, S.; Riello, P.; Boscaini, A.; Anselmi, C.; Fracasso, G.; Colombatti, M. Top-down synthesis of multifunctional iron oxide nanoparticles for macrophage labelling and manipulation. *J. Mater. Chem.* **2011**, *21*, 3803–3813. [CrossRef]
77. Vitol, E.A.; Novosad, V.; Rozhkova, E.A. Microfabricated magnetic structures for future medicine: From sensors to cell actuators. *Nanomedicine* **2012**, *7*, 1611–1624. [CrossRef]
78. Kim, D.-H.; Rozhkova, E.A.; Ulasov, I.V.; Bader, S.D.; Rajh, T.; Lesniak, M.S.; Novosad, V. Biofunctionalized magnetic-vortex microdiscs for targeted cancer-cell destruction. *Nat. Mater.* **2010**, *9*, 165. [CrossRef] [PubMed]
79. Litvinov, J.; Nasrullah, A.; Sherlock, T.; Wang, Y.-J.; Ruchhoeft, P.; Willson, R.C. High-throughput top-down fabrication of uniform magnetic particles. *PLoS ONE* **2012**, *7*, e37440. [CrossRef] [PubMed]
80. Kosiorek, A.; Kandulski, W.; Glaczynska, H.; Giersig, M. Fabrication of nanoscale rings, dots, and rods by combining shadow nanosphere lithography and annealed polystyrene nanosphere masks. *Small* **2005**, *1*, 439–444. [CrossRef] [PubMed]
81. del Campo, A.; Arzt, E. Fabrication approaches for generating complex micro-and nanopatterns on polymeric surfaces. *Chem. Rev.* **2008**, *108*, 911–945. [CrossRef] [PubMed]
82. Svetlichnyi, V.; Shabalina, A.; Lapin, I.; Goncharova, D.; Velikanov, D.; Sokolov, A. Characterization and magnetic properties study for magnetite nanoparticles obtained by pulsed laser ablation in water. *Appl. Phys. A* **2017**, *123*, 763. [CrossRef]
83. Yue, M.; Zhang, X.; Liu, J.P. Fabrication of bulk nanostructured permanent magnets with high energy density: Challenges and approaches. *Nanoscale* **2017**, *9*, 3674–3697. [CrossRef] [PubMed]
84. Bellusci, M.; Guglielmi, P.; Masi, A.; Padella, F.; Singh, G.; Yaacoub, N.; Peddis, D.; Secci, D. Magnetic Metal–Organic Framework Composite by Fast and Facile Mechanochemical Process. *Inorg. Chem.* **2018**, *57*, 1806–1814. [CrossRef]
85. Thanh, N.T.; Maclean, N.; Mahiddine, S. Mechanisms of nucleation and growth of nanoparticles in solution. *Chem. Rev.* **2014**, *114*, 7610–7630. [CrossRef]
86. Vayssieres, L.; Chanéac, C.; Tronc, E.; Jolivet, J.P. Size tailoring of magnetite particles formed by aqueous precipitation: An example of thermodynamic stability of nanometric oxide particles. *J. Colloid Interface Sci.* **1998**, *205*, 205–212. [CrossRef]
87. Roca, A.G.; Gutierrez, L.; Gavilán, H.; Brollo, M.E.F.; Veintemillas-Verdaguer, S.; del Puerto Morales, M. Design strategies for shape-controlled magnetic iron oxide nanoparticles. *Adv. Drug Deliv. Rev.* **2018**, *138*, 68–104. [CrossRef]

88. Salvador, M.; Moyano, A.; Martínez-García, J.C.; Blanco-López, M.C.; Rivas, M. Synthesis of Superparamagnetic Iron Oxide Nanoparticles: SWOT Analysis Towards Their Conjugation to Biomolecules for Molecular Recognition Applications. *J. Nanosci. Nanotechnol.* **2019**, *19*, 4839–4856. [CrossRef] [PubMed]
89. Massart, R. Preparation of aqueous magnetic liquids in alkaline and acidic media. *IEEE Trans. Magn.* **1981**, *17*, 1247–1248. [CrossRef]
90. Daffé, N.; Choueikani, F.; Neveu, S.; Arrio, M.-A.; Juhin, A.; Ohresser, P.; Dupuis, V.; Sainctavit, P. Magnetic anisotropies and cationic distribution in CoFe2O4 nanoparticles prepared by co-precipitation route: Influence of particle size and stoichiometry. *J. Magn. Magn. Mater.* **2018**, *460*, 243–252. [CrossRef]
91. Yelenich, O.; Solopan, S.; Kolodiazhnyi, T.; Tykhonenko, Y.; Tovstolytkin, A.; Belous, A. Magnetic properties and AC losses in AFe2O4 (A= Mn, Co, Ni, Zn) nanoparticles synthesized from nonaqueous solution. *J. Chem.* **2015**, *2015*, 532198. [CrossRef]
92. Nedelkoski, Z.; Kepaptsoglou, D.; Lari, L.; Wen, T.; Booth, R.A.; Oberdick, S.D.; Galindo, P.L.; Ramasse, Q.M.; Evans, R.F.; Majetich, S. Origin of reduced magnetization and domain formation in small magnetite nanoparticles. *Sci. Rep.* **2017**, *7*, 45997. [CrossRef]
93. Jovanović, S.; Spreitzer, M.; Otoničar, M.; Jeon, J.-H.; Suvorov, D. pH control of magnetic properties in precipitation-hydrothermal-derived CoFe2O4. *J. Alloys Compd.* **2014**, *589*, 271–277. [CrossRef]
94. Gomes, J.d.A.; Sousa, M.H.; Tourinho, F.A.; Aquino, R.; da Silva, G.J.; Depeyrot, J.; Dubois, E.; Perzynski, R. Synthesis of core– shell ferrite nanoparticles for ferrofluids: Chemical and magnetic analysis. *J. Phys. Chem. C* **2008**, *112*, 6220–6227. [CrossRef]
95. Pilati, V.; Cabreira Gomes, R.; Gomide, G.; Coppola, P.; Silva, F.G.; Paula, F.b.L.; Perzynski, R.G.; Goya, G.F.; Aquino, R.; Depeyrot, J. Core/shell nanoparticles of non-stoichiometric Zn–Mn and Zn–Co ferrites as thermosensitive heat sources for magnetic fluid hyperthermia. *J. Phys. Chem. C* **2018**, *122*, 3028–3038. [CrossRef]
96. Sanna Angotzi, M.; Musinu, A.; Mameli, V.; Ardu, A.; Cara, C.; Niznansky, D.; Xin, H.L.; Cannas, C. Spinel ferrite core–shell nanostructures by a versatile solvothermal seed-mediated growth approach and study of their nanointerfaces. *ACS Nano* **2017**, *11*, 7889–7900. [CrossRef]
97. Liu, X.; Liu, J.; Zhang, S.; Nan, Z.; Shi, Q. Structural, magnetic, and thermodynamic evolutions of Zn-doped Fe3O4 nanoparticles synthesized using a one-step solvothermal method. *J. Phys. Chem. C* **2016**, *120*, 1328–1341. [CrossRef]
98. Grabs, I.-M.; Bradtmöller, C.; Menzel, D.; Garnweitner, G. Formation mechanisms of iron oxide nanoparticles in different nonaqueous media. *Cryst. Growth Des.* **2012**, *12*, 1469–1475. [CrossRef]
99. Muscas, G.; Yaacoub, N.; Concas, G.; Sayed, F.; Hassan, R.S.; Greneche, J.; Cannas, C.; Musinu, A.; Foglietti, V.; Casciardi, S. Evolution of the magnetic structure with chemical composition in spinel iron oxide nanoparticles. *Nanoscale* **2015**, *7*, 13576–13585. [CrossRef] [PubMed]
100. Hemery, G.; Keyes, A.C., Jr.; Garaio, E.; Rodrigo, I.; Garcia, J.A.; Plazaola, F.; Garanger, E.; Sandre, O. Tuning sizes, morphologies, and magnetic properties of monocore versus multicore iron oxide nanoparticles through the controlled addition of water in the polyol synthesis. *Inorg. Chem.* **2017**, *56*, 8232–8243. [CrossRef] [PubMed]
101. Franceschin, G.; Gaudisson, T.; Menguy, N.; Dodrill, B.C.; Yaacoub, N.; Grenèche, J.M.; Valenzuela, R.; Ammar, S. Exchange-Biased Fe3− xO4-CoO Granular Composites of Different Morphologies Prepared by Seed-Mediated Growth in Polyol: From Core–Shell to Multicore Embedded Structures. *Part. Part. Syst. Charact.* **2018**, *35*, 1800104. [CrossRef]
102. William, W.Y.; Falkner, J.C.; Yavuz, C.T.; Colvin, V.L. Synthesis of monodisperse iron oxide nanocrystals by thermal decomposition of iron carboxylate salts. *Chem. Commun.* **2004**, 2306–2307.
103. Sun, S.; Zeng, H.; Robinson, D.B.; Raoux, S.; Rice, P.M.; Wang, S.X.; Li, G. Monodisperse mfe2o4 (m= fe, co, mn) nanoparticles. *J. Am. Chem. Soc.* **2004**, *126*, 273–279. [CrossRef]
104. Park, J.; An, K.; Hwang, Y.; Park, J.-G.; Noh, H.-J.; Kim, J.-Y.; Park, J.-H.; Hwang, N.-M.; Hyeon, T. Ultra-large-scale syntheses of monodisperse nanocrystals. *Nat. Mater.* **2004**, *3*, 891. [CrossRef]
105. Kolhatkar, A.; Jamison, A.; Litvinov, D.; Willson, R.; Lee, T. Tuning the magnetic properties of nanoparticles. *Int. J. Mol. Sci.* **2013**, *14*, 15977–16009. [CrossRef]
106. Yoo, D.; Lee, J.-H.; Shin, T.-H.; Cheon, J. Theranostic magnetic nanoparticles. *Acc. Chem. Res.* **2011**, *44*, 863–874. [CrossRef]

107. Cotin, G.; Blanco-Andujar, C.; Nguyen, D.V.; Affolter-Zbaraszczuk, C.; Boutry, S.; Anne, B.; Ronot, P.; Uring, B.; Choquet, P.; Zorn, P.E. Dendron based antifouling, MRI and magnetic hyperthermia properties of different shaped iron oxide nanoparticles. *Nanotechnology* **2019**, *30*, 37. [CrossRef]
108. Noh, S.-H.; Na, W.; Jang, J.-T.; Lee, J.-H.; Lee, E.J.; Moon, S.H.; Lim, Y.; Shin, J.-S.; Cheon, J. Nanoscale magnetism control via surface and exchange anisotropy for optimized ferrimagnetic hysteresis. *Nano Lett.* **2012**, *12*, 3716–3721. [CrossRef] [PubMed]
109. Toth, G.B.; Varallyay, C.G.; Horvath, A.; Bashir, M.R.; Choyke, P.L.; Daldrup-Link, H.E.; Dosa, E.; Finn, J.P.; Gahramanov, S.; Harisinghani, M.; et al. Current and potential imaging applications of ferumoxytol for magnetic resonance imaging. *Kidney Int.* **2017**, *92*, 47–66. [CrossRef] [PubMed]
110. Hood, M.N.; Blankholm, A.D.; Stolpen, A. The Rise of Off-Label Iron-Based Agents in Magnetic Resonance Imaging. *J. Radiol. Nurs.* **2019**, *38*, 38–41. [CrossRef]
111. Gaglia, J.L.; Harisinghani, M.; Aganj, I.; Wojtkiewicz, G.R.; Hedgire, S.; Benoist, C.; Mathis, D.; Weissleder, R. Noninvasive mapping of pancreatic inflammation in recent-onset type-1 diabetes patients. *Proc. Natl. Acad. Sci. USA* **2015**, *112*, 2139–2144. [CrossRef] [PubMed]
112. Trujillo-Alonso, V.; Pratt, E.C.; Zong, H.; Lara-Martinez, A.; Kaittanis, C.; Rabie, M.O.; Longo, V.; Becker, M.W.; Roboz, G.J.; Grimm, J. FDA-approved ferumoxytol displays anti-leukaemia efficacy against cells with low ferroportin levels. *Nat. Nanotechnol.* **2019**, *14*, 616. [CrossRef] [PubMed]
113. Huang, J.; Shu, Q.; Wang, L.; Wu, H.; Wang, A.Y.; Mao, H. Layer-by-layer assembled milk protein coated magnetic nanoparticle enabled oral drug delivery with high stability in stomach and enzyme-responsive release in small intestine. *Biomaterials* **2015**, *39*, 105–113. [CrossRef] [PubMed]
114. Shah, K. Mesenchymal stem cells engineered for cancer therapy. *Adv. Drug Deliv. Rev.* **2012**, *64*, 739–748. [CrossRef] [PubMed]
115. Qiao, L.; Xu, Z.; Zhao, T.; Zhao, Z.; Shi, M.; Zhao, R.C.; Ye, L.; Zhang, X. Suppression of tumorigenesis by human mesenchymal stem cells in a hepatoma model. *Cell Res.* **2008**, *18*, 500. [CrossRef]
116. Long, X.; Matsumoto, R.; Yang, P.; Uemura, T. Effect of human mesenchymal stem cells on the growth of HepG2 and Hela cells. *Cell Struct. Funct.* **2013**. [CrossRef]
117. Yu, Y.; Lu, L.; Qian, X.; Chen, N.; Yao, A.; Pu, L.; Zhang, F.; Li, X.; Kong, L.; Sun, B. Antifibrotic effect of hepatocyte growth factor-expressing mesenchymal stem cells in small-for-size liver transplant rats. *Stem Cells Dev.* **2009**, *19*, 903–914. [CrossRef]
118. Hu, C.; Zhao, L.; Duan, J.; Li, L. Strategies to improve the efficiency of mesenchymal stem cell transplantation for reversal of liver fibrosis. *J. Cell. Mol. Med.* **2019**, *23*, 1657–1670. [CrossRef] [PubMed]
119. Faidah, M.; Noorwali, A.; Atta, H.; Ahmed, N.; Habib, H.; Damiati, L.; Filimban, N.; Al-qriqri, M.; Mahfouz, S.; Khabaz, M.N. Mesenchymal stem cell therapy of hepatocellular carcinoma in rats: Detection of cell homing and tumor mass by magnetic resonance imaging using iron oxide nanoparticles. *Adv. Clin. Exp. Med.* **2017**, *26*, 1171–1178. [CrossRef] [PubMed]
120. Lai, L.; Chen, J.; Wei, X.; Huang, M.; Hu, X.; Yang, R.; Jiang, X.; Shan, H. Transplantation of MSCs overexpressing HGF into a rat model of liver fibrosis. *Mol. Imaging Biol.* **2016**, *18*, 43–51. [CrossRef] [PubMed]
121. Guimaraes, A.R.; Siqueira, L.; Uppal, R.; Alford, J.; Fuchs, B.C.; Yamada, S.; Tanabe, K.; Chung, R.T.; Lauwers, G.; Chew, M.L. T2 relaxation time is related to liver fibrosis severity. *Quant. Imaging Med. Surg.* **2016**, *6*, 103. [CrossRef] [PubMed]
122. Wu, W.; Wu, Z.; Yu, T.; Jiang, C.; Kim, W.-S. Recent progress on magnetic iron oxide nanoparticles: Synthesis, surface functional strategies and biomedical applications. *Sci. Technol. Adv. Mater.* **2015**, *16*, 023501. [CrossRef]
123. Li, Y.; Shang, W.; Liang, X.; Zeng, C.; Liu, M.; Wang, S.; Li, H.; Tian, J. The diagnosis of hepatic fibrosis by magnetic resonance and near-infrared imaging using dual-modality nanoparticles. *RSC Adv.* **2018**, *8*, 6699–6708. [CrossRef]
124. Zhang, C.; Liu, H.; Cui, Y.; Li, X.; Zhang, Z.; Zhang, Y.; Wang, D. Molecular magnetic resonance imaging of activated hepatic stellate cells with ultrasmall superparamagnetic iron oxide targeting integrin $\alpha v \beta 3$ for staging liver fibrosis in rat model. *Int. J. Nanomed.* **2016**, *11*, 1097.
125. Wei, Y.; Zhao, M.; Yang, F.; Mao, Y.; Xie, H.; Zhou, Q. Iron overload by superparamagnetic iron oxide nanoparticles is a high risk factor in cirrhosis by a systems toxicology assessment. *Sci. Rep.* **2016**, *6*, 29110. [CrossRef]

126. Lunov, O.; Syrovets, T.; Büchele, B.; Jiang, X.; Röcker, C.; Tron, K.; Nienhaus, G.U.; Walther, P.; Mailänder, V.; Landfester, K. The effect of carboxydextran-coated superparamagnetic iron oxide nanoparticles on c-Jun N-terminal kinase-mediated apoptosis in human macrophages. *Biomaterials* **2010**, *31*, 5063–5071. [CrossRef]
127. Kolosnjaj-Tabi, J.; Lartigue, L.; Javed, Y.; Luciani, N.; Pellegrino, T.; Wilhelm, C.; Alloyeau, D.; Gazeau, F. Biotransformations of magnetic nanoparticles in the body. *Nano Today* **2016**, *11*, 280–284. [CrossRef]
128. Yu, M.; Huang, S.; Yu, K.J.; Clyne, A.M. Dextran and polymer polyethylene glycol (PEG) coating reduce both 5 and 30 nm iron oxide nanoparticle cytotoxicity in 2D and 3D cell culture. *Int. J. Mol. Sci.* **2012**, *13*, 5554–5570. [CrossRef] [PubMed]
129. Efremova, M.V.; Naumenko, V.A.; Spasova, M.; Garanina, A.S.; Abakumov, M.A.; Blokhina, A.D.; Melnikov, P.A.; Prelovskaya, A.O.; Heidelmann, M.; Li, Z.A. Magnetite-Gold nanohybrids as ideal all-in-one platforms for theranostics. *Sci. Rep.* **2018**, *8*, 11295. [CrossRef] [PubMed]
130. Nguyen, T.; Mammeri, F.; Ammar, S. Iron oxide and gold based magneto-plasmonic nanostructures for medical applications: A review. *Nanomaterials* **2018**, *8*, 149. [CrossRef] [PubMed]
131. Martinez-Boubeta, C.; Simeonidis, K.; Serantes, D.; Conde-Leborán, I.; Kazakis, I.; Stefanou, G.; Peña, L.; Galceran, R.; Balcells, L.; Monty, C. Adjustable Hyperthermia Response of Self-Assembled Ferromagnetic Fe-MgO Core–Shell Nanoparticles by Tuning Dipole–Dipole Interactions. *Adv. Funct. Mater.* **2012**, *22*, 3737–3744. [CrossRef]
132. Lavorato, G.; Lima, E., Jr.; Vasquez Mansilla, M.; Troiani, H.; Zysler, R.; Winkler, E. Bifunctional CoFe2O4/ZnO core/shell nanoparticles for magnetic fluid hyperthermia with controlled optical response. *J. Phys. Chem. C* **2018**, *122*, 3047–3057. [CrossRef]
133. Baeza, A.; Guisasola, E.; Ruiz-Hernandez, E.; Vallet-Regí, M. Magnetically triggered multidrug release by hybrid mesoporous silica nanoparticles. *Chem. Mater.* **2012**, *24*, 517–524. [CrossRef]
134. El-Boubbou, K. Magnetic iron oxide nanoparticles as drug carriers: Clinical relevance. *Nanomedicine* **2018**, *13*, 953–971. [CrossRef]
135. Kolosnjaj-Tabi, J.; Wilhelm, C. Magnetic nanoparticles in cancer therapy: How can thermal approaches help? *Future Med.* **2017**. [CrossRef]
136. Omelyanchik, A.; Efremova, M.; Myslitskaya, N.; Zybin, A.; Carey, B.J.; Sickel, J.; Kohl, H.; Bratschitsch, R.; Abakumov, M.; Majouga, A. Magnetic and Optical Properties of Gold-Coated Iron Oxide Nanoparticles. *J. Nanosci. Nanotechnol.* **2019**, *19*, 4987–4993. [CrossRef]
137. Salvatore, A.; Montis, C.; Berti, D.; Baglioni, P. Multifunctional Magnetoliposomes for Sequential Controlled Release. *ACS Nano* **2016**, *10*, 7749–7760. [CrossRef]
138. Illés, E.; Tombácz, E. The effect of humic acid adsorption on pH-dependent surface charging and aggregation of magnetite nanoparticles. *J. Colloid Interface Sci.* **2006**, *295*, 115–123. [CrossRef] [PubMed]
139. Ungureanu, B.S.; Teodorescuv, C.-M.; Săftoiu, A. Magnetic Nanoparticles for Hepatocellular Carcinoma Diagnosis and Therapy. *J. Gastrointest. Liver Dis.* **2016**, *25*. [CrossRef]
140. Ferrucci, J.; Stark, D. Iron oxide-enhanced MR imaging of the liver and spleen: Review of the first 5 years. *AJR. Am. J. Roentgenol.* **1990**, *155*, 943–950. [CrossRef] [PubMed]
141. Giavridis, T.; van der Stegen, S.J.C.; Eyquem, J.; Hamieh, M.; Piersigilli, A.; Sadelain, M. CAR T cell-induced cytokine release syndrome is mediated by macrophages and abated by IL-1 blockade. *Nat. Med.* **2018**, *24*, 731–738. [CrossRef] [PubMed]
142. Rezvani, K.; Rouce, R.; Liu, E.; Shpall, E. Engineering Natural Killer Cells for Cancer Immunotherapy. Molecular therapy. *J. Am. Soc. Gene Ther.* **2017**, *25*, 1769–1781. [CrossRef] [PubMed]
143. Kang, J.H.; Krause, S.; Tobin, H.; Mammoto, A.; Kanapathipillai, M.; Ingber, D.E. A combined micromagnetic-microfluidic device for rapid capture and culture of rare circulating tumor cells. *Lab Chip* **2012**, *12*, 2175–2181. [CrossRef] [PubMed]
144. Liu, F.; KC, P.; Zhang, G.; Zhe, J. Microfluidic magnetic bead assay for cell detection. *Anal. Chem.* **2015**, *88*, 711–717. [CrossRef]
145. Shields, C.W., IV; Reyes, C.D.; López, G.P. Microfluidic cell sorting: A review of the advances in the separation of cells from debulking to rare cell isolation. *Lab Chip* **2015**, *15*, 1230–1249. [CrossRef]
146. Ito, A.; Takizawa, Y.; Honda, H.; Hata, K.-I.; Kagami, H.; Ueda, M.; Kobayashi, T. Tissue engineering using magnetite nanoparticles and magnetic force: Heterotypic layers of cocultured hepatocytes and endothelial cells. *Tissue Eng.* **2004**, *10*, 833–840. [CrossRef]

147. Ito, A.; Hibino, E.; Kobayashi, C.; Terasaki, H.; Kagami, H.; Ueda, M.; Kobayashi, T.; Honda, H. Construction and delivery of tissue-engineered human retinal pigment epithelial cell sheets, using magnetite nanoparticles and magnetic force. *Tissue Eng.* **2005**, *11*, 489–496. [CrossRef]
148. Omelyanchik, A.; Levada, E.; Ding, J.; Lendinez, S.; Pearson, J.; Efremova, M.; Bessalova, V.; Karpenkov, D.; Semenova, E.; Khlusov, I. Design of Conductive Microwire Systems for Manipulation of Biological Cells. *IEEE Trans. Magn.* **2018**, *54*, 1–5. [CrossRef]
149. Okochi, M.; Matsumura, T.; Honda, H. Magnetic force-based cell patterning for evaluation of the effect of stromal fibroblasts on invasive capacity in 3Dcultures. *Biosens. Bioelectron.* **2013**, *42*, 300–307. [CrossRef] [PubMed]
150. Okochi, M.; Matsumura, T.; Yamamoto, S.; Nakayama, E.; Jimbow, K.; Honda, H. Cell behavior observation and gene expression analysis of melanoma associated with stromal fibroblasts in a three-dimensional magnetic cell culture array. *Biotechnol. Prog.* **2013**, *29*, 135–142. [CrossRef] [PubMed]
151. Tanase, M.; Felton, E.J.; Gray, D.S.; Hultgren, A.; Chen, C.S.; Reich, D.H. Assembly of multicellular constructs and microarrays of cells using magnetic nanowires. *Lab Chip* **2005**, *5*, 598–605. [PubMed]
152. Rieck, S.; Heun, Y.; Heidsieck, A.; Mykhaylyk, O.; Pfeifer, A.; Gleich, B.; Mannell, H.; Wenzel, D. Local anti-angiogenic therapy by magnet-assisted downregulation of SHP2 phosphatase. *J. Controll. Release* **2019**, *305*, 155–164. [CrossRef]
153. Muthana, M.; Kennerley, A.J.; Hughes, R.; Fagnano, E.; Richardson, J.; Paul, M.; Murdoch, C.; Wright, F.; Payne, C.; Lythgoe, M.F.; et al. Directing cell therapy to anatomic target sites in vivo with magnetic resonance targeting. *Nat. Commun.* **2015**, *6*, 8009. [CrossRef]
154. Wang, X.; Ho, C.; Tsatskis, Y.; Law, J.; Zhang, Z.; Zhu, M.; Dai, C.; Wang, F.; Tan, M.; Hopyan, S. Intracellular manipulation and measurement with multipole magnetic tweezers. *Sci. Robot.* **2019**, *4*, eaav6180. [CrossRef]
155. Zamay, T.N.; Zamay, G.S.; Belyanina, I.V.; Zamay, S.S.; Denisenko, V.V.; Kolovskaya, O.S.; Ivanchenko, T.I.; Grigorieva, V.L.; Garanzha, I.V.; Veprintsev, D.V. Noninvasive Microsurgery Using Aptamer-Functionalized Magnetic Microdisks for Tumor Cell Eradication. *Nucleic Acid Ther.* **2017**, *27*, 105–114. [CrossRef]
156. Golovin, Y.I.; Gribanovsky, S.L.; Golovin, D.Y.; Klyachko, N.L.; Majouga, A.G.; Master, A.M.; Sokolsky, M.; Kabanov, A.V. Towards nanomedicines of the future: Remote magneto-mechanical actuation of nanomedicines by alternating magnetic fields. *J. Controll. Release* **2015**, *219*, 43–60. [CrossRef]
157. Du, V.; Luciani, N.; Richard, S.; Mary, G.; Gay, C.; Mazuel, F.; Reffay, M.; Menasche, P.; Agbulut, O.; Wilhelm, C. A 3D magnetic tissue stretcher for remote mechanical control of embryonic stem cell differentiation. *Nat. Commun.* **2017**, *8*, 400. [CrossRef]
158. Sun, J.; Liu, X.; Huang, J.; Song, L.; Chen, Z.; Liu, H.; Li, Y.; Zhang, Y.; Gu, N. Magnetic assembly-mediated enhancement of differentiation of mouse bone marrow cells cultured on magnetic colloidal assemblies. *Sci. Rep.* **2014**, *4*, 5125. [CrossRef] [PubMed]
159. Tseng, P.; Judy, J.W.; Di Carlo, D. Magnetic nanoparticle–mediated massively parallel mechanical modulation of single-cell behavior. *Nat. Methods* **2012**, *9*, 1113. [CrossRef] [PubMed]
160. Kollmannsberger, P.; Fabry, B. BaHigh-force magnetic tweezers with force feedback for biological applications. *Rev. Sci. Instrum.* **2007**, *78*, 114301. [CrossRef] [PubMed]
161. Lipfert, J.; Kerssemakers, J.W.; Jager, T.; Dekker, N.H. Magnetic torque tweezers: Measuring torsional stiffness in DNA and RecA-DNA filaments. *Nat. Methods* **2010**, *7*, 977. [CrossRef] [PubMed]
162. Noh, S.-H.; Moon, S.H.; Shin, T.-H.; Lim, Y.; Cheon, J. Recent advances of magneto-thermal capabilities of nanoparticles: From design principles to biomedical applications. *Nano Today* **2017**, *13*, 61–76. [CrossRef]
163. He, S.; Zhang, H.; Liu, Y.; Sun, F.; Yu, X.; Li, X.; Zhang, L.; Wang, L.; Mao, K.; Wang, G. Maximizing specific loss power for magnetic hyperthermia by hard–soft mixed ferrites. *Small* **2018**, *14*, 1800135. [CrossRef] [PubMed]
164. Riedinger, A.; Guardia, P.; Curcio, A.; Garcia, M.A.; Cingolani, R.; Manna, L.; Pellegrino, T. Subnanometer local temperature probing and remotely controlled drug release based on azo-functionalized iron oxide nanoparticles. *Nano Lett.* **2013**, *13*, 2399–2406. [CrossRef]
165. Fuller, E.G.; Sun, H.; Dhavalikar, R.D.; Unni, M.; Scheutz, G.M.; Sumerlin, B.S.; Rinaldi, C. Externally Triggered Heat and Drug Release from Magnetically Controlled Nanocarriers. *ACS Appl. Polym. Mater.* **2019**, *1*, 211–220. [CrossRef]
166. Chen, W.; Cheng, C.-A.; Zink, J.I. Spatial, Temporal, and Dose Control of Drug Delivery using Noninvasive Magnetic Stimulation. *ACS Nano* **2019**, *13*, 1292–1308. [CrossRef]

167. Tietze, R.; Zaloga, J.; Unterweger, H.; Lyer, S.; Friedrich, R.P.; Janko, C.; Pöttler, M.; Dürr, S.; Alexiou, C. Magnetic nanoparticle-based drug delivery for cancer therapy. *Biochem. Biophys. Res. Commun.* **2015**, *468*, 463–470. [CrossRef]
168. Stimphil, E.; Nagesetti, A.; Guduru, R.; Stewart, T.; Rodzinski, A.; Liang, P.; Khizroev, S. Physics considerations in targeted anticancer drug delivery by magnetoelectric nanoparticles. *Appl. Phys. Rev.* **2017**, *4*, 021101. [CrossRef]
169. Mulens, V.; Morales, M.d.P.; Barber, D.F. Development of magnetic nanoparticles for cancer gene therapy: A comprehensive review. *ISRN Nanomat.* **2013**, *2013*, 646284. [CrossRef]
170. Scialabba, C.; Puleio, R.; Peddis, D.; Varvaro, G.; Calandra, P.; Cassata, G.; Cicero, L.; Licciardi, M.; Giammona, G. Folate targeted coated SPIONs as efficient tool for MRI. *Nano Res.* **2017**, *10*, 3212–3227. [CrossRef]
171. Nielsen, M.J.; Veidal, S.S.; Karsdal, M.A.; Orsnes-Leeming, D.J.; Vainer, B.; Gardner, S.D.; Hamatake, R.; Goodman, Z.D.; Schuppan, D.; Patel, K. Plasma Pro-C3 (N-terminal type III collagen propeptide) predicts fibrosis progression in patients with chronic hepatitis C. *Liver Int.* **2015**, *35*, 429–437. [CrossRef] [PubMed]
172. Bauer, L.M.; Situ, S.F.; Griswold, M.A.; Samia, A.C.S. Magnetic particle imaging tracers: State-of-the-art and future directions. *J. Phys. Chem. Lett.* **2015**, *6*, 2509–2517. [CrossRef] [PubMed]
173. Nikitin, M.P.; Orlov, A.; Sokolov, I.; Minakov, A.; Nikitin, P.; Ding, J.; Bader, S.; Rozhkova, E.; Novosad, V. Ultrasensitive detection enabled by nonlinear magnetization of nanomagnetic labels. *Nanoscale* **2018**, *10*, 11642–11650. [CrossRef] [PubMed]
174. Haun, J.B.; Yoon, T.J.; Lee, H.; Weissleder, R. Magnetic nanoparticle biosensors. *Wiley Interdiscip. Rev. Nanomed. Nanobiotechnol.* **2010**, *2*, 291–304. [CrossRef]
175. Ehling, J.; Bartneck, M.; Fech, V.; Butzbach, B.; Cesati, R.; Botnar, R.; Lammers, T.; Tacke, F. Elastin-based molecular MRI of liver fibrosis. *Hepatology* **2013**, *58*, 1517–1518. [CrossRef]
176. Nagórniewicz, B.; Mardhian, D.F.; Booijink, R.; Storm, G.; Prakash, J.; Bansal, R. Engineered Relaxin as theranostic nanomedicine to diagnose and ameliorate liver cirrhosis. *Nanomedicine* **2019**, *17*, 106–118. [CrossRef]
177. Mardhian, D.F.; Storm, G.; Bansal, R.; Prakash, J. Nano-targeted relaxin impairs fibrosis and tumor growth in pancreatic cancer and improves the efficacy of gemcitabine in vivo. *J. Controll. Release* **2018**, *290*, 1–10. [CrossRef]
178. Tan, S.Y.; Grimes, S. Paul Ehrlich (1854-1915): Man with the magic bullet. *Singap. Med. J.* **2010**, *51*, 842–843.
179. Ledford, H. Bankruptcy filing worries developers of nanoparticle cancer drugs. *Nature* **2016**, *533*, 304–305. [CrossRef] [PubMed]
180. Autio, K.A.; Dreicer, R.; Anderson, J.; Garcia, J.A.; Alva, A.; Hart, L.L.; Milowsky, M.I.; Posadas, E.M.; Ryan, C.J.; Graf, R.P.; et al. Safety and Efficacy of BIND-014, a Docetaxel Nanoparticle Targeting Prostate-Specific Membrane Antigen for Patients With Metastatic Castration-Resistant Prostate Cancer: A Phase 2 Clinical Trial. *JAMA Oncol.* **2018**, *4*, 1344–1351. [CrossRef] [PubMed]
181. Josan, S.; Billingsley, K.; Orduna, J.; Park, J.M.; Luong, R.; Yu, L.; Hurd, R.; Pfefferbaum, A.; Spielman, D.; Mayer, D. Assessing inflammatory liver injury in an acute CCl4 model using dynamic 3D metabolic imaging of hyperpolarized [1-13C] pyruvate. *NMR Biomed.* **2015**, *28*, 1671–1677. [CrossRef] [PubMed]
182. Kanai, A.J.; Konieczko, E.M.; Bennett, R.G.; Samuel, C.S.; Royce, S.G. Relaxin and fibrosis: Emerging targets, challenges, and future directions. *Mol. Cell. Endocrinol.* **2019**, *487*, 66–74. [CrossRef]
183. Li, D.; He, L.; Guo, H.; Chen, H.; Shan, H. Targeting activated hepatic stellate cells (aHSCs) for liver fibrosis imaging. *EJNMMI Res.* **2015**, *5*, 71. [CrossRef]
184. Mederacke, I.; Hsu, C.C.; Troeger, J.S.; Huebener, P.; Mu, X.; Dapito, D.H.; Pradere, J.-P.; Schwabe, R.F. Fate tracing reveals hepatic stellate cells as dominant contributors to liver fibrosis independent of its aetiology. *Nat. Commun.* **2013**, *4*, 2823. [CrossRef]
185. Luangmonkong, T.; Suriguga, S.; Mutsaers, H.A.; Groothuis, G.M.; Olinga, P.; Boersema, M. Targeting oxidative stress for the treatment of liver fibrosis. In *Reviews of Physiology, Biochemistry and Pharmacology, Vol. 175*; Springer: Berlin, Germany, 2018; pp. 71–102.
186. Schon, H.-T.; Bartneck, M.; Borkham-Kamphorst, E.; Nattermann, J.; Lammers, T.; Tacke, F.; Weiskirchen, R. Pharmacological intervention in hepatic stellate cell activation and hepatic fibrosis. *Front. Pharmacol.* **2016**, *7*, 33. [CrossRef]

187. Ungefroren, H.; Gieseler, F.; Kaufmann, R.; Settmacher, U.; Lehnert, H.; Rauch, B. Signaling crosstalk of TGF-β/ALK5 and PAR2/PAR1: A Complex regulatory network controlling fibrosis and cancer. *Int. J. Mol. Sci.* **2018**, *19*, 1568. [CrossRef]
188. Palomer, X.; Barroso, E.; Pizarro-Delgado, J.; Peña, L.; Botteri, G.; Zarei, M.; Aguilar, D.; Montori-Grau, M.; Vázquez-Carrera, M. PPARβ/δ: A key therapeutic target in metabolic disorders. *Int. J. Mol. Sci.* **2018**, *19*, 913. [CrossRef]
189. Peng, Z.W.; Ikenaga, N.; Liu, S.B.; Sverdlov, D.Y.; Vaid, K.A.; Dixit, R.; Weinreb, P.H.; Violette, S.; Sheppard, D.; Schuppan, D. Integrin αvβ6 critically regulates hepatic progenitor cell function and promotes ductular reaction, fibrosis, and tumorigenesis. *Hepatology* **2016**, *63*, 217–232. [CrossRef] [PubMed]
190. Greupink, R.; Bakker, H.I.; van Goor, H.; de Borst, M.H.; Beljaars, L.; Poelstra, K. Mannose-6-phosphate/insulin-Like growth factor-II receptors may represent a target for the selective delivery of mycophenolic acid to fibrogenic cells. *Pharm. Res.* **2006**, *23*, 1827–1834. [CrossRef] [PubMed]
191. Bonner, J.C. Regulation of PDGF and its receptors in fibrotic diseases. *Cytokine Growth Factor Rev.* **2004**, *15*, 255–273. [CrossRef] [PubMed]
192. Bansal, R.; Prakash, J.; De Ruiter, M.; Poelstra, K. Targeted recombinant fusion proteins of IFNgamma and mimetic IFNgamma with PDGFbetaR bicyclic peptide inhibits liver fibrogenesis in vivo. *PLoS ONE* **2014**, *9*, e89878. [CrossRef]
193. van Dijk, F.; Teekamp, N.; Beljaars, L.; Post, E.; Zuidema, J.; Steendam, R.; Kim, Y.O.; Frijlink, H.W.; Schuppan, D.; Poelstra, K.; et al. Pharmacokinetics of a sustained release formulation of PDGFbeta-receptor directed carrier proteins to target the fibrotic liver. *J. Controll. Release* **2018**, *269*, 258–265. [CrossRef]
194. Gressner, A.M.; Weiskirchen, R.; Breitkopf, K.; Dooley, S. Roles of TGF-beta in hepatic fibrosis. *Front. Biosci.* **2002**, *7*, d793–d807. [CrossRef]
195. Henderson, N.C.; Arnold, T.D.; Katamura, Y.; Giacomini, M.M.; Rodriguez, J.D.; McCarty, J.H.; Pellicoro, A.; Raschperger, E.; Betsholtz, C.; Ruminski, P.G.; et al. Targeting of alphav integrin identifies a core molecular pathway that regulates fibrosis in several organs. *Nat. Med.* **2013**, *19*, 1617–1624. [CrossRef]
196. Bansal, R.; Nakagawa, S.; Yazdani, S.; van Baarlen, J.; Venkatesh, A.; Koh, A.P.; Song, W.M.; Goossens, N.; Watanabe, H.; Beasley, M.B.; et al. Integrin alpha 11 in the regulation of the myofibroblast phenotype: Implications for fibrotic diseases. *Exp. Mol. Med.* **2017**, *49*, e396. [CrossRef]
197. Samuel, C.; Royce, S.; Hewitson, T.; Denton, K.; Cooney, T.; Bennett, R. Anti-fibrotic actions of relaxin. *Br. J. Pharmacol.* **2017**, *174*, 962–976. [CrossRef]
198. Bennett, R.G.; Simpson, R.L.; Hamel, F.G. Serelaxin increases the antifibrotic action of rosiglitazone in a model of hepatic fibrosis. *World J. Gastroenterol.* **2017**, *23*, 3999. [CrossRef]
199. Feijóo-Bandín, S.; Aragón-Herrera, A.; Rodríguez-Penas, D.; Portolés, M.; Roselló-Lletí, E.; Rivera, M.; González-Juanatey, J.R.; Lago, F. Relaxin-2 in cardiometabolic diseases: Mechanisms of action and future perspectives. *Front. Physiol.* **2017**, *8*, 599. [CrossRef] [PubMed]
200. Gracia-Sancho, J.; Maeso-Diaz, R.; Fernández-Iglesias, A.; Navarro-Zornoza, M.; Bosch, J. New cellular and molecular targets for the treatment of portal hypertension. *Hepatol. Int.* **2015**, *9*, 183–191. [CrossRef] [PubMed]
201. Ng, H.H.; Leo, C.H.; Parry, L.J.; Ritchie, R.H. Relaxin as a Therapeutic Target for the Cardiovascular Complications of Diabetes. *Front. Pharmacol.* **2018**, *9*, 501. [CrossRef] [PubMed]
202. Hoy, S.M. Patisiran: First Global Approval. *Drugs* **2018**, *78*, 1625–1631. [CrossRef]
203. Bangen, J.M.; Hammerich, L.; Sonntag, R.; Baues, M.; Haas, U.; Lambertz, D.; Longerich, T.; Lammers, T.; Tacke, F.; Trautwein, C.; et al. Targeting CCl4 -induced liver fibrosis by RNA interference-mediated inhibition of cyclin E1 in mice. *Hepatology* **2017**, *66*, 1242–1257. [CrossRef]
204. Roy, S.; Benz, F.; Luedde, T.; Roderburg, C. The role of miRNAs in the regulation of inflammatory processes during hepatofibrogenesis. *Hepatobiliary Surg. Nutr.* **2015**, *4*, 24–33.

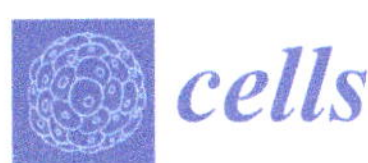

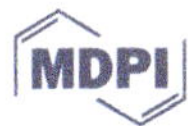

Article

The miRFIB-Score: A Serological miRNA-Based Scoring Algorithm for the Diagnosis of Significant Liver Fibrosis

Joeri Lambrecht [1], Stefaan Verhulst [1], Hendrik Reynaert [1,2] and Leo A. van Grunsven [1,*]

1 Department of Basic (Bio-)Medical Sciences, Liver Cell Biology Research Group, Vrije Universiteit Brussel, 1050 Brussels, Belgium

2 Department of Gastroenterology and Hepatology, University Hospital Brussels (UZ Brussel), B-1090 Brussels, Belgium

* Correspondence: lvgrunsv@vub.be

Received: 30 July 2019; Accepted: 27 August 2019; Published: 29 August 2019

Abstract: Background: The current diagnosis of early-stage liver fibrosis often relies on a serological or imaging-based evaluation of the stage of fibrosis, sometimes followed by an invasive liver biopsy procedure. Novel non-invasive experimental diagnostic tools are often based on markers of hepatocyte damage, or changes in liver stiffness and architecture, which are late-stage characteristics of fibrosis progression, making them unsuitable for the diagnosis of early-stage liver fibrosis. miRNAs control hepatic stellate cell (HSC) activation and are proposed as relevant diagnostic markers. **Methods**: We investigated the possibility of circulating miRNAs, which we found to be dysregulated upon HSC activation, to mark the presence of significant liver fibrosis ($F \geq 2$) in patients with chronic alcohol abuse, chronic viral infection (HBV/HCV), and non-alcoholic fatty liver disease (NAFLD). **Results**: miRNA-profiling identified miRNA-451a, miRNA-142-5p, Let-7f-5p, and miRNA-378a-3p to be significantly dysregulated upon in vitro HSC activation, and to be highly enriched in their extracellular vesicles, suggesting their potential use as biomarkers. Analysis of the plasma of patients with significant liver fibrosis ($F \geq 2$) and no or mild fibrosis ($F = 0$–1), using miRNA-122-5p and miRNA-29a-3p as positive control, found miRNA-451a, miRNA-142-5p, and Let-7f-5p, but not miRNA-378a-3p, able to distinguish between the two patient populations. Using logistic regression analysis, combining all five dysregulated circulating miRNAs, we created the miRFIB-score with a predictive value superior to the clinical scores Fibrosis-4 (Fib-4), aspartate aminotransferase/alanine aminotransferase (AST/ALT) ratio, and AST to platelet ratio index (APRI). The combination of the miRFIB-score with circulating PDGFRβ-levels further increased the predictive capacity for the diagnosis of significant liver fibrosis. **Conclusions**: The miRFIB- and miRFIB^{P}-scores are accurate tools for the diagnosis of significant liver fibrosis in a heterogeneous patient population.

Keywords: biomarker; NAFLD; viral liver disease; alcoholic liver disease; microRNA; hepatic stellate cell; fibrosis; diagnosis; liquid biopsy

1. Introduction

Liver fibrosis and subsequent cirrhosis result in over one million deaths per year worldwide, making it the eleventh most common cause of death in adults [1]. The three most important causes for the development of liver fibrosis are chronic alcohol abuse, chronic infection with the hepatitis B (HBV) or C (HCV) virus, and metabolic syndrome, which can result in non-alcoholic fatty liver disease (NAFLD) and non-alcoholic steatohepatitis (NASH) [2]. Upon the chronic presence of such liver injury-causing circumstances, inflammatory signals within the liver will induce hepatocyte-damage and the activation of liver-resident hepatic stellate cells (HSCs) towards a myofibroblastic phenotype.

This activation process is marked by an excessive production and deposition of extracellular matrix [3]. The early development of fibrosis, and its progression towards cirrhosis, can be halted and even reverted upon suitable treatment, such as the administration of anti-viral drugs, or significant life-style changes [4]. Importantly, overall disease outcome improves when the treatment is started as early as possible in the disease process [5].

To date, liver biopsy remains the gold standard for grading and staging liver fibrosis. Unfortunately, this technique is associated with sampling and interpretation variability [6], doubtable cost–benefit ratios [7], and a risk of pain and bleeding [8]. These drawbacks limit the use of liver biopsy as a tool for screening or follow-up. Various non-invasive diagnostic tools have been developed, of which some have made their way into clinical practice, including serological scoring tools, such as the enhanced liver fibrosis (ELF) test, aspartate aminotransferase/alanine aminotransferase (AST/ALT) ratio, Fibrosis-4 (Fib-4) score, and the AST to platelet ratio index (APRI), and imaging-based tools, such as transient elastography (FibroScan®), shear wave elastography (SWE), and acoustic radiation force impulse (ARFI) [9]. However, these non-invasive techniques have not yet led to full redundancy of the liver biopsy, especially due to their limited sensitivity and specificity for the detection of early stages of liver fibrosis.

MicroRNAs (miRNAs) are non-coding, single-stranded RNA structures of approximately 22 nucleotides long, and function as posttranscriptional gene regulators. More specifically, through binding to the 3′ untranslated regions of target messenger RNAs (mRNA), they can induce their cleavage, or prevent their translation into proteins [10]. Some miRNAs are known to be expressed in a cell- or tissue-specific manner. miRNAs are found in almost all body fluids, where they obtain stability by packaging into extracellular vesicles, or association to Argonaute2 or high-density lipoproteins [11]. Recent research has identified the potential of miRNAs to be used as diagnostic tools for specific subsets of liver disease, often focusing on the diagnosis of liver cirrhosis and hepatocellular carcinoma (HCC) [12,13]. However, the diagnostic value of individual miRNAs, or miRNA-panels, for the identification of early stages of liver fibrosis in heterogeneous patient populations remains to be proven.

In this study, we aimed to investigate the diagnostic value of miRNAs for the identification of significant liver fibrosis in a heterogeneous patient cohort suffering from chronic liver disease. We found that plasma levels of several individual miRNAs associated with HSC activation can distinguish between no or mild fibrosis (F0–1) and significant liver fibrosis ($F \geq 2$). More importantly, the combination of the plasma levels of five miRNAs and PDGFRβ protein levels into the miRFIB^{P}-score increased the predictive capacity for the diagnosis of significant liver fibrosis and outperformed clinical scores, such as Fib-4, the AST/ALT ratio, and APRI.

2. Materials and Methods

2.1. Animal Studies

The use and care of animals was reviewed and approved by the Ethical Committee of Animal Experimentation of the Vrije Universiteit Brussel (Brussels, Belgium) in project 16-212-2, and was carried out in accordance with European Guidelines for the Care and Use of Laboratory Animals. All mice were housed in a controlled environment with free access to water and food. Primary HSCs were isolated from male Balb/c mice aged 25 to 30 weeks (Charles River Laboratories, L'Arbresle, France), as described earlier [14,15]. Briefly, murine livers were digested by enzymatic solutions consisting of collagenase (Roche diagnostics, Mannheim, Germany) and pronase E (Merck, Darmstadt, Germany). The resulting cell suspension was centrifuged at low speed to remove hepatocytes. Hepatic stellate cells (HSCs) were purified from the non-parenchymal fraction based on their buoyancy, using an 8% Nycodenz (Axis-shield PoC AS, Dundee, Scotland) solution. Isolated HSCs were cultured on regular tissue culture dishes (Greiner Bio-One, Vilvoorde, Belgium), in Dulbecco's modified Eagle's medium (Lonza, Verviers, Belgium) supplemented with 10% foetal bovine serum (Lonza, Verviers, Belgium), 2 mM L-glutamine (Ultraglutamine 1®) (Lonza), 100 U/mL penicillin, and 100 μg/mL streptomycin

(Pen-Strep®) (Lonza), inducing in vitro myofibroblastic transdifferentiation. Cell purity was confirmed by the presence of lipid droplets and staining for HSC-specific markers.

For the in vivo induction of liver fibrosis, 10-week old mice received eight intraperitoneal injections of 15 μL carbon tetrachloride (CCl_4) diluted in 85μL mineral oil (Sigma-Aldrich, St. Louis, MO, USA) per 30 g bodyweight over a period of four weeks. Mice were sacrificed 24 h after the last injection.

2.2. Patient Cohort

Patients with liver fibrosis caused by chronic alcohol abuse and chronic viral hepatitis were recruited from the Department of Gastroenterology and Hepatology of the University Hospital of Brussels (UZ Brussel), Belgium. The extent of liver fibrosis in these patients was determined based on transient elastography (FibroScan®, Echosens, France). Patients with at least 10 valid stiffness measurements with a success rate of minimum 60% were included in the final analysis. Cut-off values used to discriminate fibrotic stages equal to or more than F2, F3, and F4 were taken at 7.2 kPa, 9.5 kPa, and 12.5 kPa [16], respectively. Patients with liver fibrosis suffering from NAFLD were recruited from the Diabetes Centre of the University Hospital of Brussels (UZ Brussel, Brussels, Belgium) in collaboration with the Department of Gastroenterology and Hepatology (UZ Brussel, Brussels, Belgium). In these patients, the extent of fibrosis was determined by use of acoustic radiation force impulse (ARFI), using cut-off values of 1.25 m/s, 1.54 m/s, and 1.84 m/s to identify a fibrotic stage equal to, or more than F2, F3, and F4, respectively. All NAFLD-patients had Diabetes Mellitus type 2. The protocol of this study was approved by the local ethical committee of the UZ Brussel and Vrije Universiteit Brussel (reference number 2015/297; B.U.N. 143201525482) and was in accordance with the Declaration of Helsinki. An informed consent was obtained from all participants, prior to inclusion in the study.

2.3. Blood Collection

Blood samples were collected by venepuncture into evacuated ethylenediaminetetraacetic acid (EDTA-KE) S-Monovette tubes (Sarstedt AG & Co, Nümbrecht, Germany) on the day of FibroScan or ARFI. All samples were subjected to haematological and biochemical analyses. Plasma was created within a maximum timespan of 2 h after collection, using a two-step centrifugation protocol of 1500 g for 10 min (4 °C), followed by 2000 g for 3 min (4 °C). Plasma was frozen at −80 °C until further use.

2.4. Serological Scoring of Fibrosis

Haematological analyses and subsequent serological scoring algorithms, such as our recently developed PRTA-score [17] and the clinical algorithms Fib-4, APRI, and the AST/ALT ratio, were used to validate the elastography-based fibrosis scoring. The PRTA-score, Fib-4, and APRI were calculated using following formulae:

$$\text{Fib-4} = \text{age} \times \text{AST[IU/L]}/(\text{thrombocytes}[10^9/\text{L}] \times (\text{ALT[IU/L]})^{1/2});$$

$$\text{APRI} = (\text{AST[IU/L]/ULN})/\text{thrombocytes}[10^9/\text{L}];$$

$$\text{PRTA-score} = (\text{sPDGFR}\beta[\text{pg/mL}] \times 100)/(\text{albumin[g/L]} \times (\text{thrombocytes}[/\text{mm}^3]/100)).$$

2.5. Messenger RNA and microRNA Analysis

miRNAs were extracted from 500 μL human- or 150 μL mouse-plasma by use of the Nucleospin® miRNA Plasma kit (Macherey-Nagel, Düren, Germany), using the manufacturer's protocol. Caenorhabditis elegans miRNA-39 (Cel-miRNA-39) (Qiagen, Hilden, Germany) was added into the plasma lysate before the start of the extraction protocol and served as an external processing control. Total RNA from liver tissue and cultured hepatic stellate cells was extracted by the TRIzol reagent (ThermoFisher scientific, Waltham, USA) and ReliaPrep™ RNA Miniprep system

(Promega, Madison, WI, USA), using the manufacturers' protocol. Messenger RNA (mRNA) was reverse-transcribed into complementary DNA (cDNA) using a mixture of hexamer random primers, Moloney murine leukemia virus reverse transcriptase (M-MLV RT) Buffer, deoxyribonucleotide triphosphate (dNTP) mix, M-MLV RT RNase (H-) Point mutant, and RNasin® Plus RNase Inhibitor (Promega). MicroRNA (miRNA) was reverse transcribed into cDNA using the miScript II RT kit (Qiagen, Hilden, Germany). The expression profiles of selected mRNA and miRNAs were analyzed by quantitative real-time polymerase chain reaction (qPCR), using the GoTaq qPCR Master Mix with BRYT green (Promega) and the miScript SYBR Green PCR kit (Qiagen), respectively, in the QuantStudio 3 real-time PCR system (ThermoFisher scientific). Obtained results were analyzed using the QuantStudio 3 Design and Analysis Software (ThermoFisher scientific). Individual gene and miRNA expression was normalized to Gapdh, RNU6, or Cel-miRNA-39, as appropriate. Relative expression was calculated using the comparative Ct method ($2^{-\Delta\Delta CT}$). miRNA- (Supplementary Table S1) and gene- (Supplementary Table S2) specific primers were produced by Integrated DNA Technologies (IDT, Leuven, Belgium).

2.6. Histological Evaluation

Four-micrometer paraffin-embedded liver tissue sections were cut, deparaffinized, and rehydrated before staining with Sirius Red/Fast Green or Hematoxyline/Eosin. The sections were then washed, dehydrated, and mounted with DPX mounting medium. Whole slide images were taken using the Aperio CS2 image capture device (Leica, Diegem, Belgium). Collagen staining was quantified using the Orbit Image Analysis software (Actelion Pharmaceuticals Ltd, Allschwil, Switzerland) [18].

2.7. Immunocytochemistry

After the isolation of primary murine hepatic stellate cells, the cells were cultured on coverslips for 24 h or 10 days. Cells were washed with PBS and fixed with formalin for 10 min. The cells were then washed three times with PBS and stored at 4 °C until further use. Prior to staining, the cells were permeabilized using PBS supplemented with 0.1% Triton-X (3 × 5 min). Afterwards, cells were incubated for 30 min with 0.1% Triton-X PBS containing 2% bovine serum albumin (BSA), to block non-specific binding sites. The cells were incubated overnight at 4 °C with anti-Desmin (1:200, RB-9014-P, ThermoFisher scientific), or anti-Vimentin (1:200, V5255, Sigma-Aldrich). Three wash-steps using 0.1% Triton-X PBS were applied, followed by incubation with donkey anti-rabbit Alexa Fluor 488 secondary antibody (1:200, A21206, ThermoFisher scientific), donkey anti-mouse Alexa Fluor 488 secondary antibody (1:200, A21202, ThermoFisher scientific), or Cy3-coupled mouse anti-αSMA primary antibody (1:100, C6198, Sigma-Aldrich) for 1.5 h. Coverslips were mounted with 4′,6-diamidino-2-phenylindole (DAPI)-containing mounting medium (Dako, Denmark). Images were taken using the EVOS FL fluorescence microscope (ThermoFisher).

2.8. Statistical Analysis

Data were analyzed using GraphPad Prism 8 (GraphPad, Palo Alto, USA). Quantitative variables are expressed as means ± standard error of the mean (SEM) or expressed as boxplots using the Tukey representation. Statistical analyses were performed using the Student's t-test, Mann–Whitney test, and One-Way ANOVA with Dunnett post hoc test, as appropriate. Categorical values were analyzed using the Chi-square test. The diagnostic accuracy and performance of the mentioned miRNAs and serological scores were determined using receiver operating characteristics (ROC) curves, and the area under the curve (AUC) was calculated. Sensitivity and specificity were calculated based on the highest Youden's index values [19]. Correlation studies were executed using the Spearman's correlation test. Logistic regression analyses were performed using MedCalc version 18 (MedCalc Software, Ostend, Belgium). The sufficiency of the sample size was confirmed by MedCalc version 18 using in house preliminary results and a type I error rate (α) of 5% and a power (1-β) of 80%. Results were considered statistically significant when $p < 0.05$.

3. Results

3.1. Identification of Candidate HSC-Linked miRNAs

As hepatic stellate cell (HSC) activation is an early event of liver fibrosis initiation and progression, we hypothesized that HSC-derived circulating miRNAs could be suitable markers for early stage liver fibrosis. In order to identify candidate miRNAs, NanoString analysis was performed on extracellular vesicles (EVs), both microvesicles and small extracellular vesicles (sEV), obtained from the conditioned medium of in vitro activating primary murine HSCs. To this end, primary mouse HSCs were plated on plastic tissue culture dishes for 10 days. The activation of cultured HSCs was verified on a protein level by the up-regulation of HSC-activation markers Desmin, α-SMA, and Vimentin (Figure 1A), and on an mRNA level by *Acta2*, *Col1a1*, and *Lox* (Figure 1B). Although the obtained miRNA counts by NanoString analysis were insufficient to compare between the quiescent and activated conditions, several miRNAs were found to be highly enriched in such EVs, as compared to the average expression level of all tested miRNAs. This list of highly shed miRNAs, and thus potential fibrosis markers, was further restricted to the miRNAs that are conserved among mouse and human, to ensure translational value, ending up with a list of nine candidate miRNAs (Supplementary Figure S1). The expression levels of these miRNAs were analyzed in the in vitro activated primary mouse HSC cultures. Expression analysis of all nine candidate miRNAs was performed by using qPCR on the cell lysate of activated HSCs, as compared to freshly isolated HSCs (Figure 1C), and identified the significant dysregulation of four miRNAs: miRNA-451a, miRNA-142-5p, Let-7f-5p, and miRNA-378a-3p (Figure 1D).

3.2. Identification of Ankrd52, Clcn5 and Peg10 as Potential Target Genes

To investigate a potential function of miRNA-451a, miRNA-142-5p, Let-7f-5p, and miRNA-378a-3p in the HSC-activation process, a bioinformatics-based target prediction was carried out, using four different predictive algorithms: TargetScan, miRDB, starBase, and miRTarBase. Of all putative targets, thirteen genes are suggested to have all four miRNAs as post-transcriptional regulators (Figure 2A). The analysis of mRNA expression in activated HSCs, compared to freshly isolated quiescent HSCs, identified three genes that remained stable during the activation process (Figure 2B), three genes that were up-regulated (Figure 2C), and seven genes that were down-regulated (Figure 2D) upon HSC-activation. The genes that were up-regulated upon HSC activation, *Ankrd52*, *Clcn5*, and *Peg10*, are of particular interest, as miRNAs are known to regulate gene expression in a dominantly negative manner.

3.3. miRNA Expression Analysis in the CCl_4-Mouse Model

Next, we analyzed the expression of miRNA-451a, miRNA-142-5p, Let-7f-5p, and miRNA-378a-3p in a well-studied mouse model of liver fibrosis, with repeated injections of carbon tetrachloride (CCl_4) [20]. When mice are exposed to the CCl_4-toxin two times a week, for four weeks, significant hepatocyte-damage and HSC-activation can be seen (Figure 3A,B). An analysis of total liver tissue from sick mice, compared to healthy controls, revealed significant changing levels for miRNA-451a, miRNA-142-5p, Let-7f-5p, and miRNA-378a-3p (Figure 3C), with overlapping expression patterns, as found in activating HSCs. The expression of two miRNAs extensively characterized in chronic liver diseases, miRNA-122-5p [21] and miRNA-29a-3p [22], was used as positive controls. Plasma obtained from the CCl_4-mouse model identified significant changing expression levels of all analyzed miRNAs (Figure 3D). Interestingly, all miRNAs had a plasma expression pattern opposite to what was found in total liver tissue or activating HSCs. Altogether, these results suggest the potential use of these circulating miRNAs, without the need to distinguish between miRNAs packaged into extracellular vesicles or bound to (lipo-)proteins, as markers for HSC activation and fibrosis progression.

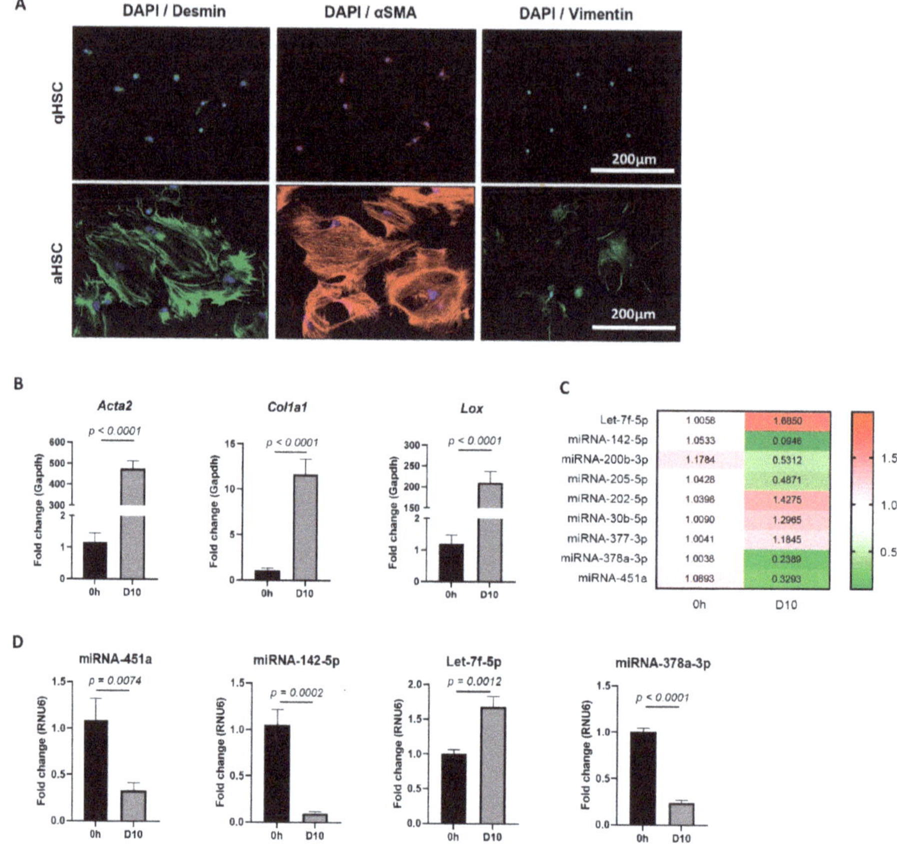

Figure 1. miRNA expression in mouse in vitro activated hepatic stellate cells (HSCs). (**A**) Immunofluorescence staining of quiescent (24 h of culture) and activated (10 days of culture) primary mouse HSCs for activation markers Desmin, αSMA, and Vimentin. 4′,6-Diamidino-2-phenylindole (DAPI) was used as nuclear staining. Representative images are shown. (**B**) mRNA expression levels determined by quantitative polymerase chain reaction (qPCR) of HSC-activation markers *Acta2*, *Col1a1*, and *Lox* in freshly isolated HSCs (0 h), as compared to HSCs activated by 10 days of culture (D10). (**C**) Heatmap of relative expression levels, as determined by qPCR, for selected candidate miRNAs in activated HSCs (D10), as compared to freshly isolated HSCs (0 h). (**D**) miRNA-451a, miRNA-142-5p, Let-7f-5p, and miRNA-378a-3p were found to be significantly dysregulated upon HSC activation. One-tailed unpaired t-test analysis was used to determine statistical significance. Results are shown as mean ± standard error of the mean (SEM); $n = 5$.

3.4. Patient Characteristics and Plasma miRNA Alterations During Liver Fibrosis Progression

Next, we investigated whether the plasma levels of these six miRNAs can be correlated to liver fibrosis severity in patients suffering from different chronic liver diseases. Patient characteristics are summarized in Table 1. A total of 208 patients were included, of which 92 patients were diagnosed with no or minimal fibrosis (F0–1) and 116 patients with significant fibrosis (F ≥ 2), as staged by elastography. Patients with various aetiologies of liver disease were recruited—chronic alcohol abuse ($n = 33$), chronic HBV/HCV infection ($n = 74$), and NAFLD ($n = 101$). Patients with chronic alcohol abuse or viral infection underwent transient elastography (FibroScan®) to distinguish significant liver fibrosis (F ≥ 2) from no or minimal fibrosis (F0–1); (median (25th; 75th percentile)) 12 (9.1; 33.6) kPa versus 5.2 (4.0;

6.1) kPa, respectively. Patients who presented with NAFLD all suffered from Diabetes Mellitus type 2 and underwent ARFI to distinguish significant liver fibrosis (F ≥ 2) from no or minimal fibrosis (F0–1); (median (25th; 75th percentile)) 1.525 (1.30; 1.68) m/s versus 1.15 (1.12; 1.20) m/s, respectively. Various clinical scoring algorithms, such as the AST/ALT ratio, Fib-4 score, APRI, and the recently developed PRTA-score [17], were calculated. All liver-related laboratory parameters, except for ALT and Creatinine values, and all fibrosis scoring tools are significantly different between the F0–1 and F ≥ 2 patient cohorts, validating the early- or late disease character of the included patients (Table 1).

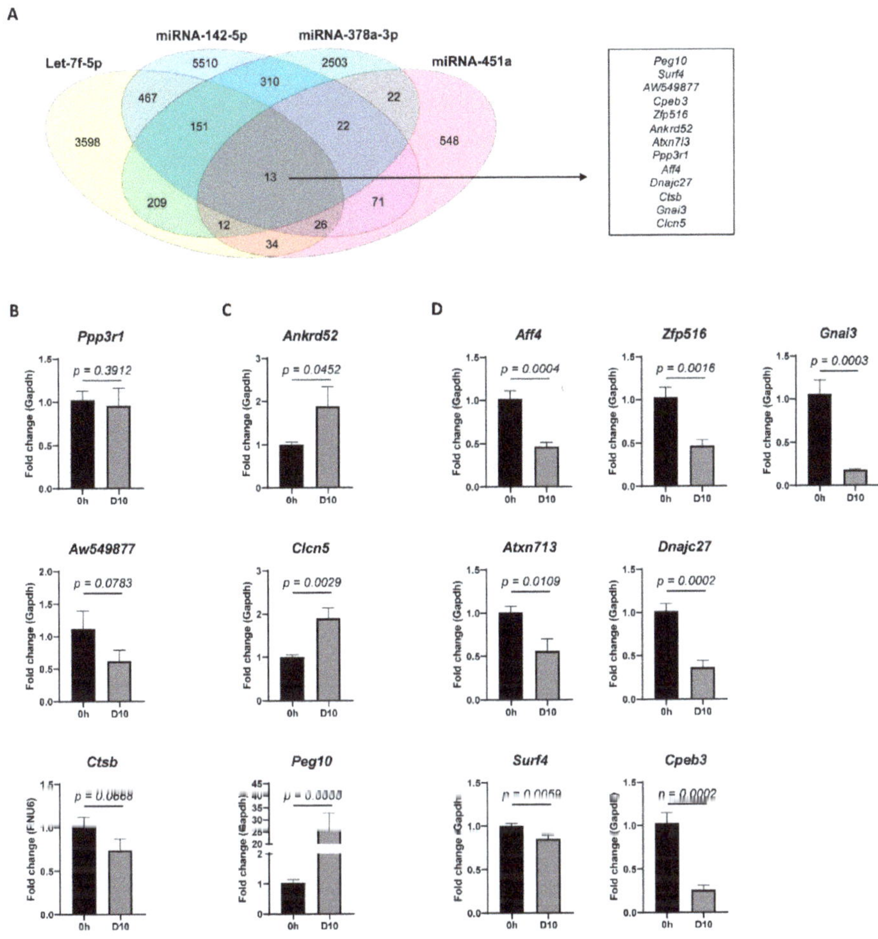

Figure 2. miRNA target prediction. Bioinformatics-based target prediction was carried out, using four different predictive algorithms: TargetScan, miRDB, starBase, and miRTarBase. (**A**) Venn diagram showing putative target genes for the differentially expressed miRNAs in culture activated primary mouse HSCs. A list of target genes mutual among all four miRNAs is shown. mRNA expression analysis of the identified mutual target genes in activated (D10) versus quiescent (0 h) HSCs identified (**B**) three genes with no significant difference, (**C**) three genes to be significantly up-regulated, and (**D**) seven genes to be significantly down-regulated. One-tailed unpaired t-test analysis was used to determine statistical significance. Results are shown as mean ± SEM; $n = 5$.

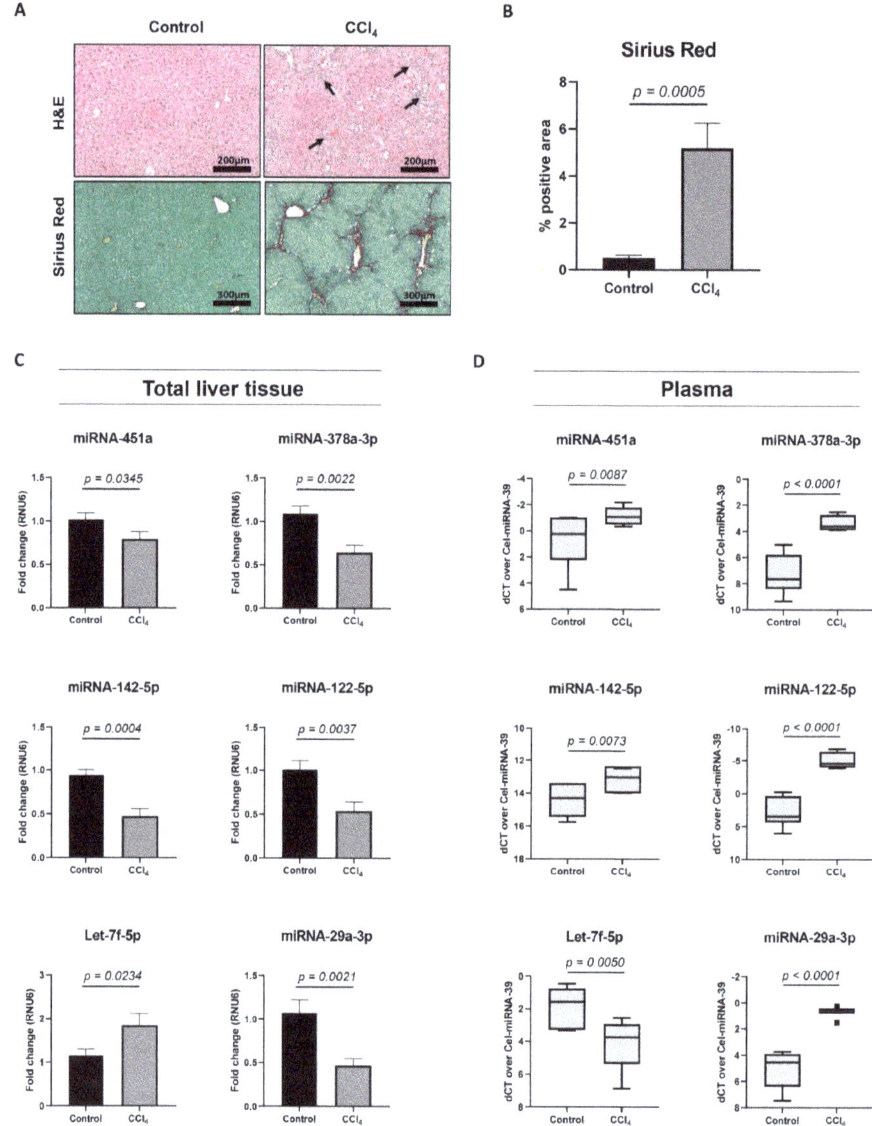

Figure 3. miRNA expression analysis in a CCl_4-induced mouse model of liver fibrosis. (**A**) Total liver tissue of mice that received CCl_4-injections two times a week, for a period of four weeks, and healthy controls, was used to visualize hepatocyte damage and inflammation (H&E), and cross-linked collagen deposition (Sirius Red). Arrows indicate infiltrated inflammatory cells. Representative images are shown. (**B**) The area of Sirius Red positive staining was calculated using Orbit analysis software and is plotted as percentage of the total area ($n = 7$ mice per group). (**C**) miRNA expression analysis of total liver tissue extracted from CCl_4-injected mice, as compared to healthy controls ($n = 7$ mice per group). Results are shown as mean ± SEM. (**D**) Tukey boxplots represent miRNA expression values in plasma obtained from CCl_4-injected mice, as compared to healthy controls ($n = 7$ mice per group). Obtained Ct levels were normalized by use of spiked-in Cel-miRNA-39. One-tailed unpaired t-test analysis was used to determine statistical significance.

Table 1. Baseline characteristics of the patient cohort.

Patient Cohorts	F0–1	F2–4	*p* Value
Individuals, *n*	92	116	
Disease aetiology: *n* (%)			
Alcoholic liver disease	6 (7%)	27 (23%)	
Viral liver disease	46 (50%)	28 (24%)	
NAFLD	40 (43%)	61 (53%)	
Characteristics			
Age (years): median (IQR)	52 (42–63)	57 (51–65)	0.0003
Male, *n* (%)	52 (57%)	84 (72%)	0.0267
BMI (kg/m^2): median (IQR)	27.44 (24.16–32.35)	29.96 (25.18–34.23)	ns
Laboratory parameters: median (IQR)			
AST (IU/L)	34 (24–48)	40 (28–67)	0.0048
ALT (IU/L)	43 (34–62)	48 (32–71)	ns
Alk Phos (IU/L)	68 (54–87)	87 (66–130)	<0.0001
GGT (IU/L)	39 (23–83)	71 (40–154)	<0.0001
Total bilirubin (mg/dL)	0.60 (0.47–0.79)	0.76 (0.57–1.20)	0.0005
Albumin (g/L)	43 (41–46)	42 (39–45)	0.0035
Thrombocytes (×10^3/mm^3)	231 (202–277)	202 (149–255)	0.0006
Creatinine (mg/dL)	0.85 (0.70–1.02)	0.87 (0.74–1.04)	ns
Fibrosis scoring: median (IQR)			
AST/ALT ratio	0.76 (0.62–0.87)	0.82 (0.67–1.18)	0.0211
APRI	0.35 (0.24–0.57)	0.56 (0.32–0.88)	0.0005
Fib-4	1.13 (0.83–1.49)	1.67 (1.08–2.80)	<0.0001
PRTA-score	7.18 (4.49–9.87)	11.63 (7.95–20.40)	<0.0001

n: number; NAFLD: non-alcoholic fatty liver disease; IQR: interquartile range; BMI: body mass index; AST: aspartate aminotransferase; ALT: alanine aminotransferase; Alk Phos: alkaline phosphatase; GGT: gamma-glutamyl transferase; AST/ALT ratio: aspartate aminotransferase/alanine aminotransferase ratio; APRI: AST to platelet ratio index; Fib-4: Fibrosis-4; PRTA-score: PDGFRβ-thrombocytes-albumin score; ns: not significant.

Analysis of the plasma of these patients showed that miRNA-451a and miRNA-142-5p were significantly up-regulated, while Let-7f-5p was significantly down-regulated, in patients with significant liver fibrosis ($F \geq 2$). miRNA-378a-3p remained stable during fibrosis progression (Figure 4A). Area under receiver operating characteristic (AUROC) analysis identified comparable diagnostic utility among miRNA-451a (AUC = 0.6065), miRNA-142-5p (AUC = 0.6220), and Let-7f-5p (AUC = 0.6485) (Figure 4A and Supplementary Table S3). Late-stage fibrosis markers miRNA-122-5p (AUC = 0.5969) and miRNA-29a-3p (AUC = 0.5922) (Figure 4B,C and Supplementary Table S3) were found to have lower diagnostic utility. While APRI (AUC = 0.6481) and AST/ALT (AUC = 0.5956) were comparable to or were outperformed by the analyzed miRNAs, FIB-4 (AUC = 0.6879) and the PRTA-score (AUC = 0.7732) remained superior for the diagnosis of significant liver fibrosis (Figure 4D and Supplementary Table S3).

3.5. Association of Circulating miRNAs With Clinical Variables

We next examined the association between miRNA expression levels and clinical-pathological variables of the patient cohort. The levels of miRNA-451a (r = −0.2118), miRNA-142-5p (r = −0.2074), Let-7f-5p (r = 0.3426), miRNA-122-5p (r = 0.2193), and miRNA-29a-3p (r = 0.2413) were correlated with fibrosis severity, as determined by elastography (Supplementary Table S4 and Figure S2). Let-7f-5p was correlated with various fibrosis-linked parameters, such as decreasing albumin levels (r = −0.2031) and platelet counts (r = −0.3778), and to the fibrosis-scores Fib-4 (r = 0.3215), APRI (r = 0.2820), and PRTA-score (r = 0.4332), suggesting its association with hepatic fibrosis severity. As expected, miRNA-122-5p was strongly associated with AST (r = −0.2625) and ALT (r = −0.4093) levels, and thus marks hepatocyte damage. miRNA-142-5p (r = −0.1602), Let-7f-5p (r = 0.1416), and miRNA-122-5p (r = 0.2628) were associated with age, while Let-7f-5p (r = −0.1563) and miRNA-29a-3p (r = −0.2161) were associated with body mass index (Table 2).

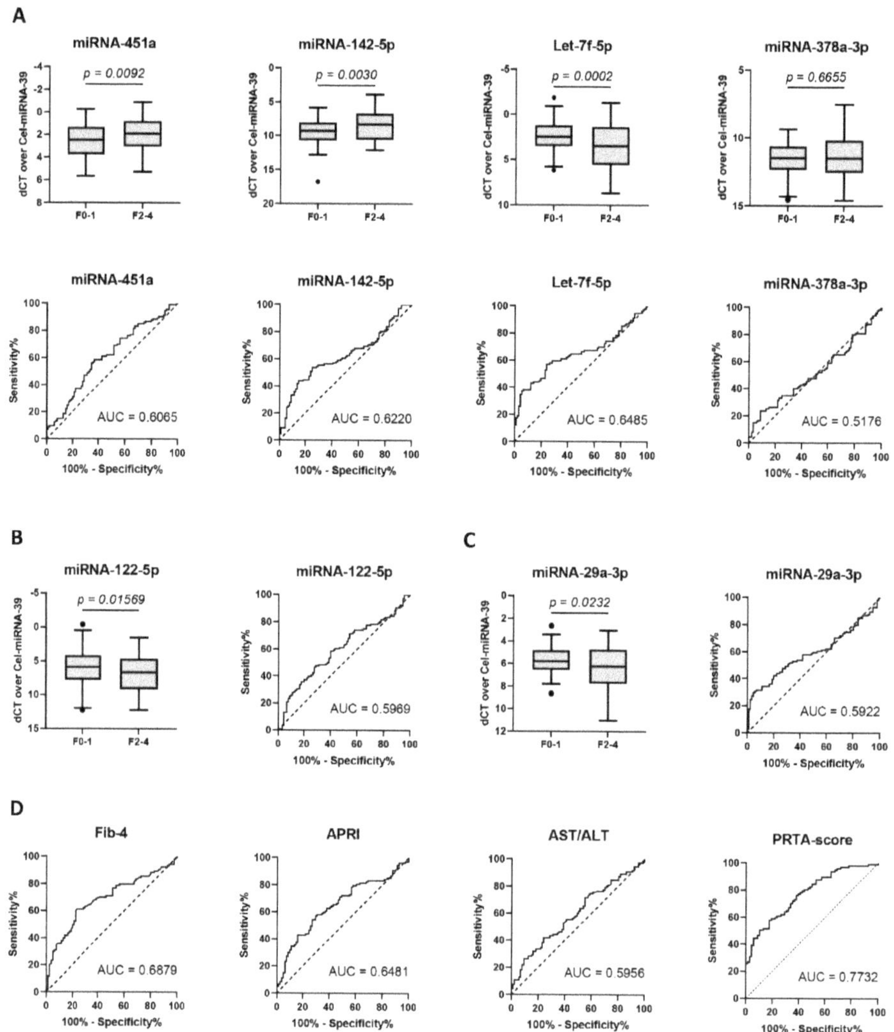

Figure 4. Evidence of significant liver fibrosis by the plasma levels of individual miRNAs. Expression analysis of circulating miRNAs in patients (n = 208) with chronic alcohol abuse, viral infection, and non-alcoholic fatty liver disease (NAFLD), with (F2–4) or without (F0–1) significant liver fibrosis. p-values were calculated using the Mann–Whitney U-test. Data is presented as Tukey boxplots. Receiver operating characteristic curve analysis was performed, and area under the curve (AUC) values were calculated to quantify the diagnostic value. The discriminative capacity of (**A**) candidate miRNAs was compared to (**B**) miRNA-122-5p and (**C**) miRNA-29a-3p and to (**D**) the serological scoring algorithms Fib-4, APRI, AST/ALT, and PRTA.

3.6. Discrimination of Significant Liver Fibrosis by the miRFIB-Score

To investigate whether a combination of the evaluated miRNAs could be used to diagnose significant ($F \geq 2$) liver fibrosis with a higher predictive value than the individual miRNAs, we created an miRNA-algorithm using logistic regression analysis. Here, the total patient cohort ($n = 208$) was randomly divided (Excel, Microsoft, WA, USA) into a derivation ($n = 143$) and validation ($n = 65$) cohort. Considering the lack of association between miRNA-378a-3p and fibrosis severity (Figure 3 and Supplementary Table S4), we chose to exclude this miRNA from the score. Combination of the other miRNA-variables generated the miRFIB-score:

$$\text{miRFIB} = 4.3799 + (0.70824 \times \text{Let-7f-5p (dCT)}) - (0.090912 \times \text{miRNA-122-5p (dCT)}) \\ - (0.26149 \times \text{miRNA-142-5p (dCT)}) - (0.53602 \times \text{miRNA-29a-3p (dCT)}) \\ - (0.041140 \times \text{miRNA-451a (dCT)}).$$

Table 2. Correlations of circulating miRNA expression levels with clinical parameters.

	miRNA-451a		miRNA-142-5p		Let-7f-5p		miRNA-378a-3p		miRNA-122-5p		miRNA-29a-3p	
	r	*p*	*r*	*p*	*r*	*p*	*r*	*p*	*r*	*p*	*r*	*p*
Age	−0.0409	ns	−0.1602	0.0234	0.1416	0.0413	0.0905	ns	0.2628	0.0001	0.0096	ns
BMI	0.0280	ns	−0.0397	ns	−0.1563	0.0287	−0.1037	ns	−0.0667	ns	−0.2161	0.0025
AST	−0.1554	0.0318	0.0076	ns	0.1371	ns	−0.1038	ns	−0.2625	0.0002	0.1150	ns
ALT	−0.0727	ns	0.0207	ns	0.0534	ns	−0.1412	0.0484	−0.4093	<0.0001	−0.0166	ns
Alk Phos	−0.0022	ns	−0.0804	ns	0.2027	0.0050	−0.0047	ns	0.2059	0.0046	0.1600	0.0287
GGT	−0.1372	ns	−0.1756	0.0174	0.1730	0.0163	−0.0621	ns	0.0060	ns	0.0899	ns
Bilirubin	−0.0609	ns	−0.0237	ns	0.3194	<0.0001	0.1295	ns	0.1213	ns	0.2790	0.0001
Albumin	−0.1064	ns	0.0365	ns	−0.2031	0.0067	−0.0148	ns	−0.2394	0.0014	−0.1747	0.0207
Platelet count	0.1243	ns	−0.1139	ns	−0.3778	<0.0001	−0.1629	0.0255	−0.1050	ns	−0.3514	<0.0001
Creatinine	−0.0419	ns	−0.0399	ns	0.0054	ns	−0.0094	ns	0.0652	ns	−0.0257	ns
AST/ALT	−0.1026	ns	−0.0126	ns	0.0756	ns	0.0311	ns	0.1920	0.0072	0.1627	0.0234
Fib-4	−0.1223	ns	0.0439	ns	0.3215	<0.0001	0.1400	ns	0.0607	ns	0.2852	0.0001
APRI	−0.1551	0.0365	0.1039	ns	0.2820	<0.0001	0.0321	ns	−0.1573	0.0321	0.2551	0.0005
PRTA-score	−0.0559	ns	0.0266	ns	0.4332	<0.0001	0.1479	ns	0.2401	0.0020	0.3447	<0.0001

Correlations were evaluated by the Pearson's correlation coefficient (r). ns: not significant; BMI: body mass index; AST: aspartate aminotransferase; ALT: alanine aminotransferase; Alk Phos: alkaline phosphatase; GGT: gamma-glutamyl transferase; AST/ALT ratio: aspartate aminotransferase/alanine aminotransferase ratio; APRI: AST to platelet ratio index; Fib-4: Fibrosis-4; PRTA-score: PDGFRβ-thrombocytes-albumin score.

The diagnostic value of the miRFIB-score to diagnose significant liver fibrosis in the derivation cohort was superior (AUC = 0.7251) to the clinical scores AST/ALT, APRI, and Fib-4 (AUC of 0.5936, 0.6273, and 0.6773, respectively). The diagnostic value of the miRFIB-score was confirmed in the validation cohort (AUC = 0.8173) and total cohort (AUC = 0.7558) (Table 3 and Figure 5). Additionally, the miRFIB-score was found to be significantly correlated with fibrosis severity (r = 0.4365) (Supplementary Table S4) and was able to differentiate patients with specific stage F2 from patients with stage F0–1 ($p < 0.0001$) (Supplementary Figure S2).

3.7. Inclusion of PDGFRβ Improves the Diagnostic Power of the miRFIB-Score

We previously reported the diagnostic utility of circulating PDGFRβ protein levels to detect significant liver fibrosis [17]. Thus, we performed logistic regression analysis on the derivation cohort, combining PDGFRβ levels with our five-miRNA panel. This generated the miRFIB^{P}-score, which was calculated as follows:

$$\text{miRFIB}^{P}\text{-score} = (0.97229 \times \text{miRFIB-score}) + (0.00021150 \times \text{PDGFR}\beta \text{ (pg/mL)}) - 1.8678.$$

The score had an increased diagnostic value for the identification of significant liver fibrosis in the derivation cohort (AUC = 0.7912; sensitivity = 80.82%; specificity = 70.37%), validation cohort (AUC = 0.8009; sensitivity = 68.75%; sensitivity = 81.48%), and total cohort (AUC = 0.7970; sensitivity = 79.05%; sensitivity = 69.51%) (Table 3 and Figure 5). The inclusion of PDGFRβ into the miRFIB-score further improved the correlation with fibrosis severity (r = 0.4847) (Supplementary Table S4), with a persistent possibility to differentiate patients with specific stage F2 liver fibrosis from patients with stage F0–1 fibrosis ($p < 0.0001$) (Supplementary Figure S2).

Table 3. Performance of the miRFIB- and miRFIB^{P}-score, as compared to the AST/ALT, APRI, Fib-4, and PRTA scoring algorithms, for the detection of significant liver fibrosis (F ≥ 2).

	AUC	95% CI	Optimal Cut-Off	Sensitivity (%)	Specificity (%)	PPV	NPV
AST/ALT							
Derivation	0.5936	0.4986–0.6886	0.6948	73.68	45.16	62.87	58.65
Validation	0.5988	0.4546–0.7430	1.025	38.24	84.00	75.08	51.90
Total	0.5956	0.5166–0.6747	0.8725	41.82	75.86	68.59	50.85
APRI							
Derivation	0.6273	0.5313–0.7234	0.4928	59.46	68.97	70.72	57.44
Validation	0.7128	0.5773–0.8482	0.7531	45.45	95.65	92.94	58.18
Total	0.6481	0.5696–0.7267	0.4928	57.01	70.37	70.80	56.49
Fib-4							
Derivation	0.6773	0.5847–0.7698	1.505	61.11	73.68	74.53	60.05
Validation	0.7083	0.5692–0.8474	1.520	58.06	86.96	84.88	62.19
Total	0.6879	0.6112–0.7647	1.505	60.19	77.50	77.13	60.70
PRTA-score							
Derivation	0.7399	0.6525–0.8272	10.36	59.15	81.63	80.23	61.32
Validation	0.7912	0.6566–0.9258	7.842	86.21	72.22	79.64	80.60
Total	0.7732	0.7033–0.8431	11.59	50.52	89.71	86.09	58.99
miRFIB							
Derivation	0.7251	0.6393–0.8110	0.1109	77.33	61.40	71.63	68.24
Validation	0.8173	0.7112–0.9235	0.3412	65.71	92.86	92.06	68.24
Total	0.7558	0.6887–0.8229	0.1404	78.38	62.35	72.41	69.59
miRFIB^{P}							
Derivation	0.7912	0.7120–0.8704	0.0673	80.82	70.37	77.47	74.43
Validation	0.8009	0.6844–0.9175	0.3840	68.75	81.48	82.39	67.41
Total	0.7970	0.7329–0.8611	0.1043	79.05	69.51	76.57	72.47

AST/ALT ratio: aspartate aminotransferase/alanine aminotransferase ratio; APRI: AST to platelet ratio index; Fib-4: Fibrosis-4; PRTA-score: PDGFRβ-thrombocytes-albumin score; AUC: area under the curve; CI: confidence interval; PPV: positive predictive value; NPV: negative predictive value.

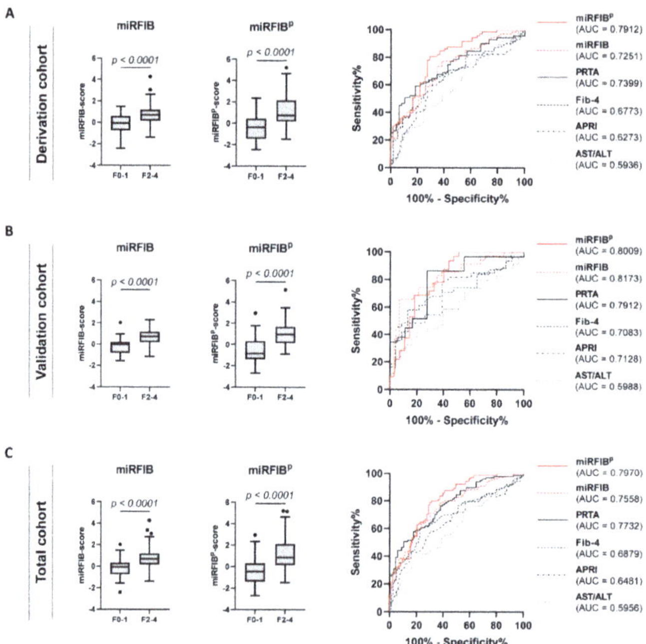

Figure 5. Diagnostic performance of the miRFIB- and the miRFIB^{P}-score for significant liver fibrosis. Performance comparison of the miRFIB-, the miRFIB^{P}-score, and commonly used validated diagnostic algorithms for the diagnosis of significant liver fibrosis (F2–4) in (**A**) the derivation, (**B**) validation, and (**C**) total patient cohort.

4. Discussion

Studies concerning the identification of novel non-invasive diagnostic tools suitable for the screening and monitoring of liver fibrosis in a general patient population remain limited. However, they are highly needed, as an accurate diagnosis of liver fibrosis has been shown to be a critical determinant of patient outcome [23,24]. Serological scoring tools, such as Fib-4, APRI, and AST/ALT, have been integrated into clinical practice, but lack accuracy for the identification of early stages of, and minor changes in, liver fibrosis [25–27]. Therefore, they are often only used as an indicator of the need for liver biopsy. The need for liver biopsy in current clinical practice thus remains. The identification of an adequate, sensitive, and specific serological marker for liver fibrosis would be of great value, as it could be used as an efficient first-line diagnostic step in screening at-risk patients [28], provide an easy tool for monitoring patients with fibrosis, and be of use in clinical trials evaluating fibrosis.

In the present study, we assessed the diagnostic utility of miRNAs differentially expressed during the activation of in vitro cultured primary HSCs, to identify significant liver fibrosis in a heterogeneous patient cohort with chronic viral infection, chronic alcohol abuse, and NAFLD. We identified an increased expression of miRNA-451a and miRNA-142-5p in the plasma of patients with significant liver fibrosis versus patients with no or mild fibrosis, whereas Let-7f-5p expression was decreased (Figure 4A). The observed down-regulation of miRNA-451a in total liver tissue of CCl_4-injected mice (Figure 3C) mimics their down-regulated expression in livers of NASH patients, compared to patients with simple steatosis [29]. Additionally, its enhanced circulating expression, observed in our patient cohort with significant liver fibrosis (Figure 4A), was also seen when comparing the serum of NAFLD patients with healthy controls [30]. In contrast, one study identified a down-regulation of miRNA-451a in the plasma of cirrhotic HBV patients, compared to healthy controls [31]. These results could not be confirmed in our patient cohort with chronic viral infection. Differences in miRNA-451a expression between HBV and HCV patients should further be investigated. Su et al [32] identified the inflammatory signals IL4 and IL13 to increase miRNA-142-5p expression in macrophages, activating them towards a pro-fibrogenic character. Furthermore, they identify its up-regulation in liver tissue of six-weeks CCl_4-treated C57BL/6J mice. This is in contrast to the down-regulation we observed in the liver tissue of four-weeks CCl_4-treated Balb/c mice (Figure 3C). Differences in fibrosis progression or in miRNA expression between mouse strains could be the cause of such discrepancy. Our results concerning liver miRNA-142-5p expression seem to mimic the down-regulation seen in the liver tissue of cirrhotic HCV patients [33]. While decreasing levels of circulating Let-7a-5p, Let-7c-5p, and Let-7d-5p are correlated with fibrosis severity in patients with chronic HCV infection [34], the diagnostic utility of Let-7f-5p was not investigated in these studies. We show that circulating Let-7f-5p has the highest diagnostic value of all candidate miRNAs (Figure 4A and Supplementary Table S3) for the identification of significant liver fibrosis. Additionally, from the candidate miRNA panel, Let-7f-5p was the only miRNA to be correlated with the Fib-4, APRI, and PRTA-scoring tools (Table 2), what further underlines its diagnostic potential.

In the search for the ideal diagnostic miRNA-based algorithm, we supplemented our candidate miRNA panel with the well-studied miRNA-122-5p and miRNA-29a-3p. miRNA-122-5p is the most abundant miRNA in the liver, with dominant expression in the hepatocytes (Supplementary Figure S3) [35], where it is involved in cholesterol synthesis [36]. The elevated levels of circulating miRNA-122-5p in patients with early stage fibrosis (F1–2) as compared to healthy controls are suggested to represent miRNA-release from injured hepatocytes. On the other hand, the decreased circulating miRNA-122-5p levels during later stages of fibrosis (F3–4) would be caused by the progressive loss of functional hepatocytes in the injured liver [37]. Its diagnostic utility for late-stage liver fibrosis and cirrhosis has already been suggested in various liver disease aetiologies [38–43]. Our study shows that while miRNA-122-5p has little diagnostic value on its own for significant fibrosis (Figure 4B), its contribution is essential to the miRFIB-score (Figure 5). In contrast to the hepatocyte-specificity of miRNA-122-5p, miRNA-29a-3p shows the highest expression in HSCs (Supplementary Figure S3), undergoing down-regulation upon in vitro and in vivo activation [22]. Its potential use as a therapeutic target has been elaboratively reported by the group of Y.H. Huang et al. using various mouse models of liver disease [44–47]. The negative correlation of circulating miRNA-29a-3p levels with fibrosis/cirrhosis severity has been shown in patients with NAFLD [48], HBV [49], HCV, alcohol abuse, and biliary disease [22].

Individually, all of the analyzed significantly dysregulated miRNAs had low predictive values for the diagnosis of significant liver fibrosis, with AUC values ranging from 0.59 to 0.64 (Figure 4A–C and Supplementary Table S3). However, using logistic regression analysis, we generated an algorithm, the miRFIB-score, consisting of miRNA-142-5p, miRNA-451a, Let-7f-5p, miRNA-122-5p, and miRNA-29a-3p, with a predictive value superior to the clinical scoring systems Fib-4, APRI, and AST/ALT (Figure 5 and Table 3). As we recently reported the highly discriminative potential of circulating PDGFRβ-levels for significant liver fibrosis in patients with various aetiologies of liver disease [17], we generated a second diagnostic algorithm combining the miRFIB-score with such circulating PDGFRβ-levels, the miRFIB^P-score. A marked improvement in diagnostic values was observed for this combinatory algorithm (Figure 5 and Table 3).

An unexpected finding was the discrepancy between the enhanced expression of miRNA-122-5p and miRNA-29a-3p in the plasma of mice treated with CCl_4 (Figure 3D), and their lowered expression levels in the plasma of patients with significant fibrosis (Figure 4C). All other tested miRNAs seem to have an overlapping expression pattern between mouse and human subjects. In our experiments, Balb/c mice underwent only four weeks of CCl_4-injections, which is thought to represent early-stage fibrosis. To induce late-stage fibrosis, or cirrhosis, 8–20 weeks of CCl_4-injections should be performed [20]. However, the enhanced expression of miRNA-122-5p in the plasma of CCl_4-injected mice is in line with our previous results comparing the plasma of patients with early-stage fibrosis to healthy subjects [14]. Alternatively, the enhanced expression of miRNA-122-5p in the plasma of mice treated with CCl_4 could reflect the hepatocyte damage caused by the last CCl_4-injection, since samples were taken only 24 h later. For miRNA-29a-3p, this is likely not the case, since this miRNA has thus far not been associated with hepatocyte damage. To further investigate this, healthy individuals should be included in future studies.

miRNA-451a, miRNA-142a-5p, Let-7f-5p, and miRNA-378a-3p were found to be significantly dysregulated in activated HSCs, as compared to quiescent controls (Figure 1D), which suggests a role in the HSC activation process. To further investigate this, target prediction was performed, and we focused on the target genes regulated by all four HSC-activation linked miRNAs. Of the predicted 13 overlapping miRNA targets (Figure 2A), three genes (*Ankrd52*, *Clcn5*, and *Peg10*), were found to be significantly up-regulated upon HSC activation (Figure 2C). As miRNAs negatively regulate gene expression by mRNA decay or inhibition of translation [50], and due to the dominantly down-regulated expression of the selected miRNAs, we hypothesize *Ankrd52*, *Clcn5*, and *Peg10* to be regulated by the selected miRNAs. However, to confirm this, further functional studies should be performed. While the roles of *Ankrd52* and *Clcn5* in liver disease remain unclear, *Peg10* has been widely studied in hepatocellular carcinoma (HCC) pathology. More specifically, *Peg10* expression levels are elevated in HCC [51], where it is found to inhibit the pro-apoptotic mediator *Siah1* [52], and stimulate cell proliferation by association with c-MYC [53]. Additionally, *Peg10* tissue mRNA levels mark HCC progression and poor survival [54,55]. Due to its high expression in activated HSCs (Figure 2C), and its important functionality in HCC, it would be of interest to investigate its role in liver fibrogenesis. As it cannot be excluded that a target gene is dominantly regulated by just one specific miRNA, it is possible that the increasing Let-7f-5p levels found upon HSC activation lead to the identified down-regulation of multiple predicted target genes (Figure 2D). Among these, *Cpeb3* and *Gnai3* have proven functionality as tumor suppressors in HCC. Both genes are found to undergo negative regulation by miRNAs, *Cpeb3* by miRNA-452-3p and miRNA-107 [56,57], and *Gnai3* by miRNA-222 [58]. However, their role during liver fibrosis remains to be determined.

Whether a miRFIB- or miRFIB^P-score can be integrated into the clinical practice will depend on future technical developments. Currently, a combination of protein and miRNA detection from the same plasma sample is not standard practice in hospital settings. Due to this more complex character, we expect the miRFIB^{P}-score to have a more important financial cost, compared to the miRFIB-score. However, our analysis identified the miRFIB^{P}-score to have superior diagnostic value for the identification of significant liver fibrosis and an in-depth cost–benefit analysis should determine if this diagnostic superiority outweighs the additional costs. Furthermore, the manipulation of blood samples should be performed with great care, since hemolysis of red blood cells may result in the release of their cytoplasmic miRNAs, such as miRNA-451a [59,60], and thus influence the results of the miRNA-based diagnostic algorithms. Additionally, the time interval between blood sampling and plasma storage should be kept as short as possible, as specific miRNAs, including miRNA-122-5p, can undergo a time-dependent decline in stability when the sample is kept at room temperature [61].

There were a number of limitations with the current study. The patient cohort size was relatively small and contained an imbalance in the presence of liver disease aetiologies. Although recent research has reported substantial differences in miRNA expression values in the plasma of patients with HBV infection versus patients with HCV infection [62], due to insufficient patient numbers we were unable to make any claims regarding such differences in our patient cohort. Furthermore, due to the cross-sectional character of the study, we did not possess any clinical follow-up material of the included patients. We were thus unable to test the prognostic ability of the miRFIB- and miRFIB^{P}-score. Finally, all included patients were staged for liver fibrosis by use of elastography. Future studies should focus on the validation of our results using plasma obtained from biopsy-staged patients. Moreover, the score should be tested during treatment to study if the scores can be used to evaluate early changes in fibrosis, and possibly predict the outcome.

In conclusion, we have identified five miRNAs that, when combined into the predictive miRFIB-signature, had high diagnostic values for significant liver fibrosis in a heterogeneous patient population with chronic alcohol abuse, viral infection, and NAFLD. Combining the miRFIB-score with circulating PDGFRβ-levels increased its diagnostic utility. Although these proposed scores require further validation, they may provide crucial information regarding liver fibrosis severity and evolution. Thanks to their non-invasive character, the scores would allow repeated measures and objective interpretation, at a relatively low financial cost. Additionally, functional studies could unravel the importance of the selected miRNAs during fibrogenesis and fibrolysis, and their potential utility as therapeutic targets.

Supplementary Materials: The following are available online at http://www.mdpi.com/2073-4409/8/9/1003/s1; **Supplementary Materials and Methods**: Extracellular vesicle isolation and RNA extraction, Nanostring miRNA analysis, Simultaneous isolation of different liver cell types. **Supplementary Figures and Tables**: Figure S1: Top enriched miRNAs in EVs derived from activating HSCs, Figure S2: Fibrosis-stage specific presence of circulating miRNAs, Figure S3: miRNA expression analysis in liver cell types, Table S1: miRNA primers, Table S2: mRNA primers, Table S3: Performance of individual plasma miRNAs, as compared to the AST/ALT, APRI, Fib-4, and PRTA scoring algorithms, for the detection of significant liver fibrosis ($F \geq 2$), Table S4: Correlation of circulating miRNA expression levels with fibrosis stage.

Author Contributions: J.L. study concept and design; acquisition of data; analysis and interpretation of data; statistical analysis; writing of the manuscript. S.V. analysis and interpretation of data. H.R. provision of samples; interpretation of data; critical revision of the manuscript. L.A.v.G. study concept and design; interpretation of data; critical revision of the manuscript.

Funding: This research received funding by the Vrije Universiteit Brussel (VUB), the Institute for the Promotion of Innovation through Science and Technology in Flanders (IWT-Flanders) (HILIM-3D; SBO140045), the Fund of Scientific Research Flanders (FWO), and the Gilead Sciences BeLux Fellowship Programme 2018 (awarded to H.R.).

Acknowledgments: We would like to acknowledge Daniella Blyweert, Nathalie Eysackers, Aneta Kozyra, Iona De Mol, and Christella Ukunda for technical support.

Conflicts of Interest: The authors declare no conflict of interest.

References

1. World Health Organization. Global Health Estimates for Cause Specific Mortality. 2016. Available online: https://www.who.int/healthinfo/global_burden_disease/estimates/en/ (accessed on 11 July 2019).
2. Tsochatzis, E.A.; Bosch, J.; Burroughs, A.K. Liver cirrhosis. *Lancet* **2014**, *383*, 1749–1761. [CrossRef]
3. Tsuchida, T.; Friedman, S.L. Mechanisms of hepatic stellate cell activation. *Nat. Rev. Gastroenterol. Hepatol.* **2017**, *14*, 397–411. [CrossRef] [PubMed]
4. Lee, Y.A.; Wallace, M.C.; Friedman, S.L. Pathobiology of liver fibrosis: A translational success story. *Gut* **2015**, *64*, 830–841. [CrossRef] [PubMed]
5. Brenner, D.A. Reversibility of liver fibrosis. *Gastroenterol. Hepatol.* **2013**, *9*, 737–739.
6. Regev, A.; Berho, M.; Jeffers, L.J.; Milikowski, C.; Molina, E.G.; Pyrsopoulos, N.T.; Feng, Z.Z.; Reddy, K.R.; Schiff, E.R. Sampling error and intraobserver variation in liver biopsy in patients with chronic HCV infection. *Am. J. Gastroenterol.* **2002**, *97*, 2614–2618. [CrossRef] [PubMed]
7. Pasha, T.; Gabriel, S.; Therneau, T.; Dickson, E.R.; Lindor, K.D. Cost-effectiveness of ultrasound-guided liver biopsy. *Hepatology* **1998**, *27*, 1220–1226. [CrossRef] [PubMed]
8. Cadranel, J.F.; Rufat, P.; Degos, F. Practices of liver biopsy in France: Results of a prospective nationwide survey. For the Group of Epidemiology of the French Association for the Study of the Liver (AFEF). *Hepatology* **2000**, *32*, 477–481. [CrossRef] [PubMed]
9. Lambrecht, J.; Verhulst, S.; Mannaerts, I.; Reynaert, H.; van Grunsven, L.A. Prospects in non-invasive assessment of liver fibrosis: Liquid biopsy as the future gold standard? *Biochim. Biophys. Acta Mol. Basis Dis.* **2018**, *1864*, 1024–1036. [CrossRef] [PubMed]
10. Lambrecht, J.; Mannaerts, I.; van Grunsven, L.A. The role of miRNAs in stress-responsive hepatic stellate cells during liver fibrosis. *Front. Physiol.* **2015**, *6*, 209. [CrossRef] [PubMed]
11. Turchinovich, A.; Weiz, L.; Burwinkel, B. Extracellular miRNAs: The mystery of their origin and function. *Trends Biochem. Sci.* **2012**, *37*, 460–465. [CrossRef] [PubMed]
12. Loosen, S.H.; Schueller, F.; Trautwein, C.; Roy, S.; Roderburg, C. Role of circulating microRNAs in liver diseases. *World J. Hepatol.* **2017**, *9*, 586–594. [CrossRef] [PubMed]
13. Hayes, C.N.; Chayama, K. MicroRNAs as Biomarkers for Liver Disease and Hepatocellular Carcinoma. *Int. J. Mol. Sci.* **2016**, *17*, 280. [CrossRef] [PubMed]
14. Lambrecht, J.; Jan Poortmans, P.; Verhulst, S.; Reynaert, H.; Mannaerts, I.; van Grunsven, L.A. Circulating ECV-Associated miRNAs as Potential Clinical Biomarkers in Early Stage HBV and HCV Induced Liver Fibrosis. *Front. Pharmacol.* **2017**, *8*, 56. [CrossRef] [PubMed]
15. Guimaraes, E.L.; Empsen, C.; Geerts, A.; van Grunsven, L.A. Advanced glycation end products induce production of reactive oxygen species via the activation of NADPH oxidase in murine hepatic stellate cells. *J. Hepatol.* **2010**, *52*, 389–397. [CrossRef] [PubMed]
16. Friedrich-Rust, M.; Ong, M.F.; Martens, S.; Sarrazin, C.; Bojunga, J.; Zeuzem, S.; Herrmann, E. Performance of transient elastography for the staging of liver fibrosis: A meta-analysis. *Gastroenterology* **2008**, *134*, 960–974. [CrossRef] [PubMed]
17. Lambrecht, J.; Verhulst, S.; Mannaerts, I.; Sowa, J.P.; Best, J.; Canbay, A.; Reynaert, H.; van Grunsven, L.A. A PDGFRbeta-based score predicts significant liver fibrosis in patients with chronic alcohol abuse, NAFLD and viral liver disease. *EBioMedicine* **2019**, *43*, 501–512. [CrossRef] [PubMed]
18. Seger, S.; Stritt, M.; Vezzali, E.; Nayler, O.; Hess, P.; Groenen, P.M.A.; Stalder, A.K. A fully automated image analysis method to quantify lung fibrosis in the bleomycin-induced rat model. *PLoS ONE* **2018**, *13*, e0193057. [CrossRef] [PubMed]
19. Youden, W.J. Index for rating diagnostic tests. *Cancer* **1950**, *3*, 32–35. [CrossRef]
20. Scholten, D.; Trebicka, J.; Liedtke, C.; Weiskirchen, R. The carbon tetrachloride model in mice. *Laboratory Animals* **2015**, *49*, 4–11. [CrossRef] [PubMed]
21. Li, J.; Ghazwani, M.; Zhang, Y.; Lu, J.; Li, J.; Fan, J.; Gandhi, C.R.; Li, S. miR-122 regulates collagen production via targeting hepatic stellate cells and suppressing P4HA1 expression. *J. Hepatol.* **2013**, *58*, 522–528. [CrossRef]
22. Roderburg, C.; Urban, G.W.; Bettermann, K.; Vucur, M.; Zimmermann, H.; Schmidt, S.; Janssen, J.; Koppe, C.; Knolle, P.; Castoldi, M.; et al. Micro-RNA profiling reveals a role for miR-29 in human and murine liver fibrosis. *Hepatology* **2011**, *53*, 209–218. [CrossRef] [PubMed]

23. Ekstedt, M.; Hagstrom, H.; Nasr, P.; Fredrikson, M.; Stal, P.; Kechagias, S.; Hultcrantz, R. Fibrosis stage is the strongest predictor for disease-specific mortality in NAFLD after up to 33 years of follow-up. *Hepatology* **2015**, *61*, 1547–1554. [CrossRef] [PubMed]
24. Angulo, P.; Kleiner, D.E.; Dam-Larsen, S.; Adams, L.A.; Bjornsson, E.S.; Charatcharoenwitthaya, P.; Mills, P.R.; Keach, J.C.; Lafferty, H.D.; Stahler, A.; et al. Liver Fibrosis, but No Other Histologic Features, Is Associated With Long-term Outcomes of Patients With Nonalcoholic Fatty Liver Disease. *Gastroenterology* **2015**, *149*, 389–397. [CrossRef] [PubMed]
25. Mato, J.M.; Lu, S.C. Where are we in the search for noninvasive nonalcoholic steatohepatitis biomarkers? *Hepatology* **2011**, *54*, 1115–1117. [CrossRef] [PubMed]
26. Kim, W.R.; Berg, T.; Asselah, T.; Flisiak, R.; Fung, S.; Gordon, S.C.; Janssen, H.L.; Lampertico, P.; Lau, D.; Bornstein, J.D.; et al. Evaluation of APRI and FIB-4 scoring systems for non-invasive assessment of hepatic fibrosis in chronic hepatitis B patients. *J. Hepatol.* **2016**, *64*, 773–780. [CrossRef] [PubMed]
27. Xiao, G.; Yang, J.; Yan, L. Comparison of diagnostic accuracy of aspartate aminotransferase to platelet ratio index and fibrosis-4 index for detecting liver fibrosis in adult patients with chronic hepatitis B virus infection: A systemic review and meta-analysis. *Hepatology* **2015**, *61*, 292–302. [CrossRef]
28. Ampuero, J.; Romero-Gomez, M. Editorial: Looking for patients at risk of cirrhosis in the general population-many needles in a haystack. *Aliment. Pharmacol. Ther.* **2018**, *47*, 692–694. [CrossRef]
29. Hur, W.; Lee, J.H.; Kim, S.W.; Kim, J.H.; Bae, S.H.; Kim, M.; Hwang, D.; Kim, Y.S.; Park, T.; Um, S.J.; et al. Downregulation of microRNA-451 in non-alcoholic steatohepatitis inhibits fatty acid-induced proinflammatory cytokine production through the AMPK/AKT pathway. *Int. J. Biochem. Cell Biol.* **2015**, *64*, 265–276. [CrossRef]
30. Yamada, H.; Suzuki, K.; Ichino, N.; Ando, Y.; Sawada, A.; Osakabe, K.; Sugimoto, K.; Ohashi, K.; Teradaira, R.; Inoue, T.; et al. Associations between circulating microRNAs (miR-21, miR-34a, miR-122 and miR-451) and non-alcoholic fatty liver. *Clin. Chim. Acta* **2013**, *424*, 99–103. [CrossRef]
31. Jin, B.X.; Zhang, Y.H.; Jin, W.J.; Sun, X.Y.; Qiao, G.F.; Wei, Y.Y.; Sun, L.B.; Zhang, W.H.; Li, N. MicroRNA panels as disease biomarkers distinguishing hepatitis B virus infection caused hepatitis and liver cirrhosis. *Sci. Rep.* **2015**, *5*, 15026. [CrossRef]
32. Su, S.; Zhao, Q.; He, C.; Huang, D.; Liu, J.; Chen, F.; Chen, J.; Liao, J.Y.; Cui, X.; Zeng, Y.; et al. miR-142-5p and miR-130a-3p are regulated by IL-4 and IL-13 and control profibrogenic macrophage program. *Nat. Commun.* **2015**, *6*, 8523. [CrossRef] [PubMed]
33. Tsang, F.H.; Au, S.L.; Wei, L.; Fan, D.N.; Lee, J.M.; Wong, C.C.; Ng, I.O.; Wong, C.M. MicroRNA-142-3p and microRNA-142-5p are downregulated in hepatocellular carcinoma and exhibit synergistic effects on cell motility. *Front. Med.* **2015**, *9*, 331–343. [CrossRef] [PubMed]
34. Matsuura, K.; De Giorgi, V.; Schechterly, C.; Wang, R.Y.; Farci, P.; Tanaka, Y.; Alter, H.J. Circulating let-7 levels in plasma and extracellular vesicles correlate with hepatic fibrosis progression in chronic hepatitis C. *Hepatology* **2016**, *64*, 732–745. [CrossRef] [PubMed]
35. Schueller, F.; Roy, S.; Trautwein, C.; Luedde, T.; Roderburg, C. miR-122 expression is not regulated during activation of hepatic stellate cells. *J. Hepatol.* **2016**, *65*, 865–867. [CrossRef] [PubMed]
36. Esau, C.; Davis, S.; Murray, S.F.; Yu, X.X.; Pandey, S.K.; Pear, M.; Watts, L.; Booten, S.L.; Graham, M.; McKay, R.; et al. miR-122 regulation of lipid metabolism revealed by in vivo antisense targeting. *Cell Metab.* **2006**, *3*, 87–98. [CrossRef] [PubMed]
37. Trebicka, J.; Anadol, E.; Elfimova, N.; Strack, I.; Roggendorf, M.; Viazov, S.; Wedemeyer, I.; Drebber, U.; Rockstroh, J.; Sauerbruch, T.; et al. Hepatic and serum levels of miR-122 after chronic HCV-induced fibrosis. *J. Hepatol.* **2013**, *58*, 234–239. [CrossRef] [PubMed]
38. Wang, T.Z.; Lin, D.D.; Jin, B.X.; Sun, X.Y.; Li, N. Plasma microRNA: A novel non-invasive biomarker for HBV-associated liver fibrosis staging. *Exp. Ther. Med.* **2019**, *17*, 1919–1929. [CrossRef] [PubMed]
39. Ye, D.; Zhang, T.; Lou, G.; Xu, W.; Dong, F.; Chen, G.; Liu, Y. Plasma miR-17, miR-20a, miR-20b and miR-122 as potential biomarkers for diagnosis of NAFLD in type 2 diabetes mellitus patients. *Life Sci.* **2018**, *208*, 201–207. [CrossRef]
40. Shaker, O.G.; Senousy, M.A. Serum microRNAs as predictors for liver fibrosis staging in hepatitis C virus-associated chronic liver disease patients. *J. Viral. Hepat.* **2017**, *24*, 636–644. [CrossRef]

41. Miyaaki, H.; Ichikawa, T.; Kamo, Y.; Taura, N.; Honda, T.; Shibata, H.; Milazzo, M.; Fornari, F.; Gramantieri, L.; Bolondi, L.; et al. Significance of serum and hepatic microRNA-122 levels in patients with non-alcoholic fatty liver disease. *Liver Int.* **2014**, *34*, e302–e307. [CrossRef]
42. Waidmann, O.; Koberle, V.; Brunner, F.; Zeuzem, S.; Piiper, A.; Kronenberger, B. Serum microRNA-122 predicts survival in patients with liver cirrhosis. *PLoS ONE* **2012**, *7*, e45652. [CrossRef] [PubMed]
43. Zhang, Y.; Jia, Y.; Zheng, R.; Guo, Y.; Wang, Y.; Guo, H.; Fei, M.; Sun, S. Plasma microRNA-122 as a biomarker for viral-, alcohol-, and chemical-related hepatic diseases. *Clin. Chem.* **2010**, *56*, 1830–1838. [CrossRef] [PubMed]
44. Yang, Y.L.; Wang, F.S.; Li, S.C.; Tiao, M.M.; Huang, Y.H. MicroRNA-29a Alleviates Bile Duct Ligation Exacerbation of Hepatic Fibrosis in Mice through Epigenetic Control of Methyltransferases. *Int. J. Mol. Sci.* **2017**, *18*, 192. [CrossRef] [PubMed]
45. Huang, Y.H.; Kuo, H.C.; Yang, Y.L.; Wang, F.S. MicroRNA-29a is a key regulon that regulates BRD4 and mitigates liver fibrosis in mice by inhibiting hepatic stellate cell activation. *Int. J. Med. Sci.* **2019**, *16*, 212–220. [CrossRef] [PubMed]
46. Yang, Y.L.; Kuo, H.C.; Wang, F.S.; Huang, Y.H. MicroRNA-29a Disrupts DNMT3b to Ameliorate Diet-Induced Non-Alcoholic Steatohepatitis in Mice. *Int. J. Mol. Sci.* **2019**, *20*, 1499. [CrossRef] [PubMed]
47. Li, S.C.; Wang, F.S.; Yang, Y.L.; Tiao, M.M.; Chuang, J.H.; Huang, Y.H. Microarray Study of Pathway Analysis Expression Profile Associated with MicroRNA-29a with Regard to Murine Cholestatic Liver Injuries. *Int. J. Mol. Sci.* **2016**, *17*, 324. [CrossRef] [PubMed]
48. Jampoka, K.; Muangpaisarn, P.; Khongnomnan, K.; Treeprasertsuk, S.; Tangkijvanich, P.; Payungporn, S. Serum miR-29a and miR-122 as Potential Biomarkers for Non-Alcoholic Fatty Liver Disease (NAFLD). *Microrna* **2018**, *7*, 215–222. [CrossRef]
49. Bao, S.; Zheng, J.; Li, N.; Huang, C.; Chen, M.; Cheng, Q.; Yu, K.; Chen, S.; Zhu, M.; Shi, G. Serum MicroRNA Levels as a Noninvasive Diagnostic Biomarker for the Early Diagnosis of Hepatitis B Virus-Related Liver Fibrosis. *Gut Liver* **2017**, *11*, 860–869. [CrossRef]
50. Gebert, L.F.R.; MacRae, I.J. Regulation of microRNA function in animals. *Nat. Rev. Mol. Cell Biol.* **2019**, *20*, 21–37. [CrossRef]
51. Dong, H.; Ge, X.; Shen, Y.; Chen, L.; Kong, Y.; Zhang, H.; Man, X.; Tang, L.; Yuan, H.; Wang, H.; et al. Gene expression profile analysis of human hepatocellular carcinoma using SAGE and LongSAGE. *BMC Med. Genomics* **2009**, *2*, 5. [CrossRef]
52. Okabe, H.; Satoh, S.; Furukawa, Y.; Kato, T.; Hasegawa, S.; Nakajima, Y.; Yamaoka, Y.; Nakamura, Y. Involvement of PEG10 in human hepatocellular carcinogenesis through interaction with SIAH1. *Cancer Res.* **2003**, *63*, 3043–3048. [PubMed]
53. Li, C.M.; Margolin, A.A.; Salas, M.; Memeo, L.; Mansukhani, M.; Hibshoosh, H.; Szabolcs, M.; Klinakis, A.; Tycko, B. PEG10 is a c-MYC target gene in cancer cells. *Cancer Res.* **2006**, *66*, 665–672. [CrossRef] [PubMed]
54. Ip, W.K.; Lai, P.B.; Wong, N.L.; Sy, S.M.; Beheshti, B.; Squire, J.A.; Wong, N. Identification of PEG10 as a progression related biomarker for hepatocellular carcinoma. *Cancer Lett.* **2007**, *250*, 284–291. [CrossRef] [PubMed]
55. Bang, H.; Ha, S.Y.; Hwang, S.H.; Park, C.K. Expression of PEG10 Is Associated with Poor Survival and Tumor Recurrence in Hepatocellular Carcinoma. *Cancer Res. Treat.* **2015**, *47*, 844–852. [CrossRef] [PubMed]
56. Zou, C.D.; Zhao, W.M.; Wang, X.N.; Li, Q.; Huang, H.; Cheng, W.P.; Jin, J.F.; Zhang, H.; Wu, M.J.; Tai, S.; et al. MicroRNA-107: A novel promoter of tumor progression that targets the CPEB3/EGFR axis in human hepatocellular carcinoma. *Oncotarget* **2016**, *7*, 266–278. [CrossRef] [PubMed]
57. Tang, H.; Zhang, J.; Yu, Z.; Ye, L.; Li, K.; Ding, F.; Feng, X.; Meng, W. Mir-452-3p: A Potential Tumor Promoter That Targets the CPEB3/EGFR Axis in Human Hepatocellular Carcinoma. *Technol. Cancer Res. Treat.* **2017**, *16*, 1136–1149. [CrossRef] [PubMed]
58. Zhang, Y.; Yao, J.; Huan, L.; Lian, J.; Bao, C.; Li, Y.; Ge, C.; Li, J.; Yao, M.; Liang, L.; et al. GNAI3 inhibits tumor cell migration and invasion and is post-transcriptionally regulated by miR-222 in hepatocellular carcinoma. *Cancer Lett.* **2015**, *356*, 978–984. [CrossRef] [PubMed]
59. Pritchard, C.C.; Kroh, E.; Wood, B.; Arroyo, J.D.; Dougherty, K.J.; Miyaji, M.M.; Tait, J.F.; Tewari, M. Blood cell origin of circulating microRNAs: A cautionary note for cancer biomarker studies. *Cancer Prev. Res.* **2012**, *5*, 492–497. [CrossRef] [PubMed]

60. Kirschner, M.B.; Kao, S.C.; Edelman, J.J.; Armstrong, N.J.; Vallely, M.P.; van Zandwijk, N.; Reid, G. Haemolysis during sample preparation alters microRNA content of plasma. *PLoS ONE* **2011**, *6*, e24145. [CrossRef] [PubMed]
61. Koberle, V.; Pleli, T.; Schmithals, C.; Augusto Alonso, E.; Haupenthal, J.; Bonig, H.; Peveling-Oberhag, J.; Biondi, R.M.; Zeuzem, S.; Kronenberger, B.; et al. Differential stability of cell-free circulating microRNAs: Implications for their utilization as biomarkers. *PLoS ONE* **2013**, *8*, e75184. [CrossRef] [PubMed]
62. Appourchaux, K.; Dokmak, S.; Resche-Rigon, M.; Treton, X.; Lapalus, M.; Gattolliat, C.H.; Porchet, E.; Martinot-Peignoux, M.; Boyer, N.; Vidaud, M.; et al. MicroRNA-based diagnostic tools for advanced fibrosis and cirrhosis in patients with chronic hepatitis B and C. *Sci. Rep.* **2016**, *6*, 34935. [CrossRef] [PubMed]

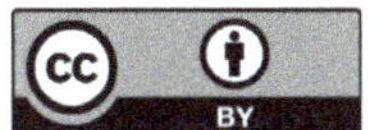

MDPI
St. Alban-Anlage 66
4052 Basel
Switzerland
Tel. +41 61 683 77 34
Fax +41 61 302 89 18
www.mdpi.com

Cells Editorial Office
E-mail: cells@mdpi.com
www.mdpi.com/journal/cells

www.ingramcontent.com/pod-product-compliance
Lightning Source LLC
LaVergne TN
LVHW070150170726
843515LV00007B/1887